# Anaphylaxis and Hypersensitivity Reactions

Mariana C. Castells, MD
Editor

# Anaphylaxis and Hypersensitivity Reactions

Humana Press

*Editor*
Mariana C. Castells, MD
Brigham and Women's Hospital
Harvard Medical School
Boston, MA USA
mcastells@partners.org

ISBN 978-1-4939-6148-1 ISBN 978-1-60327-951-2 (eBook)
DOI 10.1007/978-1-60327-951-2
Springer New York Dordrecht Heidelberg Londont



Printed on acid-free paper

Humana Press is part of Springer Science+Business Media (www.springer.com)

# Preface

A 2007 National Electronic Injury Surveillance System (NEISS) indicated that in the USA, 10% of the emergency room visits were due to anaphylaxis. The median age of the patients was 26 years, and 24% of the visits involved children less than 5 years of age who reacted to peanut or tree nuts. Only 19% of the patients received epinephrine and 57% of the patients presenting symptoms compatible with anaphylaxis were not recognized as having anaphylaxis upon discharge. Anaphylaxis is a recognized public health problem with increased prevalence, and yet because of its acute onset and the lack of specific biochemical markers, underrecognized and underdiagnosed. Anaphylaxis is defined as the most severe of the allergic reactions, with a rapid onset and which may cause death if prompt treatment is not installed. It occurs after exposure to an allergen in a previously healthy individual and can involve most organ systems in minutes, including the skin, gastrointestinal, respiratory, and cardiovascular systems. Death can be caused by cardiovascular collapse or laryngeal edema and asphyxiation. Allergens most commonly associated include foods with peanuts and nuts being the most frequent in children, and medications including antibiotics, monoclonals, and chemotherapy drugs such as platins and taxenes. Hymenoptera stings and exercise are well-recognized treatable causes of anaphylaxis. Mastocytosis and mast cell activation syndromes can present as anaphylaxis, and their diagnosis requires a high index of suspicion from clinicians. Recently, contaminants in pharmaceutical products have been recognized as likely triggers of hypersensitivity reactions and anaphylaxis.

The mechanisms leading to anaphylaxis relate to an individual's sensitization and the presence of specific IgE antibodies against an allergen, which can activate mast cells and basophils and release powerful inflammatory mediators. More recently, anaphylaxis has been recognized in the absence of an IgE-recognized mechanism but with identical clinical symptoms and severity such as during complement activation, kinins and bradykinins generation, and direct mast cell/basophil activation. This is important in hypersensitivity reactions to chemotherapy and monoclonal antibodies and other biological agents in which the mechanisms leading to anaphylaxis have not been elucidated. Although tryptase immunoassays have been available since 1987, they have been underutilized in emergency rooms and faster mediator assays are not available. New mediators such as PAF have been measured in patients suffering from severe peanut-induced anaphylaxis and its increased levels associated to the decrease in PAF acetyl hydrolase. A study of postmortem tryptase levels in patients who died of unidentified causes showed that in at least 20% of the cases tryptase was elevated indicating that anaphylaxis was a likely cause of death. Recognition of the early symptoms and prompt treatment with epinephrine are key to decreasing its morbidity and mortality, and anti-IgE therapy has shown to decrease the sensitivity of food allergic individuals.

The aim of this book is to fill the gaps in the recognition of the clinical presentation and triggers of anaphylaxis, the understanding of its natural history, its prevention, and the newest treatment options. The book provides up-to-date information elucidating some of its cellular, molecular, and genetic targets, including the description of a novel mast cell activation syndrome associated to c-kit

D816V mutation. Rapid desensitizations for the treatment of anaphylactic reactions to antibiotics, chemotherapy, and monoclonal antibodies is described here as the new frontier in providing first-line therapy for patients with cancer, cystic fibrosis, and other life-threatening conditions.

The audience includes clinicians, translational researchers, as well as basic researchers. The development of better diagnostic assays, less allergenic medications and biological agents, and the understanding of the pathophysiology of anaphylaxis will contribute to reduced morbidity and mortality.

Boston, MA Mariana C. Castells, MD

# Foreword

Anaphylaxis is a rapidly progressive, potentially lethal event that can affect patients of all ages and that requires immediate recognition and intervention. It can be induced by a diverse range of mechanisms, including classical IgE-dependent reactions to allergens (drugs, stinging insects, foods), idiosyncratic reactions to medications (aspirin, contrast dyes), and responses to physical stimuli (exercise, cold air) in predisposed individuals. In many such instances, the concomitant diagnosis of asthma is associated with a higher incidence of poor outcome. Additionally, certain individuals experience repeated anaphylaxis without a clear precipitating cause (idiopathic anaphylaxis). Clonal abnormalities of mast cell development may be associated with the latter group. The rising prevalence of allergic diseases worldwide, combined with the introduction and increasing use of potentially allergenic biologic agents for the treatment of cancer and autoimmunity make it likely that anaphylaxis will only become more frequent.

Regardless of the initiating cause, anaphylaxis results from the pathophysiologic effects of potent mediators, most of all of which derive from mast cells (and perhaps basophils), which act at vascular and airway smooth muscle to induce changes in tone and permeability. These changes, if generalized or dysregulated, can rapidly produce airway obstruction and cardiovascular collapse that can be lethal. Although the manifestations of an anaphylactic episode can be reversed by rapid administration of epinephrine, this modality remains underutilized, even in emergency departments. Thousands of individuals die or suffer unnecessarily due to underrecognition and undertreatment of anaphylaxis. Animal models of anaphylaxis do not reflect the major target organs in humans, namely, the bronchial tree, the larynx, and the cardiovascular system; therefore mediators and tissue targets have to be studied in humans.

This text, aimed at practitioners from all specialties, provides a superb overview of pathophysiology, epidemiology, causes, underlying predisposing conditions, and treatment of anaphylaxis. It is carefully compiled and edited by Dr. Mariana Castells, an acclaimed expert in the diagnosis and management of anaphylaxis. The topic list is comprehensive. The contributors are among the world authorities in each topic area. Each chapter is easily readable, with a thorough and up-to-date bibliography. The life-threatening nature of anaphylaxis, the broad age range of susceptible patients, and the myriad of underlying causes and predisposing factors make it essential for all physicians and providers to gain competence in the diagnosis and management of anaphylaxis. This textbook provides an essential step toward that end.

Bostan, MA Joshua A. Boyce

# Contents

# Contributors

**Cem Akin**
Harvard Medical School, Brigham and Women's Hospital, Boston, MA, USA

**Aleena Banerji**
Harvard Medical School, Brigham and Women's Hospital, Boston, MA, USA

**David I. Bernstein**
University of Cincinnati College of Medicine, Cincinnati, OH, USA

**Philippe Jean Bousquet**
Hôpital Arnaud de Villeneuve, University Hospital Montpellier, Montpellier, France

**Joshua A. Boyce**
Harvard Medical School, Brigham and Women's Hospital, Boston, MA, USA

**Patrick Brennan**
Harvard Medical School, Brigham and Women's Hospital, Boston, MA, USA

**A. Wesley Burks**
Duke University Medical Center, Durham, NC, USA

**Joseph H. Butterfield**
Mayo Clinic, Rochester, MN, USA

**Mariana C. Castells**
Harvard Medical School, Brigham and Women's Hospital, Boston, MA, USA

**George H. Caughey**
University of California at San Francisco, Medicine and Cardiovascular Research Institute, San Francisco, CA, USA

**Scott P. Commins**
University of Virginia Health System, Charlottesville, VA, USA

**Pascal Demoly**
Hôpital Arnaud de Villeneuve, University Hospital of Montpellier, Montpellier, France

**Pascale Dewachter**
Hôpital Necker-Enfants Malades, AP-HP, Université Paris-Descartes, Paris, France

**Luis Escribano**
Centro de Estudios de Mastocitosis de Castilla La Mancha, Hospital Virgen del Valle, Toledo, Spain

**Anna M. Feldweg**
Harvard Medical School, Brigham and Women's Hospital, Boston, MA, USA

**Fred D. Finkelman**
University of Cincinnati College of Medicine, Cincinnati, OH, USA

**Stephen J. Galli**
Professor of Pathology and of Microbiology and Immunology Department of Pathology, Stanford Universtiy School of Medicine, Stanford, CA, USA

**Leslie C. Grammer**
Northwestern University, Feinberg School of Medicine, Chicago, IL, USA

**David L. Hepner**
Harvard Medical School, Brigham and Women's Hospital, Boston, MA, USA

**Paul Hesterberg**
Massachusetts General Hospital, Boston, MA, USA

**F. Ida Hsu**
Harvard Medical School, Brigham and Women's Hospital, Boston, MA, USA

**Karen Hsu Blatman**
Northwestern University, Feinberg School of Medicine, Chicago, IL, USA

**Kirsi M. Järvinen-Seppo**
Mount Sinai School of Medicine, New York, NY, USA

**Stephen F. Kemp**
University of Mississippi Medical Center, Jackson, MS, USA

**Peter Korosec**
University Clinic of Respiratory and Allergic Diseases, Golnik, Slovenia

**Mitja Kosnik**
University Clinic of Respiratory and Allergic Diseases, Golnik, Slovenia

**Tanya M. Laidlaw**
Harvard Medical School, Brigham and Women's Hospital, Boston, MA, USA

**Henry J. Legere III**
Allergy and Immunology, Texas A&M School of Medicine, TX, USA

**Phil Lieberman**
College of Medicine, University of Tennessee, Memphis, TN, USA

**Richard F. Lockey**
University of South Florida, College of Medicine, Tampa, FL, USA

**Donald MacGlashan**
Johns Hopkins University, Asthma and Allergy Center, Baltimore, MD, USA

**Dean D. Metcalfe**
National Institutes of Health, National Institute of Allergy and Infectious Diseases, Bethesda, MD, USA

**Anna Nowak-Węgrzyn**
Mount Sinai School of Medicine, New York, NY, USA

**Eyal Oren**
North Shore Medical Center, Salem, MA, USA

**Alberto Orfao**
Servico Central de Citometria, Centro de IN Vestigación del Cáncer (CIC), Salamanca, Spain

**Ross I. Palis**
Washington University School of Medicine, Barnes-Jewish Hospital, St. Louis, MO, USA

**Thomas A.E. Platts-Mills**
University of Virginia Health System, Charlottesville, VA, USA

**Richard S.H. Pumphrey**
Honorary Consultant Immunologist, Department of Immunology, Manchester Royal Infirmary, Manchester, UK M13 9WL

**Antonino Romano**
Complesso Integrato Columbus, Rome, Italy

**Tito Rodriguez Bouza**
Harvard Medical School, Brigham and Women's Hospital,
Boston, MA, USA

**Albert L. Sheffer**
Harvard Medical School, Brigham and Women's Hospital, Boston, MA, USA

**David E. Sloane**
Rheumatology, Immunology, and Allergy Brigham and Women's Hospital Smith Building
1 Jimmy Fund Way Room 636, Boston, MA, 02115

**Mindy Tsai**
Stanford Universtiy School of Medicine, Stanford, CA, USA

**Pooja Varshney**
Duke University Medical Center, Durham, NC, USA

**Andrew A. White**
Allergy, Asthma and Immunology Department, Scripps Clinic and Scripps Green Hospital, San Diego, CA, USA

**Katharine Woessner**
Allergy, Asthma and Immunology Department, Scripps Clinic and Scripps Green Hospital, San Diego, CA, USA

# Chapter 1
# Definition and Criteria for the Diagnoses of Anaphylaxis

**Phil Lieberman**

**Abstract** It seems anti-intuitive that a phenomenon such as anaphylaxis, with explosive manifestations and distinct symptoms, should be difficult to define. However, since its discovery as a medical event in humans, there have been numerous different definitions. These definitions have evolved over approximately one century since the first demonstration of an anaphylactic event in an animal model.

Although we clearly understand the mechanism of production of anaphylactic events, and a successful treatment paradigm has been discovered, there is still debate as to the proper definition of the term "anaphylaxis." This debate has revolved around the different mechanisms of production, specifically whether the event in question is mediated by IgE, other immunologic mechanisms, or is non-immunologic. The discussion has also revolved around the clinical manifestations required to clearly establish the presence of an anaphylactic event, versus, for example, an immediate hypersensitivity disorder not reaching the requirements for an anaphylactic episode.

Thus, a number of meetings have been called and a number of physician statements have been published over the years in an attempt to refine the definition of anaphylaxis and to gather a consensus as to all it includes. This chapter traces the history of the various definitions of this condition, and focuses on those that have more recently appeared in the literature. It also briefly discusses the mechanism of production of these events and their clinical manifestations that have prompted the various definitions in question.

**Keywords** Anaphylactoid • Anaphylaxis • Angioedema • Basophil • Biphasic anaphylaxis • Carboxypeptidase • Cramping abdominal pain • Flush • Hypersensitivity reaction • IgE • Intravascular coagulation • Mast cell • Mastocytosis • National Institute of Health/Food Allergy and Anaphylaxis Network Symposium • Non-IgE-mediated • Platelet-activating factor • Protracted anaphylaxis • Scombroidosis • Shock • Shortness of breath • Syncopal episode • Tryptase • Urinary histamine • Urticaria • Vasodepressor • Vasovagal • Wheeze

## 1.1 Introduction

It seems almost counterintuitive that we would require deliberations as to what the definition of an anaphylactic event would be. Counterintuitive because such events are dramatic in presentation, and certainly are easily recognized by any physician who has dealt with the management of these events.

---

P. Lieberman (✉)
College of Medicine, University of Tennessee, 6139 Chapelle Circle West, Memphis, TN 38120, USA
e-mail: philleberman@hotmail.com

M.C. Castells (ed.), *Anaphylaxis and Hypersensitivity Reactions*,
DOI 10.1007/978-1-60327-951-2_1, 

Nonetheless, the definition of this term has been elusive since its discovery, and in the last decade, two large gatherings have been convened to discuss the criteria necessary to make a diagnosis and to establish appropriate terminology and a definition which would be suitable for all episodes.

The intent of this chapter is to discuss the evolution of the definition of anaphylaxis, the controversies regarding the nomenclature referring to anaphylactic events, and the criteria to establish a diagnosis.

## 1.2 History

In order to fully understand the present-day debate over the definition of the term "anaphylaxis" and the criteria necessary to establish its diagnosis, one must first become familiar with the history behind the development of the term.

The term "anaphylaxis" was coined in 1901 by Charles Richet and Paul Portier to describe a phenomenon they discovered while experimenting with the injection of aqueous glycerin extracts of the filaments of a species of sea anemone, *Physalia.* They first employed ducks and rabbits, and later dogs, as their experimental animals. The original experiments were conducted during a cruise on the yacht of Prince Albert of Monaco. The first experiments were carried out with *Physalia*, on the yacht utilizing ducks and rabbits. Later, upon return to France, a species of anemone, *Actinaria*, which was related to *Physalia*, but which was more readily available, was substituted, and the experiments were further carried out in dogs.

It was their intent to "immunize" the animals to the venom of these sea anemone species, but they found that the "opposite" was produced. That is, the dogs developed an *increased sensitivity* to the venom upon re-administration after a course of "immunization" injections. That is, they experienced fatal reactions to a far lower dose than occurred prior to immunization. In addition, the mode of death was different than that experienced after the administration of *toxic* fatal doses. They thus realized they were witnessing a new phenomenon. Because they produced the opposite of their original intent, prophylaxis, they called this phenomenon "anaphylaxis" ("ana" being Greek for "against" or "opposite," "phylaxis" being Greek for "protection") [1, 2]. These seminal experiments later resulted in the award of the Nobel Prize to Charles Richet in 1913.

The term anaphylaxis gained rapid clinical recognition, and, by 1925, Arthur Coca devoted a chapter to this condition in his immunology text [3]. At that time, however, our knowledge of this phenomenon was almost entirely limited to animal models, and there was some question as to whether humans belonged "in the group of animals that are 'refractory' to anaphylactic sensitization" [3]. It was also stated that at that time "no fatal sensitiveness in human beings has been recorded as a result of injections given subcutaneously, although such injections must have been given in innumerable instances at an interval of 10 days or more."

With the increased use of medications, however, it became evident that anaphylactic reactions could readily occur in human beings, and in 1945, Robert Cooke [4] defined anaphylaxis as "a special or particular immunologic type of induced protein (or hapten) sensitivity in man or experimental animals and may properly be considered as a subdivision of Allergy."

With the explosion of the number of new drugs and the utilization of polypharmacy, the incidence of anaphylactic events increased proportionally. And with the discovery of IgE, it became apparent that anaphylactic reactions were in many instances mediated via this antibody. However not all episodes could be attributed to an IgE-mediated mechanism. Thus, it was realized that the clinical expression characteristic of an anaphylactic episode had more than one mechanism of production, and the term "anaphylactoid reaction" was introduced to describe events that were clinically similar but not IgE-mediated [1]. At that time (the 1970s), the definition of anaphylaxis became "a systemic, immediate hypersensitivity reaction caused by IgE-mediated immunologic

**Table 1.1** A comparison of present-day definitions of anaphylaxis

| Term | World Allergy Organization suggested definition | Previous terminology |
|---|---|---|
| Anaphylaxis | May be immunologic or non-immunologic; used to refer to all episodes | Limited to IgE-mediated events |
| Anaphylactoid | Not used | Any event not IgE-mediated |
| Examples: | | |
| IgG or IgM related transfusion reaction | Would be classified as immunologic, non-IgE-mediated anaphylaxis | Would be classified as an anaphylactoid reaction |
| Radiocontrast (direct histamine release) | Would be classified as non-immunologic anaphylaxis | Would be classified as an anaphylactoid reaction |
| Event due to shrimp ingestion | Immunologic anaphylaxis, IgE-mediated | Anaphylaxis |

release of mediators from mast cells and basophils." The recognition that non-IgE-mediated mechanisms could produce a clinically similar event spawned the descriptor "anaphylactoid." Thus, "the term 'anaphylactoid reaction' referred (and still does refer) to a clinically similar event not mediated by immunoglobulin E."

There were objections to this terminology, however, and, in 2003, the World Allergy Organization suggested that the term "anaphylactoid" be abandoned and all such events, regardless of the mechanism of production, be called "anaphylactic episodes." They further suggested that these episodes be divided into immunologic and non-immunologic events. The non-immunologic anaphylactic events could be considered synonymous with the term "anaphylactoid," and the immunologic events were further subcategorized as IgE- and non-IgE-mediated [5, 6]. However, there are also problems with this terminology, and, to date, the term "anaphylactoid," which had become embedded in our lexicon, still remains in use. A comparison of the "anaphylaxis/anaphylactoid" classification versus the World Allergy Organization suggested change in terminology is seen in Table 1.1.

In spite of this intense and well-meaning debate over the definition of anaphylaxis, problems still haunted our efforts to find a completely acceptable terminology. For example, idiopathic anaphylaxis, which is responsible for a significant number of cases [7], is not easily accounted for utilizing either of these two presently accepted definitions. Therefore, Simons has proposed a separate category that is neither immunologic nor non-immunologic to refer to "idiopathic" events [8].

## 1.3 Issues Surrounding the Definition Today

It became obvious that another definition of anaphylaxis, perhaps established by a consensus panel, was needed. There was much disagreement over the meaning of the term "anaphylaxis," especially between physicians belonging to different specialties engaged in treating the acute event. For example, a patient manifesting only urticaria after an allergy injection administered in an allergist's office was considered by the allergist to have anaphylaxis in its first stages and therefore became a candidate for the injection of epinephrine. On the contrary, a patient presenting only with acute urticaria to an emergency department physician might not be considered by the emergency department doctor to have anaphylaxis but rather only acute urticaria. Therefore, patients presenting with identical complaints, in two different venues, were diagnosed differently. These differences in approach to the patient with a potential anaphylactic reaction might appear insignificant at first glance. However, they proved not to be because studies revealed that patients treated in emergency departments for anaphylactic events often failed to receive epinephrine, the drug of choice [9–13]. The problem was even more complex because the only diagnostic code for anaphylaxis was (and still is at the time of this writing) "anaphylactic shock" (ICD 995.0). This code does not account for patients with an obvious anaphylactic event presenting with, for example, urticaria, angioedema, wheeze, shortness of breath, and cramping abdominal pain. This ICD coding problem most certainly affects the way in which we interpret findings and code our diagnoses on a daily basis.

Because of these difficulties, an international panel of physicians with strong interests in anaphylaxis was recruited by the National Institute of Health (NIH) and the Food Allergy and Asthma Network (FAAN) to establish a more consistent, clinically relevant set of criteria that would be acceptable not only to the allergy community but to all physicians managing this disorder to diagnose this condition. The panel consisted of allergist–immunologists, emergency department physicians, intensive care physicians, pediatricians, internists, and a pathologist. There were also lay representatives from FAAN. Members were from three continents – North America, Europe, and Australia – and many were appointed as representatives of the various governing bodies of their respective specialties and subspecialties. They had two consecutive meetings, each lasting 2 days, to conduct their deliberations, and the end result was two publications: one in 2005 [14], and the other in 2006 [15].

This panel perhaps did not produce a classic definition of anaphylaxis viewed from a mechanistic perspective, but they clearly delineated the clinical characteristics that would establish a diagnosis and thus mandate treatment with epinephrine. This classification highlights a two-system involvement to make anaphylaxis highly likely even though a known allergen had not been encountered, and a one-system event (shock) if a known allergen had been encountered. The details of the classification are noted in Table 1.2.

The symposium not only developed the system seen in Table 1.2, but also felt it important to construct a short, pithy definition that would serve a clinical useful purpose not only for specialists but for all physicians faced with the diagnosis and management of a patient with anaphylaxis.

To quote: "Anaphylaxis is a severe, potentially fatal, systemic allergic reaction that occurs suddenly after contact with an allergy-causing substance."

Participants at the symposium agreed that a brief, broad definition of anaphylaxis that reflected its course and potential severity would be most useful to both the medical and lay community and recommended the following for a lay audience:

"Anaphylaxis is a serious allergic reaction that is rapid in onset and may cause death."

Even though this international panel was satisfied with their deliberations, they realized that, in truth, no established consensus criteria would provide 100% sensitivity and specificity. However, it

**Table 1.2** Critical criteria for diagnosing anaphylaxis [15]

| Anaphylaxis is highly likely when any one of the following three criteria is fulfilled: |
|---|
| 1. Acute onset of an illness (minutes to several hours) with involvement of the skin, mucosal tissues, or both (e.g., generalized hives; pruritus or flushing; swollen lips, tongue, uvula), *and at least one of the following*: |
| (a) Respiratory compromise (e.g., dyspnea, wheeze-bronchospasm, stridor, reduced PEF, hypoxemia) |
| (b) Reduced BP or associated symptoms of end-organ dysfunction (e.g., hypotonia [collapse], syncope, incontinence) |
| 2. Two or more of the following that occur rapidly after exposure to a *likely allergen for that patient* (minutes to several hours): |
| (a) Involvement of the skin-mucosal tissue (e.g., generalized hives, itch, flush, swollen lips, tongue, uvula) |
| (b) Respiratory compromise (e.g., dyspnea, wheeze-bronchospasm, stridor, reduced PEF, hypoxemia) |
| (c) Reduced BP or associated symptoms of end-organ dysfunction (e.g., hypotonia [collapse], syncope, incontinence) |
| (d) Persistent gastrointestinal symptoms (e.g., crampy abdominal pain, vomiting) |
| 3. Reduced BP after exposure to known allergen for that patient (minutes to several hours): |
| (a) Infants and children: Low systolic BP (age specific) or greater than 30% decrease in systolic BP[a] |
| (b) Adults: Systolic BP of less than 90 mmHg or greater than 30% decrease from their baseline |

*PEF* peak expiratory flow, *BP* blood pressure

[a] Low systolic BP for children is defined as less than 70 mmHg from 1 month to 1 year, less than 70 mmHg + 2x age from 1 to 10 years, and less than 90 mmHg from 11 to 17 years

was felt that the definition proposed and the criteria used to establish a diagnosis would be more than likely able to capture more than 95% of the cases.

Since the development of these criteria and the definition that they proposed, no further attempts have been made to establish diagnostic criteria or a more definitive definition.

There is little question that the deliberations of this committee have improved upon the definition of anaphylaxis because they have established a mutually acceptable definition suitable for the allergy specialist as well as other medical disciplines involved in the management of patients with anaphylaxis. However, from the standpoint of the specialist in allergy–immunology, a mechanistic definition is still important, and the author favors the definition cited above to classify anaphylactic reactions mechanistically. This definition again is: "A systemic, immediate hypersensitivity reaction caused by IgE-mediated immunologic release of mediators from mast cells and basophils." The debate as to whether all clinically similar events, not mediated by IgE, should also be referred to as *anaphylactic* as suggested by the World Allergy Organization or called *anaphylactoid* reactions still rages on.

## 1.4 The Basis for the Definition of and Criteria for the Diagnosis of Anaphylaxis

The criteria for the diagnosis of anaphylaxis that underlie its definition have been established by observational studies of the clinical manifestations of anaphylactic episodes [7, 16–36]. These series and case reports contain more than 2,000 patients and give us a fairly comprehensive picture of the frequency of the various clinical manifestations of anaphylactic events (Table 1.3).

As one can see from this table, cutaneous and subcutaneous manifestations (pruritus, flush, urticaria, and angioedema) are by far the most common in occurrence. Following cutaneous and

**Table 1.3** Frequency of occurrence of signs and symptoms of anaphylaxis[a]

| Signs and symptoms | Percentage of cases[b] |
|---|---|
| *Cutaneous* | >90 |
| Urticaria and angioedema | 85–90 |
| Flush | 45–55 |
| Pruritus without rash | 2–5 |
| *Respiratory* | 40–60 |
| Dyspnea, wheeze | 45–50 |
| Upper airway angioedema | 50–60 |
| Rhinitis | 15–20 |
| *Dizziness, syncope, hypotension* | 30–35 |
| *Abdominal* | |
| Nausea, vomiting, diarrhea cramping pain | 25–30 |
| *Miscellaneous* | |
| Headache | 5–8 |
| Substernal pain | 4–6 |
| Seizure | 1–2 |
| *Rare* | |
| Disseminated intravascular coagulation | |

[a]Based on a compilation of 2,014 patients reviewed in [7, 16–36]

[b]Percentages are approximations (see text)

subcutaneous manifestations are respiratory, cardiovascular, and gastrointestinal. These frequencies of occurrence support the suggestion by the consensus committee [14, 15] that "skin plus another manifestation" is necessary to establish the diagnosis except when shock as a single manifestation occurs in the face of exposure to a known allergen.

It is well established that cardiovascular collapse with shock can occur immediately without any cutaneous or respiratory symptoms. In a series of 27 severe episodes [29], only 70% of patients with circulatory and/or cardiovascular collapse demonstrated cutaneous manifestations. Thirty percent of these had gastrointestinal symptoms, and 85% had neurologic symptoms (seizures, impaired consciousness, and muscle spasm). The relative paucity of cutaneous manifestations may be contributed to the fact that data were recorded only from signs observed after the arrival of emergency personnel. However, another possibility is that the lack of cutaneous symptoms in these cases may have been due to sequestration of blood in the third space, leaving none available to reach the skin and cause flush or urticaria.

There are other subtleties contained within a review of these articles that do not appear from a review of the table alone. For example, although cutaneous symptoms are common manifestations of food allergy, double-blind, placebo-controlled food challenges, for reasons that have not been determined, often show a lower incidence of cutaneous reactions than has been recorded in random series. For example, Sampson [37], in an evaluation of 100 children with food allergy, employing oral food challenges, found skin symptoms occurred in only approximately 84% of subjects.

In addition, Braganza, et al., recorded a series of 57 children presenting to the emergency department with anaphylaxis. In this series, cutaneous symptoms were far less frequent than reported as a whole. Pruritus occurred in 40%, generalized erythema in 26%, and on examination, urticaria in 54%, and angioedema in 12% [32]. The overall percentage with cutaneous manifestations was 82%. The incidence of cutaneous features in this report may have been reduced because of the time between the onset of symptoms and the presentation to the emergency department. In contrast, in a larger series of anaphylaxis in children reported by Simons et al., cutaneous symptoms were clearly predominant [31].

From the studies described above, it can be seen that the definition and criteria established by the NIH/FAAN-sponsored symposium is supported by published literature. However anaphylactic episodes can manifest in unusual ways.

## 1.5 Less Common Presentations of Anaphylaxis

The symptoms of most anaphylactic events begin within 5–30 min after exposure to antigen by injection. When antigen has been ingested, symptoms usually occur within the first 2 h after ingestion. Occasionally there can be a delay for several hours. It is thought that the more rapidly they appear after exposure to antigen, the more severe the attack.

An episode can abate and then exhibit a recurrence several hours after the disappearance of the original manifestations. Such events have been termed "biphasic anaphylactic episodes." In addition, attacks can be prolonged, persisting for several days without interruption in symptoms. Protracted shock and adult respiratory distress syndrome can occur despite appropriate therapy. The exact incidence of biphasic reactions is unknown. However, series have demonstrated them to occur from as low as 1% to as high as 20% of episodes [38].

The severity of the second response is variable. Events have ranged from mild to severe. Fatalities have been reported during biphasic episodes.

Cardiac manifestations of anaphylaxis can be highly varied. Characteristically, anaphylaxis is associated with a compensatory tachycardia occurring in response to a decreased effective vascular volume. Additionally, the tachycardia has been used to differentiate an anaphylactic event from a vasodepressor (vasovagal) reaction. However, bradycardia, presumably caused by increased vagal reactivity, can also occur in anaphylaxis. The mechanism appears to be mediated via the Bezold–Jarisch reflex. The reflex is cardioinhibitory. It has its origin in sensory receptors in the inferoposterior wall of the left ventricle. It is carried by unmyelinated vagal C fibers activated by ischemia. Brown et al. [33] reported bradycardia in a study of anaphylaxis provoked by deliberate insect stings in a controlled setting is not uncommon. Bradycardia, accompanied by hypotension, occurred in a significant number of subjects. Usually the bradycardia was preceded by a tachycardia.

Anaphylaxis can present with unusual features making a diagnosis difficult. Syncope without other manifestations has been reported after fire ant sting, mastocytosis, and exercise [25]. Individuals experiencing syncope alone can present with a seizure or simply spontaneous loss of consciousness. This form of presentation oftentimes results in unnecessary cardiovascular and neurological evaluation before the diagnosis of anaphylaxis is established. In toddlers and infants who present with anaphylactic episodes, the major manifestation may mimic foreign body aspiration [25]. Vomiting without aspiration minutes after the ingestion of an allergenic food is also a common initial presentation in this age group.

Anaphylaxis has been known to cause adrenal hemorrhage, and present with hypotension and symptoms of adrenal insufficiency [1].

Profound anaphylactic episodes with hypotension can result in disseminated intravascular coagulation. These events may be both IgE- and non-IgE-mediated [35].

## 1.6 Conditions with Similar Manifestations: The Differential Diagnosis of Anaphylaxis

Any chapter dealing with the manifestations of anaphylaxis would not be complete without a mention of those conditions that express similar manifestations, and therefore should be considered in the differential diagnosis of anaphylactic events (Table 1.4).

Perhaps the most common condition mimicking anaphylaxis is the vasodepressor (vasovagal) response. The vasodepressor reaction is characterized by a fall in blood pressure, pallor, weakness, nausea, vomiting, and diaphoresis. There may be loss of consciousness. Such reactions can result from a threatening event or emotional trauma. There is a characteristic bradycardia that has been used as a differential diagnostic factor, but as noted above, bradycardia can also occur during anaphylaxis. Therefore, important distinguishing features are the lack of urticaria, angioedema, or flush in vasodepressor responses.

Entities causing flush should also be considered in the differential diagnosis. A number of ingested substances including niacin, nicotine, catecholamines, angiotensin converting enzyme (ACE) inhibitors, and alcohol can produce flushing. Flushing can also be seen in association with carcinoid syndrome, pancreatic tumors, medullary carcinoma of the thyroid, hypoglycemia, rosacea, pheochromocytoma, menopause, autonomic epilepsy, panic attacks, and systemic mastocytosis [1]. Scombroidosis, histamine poisoning, is also considered in a differential diagnosis. It is due to the ingestion of spoiled fish and is increasing in frequency. Histamine is the major chemical involved in the production of symptoms, but these symptoms cannot be explained entirely by the ingestion of histamine alone [1]. The ingestion of histamine-contaminated spoiled fish is more toxic than the ingestion of equal amounts of pure histamine by mouth. Cis-urocanic acid, an imidazole compound similar to histamine that is derived from histidine in spoiled fish, might be partially responsible for the manifestations of Scombroidosis [1].

The features of scombroidosis are very similar to those of anaphylaxis and include cardiovascular, gastrointestinal, cutaneous, and neurologic manifestations. They occur a few minutes to several hours after ingestion of fish and can last for a few hours to several days. They include urticaria, flush,

**Table 1.4** Differential diagnosis of anaphylaxis

| |
|---|
| *Anaphylaxis due to exogenously administered agents, e.g., drugs and foods* |
| *Anaphylaxis due to physical factors* |
| Exercise |
| Cold |
| Heat |
| Sunlight |
| *Idiopathic anaphylaxis* |
| *Vasodepressor reactions* |
| *Flush syndromes* |
| Carcinoid |
| Postmenopausal |
| Alcohol |
| Drugs |
| Niacin |
| Vasointestinal polypeptide secreting tumors |
| Medullary carcinoma thyroid |
| *Other forms of shock* |
| Hemorrhagic |
| Cardiogenic |
| Endotoxic |
| "*Restaurant syndromes*" |
| Monosodium glutamate (MSG) |
| Sulfites |
| Scombroidosis |
| *Excess endogenous production of histamine syndromes* |
| Systemic mastocytosis |
| Urticaria pigmentosa |
| Basophilic leukemia |
| Acute promyelocytic leukemia (tretinoin treatment) |
| Hydatid cyst |
| *Non-organic disease* |
| Panic attacks |
| Münchhausen stridor |
| Vocal cord dysfunction syndrome |
| Globus hystericus |
| Undifferentiated somatoform anaphylaxis |
| *Miscellaneous* |
| Hereditary angioedema |
| "Progesterone" anaphylaxis |
| Urticarial vasculitis |
| Pheochromocytoma |
| Hyperimmunoglobulin E, urticaria syndrome |
| Neurologic (seizure, stroke) |
| Pseudoanaphylaxis |
| Red man syndrome (vancomycin) |
| Capillary leak syndrome |

angioedema, nausea, vomiting, diarrhea, and hypotension. Neurological findings and wheezing can also occur. Flushing of the face and neck is the most common manifestation. The rash itself is usually more similar to sunburn than urticaria. Scombroidosis can be distinguished from anaphylaxis by the nature of cutaneous symptoms and the presence of elevated amounts of plasma histamine and 24-h urinary histamine metabolites in the absence of elevation of serum tryptase. Also, in scombroidosis, several members at the dinner table may experience symptoms simultaneously.

## 1.7 The Need for a Biomarker

As one can see from the above comments, it would be highly desirable to have a biomarker to increase the sensitivity and specificity of efforts to establish a definitive diagnosis of anaphylaxis. This biomarker ideally would be highly specific and extremely sensitive. To date, we have reasonably good specificity with our biomarkers, but less than desirable sensitivity.

The biomarkers that have been best studied are plasma histamine, 24-h urinary histamine and/or its metabolites, serum tryptase, serum carboxypeptidase, and platelet-activating factor.

### *1.7.1 Tryptase*

The most widely employed biomarker to confirm a diagnosis of anaphylaxis consists of the measurement of total tryptase. It is more valuable in terms of its specificity than its sensitivity, and, therefore, a negative total tryptase cannot be used by itself to exclude the diagnosis. The optimal time to obtain a total serum tryptase is within 3 h of the onset of symptoms [6]. Normal values usually range from 1 to 11.4 ng/mL.

Not only does an elevated level of tryptase measured during an episode support a diagnosis of anaphylaxis, baseline levels between episodes may also be helpful as a screening test for systemic mastocytosis as a cause for anaphylactic episodes. In this regard, they have a very high specificity but the sensitivity is probably around 85% [6].

Also there are some vagaries that are poorly understood regarding the measurement of serum tryptase. One of these is the fact that food-induced anaphylactic episodes are less likely to be associated with elevated levels. The cause for this is unclear, but it has been hypothesized that tryptase released by mucosal mast cells is less likely to produce elevated serum levels than that produced by connective tissue (perivascular) mast cells. Mucosal mast cells contain less tryptase, and theoretically tryptase from mucosal surface mast cells may enter the circulation less efficiently than that produced by cells located in connective tissue [39].

In addition, total tryptase levels can be elevated in other conditions including acute monocytic leukemia, hypereosinophilic syndrome associated with the FIP1L1-PDGFRA mutation, end-stage renal disease, and various myelodysplastic syndromes.

### *1.7.2 Plasma Histamine and Urinary Histamine*

Perhaps the second most common test ordered to substantiate the diagnosis of anaphylaxis is a measurement of either plasma histamine or 24-h urinary histamine metabolites. Because histamine has a very short half-life in blood, it must be measured within 60 min of the onset of symptoms to obtain optimal results. When measured at that time, plasma histamine levels may be more likely to be elevated than serum tryptase [39].

Because it is rare that plasma histamine levels can be obtained shortly after the onset of symptoms, urinary histamine metabolites collected over a 24-h period have been utilized.

### 1.7.3 Carboxypeptidase A

Carboxypeptidase A3 can be measured in serum or plasma and has been investigated as a marker for anaphylactic episodes. In some studies, it has been shown to be superior to tryptase as a diagnostic marker. Mast cell carboxypeptidase A and tryptase have different pharmacokinetics and times of appearance and disappearance in the serum and do not necessarily correlate with each other. Carboxypeptidase A levels usually remain elevated longer than total serum tryptase and have been detected in patients with anaphylaxis who did not demonstrate elevated total tryptase levels [39].

### 1.7.4 Platelet-Activating Factor

Platelet-activating factor is secreted by numerous cells including basophils, mast cells, macrophages, and monocytes. It has been shown to be elevated in patients experiencing anaphylactic episodes and levels have been shown in at least one study to correlate with the severity of the disease [40].

## 1.8 Conclusions

The definition of anaphylaxis has evolved considerably since the first description by Richet and Portier. There is no perfect definition of this disorder, but the definition and criteria established by the NIH/FAAN Symposium appears to be the best to date, establishing the clinical manifestations necessary to make the diagnosis of an anaphylactic event. Most importantly, these criteria can be considered to define the manifestations necessary for the administration of epinephrine.

In addition, this symposium put forth simple definitions for both the lay public and for physicians including specialists and nonspecialists. However, the symposium did not offer a definition based upon mechanism. In addition, this symposium did not definitively address the issues involved as to terminology, namely as to whether or not, as suggested by the World Allergy Organization, the term "anaphylactoid reaction" be no longer used.

Thus, in summary, there still remain several possible definitions to refer to an anaphylactic event as follows:

1. The mechanistic definition: "Anaphylaxis is a systemic, immediate hypersensitivity reaction caused by IgE-mediated immunologic release of mediators from mast cells and basophils."
2. A definition suitable for physicians of all specialties and subspecialties that is not concerned with mechanisms, but designed for simplicity: "Anaphylaxis is a severe, potentially fatal, systemic allergic reaction that occurs suddenly after contact with an allergy causing substance."
3. A definition mainly designed for the lay public: "Anaphylaxis is a serious allergic reaction that is rapid in onset and may cause death."

The issue of terminology then still persists. According to the classic terminology, anaphylaxis is distinguished from anaphylactoid events based upon the mechanism of action underlying the event. In the "classic" definition, an anaphylactoid event would be defined as follows: "An anaphylactoid event refers to an event clinically similar to anaphylaxis not mediated by immunoglobulin E activated degranulation of mast cells and basophils."

In the World Allergy Organization suggestion for terminology, all such events would be "anaphylactic," further subdivided as to whether they are immunologically mediated by IgE, immunologically medicated by other mechanisms, or due to non-immunologic direct histamine release.

## References

1. Lieberman P. Anaphylaxis and anaphylactoid reactions. In: Middleton E, Ellis EF, Yunginger JW, Reed CE, Adkinson NF, Busse WW, eds. *Allergy: Principles and Practice.* 5th ed., Vol. II. St. Louis, MO: Mosby-Year Book, Inc.; 1998:1079–1092.
2. Samter M. *Excerpts from Classics in Allergy.* Columbus, OH: Ross Laboratories; 1969:32–33. Library of Congress Catalog Number 70-77908. Published for the 25th Anniversary of the American Academy of Allergy.
3. Coca AF. *Essentials of Immunology for Medical Students.* Baltimore, MD: The Williams and Wilkins Company; 1925:63.
4. Cooke RA. *Allergy in Theory and Practice.* Philadelphia, PA: W. B. Saunders Company; 1945:5.
5. Johansson SJO, Bieber T, Dahl R, et al. Revised nomenclature for allergy for global use: report of the nomenclature review committee of the World Allergy Organization, October 2003. *J Allergy Clin Immunol.* 2004;113:832–836.
6. Lieberman P. Anaphylaxis. In: Atkinson F, Bochner B, Busse W, Holgate S, Lemanske R, Simons FER, eds. *Allergy: Principles and Practice.* 7th ed. Philadelphia, PA: Mosby; 2009:1027–1051.
7. Webb L, Lieberman P. Anaphylaxis: a review of 601 cases. *Ann Allergy, Asthma, Immunol.* 2006;97(1):39–43.
8. Simons FER. Anaphylaxis, killer allergy: long-term management in the community. *J Allergy Clin Immunol.* 2006;117:367–377.
9. Oren E, Banerji A, Clark S, Camargo C. Food-induced anaphylaxis and repeated epinephrine treatments. Ann. Allergy Asthma Immunol. November 2007;99(5):429–432.
10. Lieberman P, Decker W, Camargo CA Jr, Oconnor R, Oppenheimer J, Simons FE. SAFE, a multidisciplinary approach to anaphylaxis education in the emergency department. *Ann Allergy Asthma Immunol.* 2007;98(6):519–523.
11. Clark S, Camargo CA Jr. Emergency treatment and prevention of insect sting anaphylaxis. *Curr Opin Allergy Clin Immunol.* 2006; 6(4):279–283.
12. Clark S, Long AA, Gaeta TJ, Camargo CA Jr. Multicenter study of emergency department visits for insect sting allergy. *J Allergy Clin Immunol.* 2005;116(3):643–649.
13. Clark S, Bock SA, Gaeta TJ, Brenner BE, Cydulka RK, Camargo CA. Multicenter study of emergency department visits for food allergy. *J Allergy Clin Immunol.* 2004;113(2):347–352.
14. Sampson HA, Munoz-Furlong A, Bock SA, et al. Symposium on the definition and management of anaphylaxis: summary report. *J Allergy Clin Immunol.* 2005;115:584–592.
15. Sampson HA, Munoz-Furlong A, Campbell RL, et al. Second symposium on the definition and management of anaphylaxis: summary report – Second National Institute of Allergy and Infectious Disease/Food Allergy and Anaphylaxis Network Symposium. *J Allergy Clin Immunol.* 2006;117:391–397.
16. Yocum MW, Butterfield J, Klein J, et al. Epidemiology of anaphylaxis in Olmstead County, A population-based study. *J Allergy Clin Immunol.* 1999;104:452–456.
17. Yocum MW, Khan DA. Assessment of patients who have experienced anaphylaxis: a three year survey. *Mayo Clin Proc.* 1994;69:16–23.
18. Perez C, Tejedor MA, Hoz A, Puras V. Anaphylaxis: a descriptive study of 182 patients (abstract). *J Allergy Clin Immunol.* 1995;95:368.
19. Coghlan-Johnston M, Lieberman P. Demographic and clinical characteristics of anaphylaxis (abstract). *J Allergy Clin Immunol.* 2001;107:557.
20. Lee JM, Greenes DS. Biphasic anaphylactic reactions in pediatrics. *Pediatrics.* 2000;106:762.
21. Wade JP, Liang MH, Sheffer AL. Exercise-induced anaphylaxis: epidemiological observations. *Prog Clin Biol Res.* 1989;297:175.
22. Ditto A, Harris K, Krasnick J, et al. Idiopathic anaphylaxis: a series of 335 cases. *Ann Allergy Asthma Immunol.* 1996;77:285–291.
23. Wiggins CA. Characteristics and etiology of 30 patients with anaphylaxis. *Immun Allergy Pract.* 1991;13(8):313–316.
24. Perez C, Tejdor M, de la Hoz B, et al. Anaphylaxis: a descriptive study of 182 patients (abstract). *J Allergy Clin Immunol.* 1995;95:368.
25. Lieberman P. Unique clinical presentations of anaphylaxis. *Immunol Allergy Clin North Am.* 2001;21:813.
26. Cianferoni A, Novembre E, Lombardi E, et al. Clinical features of severe acute anaphylaxis in patients admitted to a university hospital: an 11 year retrospective review. *J Allergy Clin Immunol.* 2001;107:S57.
27. Dibs SD, Baker SD. Anaphylaxis in children: a 5 year experience (abstract). *Pediatrics.* 1997;99:118.
28. Viner NA, Rhamy RK. Anaphylaxis manifested by hypotension alone. *J Urol.* 1975;113:108.
29. Soreide E, Buxrud T, Harboe S. Severe anaphylactic reactions outside hospital: etiology, symptoms and treatment. *Acta Anaesthesiol Scand.* 1988;32:339.
30. Sampson HA. Food allergy, part II: diagnosis and management. *J Allergy Clin Immunol.* 1999;103:981.

31. Simons FER, Chad ZH, Gold M. Anaphylaxis in children. *Allergy Clin Immunol Int.* 2004;1(Suppl):242–244.
32. Braganza SC, Acworth JP, Mckinnon DR, et al. Pediatric emergency department anaphylaxis: different patterns from adults. *Arch Dis Child.* 2006;91:159–163.
33. Brown SG, Blackman KE, Stenlake V, et al. Insect sting anaphylaxis; prospective evaluation of treatment with intravenous adrenaline and volume resuscitation. *Emerg Med J.* 2004;21:149–154.
34. Kounis NG. Kounis syndrome (allergic angina and allergic myocardial infarction): a natural paradigm. *Int J Cardiology.* 2006;110:7–14. (Epub 2005, October 24)
35. DeSouza RL, Short T, Warman GR, et al. Anaphylaxis associated with fibrinolysis, reversed with tranexamic acid and demonstrated by thromboelastography. *Anaesth Intensive Care.* 2004;32:580–587.
36. Alangari AA, Twarog FJ, Shih M-C, Schneider LC. Clinical features and anaphylaxis in children with cold urticaria. *Pediatrics.* 2004;113(4):e313–e317. Available at http://www.pediatrics.org/cgi/content/full/113/4/e313. Accessed January 2009.
37. Sampson HA. Utility of food-specific IgE concentrations in predicting symptomatic food allergy. *J Allergy Clin Immunol.* 2001;107:891–896.
38. Lieberman P. Biphasic anaphylactic reactions. *Ann Allergy Asthma Immunol.* 2005;95:217–228.
39. Simons FER, Frew AJ, Ansotequi IJ, et al. Risk assessment in anaphylaxis: current and future approaches. *J Allergy Clin Immunol.* 2007;120(1):S2–S24.
40. Vadas P, Gold M, Perelman B, et al. Platelet-activating factor, PAF acetyl hydrolase, and severe anaphylaxis. *N Engl J Med.* 2008;358:28.

# Chapter 2
# An Epidemiological Approach to Reducing the Risk of Fatal Anaphylaxis

**Richard S.H. Pumphrey**

**Abstract** Estimates of the population prevalence of anaphylaxis range from 0.03% to 0.95% with immediately-life-threatening reactions affecting <0.1% of the population; wide differences in published statistics are due to differing inclusion criteria and imprecise use of terms such as incidence and prevalence. Expected symptoms in anaphylaxis vary according to the trigger and population studied. The severity of reactions is determined by interaction between genetic and environmental factors and cannot yet be predicted accurately. Whether a reaction is fatal or not depends as much on comorbidity such as asthma or heart disease as it does on severity of allergy or dose and route of exposure to the trigger.

The UK fatal anaphylaxis register is the longest-running and most comprehensive attempt at epidemiology of fatal anaphylaxis; it has recorded around 1 anaphylactic death per 3 million population each year since 1992, about half of these were iatrogenic (predominantly older people) and the rest divided between sting reactions and (mostly in younger people) food allergy. Most deaths were first reactions: fatal recurrent reactions occurred through avoidance failure combined with failure of rescue treatment – lessons from these failures can teach how to reduce future fatalities.

**Keyword** Epidemiology fatal anaphylaxis

## 2.1 Introduction

Epidemiology is the "who, what, why, where, and when?" of a disease; it is essential for the development of logical management strategies. In the case of anaphylaxis it asks "Who is affected? What triggers their reactions? Why, where, and when do they become exposed to the trigger for their reactions?" Although it is generally an observational rather than interventional science, it can nevertheless study outcomes of different management strategies, for instance by asking "How many of those dying had been prescribed self-injectible epinephrine and why had this failed to save them?"

But epidemiology depends on clear and simple definition of the population to be studied and here anaphylaxis presents a problem: allergic reactions have a continuous spectrum of severity (Fig. 2.1) [1–3] and manifold combinations of symptoms contributing to this severity. Non-life-threatening reactions may have dramatic presentation with many severe symptoms and fatal reactions may show little before cardiac or respiratory arrest.

R.S.H. Pumphrey (✉)
Honorary Consultant Immunologist, Department of Immunology,
Manchester Royal Infirmary, Manchester, UK M13 9WL
e-mail: richard.pumphrey@nhs.net

M.C. Castells (ed.), *Anaphylaxis and Hypersensitivity Reactions*,
DOI 10.1007/978-1-60327-951-2_2, © Springer Science+Business Media, LLC 2011

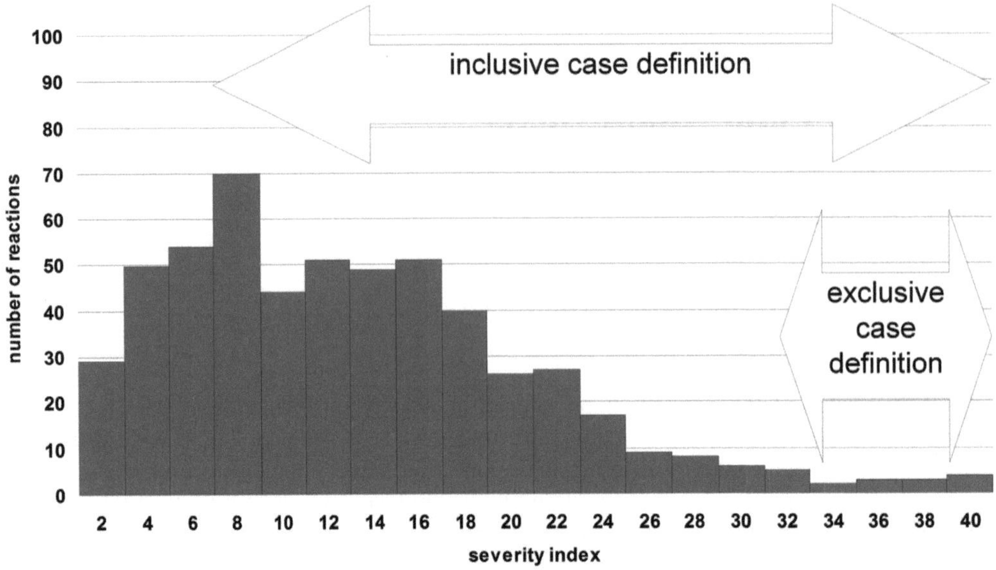


**Fig. 2.1** Distribution of severity of 720 reactions in 320 Manchester clinic patients using a weighted symptom score described in reference [1]. Applying different case definitions from published studies such as reference [2] or reference [3], there could be as much as a thirty-fold difference in numbers of the population included in the study

A variety of definitions have been proposed for anaphylaxis, all including descriptions such as "allergic reaction," "severe, generalized," "life-threatening." None of these is perfect because not all anaphylaxis is allergic [4], most authors include cases that did not endanger life, and acute allergic reactions can kill without being generalized.

Whatever the definition, there is general agreement that anaphylactic reactions are best treated by epinephrine [5, 6], and that the first dose should be given early during the course of the reaction. Because the evolution of such reactions is unpredictable, consensus groups have moved away from a bald definition towards detailed descriptions of symptom complexes that are characteristic of allergic reactions that *might* progress to anaphylaxis. A leading example is shown in Table 2.1. The authors [7] estimate it will identify 95% of all cases that will progress to anaphylaxis (i.e., its sensitivity is 0.95) but give no estimate of the definition's specificity (the fraction of allergic reactions that will not progress to anaphylaxis that are excluded by the Table 2.1 description). Clinical experience and data such as Figure 2.1 suggest that the specificity will be low because so few patients fulfilling the criteria in Table 2.1 would progress to respiratory or cardiac arrest if given no treatment. A low specificity may be unimportant if the objective is to make sure that every case that might need epinephrine is given it early in the reaction, but epidemiology needs a specific definition as much as it needs a sensitive one.

Further discussion of sensitivity and specificity of definitions for anaphylaxis can be found in the publications of the Brighton Collaboration, whose focus is specifically on recording adverse reactions to vaccines [8]. Accepting the inverse relationship between specificity and sensitivity, they resorted to using three levels of certainty: level 1 with highest specificity but lowest sensitivity, and level 3 with highest sensitivity but lowest specificity. Numerical estimates for sensitivity (approximately 0.6–0.7) and specificity (approximately 0.7–0.8) of these definitions have recently been published [9]. Because there is no gold standard for the definition of anaphylaxis, these estimates are based on physician diagnosis and therefore reflect the physician's opinion about what anaphylaxis is. Such opinion is typically colored by confusion between a *definition* of anaphylaxis and *descriptions of symptom complexes that might progress to anaphylaxis*, resulting in inclusions of non-anaphylactic reactions with symptoms of the type that occur in reactions that might progress to anaphylaxis.

**Table 2.1** Anaphylaxis is likely when any one of these three criteria is fulfilled. Note that this is *not a definition of anaphylaxis* but, rather, is a description of symptom complexes that might progress to anaphylaxis

1. Acute onset of an illness (minutes to several hours) with involvement of the skin, mucosal tissue, or both (e.g., generalized hives, pruritus or flushing, swollen lips/tongue/uvula) *and at least one of the following*:
   (a) Respiratory compromise (e.g., dyspnea, wheeze–bronchospasm, stridor, reduced PEF [peak expiratory flow], hypoxemia)
   (b) Reduced BP (blood pressure) or associated symptoms of end-organ dysfunction (e.g., hypotonia [collapse], syncope, incontinence)
2. Two or more of the following that occur rapidly after exposure to a likely allergen for that patient (minutes to several hours):
   (a) Involvement of the skin-mucosal tissue (e.g., generalized hives, itch–flush, swollen lips/tongue/uvula)
   (b) Respiratory compromise (e.g., dyspnea, wheeze–bronchospasm, stridor, reduced PEF, hypoxemia)
   (c) Reduced BP or associated symptoms (e.g., hypotonia [collapse], syncope, incontinence)
   (d) Persistent gastrointestinal symptoms (e.g., crampy abdominal pain, vomiting)
3. Reduced BP after exposure to known allergen for that patient (minutes to several hours):
   (a) Infants and children: low systolic BP (age specific) or greater than 30% decrease in systolic BP [Low systolic blood pressure for children is defined as less than 70 mm Hg from 1 month to 1 year, less than (70 mm Hg + [2 x age]) from 1 to 10 years, and less than 90 mm Hg from 11 to 17 years]
   (b) Adults: systolic BP of less than 90 mm Hg or greater than 30% decrease from that person's baseline

## 2.2 Prevalence and Incidence of Anaphylaxis

The imprecise use of the terms incidence and prevalence by some reports on the epidemiology of anaphylaxis may cause confusion. The *incidence* of a condition is *the rate of appearance of new cases.* Incidence is a fractional rate with units $t^{-1}$; it is usually quoted as cases per 100,000 (or similar fraction) per year (or similar interval). Studies of incidence of anaphylaxis have generally reported the incidence of reactions, not of new cases: those studies that have asked the appropriate question have recorded that most of those presenting with an acute reaction have a history of previous reactions and are therefore not new cases.

In a defined population, at a given time, the *prevalence* of a condition is *the probability that an individual chosen at random will have the condition.* Prevalence is a dimensionless number in the range 0–1. It is usually quoted as a percentage or cases per 100,000. Anaphylactic reactions occur when someone with the underlying hypersensitivity state is exposed to the appropriate trigger in a way that will cause an anaphylactic reaction. Epidemiology of anaphylaxis measures the prevalence of *reactions*, not the underlying hypersensitivity state. Thus the observed prevalence is the product of the prevalence of the hypersensitivity state and the probability of exposure to a sufficient dose of provoking agent by an appropriate route to cause an anaphylactic reaction. The prevalence of anaphylactic hypersensitivity in the general population might be as high as 15% if one worked at finding the optimal dose and route for the allergen – e.g., an intravenous injection of grass pollen extract in people with hay fever, or restinging everyone who had a wasp sting 3–8 weeks after their sting. Fortunately, the probability of exposure is low and kept low by self-preservation. After a mild allergic reaction to nuts, most people carefully avoid nuts. One study [10] found within a median interval of 5.4 years following the initial peanut reaction, 55% had 1–5 (average 2) accidental re-exposures.

## 2.3 Epidemiological Studies of Nonfatal Anaphylaxis

The Brighton Collaboration definition of anaphylaxis (or more exactly, description of symptom complexes that might occur in anaphylaxis) may be the best achievable for epidemiological recording but is too elaborate for most retrospective studies. An approximation to the prevalence and incidence of anaphylaxis is known from a variety of approaches that settle for lower sensitivity and specificity such as analysis of prescribing of self-injectible epinephrine [11, 12], coding of hospital admissions [13] or discharges [14], or cases developing in those already admitted to hospital [15], general practitioner records[16], referrals to emergency medicine departments [17, 18] or allergy clinics [1, 19, 20], or self-reported anaphylaxis from a sample population by questionnaire [21].

When the case definition is based on self-injectible epinephrine prescriptions, there is an assumption that anaphylaxis has been adequately diagnosed by the prescribing doctor. An unpublished audit of referrals to anaphylaxis clinics in Manchester, UK, suggested the diagnosis was correct for around half the patients. Because it is impossible to predict which reactions will become dangerous, epinephrine must be given for any reaction with the characteristics in Table 2.1 if it is to have a chance of preventing 95% of evolving allergic reactions becoming life-threatening. Depending on our degree of caution, from 0.1% to 100% of those with a history of acute allergic reaction might benefit by carrying epinephrine in the sense that it would attenuate the severity of a recurrence of their reaction. These considerations indicate that estimates of anaphylaxis prevalence based on self-injectible epinephrine prescriptions may have a tenuous link to the actual prevalence.

When the case definition is based on the diagnostic code, the assumption is both that the diagnosis (usually by a nonspecialist) was correct, and that the condition has been correctly coded. While common conditions are accurately coded, rare conditions such as anaphylaxis are frequently coded incorrectly. It should also be pointed out that most cases of anaphylaxis treated in the emergency department do not get admitted to hospital; unpublished audit of admissions in Central Manchester, UK, suggest that a majority of cases admitted and coded as anaphylaxis were not. Examples include idiopathic angioedema that was dramatic but not life-threatening, gross angioedema of the tongue unresponsive to epinephrine, angiotensin converting enzyme inhibitor (ACEI)-induced angioedema and one patient with acquired C1 esterase inhibitor who was admitted seven times with upper airways angioedema unresponsive to epinephrine before the correct diagnosis was made.

These limitations mean that the statistics presented in the tables here can only give the broadest-brush picture of anaphylaxis around the world. In summary:

1. The continuous spectrum of severity of allergic reactions leads to wide variations in estimates of the prevalence of anaphylaxis (Fig. 2.1). A recent expert review [22] reckoned that the best estimates of population prevalence ranged from 0.03% to 0.95% with one estimate of 1.2–16.8% [2]. This implies that immediately life-threatening reactions (those causing a dangerous degree of shock or severe respiratory difficulty) affect <0.1% of the population, consistent with data in the UK fatal anaphylaxis register indicating 0.005–0.01% of UK deaths were due to anaphylaxis during 1992–2005.
2. Expected symptoms in anaphylaxis vary according to the trigger and population studied (Table 2.2) [1–5].
3. Common triggers for severe reactions comprise iatrogenic, stings, food, and latex; for some reactions no trigger was found – maybe because the patient was underinvestigated or maybe because it was an idiopathic reaction. The relative frequency of each class of trigger and of individual triggers within each class depends on the population studied (Table 2.3). Infants and young children are most likely to have severe reactions to milk and eggs; older children and adolescents to nuts or seafood; and adults to iatrogenic triggers, stings, and foods such as nuts and seafood. When only reactions that caused respiratory or cardiac arrest are considered, iatrogenic causes outweigh stings and foods in most studies that include all three classes in an unbiased way. For food allergy in particular, mild to moderate reactions are so much more common than immediately life-threatening reactions that wide differences in estimates of the dominant causes of anaphylaxis have been reported, depending on the cut-off taken between acute allergic reaction and anaphylaxis.

**Table 2.2** The probability of various symptoms/signs in anaphylaxis. Frequencies in different publications reflect different concepts of "anaphylaxis" and different catchment populations. Each study omitted frequencies for some symptoms; none mentioned common symptoms such as a sense of impending doom or important symptoms seen occasionally in severe reactions such as fitting or pink froth from the mouth due to pulmonary edema. Each individual symptom/sign has moderate to low sensitivity and most have low specificity, even in the case of a rapidly evolving illness

| | Med Rec [23] | Adult ED [24] | Ped ED [25] | Perioperative [26] | Drug induced [27] |
|---|---|---|---|---|---|
| Pruritus | 0.55 | 0.56 | 0.40 | – | 0.34 |
| Difficulty breathing | 0.43 | 0.43 | 0.54 | – | |
| Faintness | 0.15 | 0.15 | 0.04 | – | |
| Sneezing/rhinitis | 0.17 | 0.06 | [<0.11] | – | [<0.1] |
| Chest pain | 0.03 | | | – | |
| Abdominal pain | 0.08 | | | – | 0.06 |
| Nausea/vomiting | 0.09 | 0.19 | 0.21 | – | 0.19 |
| Urgent bowel action | 0.01 | | | – | 0.05 |
| Erythema | 0.36 | 0.07 | 0.25–0.35 | [<0.72/<0.93] | 0.64 |
| Urticaria | 0.55 | 0.49 | 0.54 | [<0.72/<0.93] | 0.29 |
| Angioedema (unspecified) | 0.56 | 0.40 | 0.32 | 0.12/0.08 | 0.55 |
| Angioedema tongue | 0.15 | | | | [<0.1] |
| Upper airway Angioedema | 0.07 | 0.11 | 0.18 | | 0.07 |
| Bronchospasm/wheeze | 0.26 | 0.18/0.35 | 0.19 | 0.40/0.19 | 0.51 |
| Stridor | | 0.01 | 0.01 | | |
| Conjunctivitis | 0.23 | [<0.06] | [<0.11] | | 0.10 |
| Tachycardia | 0.27 | | | | 0.24 |
| Bradycardia | 0.02 | | | 0.01/0.01 | 0.09 |
| Collapse | 0.03 | 0.02 | 0 | 0.51/0.11 | 0.35 |
| Shock/hypotension | 0.05 | 0.09 | 0 | 0.17/0.18 | 0.55 |

4. Geographical differences in anaphylaxis are complex and depend on many factors, ranging from prescribing habits [28], stinging insect populations [29], pollen exposure [30], food ingredient prevalence [31], to ethnic [32] and racial genetic characteristics.
5. As well as seasonal variation [33], studies of time trends indicate that anaphylaxis is getting more common [12, 34].

## 2.4 Factors Determining the Severity of Acute Allergic Reactions

What factors underlie the range of severity of acute allergic reactions seen in Figure 2.1? Broadly we might expect the severity of a reaction to be a product of the degree of allergy and the dose of allergen. Those who regularly perform challenge tests will be familiar with the unpredictable way in which reactions become more severe with increasing challenge dose once the threshold for reacting has been passed. The threshold dose for a reaction may change from day to day and can be affected by the process of challenge: thus cautiously increasing repeated doses during a challenge may be similar in effect to ultra-rush immunotherapy induction and raise the threshold for a reaction. Conversely, a negative sting challenge may be followed by a reaction to a subsequent sting [35], maybe through naturally occurring fluctuations in the reaction threshold or because the challenge sting sensitized the patient.

Allergy tests do not tell us how severe a reaction will be. Although there is good correlation between *negative* specific IgE and/or skin prick tests and *lack of clinical sensitivity*, neither specific IgE level nor skin prick test weal diameter relate closely to the severity of reactions and even the

**Table 2.3** Relative frequency of major groups of supposed trigger for anaphylaxis

| Source | Cases | Drug (%) | Common drugs | Stings (%) | Food (%) | Common foods | Other (%) | Other= | Idiopathic (%) |
|---|---|---|---|---|---|---|---|---|---|
| ED Hong Kong[18] | 282 | 40 | NSAID, antibiotics, Chinese medicines | 7 | 50 | Seafood | | | 1 |
| *clinic Switzerland [20] | 226 | 18 | NSAID > antibiotics > others | 59 | 10 | Celeriac > all others | 3 | Latex | 5 |
| Adult ED Australia [24] | 142 | 28 | Antibiotics > NSAID > others | 17 | 17 | Seafood > nuts | | | 17 |
| Ped ED Australia [25] | 57 | 5 | Antibiotics | 5 | 32 | Egg, milk > nuts | 1 | Latex | 32 |
| Clinic Australia[19] | 432 | 8 | NSAID > antibiotic > others | 20 | 61 | Nuts > egg > others | 1 | | 8 |
| †OR France[26] | 4904 | 86 | NMBA > antibiotics > others | 0 | 0 | | 14 | Latex | 0 |
| Ped Hospital code USA[14] | 6457 | 28 + 25 | Immunization/ serum + others | Excluded | 32 | ? | 14 | Unspecified | |
| Hospital codes Holland[27] | 391 | 35 | Glafenine > antibiotics > others | 55 | 9 | | 1 | | |

*anaphylaxis defined as including shock.

†compiled from a table of IgE-mediated perioperative reactions 1984–2002: the original table demonstrates strong time trends in the relative frequency of the causative agents.

Double Blind Placebo Controlled Food Challenge (DBPCFC) response only correlated weakly [36]. So what are the other factors that determine severity?

Data from patients in Manchester, UK [37], suggested the severity of coexisting atopic diseases predicted which patients were most likely to develop life-threatening allergic reactions to peanuts and tree nuts. A previous history of atopic eczema correlated with shock during anaphylaxis, rhinitis with upper airway angioedema, and asthma with a principally asthmatic mode of anaphylaxis. Additionally, patients with the lowest serum angiotensin converting enzyme (ACE) concentrations were more likely to develop life-threatening pharyngeal edema, suggesting that this type of reaction may be partly mediated by bradykinin. There was also a relationship between allergen and mode of reaction; for example, pharyngeal edema was more likely with tree nuts (particularly Brazil nuts) than with peanuts. The low ACE levels found in some patients in this study of nut allergy contrasts with the findings in sting anaphylaxis where plasma angiotensinogen levels were lower in those with a history of sting reactions when compared with controls but ACE levels were similar in both groups [38].

Platelet activating factor (PAF) is another mediator with established importance in animal models of anaphylaxis [39, 40]. In human reactions to peanuts, high PAF levels correlated with severity as did low serum levels of PAF-acteylhydrolase (PAF-AH) [41]. In particular, PAF-AH levels were low in serum samples from those dying from fatal peanut reactions; PAF-AH is a major pathway for inactivation of PAF; thus, low levels are associated with enhanced PAF activity. Fatal peanut anaphylaxis typically has a dominant asthmatic component leading to primary respiratory arrest, but PAF-AH levels were not significantly different in life-threatening and non-life-threatening asthma from other causes, indicating specificity for asthmatic anaphylaxis rather than asthma from other causes.

It seems likely that many other allotypic variations will be found that determine which organ system is most affected by anaphylaxis and which mediators cause the most profound effects during anaphylactic reactions, but whether a reaction is fatal or not may be determined as much by comorbidity of coronary artery disease, bronchial hyperreactivity and vascular sensitivity, which in turn have genetic predispositions and may be modulated by cytokines.

## 2.5 Epidemiology of Fatal Anaphylaxis

There are good reasons to study fatal anaphylaxis. Experimental animal anaphylaxis differs in important respects from that in humans, and experimentation on humans could never be acceptable. We must therefore make the best of whatever observations we can to find who may be affected, what triggers their reactions, the circumstances leading to the reaction, and why whatever treatment was applied had failed. In cases where the fatal reaction was not the first indication of a severe allergy, we can also study why allergen avoidance failed.

While epidemiology of fatal anaphylaxis avoids the problem of deciding whether the reaction was severe enough to be classified as anaphylaxis, it leaves two key uncertainties: whether death was really due to anaphylaxis and whether the suggested trigger agent was really what caused the reaction.

Estimating the likelihood death was due to anaphylaxis is not simple because underlying pathology contributes so much to the lethality of the reaction. For example, when shock and coronary artery spasm lead to myocardial infarction because the coronary arteries were already partly occluded by atheroma, it may be difficult to prove whether sudden death following a dose of antibiotics was due to anaphylaxis or non-anaphylactic myocardial infarction. Similarly, there may be little difference between fatal asthma and fatal anaphylaxis, particularly with food allergy reactions; it may even be meaningless to make such a distinction, particularly if we think of anaphylaxis as an acute allergic reaction that would benefit by treatment with epinephrine.

Nor is it easy to determine what triggered a fatal reaction. With clinic patients, skin prick and challenge tests can be used in an attempt to prove the cause; but in fatal cases, challenge tests and skin prick tests are clearly impossible. Assessment of mast cell tryptase and IgE antibodies to the supposed trigger is possible only when a suitable sample has been retained and even then, insight into the limitations of these investigations is needed for accurate interpretation of the results [42]. Urgent retrieval of samples for these investigations before they are discarded is vital to ascertain the cause of death.

## 2.6 Fatal Anaphylaxis Around the World

Eighty-nine deaths in Florida 1996–2005 were identified as due to anaphylaxis by diagnostic codes on the death certificate; 41 had autopsies and the autopsy reports were available for 34. But beyond this, the cause of death was not verified by scrutiny of the medical records or details of events surrounding the death [43]. The reaction trigger was identified in 44 deaths: of these, 64% were iatrogenic, 16% triggered by food allergy, and 20% by stings.

A detailed study of 26 deaths attributed to anaphylaxis in a register of all fatalities in Cook County, Chicago 1989–2001 highlighted the role of comorbidity in fatal anaphylaxis [44]. Of these, the authors considered 15 were consistent with anaphylaxis, 8 probably consistent and 2 possibly consistent, recognizing the difficulty in validating the cause of death in a register of this type. Out of 23 with autopsy findings available, 15 had coronary arterial disease and 5 had chronic obstructive airways disease that may have contributed to the lethality of the reaction.

An unpublished Canadian study [45] identified 63 anaphylactic deaths from the records of the chief coroner for Ontario, 32 related to food allergy. Of these 32, 11 were under 18 (two of them 17 years old). Nine of the 11 were known to have been asthmatic, the remaining 2 may have been. The population of Ontario is around 12.5 million, giving a death rate of one child in a 20 million population each year – comparable to the UK rate.

The French anaphylaxis network (Réseau d'Allergo Vigilance) has a register of severe anaphylactic reactions [46] but has not focused on fatal reactions, only four of which (three due to food allergy) were recorded 2002–2003 from a population of 60M [47].

In New South Wales, Australia, 10 fatal reactions to food were recorded 1999–2008 (R Loblay and J Ruhno, personal communications, 2009). Five were attributed to peanuts, three to Chinese food, and two to milk. Eight of these were in children (four male, four female) and at least five of the children had asthma. This gives a death rate of one each year for 6 million population, substantially higher than the UK rate for fatal reactions to food in childhood. One of these cases was widely publicized and details are interesting in that they highlight some of the problems of children with peanut allergy [48]. During a "trivia challenge" at a school camp, this 13-year-old boy had to eat a spoonful of peanut butter as fast as possible. Within seconds of contact, he spat out the food, vomited, developed intense itch, rapid lip and tongue swelling, wheeze, and choking. The first epinephrine was given 13 min after his collapse: resuscitation was unsuccessful. He had had a minor reaction to a sweet containing peanut some months before this and a history of other food allergy, eczema, and asthma. Contributory factors may have included peer pressure to participate in the challenge.

Seven fatal food reactions in Sweden (population 9M) were identified 1993–1996 [49]. Of these deaths two were caused by peanut, three by soy, one by tree nut, and one of unknown food (T Foucard, personal communication, 2008). Subsequently, during 1997–2003 there were two deaths caused by peanuts, one by tree nuts, none by soy and two by unknown food [50]. The authors speculated that the change in incidence might be due to increased awareness of the risk of soy allergy.

## 2.7 The UK Fatal Anaphylaxis Register

Given the difficulty devising prospective trials of anaphylaxis management, it seemed that studying a large number of fatal reactions might give insight into why prevention and treatment had failed. With this in mind, a register of all fatal anaphylactic reactions in the UK since 1992 was established. The register holds detailed information about the deceased, their medical history, the events leading up to the reaction, the reaction itself, and, where the evidence is sufficient, estimates of the likelihood the cause of death was anaphylaxis and the likelihood for one or more possible trigger factors. This has provided a wealth of data and has taught important lessons for the management of anaphylaxis [51].

There seemed a strong chance that searches for the register might miss cases, particularly deaths attributed to asthma rather than anaphylaxis in asthmatics with food allergy or aspirin sensitivity, deaths due to antibiotics taken by patients at home and sting deaths in older people where the sudden death was most likely to be blamed on myocardial infarction. Retrospective re-investigation of asthma deaths proved futile. Cases in the register suggested that asthma deaths age 0–32 were the ones most likely to have been attacks triggered by food allergy; this led to a year-long prospective study of fatal asthma in this age group. The outcome suggested that most of the food allergy-related acute asthmatic deaths had already been identified through the diligent surveillance of the UK Anaphylaxis Campaign, and that it was unlikely that many cases had been missed. Nevertheless the findings strongly suggest that young people who go into respiratory arrest within an hour of the start of a sudden attack of asthma should be investigated for anaphylaxis. If they have a history of food allergy, this should include examination of their gastric contents for food they were not seen to eat, such as a recent UK case where the stomach contained sesame seeds, pumpkin seeds, linseed, and poppy seeds in a boy with known sesame allergy who had not been seen to eat any such food. Sadly most cases like this are still diagnosed as due to asthma, the verdict is given as "death from natural causes" and no further investigation is undertaken; retrospective surveys then have no hope of deciding whether the asthma attack had an intrinsic or extrinsic trigger.

More recently the searches of the UK death register have been expanded to include all asphyxia deaths due to upper airways angioedema; this retrieved a few further cases of probable anaphylactic death that the original searches had missed and consolidated data on fatal ACE inhibitor-related angioedema and hereditary angioedema. Some such deaths had already been retrieved because of an improbable diagnosis of anaphylaxis. Amniotic fluid embolus deaths are also under study because the differential diagnosis for some cases included antibiotic or anesthetic anaphylaxis.

There are 536 UK fatalities in the register and following detailed investigation of 345, 272 seem more likely than not due to anaphylaxis while the remaining 73 have more likely other causes of death including at least 2 directly due to epinephrine overdose, 11 with ACEI-related angioedema and no evidence of an allergic trigger, and 4 following insertion of bone cement. Data to assess the remaining 191 is still being collected; from information on the death certificate it is likely that over 100 will prove to have been due to anaphylaxis.

### 2.7.1 *What Has Triggered Fatal Reactions?*

Over the last 16 years in the UK, around 20 deaths each year were most probably due to anaphylaxis; about half of these were iatrogenic and the rest divided between sting reactions and food allergy deaths. A small number were triggered by less common agents, including latex, hair dye, and hydatid cyst rupture (Fig. 2.2, Table 2.4). It seems likely that the rate of fatal anaphylaxis in the UK has remained largely unchanged 1992–2005.

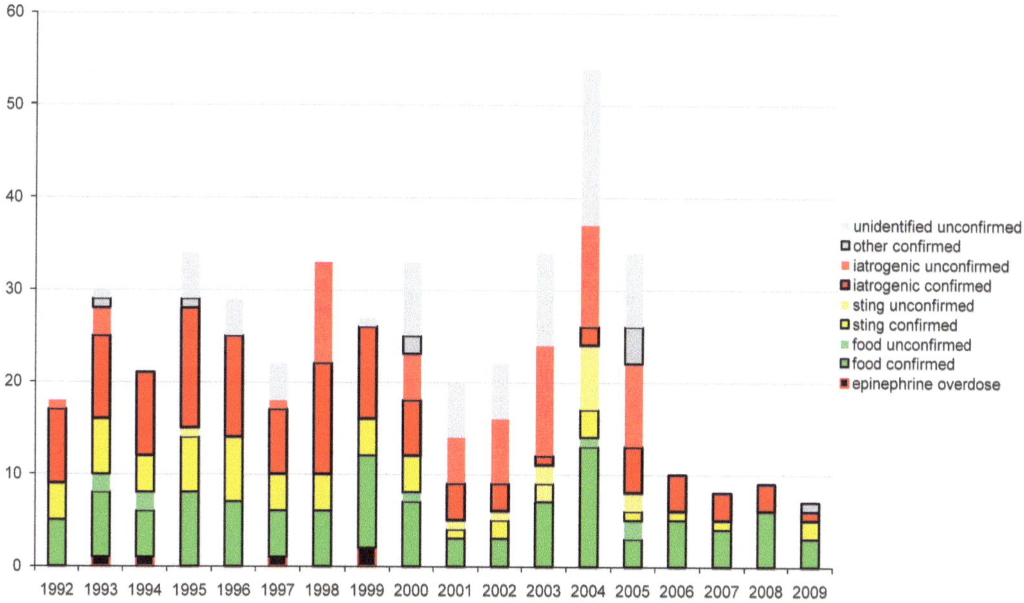


**Fig. 2.2** Yearly totals for fatal anaphylaxis in the UK. Confirmed cases have been studied in detail; for some of the unconfirmed cases, anaphylaxis may seem an unlikely cause of death once they have been studied in more detail and so the final numbers will be lower. Extrapolating from the cases reviewed so far, most of the "unidentified, unconfirmed" cases 2003–2005 will have been diagnosed as anaphylaxis on the basis of serum tryptase levels at autopsy and will be found to have low probability of anaphylaxis. The England & Wales Death Register has not yet been searched for 2006–2009; thus, the entries for these years are mainly cases studied in detail immediately following death

**Table 2.4** Dominant mode of death in fatal anaphylaxis. The data are taken from the UK Fatal Anaphylaxis Register. The dominant mode of death depends on age and the reaction trigger. At higher resolution, the nature of the food (milk, peanut, tree nut, fish, etc.) or the nature of the iatrogenic intervention (contrast medium, antibiotic, muscle relaxant, NSAID, etc.) also have different modes and age distributions

| | | | | | | | | | |
|---|---|---|---|---|---|---|---|---|---|
| *110 Fatal food reactions* | | | | | | | | | |
| Age | 0–9 | 10–19 | 20–29 | 30–39 | 40–49 | 50–59 | 60–69 | 70–79 | >80 |
| Asthma | 8 | 24 | 8 | 4 | 3 | 2 | 1 | | |
| Breathing difficulty | 1 | 8 | 8 | 5 | 1 | 1 | | | |
| Upper airway swelling | | 1 | 4 | 2 | | 2 | 1 | | 1 |
| Shock and dib | 1 | 4 | 7 | 1 | | 1 | | | |
| Shock | | 1 | 2 | 1 | | | | | |
| Other | 1 EpiOD | 2 DIC EpiOD | 2 DIC inhV | 1 EpiOD | | | | | 1 inhV |
| *48 Fatal sting reactions* | | | | | | | | | |
| Asthma | | | 1 | | | 1 | | 1 | |
| Breathing difficulty | | | | | 1 | 2 | 2 | | |
| Upper airway swelling | | | | | 3 | 1 | 1 | 3 | 1 |
| Shock and dib | | | | 1 | 1 | | | 1 | 2 |
| Shock | | | 1 | 2 | 4 | 6 | 6 | 3 | 1 |
| Other | | | | | | 1 inhV | 1 Epil | 1 MI | |
| *94 Fatal iatrogenic reactions* | | | | | | | | | |
| Asthma | | 2 | | 2 | | 2 | 3 | | |
| Breathing difficulty | | | 1 | | 2 | | 2 | | 2 |
| Upper airway swelling | | | 1 | 1 | 1 | 2 | | 2 | |
| Shock and dib | | 1 | 2 | 1 | 2 | 5 | 10 | 6 | 2 |
| Shock | 2 | | | 3 | 4 | 3 | 8 | 8 | 2 |
| Other | | | 2 DIC EpiOD | 1 Bowel infarct | | 1 DIC | 3 2xDIC Bowel infarct | 4 3xMI Infected line | 1 EpiOD |

EpiOD = overdose of epinephrine. DIC = disseminated intravascular coagulation (but in every case there was also cerebral infarction) MI = myocardial infarction. The cause of the infarcted bowel is unknown but speculation included vasospasm from epinephrine or prolonged shock. Epil = epilepsy following shock/cerebral anoxia. inhV = inhaled vomit during reaction thought to be the cause of respiratory arrest.

## 2.7.2 *Who Died from Anaphylaxis?*

There are clear differences in the profiles of those dying from anaphylaxis triggered by different agents, with iatrogenic deaths mostly in older patients, while foods affected a higher proportion of young people (Table 2.4). Most of those dying from food allergy were atopic but iatrogenic and sting deaths did not show this tendency. Overall there were approximately equal numbers of male and female; for food allergy there was a male predominance in childhood and female in early adulthood, similar to patterns of epinephrine pen prescribing [11]. There was a male predominance in sting reactions and fatal contrast medium reactions, contrasting with the female predominance for nonfatal contrast medium reactions. All races were represented but there was a remarkable excess of boys with milk allergy with one or both parents from Africa, the Middle-East, or Far-East: it is not known whether this was for genetic or cultural reasons.

### 2.7.3 When Did They Die?

Fatal reactions showed both circadian and annual variation; both seem most likely to depend simply on the chance of exposure. For example, fatal sting reactions occurred May–November peaking in August when wasp populations are highest, and food reactions were highest in December, probably associated with festive eating.

### 2.7.4 How Did They Die?

Acute allergic reactions can kill by shock or respiratory arrest (Table 2.4). Those resuscitated from the acute reaction died later (median 60 h post-reaction) from a variety of reasons, related to cerebral infarction, adult respiratory distress syndrome, infections, infarction of the bowel, or bleeding due to disseminated intravascular coagulation. Two additional patients died shortly after anaphylaxis during surgery, but there seemed a more likely cause for their death than the after-effects of the reaction.

Anaphylactic shock is not caused by the same process in every patient. It may be cardiogenic due to the direct effect of the reaction and its mediators on the heart muscle (more typical of older patients with diseased hearts) or peripheral due to vasodilatation and/or fluid leakage from intravascular to extravascular compartments (more typical of younger patients with healthy hearts), or a combination of both. Death outside hospital from peripheral shock has typically followed a change to a more upright posture, highlighting the need to keep shocked patients lying flat [52]; there may be further advantage in raising the legs to help maintain venous return to the heart [53].

Anaphylactic shock causes myocardial ischemia and sometimes infarction. Reduced pulse pressure leads to reduced flow through the coronary arteries: this is made more dangerous if the coronary arteries are narrowed by disease or undergo spasm as part of the reaction. Allergic angina (Kounis syndrome [54]) due to vasospasm in allergic reactions is more likely in hearts with existing arterial disease because of the increased numbers of mast cells. Caution in the use of epinephrine has been urged in such cases (typically middle-aged men developing angina, maybe with a rash and breathing difficulty, within 30 min of starting a drug such as a beta-lactam antibiotic) [55]. Transient left ventricular dysfunction has been described in anaphylaxis, possibly due to multi-vessel epicardial coronary spasm or coronary microvascular impairment or maybe a direct effect on the myocardium of catecholamines released or injected during the reaction; recently a case report emphasized the role of injected epinephrine in myocardial stunning leading to transient left ventricular dysfunction [56].

Primary respiratory arrest in anaphylaxis has a variety of causes: these comprise upper airways angioedema, bronchospasm (often with mucus plugging), inhaled vomit, and pulmonary edema. Upper airway occlusion by angioedema may be part of a generalized reaction, such as following a sting, or a local mucosal reaction from food such as Brazil nuts. Lower airway occlusion by bronchospasm is most commonly due to an acute asthma attack in someone taking daily asthma medication, with or without other indications of an allergic reaction such as urticaria or angioedema. Upper and lower airway occlusion may occur together, such as in a case where tracheostomy was performed because of pharyngeal edema in a Brazil nut reaction, only to find the lungs could not be ventilated because of bronchospasm and mucus plugging. Inhalation of vomit can be fatal in the absence of allergy but is also a possible outcome of an acute allergic gastric reaction in someone with food allergy. Pulmonary edema with shock results from sudden left ventricular failure, and while this may be due to massively severe anaphylaxis, in the UK register it has perhaps more commonly resulted from intravenous bolus injection of epinephrine.

Although anaphylaxis can kill fit and healthy people, most deaths in the UK register resulted from existing pathology made fatal by a relatively mild allergic reaction. Thus an allergic reaction to milk may cause a fatal attack of asthma in a child with poorly controlled asthma, particularly if the asthma is already exacerbated by a rhinovirus infection. Most fatal allergic reactions to food have been of this type. Optimal daily control of asthma is crucial in reducing the risk of a fatal reaction in those with food allergy [57]. Similarly, a sting reaction that would otherwise be mild may be fatal in someone with systemic mastocytosis. Raised background tryptase levels have been found in many of those presenting with sting anaphylaxis and may be due to clonal mast cell proliferation [58]. Existing coronary artery disease is frequently found at autopsy in those dying from iatrogenic anaphylaxis.

Drugs used to treat asthma, hypertension, arrhythmia, and various other conditions may also enhance the effects of anaphylaxis or make its management more difficult. A recent history of high daily dosage of beta-2 agonists was found in several of those dying from food-allergy-related anaphylaxis/asthma who failed to respond to epinephrine: whether the failure of epinephrine to rescue the patient was because the asthma was very severe or because the excessive beta-2 agonist use reduced the effectiveness of epinephrine by tachyphylaxis is not known. When an anaphylaxis patient with arrhythmia might benefit from treatment with a beta-adrenergic blocking drug, it will be helpful for the cardiologist and allergist to discuss which condition poses the greater risk to the patient and what the optimal management plan might be. Because ACE is the major pathway for bradykinin inactivation, ACE inhibitors may augment the severity of anaphylaxis, in some patients by increasing the likelihood of angioedema, in others by blocking formation of angiotensin II which is one of the homeostatic pathways opposing shock in anaphylaxis [59]. As well as ACE inhibitors, NSAID, aspirin, and beta-blockers were associated with severe reactions to foods [60].

## 2.8 Fatal First Reactions: Why Was Rescue Treatment Unsuccessful?

For those whose previous history is adequately known, the fatal reaction was thought to be their first for 19 out of 32 antibiotic, 17 out of 20 muscle relaxant, 7 out of 13 nonsteroidal anti-inflammatory drug, 13 out of 13 other drug, 10 out of 10 contrast media-related, and 22 out of 38 insect sting anaphylactic deaths [61]. Most patients had been exposed to the causative drug or been stung previously without reaction. For such patients, management is limited to what can be done at the time of their first reaction and this will depend on where the reaction occurs (Table 2.5).

The commonest place for iatrogenic reactions is the operating room, and this will be fully equipped to provide appropriate emergency care. The main problem here has been recognizing that the sudden change in the patient's condition was due to anaphylaxis in time to prevent progression.

**Table 2.5** Circumstances of 278 fatal anaphylactic reactions

| Food | | Iatrogenic | | Sting | | |
|---|---|---|---|---|---|---|
| Home | 31 | Home | 30 | Home | 18 | 2 in bed |
| School | 7 | School | 1 | | | |
| Work | 5 | Work | 1 | Work | 6 | 5 outdoors labor, 1 driving truck |
| Out /about | 6 | | | Out /about | 11 | 2 driving, 1 cycling, 4 walking, 4 sitting, 1 sport |
| Friend's house | 13 | OR | 60 | Orchard/garden | 15 | |
| Relative's house | 8 | ER | 2 | By bee hives | 2 | |
| Restaurant | 23 | Ward/department | 22 | | | |
| Takeaway | 6 | | | | | |
| Wedding | 2 | Dentist | 2 | | | |
| Abroad | 4 | GP | 1 | | | |
| Camping | 2 | | | | | |

In this situation, the median time to first arrest has been 5 min and for a few the time was less than a minute. The first drug used in treatment has usually not been epinephrine but rather alpha adrenergic agonists such as metaraminol or norepinephrine for hypotension or salbutamol for increased airways resistance. There are case reports that could be taken as supporting either approach [62, 63] but in general the consensus is that epinephrine is the preferred drug for initial treatment of anaphylactic reactions in the OR [64, 65].

## 2.9 Fatal Recurrent Reactions

### *2.9.1 Reducing the Likelihood of a Severe Recurrence*

For the other patients who had a previous reaction, even if this was mild (as was the case for the majority of anaphylactic deaths attributed to food allergy) there is an opportunity to protect the patient against the worst effects of a recurrence. Allergen-specific immunotherapy and other more recently devised methods of attenuating or eliminating the allergic response to allergen exposure are discussed elsewhere in this book. Optimal daily management of asthma, hypertension, and arrhythmia has been discussed above a way of avoiding factors that will increase the severity of a recurrent reaction.

### *2.9.2 Why Did Avoidance Fail?*

For the minority of patients who had a previous reaction and knew what caused it, allergen avoidance failed for a variety of reasons. Iatrogenic fatal recurrent anaphylaxis was largely due to beta-lactam antibiotics and NSAID. Reasons for avoidance failure include:

1. Ignoring a patient's claim of penicillin allergy. Most of the many patients who claim "penicillin allergy" will not react if given penicillin because their allergy was a rash on the second to fourth day of amino-penicillin treatment for a sore throat. If on the other hand their allergy was rapidly developing symptoms following the first dose of a new course, the chance of anaphylaxis on re-exposure is high. Patients commonly do not remember the reaction that led to their label of "penicillin allergy" making it difficult to conclude whether penicillin treatment might be dangerous; fatal reactions have resulted from the decision to treat in the face of such a claim of penicillin allergy. There is evidence in some such cases that the penicillin allergy was side-chain specific and previous treatment with a different beta-lactam antibiotic without a reaction made the doctor discount the earlier history of a severe reaction. Doctors should take a history of penicillin allergy seriously and, if they are uncertain whether it is significant, should err on the side of caution.
2. Bypassing protocols intended to protect patients with drug allergy. Patients have been classified as penicillin allergic and given a red armband warning of their allergy, which was not seen when the antibiotic was injected in the other arm. Penicillin allergy warnings on treatment sheets or GP records have frequently been overlooked or not transferred from old handwritten records to new computer records. Patients have repeatedly detected and rejected inappropriate prescriptions for a drug they thought they were allergic to only to be caught out subsequently when the same drug was prescribed with a different name.
3. Of 16 patients dying from cephalosporin anaphylaxis, five had previously reacted to a penicillin; three died following cefaclor given because of previous amoxicillin reactions on the grounds that only one in ten patients with penicillin allergy react to cephalosporins.

Fatal repeat anaphylaxis to NSAID have followed avoidance failure for reasons such as the patient not recognizing that the new prescription was a potentially cross-reacting drug or the same drug with a different name, or the doctor having been given the records of a patient with similar name and age who was not NSAID allergic and so was not warned of the allergy.

The previous sting history is known for 38 fatal sting reactions on the register: 16 had a previous acute reaction. None of these had had venom-specific immunotherapy. Despite advice that a 3–5 year course of specific immunotherapy is optimal management of proven sting allergy, some patients preferred to rely on sting avoidance and self-injectible epinephrine, especially where there was difficulty attending for specific immunotherapy. Five had self-injectible epinephrine that failed to save them (see below for details). It is not known how many had adopted a diligent sting avoidance strategy. While even obsessive avoidance cannot be totally successful, the risk of being stung can be substantially reduced by a few simple rules. Advice for each region is available on the internet.

We recently reported 48 additional food-allergy deaths in the UK [66]. The food blamed for fatal reactions was catered (18), domestically prepared (6), packaged/labeled (16), sold loose/unlabelled (2), whole nuts (3), and unknown (3). Fourteen were thought not to have been avoiding the culprit food; avoidance was graded as casual for 16, careful for 7, extremely careful for 6, and unknown for 5. Even with the most diligent avoidance, lapses occurred during festive eating, foreign travel, or when distracted by disruption to routine. Just as much as they need to recognize foods that will cause them to react, patients should be made aware of these potentially dangerous circumstances and be supported in assessing them and developing appropriate coping strategies with increased vigilance in hazardous situations.

## 2.10 Self-injectible Epinephrine

Since 1905, epinephrine has been known as an effective treatment for an acute attack of asthma [67] and since 1910 as an antidote to anaphylaxis [68]. It seems to have been in routine use to treat anaphylaxis by the 1930s, as demonstrated by a graphic personal account by a beekeeper of his anaphylactic reaction and the severe angina that affected him following the use of 10 minim (0.6 mL) of epinephrine in treatment of his shock and breathing difficulty [69]. Early studies of fatal and near-fatal food allergy emphasized the need for treatment with epinephrine early in the reaction [70, 71] and recommended that those at risk should carry their own epinephrine treatment. For the patient, achieving the correct dose and route was difficult [72] until the auto-injectors for self-treatment with epinephrine that had been available since 1980 [73] were used more generally.

The current widespread availability of auto-injectors has not solved all the problems. There is much we may learn from 31 food allergy and 5 sting-allergic fatalities who had been prescribed epinephrine for self-treatment:

1. In 15/36 treatment failures, an auto-injector was used early in the reaction and apparently correctly. One patient was so confident her epinephrine would save her that she bit into a chocolate knowing it might be risky. She saw the nut, rapidly developed difficulty breathing, and used her pen immediately and apparently correctly. Her symptoms did not remit; she arrested and could not be resuscitated. It must be recognized that although epinephrine is the most effective treatment for anaphylaxis if used early in the reaction, not all patients will be saved. Such failure could be speculatively attributed to a variety of causes:

   (a) Obesity preventing intramuscular injection. Epinephrine injected into the subcutaneous tissue causes intense vasospasm, and most of the epinephrine will remain there for hours without being absorbed. This, after all, is the rationale for adding epinephrine to local anesthetics to prolong their action. For optimal absorption, the injection must be intramuscular, and even then not all muscles absorb well. The anterolateral aspect of the thigh near the midpoint of its length is easy to reach and, fortunately, a good site for absorption of epinephrine when tested in active men aged 18–35 [74]. However, with the rising tide of obesity the depth of subcutaneous adiposity is frequently greater than the 16mm of needle in the EpiPen [75–77] and even more often longer than the 10mm of the Anapen. If the vasculature of older humans behaves like that of older rats [78], the absorption of epinephrine may be less effective than in young men. It is worth recording that in none of the autopsies of these cases was the auto-injector needle track dissected to establish which tissue the epinephrine was injected into: this information would have been valuable.

(b) Overuse of salbutamol for daily asthma treatment. Most of those dying from food anaphylaxis take daily treatment for asthma and it has been possible to establish for some of those whose fatal asthma was triggered by food allergy and whose self-injectible epinephrine failed to save them that the dose of short-acting beta-2 agonist was greatly in excess of the maximum recommended. In such cases epinephrine may no longer be effective at reversing bronchospasm [57].

(c) In at least one case, bisoprolol had been prescribed by a cardiologist unaware that the patient was at risk of anaphylaxis and might need epinephrine treatment. This patient had previously used his auto-injector on three occasions following stings and had symptoms of limited severity; but the next sting, after he had started taking bisoprolol, was fatal despite early use of his auto-injector. As patients with sting or food allergy get older there is an increasing risk they will develop hypertension or arrhythmia and may be prescribed a beta-blocker or angiotensin converting enzyme inhibitor (ACEI). Beta-blockers will attenuate the usefulness of epinephrine in anaphylaxis and ACEI may promote hypotension or angioedema in susceptible patients. Patients at risk of anaphylaxis, in particular those carrying their own epinephrine, should be instructed to make sure any doctor prescribing for them is fully aware of this. Ideally patients should attend for regular review and retraining; any new medication should be evaluated in the contest of their anaphylaxis rescue package. In practice however, it is my experience that many older patients decline the offer of regular follow-up even if they have used their auto-injector on a number of occasions.

(d) Extreme severity of reaction. The need for two or more doses of epinephrine may be an indicator of severity. One patient used two pens and two patients used three pens but still died; retrospective proof whether this was due to their obesity or due to the severity of the reaction is impossible.

2. The dose prescribed was too low for 2/32. One had been given an epinephrine inhaler and told not to take more than 2 puffs at a time when it was thought this treatment might be effective if 20 or more inhalations were used. The other weighed 36kg but had a junior (0.15mg) pen. A second pen had been available but was used incorrectly.
3. The injection was given late in the reaction in 5/36. One was heard by her husband to shout "anaphylaxis;" he found her collapsed with her pen on the floor; he gave the dose but she showed no improvement. Two had left pens elsewhere and had to retrieve them (of which one was time-expired); one collapsed while waiting in pharmacy queue for pen to be dispensed; for one, the reason was unknown.
4. Six failed to use their injection correctly, indicating inadequate training.

   (a) One jabbed the pen on her thigh but withdrew it immediately, spilling most of the epinephrine.
   (b) One pulled the pen apart, preventing it from activating properly.
   (c) One man was found dead with the telephone in one hand and his epinephrine injection in the other. He had a history of wasp allergy and there was a dead wasp trapped in his clothing. It seems reasonable to suppose he was uncertain how to use his epinephrine and the progress of the reaction was too swift to allow him to take the treatment.

(d) In one fatal sting reaction, the first pen is said to have failed to activate, the second and third fired while being removed from their canister, a fourth pen given by a paramedic failed to revive the patient.
(e) One had been given a pen for nut allergy but was reacting to latex and did not use it [79].
(f) It is not known why one other failed to use his pen.

5. Eight out of 36 did not have it with them at the crucial time.

(a) Three had left pen elsewhere, too far away to be retrieved in time for treatment
(b) Two had not replaced after use (one used the day before, the other several years previously)
(c) One found her epinephrine to be out of date and so went to hospital; she then died after inappropriate bolus iv injection of epinephrine 1 mg
(d) Two reason not known

The failure in these latter cases might be attributed to poor training; often the doctor prescribing the pen is unfamiliar with the device [80, 81] and fails to train the patient adequately to ensure they have the device with them when it might be needed, to use it at the correct time in a reaction with a correct injection technique [82–84].

Of 102 fatal reactions to foods, 71 had not been prescribed epinephrine for self-treatment. This is not so surprising when the severity of their worst previous reaction is taken into account – three quarters of those whose death was attributed to food anaphylaxis had never had a severe reaction previously. I have presented one such case to various audiences to see who might have recommended he should carry an epinephrine pen. In UK audiences a small minority would have recommended a pen but in Canada a large majority would have, reflecting national differences of opinion. Of the fatal cases in the UK, at least 2/71 had requested an auto-injector but their doctor refused to prescribe one.

## 2.11 Conclusion

Detailed study of fatal reactions provides insight that is vital for reducing risk and improving management. Most fatal reactions occur unexpectedly in those with no previous history of reactions; knowing the typical circumstances of fatal reactions allows better planning for training in the correct use of epinephrine and basic life support for the particular mode of anaphylaxis the patient exhibits, including posture appropriate for shock or respiratory distress. In those whose history suggests they may be at significant risk of a life-threatening reaction, the key elements of risk reduction include training in effective allergen avoidance, optimizing their daily management of conditions such as asthma, hypertension, and heart disease to use drugs that will not increase the risk from anaphylaxis or if that is not possible, to achieve a logical balance of risk between the treated condition and anaphylaxis, and lastly, provision of appropriate kit for self-treatment in the event of a reaction. The ways in which self-injectible epinephrine failed teach important lessons, not only about the need for continual review and retraining but also the provision of kit and instructions appropriate for the individual patient, according to their body mass and their attitude to their allergy.

## References

1. Pumphrey RS, Stanworth SJ. The clinical spectrum of anaphylaxis in north-west England. *Clin Exp Allergy.* 1996;26(12):1364–1370.
2. Macdougall CF, Cant AJ, Colver AF. How dangerous is food allergy in childhood? The incidence of severe and fatal allergic reactions across the UK and Ireland. *Arch Dis Child.* 2002;86:236–239.

3. Neugut AI, Ghatak AT, Miller RL. Anaphylaxis in the United States: an investigation into its epidemiology. *Arch Intern Med.* 2001;161(1):15–21.
4. Johansson SGO, Bieber T, Dahl R, et al. Revised nomenclature for allergy for global use: report of the nomenclature review committee of the World Allergy Organization, October 2003. *J Allergy Clin Immunol.* 2004;113:832–836.
5. Kemp SF, Lockey RF, Simons FER. Epinephrine: the drug of choice for anaphylaxis. A statement of the World Allergy Organization. *Allergy.* 2008;63:1061–1070.
6. Soar J, Pumphrey R, Cant A, et al. Emergency treatment of anaphylactic reactions guidelines for healthcare providers. *Resuscitation.* 2008;77:157–169.
7. Sampson HA, Muñoz-Furlong A, Campbell RL, et al. Second symposium on the definition and management of anaphylaxis: summary report – Second National Institute of Allergy and Infectious Disease/Food Allergy and Anaphylaxis Network symposium. *J Allergy Clin Immunol.* 2006;117(2):391–397.
8. Rüggeberg JU, Gold MS, Bayas JM, et al. Brighton Collaboration Anaphylaxis Working Group. Anaphylaxis: case definition and guidelines for data collection, analysis, and presentation of immunization safety data. *Vaccine.* 2007;25(31):5675–5684.
9. Erlewyn-Lajeunesse M, Dymond S, Slade I, et al. Diagnostic utility of two case definitions for anaphylaxis: a comparison using a retrospective case notes analysis in the UK. *Drug Saf.* 2010; 33(1):1–8.
10. Sicherer SH, Burks AW, Sampson-HA. Clinical features of acute allergic reactions to peanut and tree nuts in children. *Pediatrics.* 1998;102:e6
11. Simons FE, Peterson S, Black CD. Epinephrine dispensing patterns for an out-of-hospital population: a novel approach to studying the epidemiology of anaphylaxis. *J Allergy Clin Immunol.* 2002;110(4):647–651.
12. Sheikh A, Hippisley-Cox J, Newton J, Fenty J. Trends in national incidence, lifetime prevalence and adrenaline prescribing for anaphylaxis in England. *J R Soc Med.* 2008;101(3):139–143.
13. Sheikh A, Alves B. Age, sex, geographical and socio-economic variations in admissions for anaphylaxis: analysis of four years of English hospital data. *Clin Exp Allergy.* 2001;31(10):1571–1576.
14. Sheehan WJ, Graham D, Ma L, Baxi S, Phipatanakul W. Higher incidence of pediatric anaphylaxis in northern areas of the United States. *J Allergy Clin Immunol.* 2009;124(4):850–852.e2.
15. The International Collaborative Study of Severe Anaphylaxis. An epidemiologic study of severe anaphylactic and anaphylactoid reactions among hospital patients: methods and overall risks. *Epidemiology.* 1998;9(2):141–146.
16. Peng MM, Jick H. A population-based study of the incidence, cause, and severity of anaphylaxis in the United Kingdom. *Arch Intern Med.* 2004;164(3):317–319.
17. Stewart AG, Ewan PW. The incidence, aetiology and management of anaphylaxis presenting to an accident and emergency department. *QJM.* 1996;89(11):859–864.
18. Smit DV, Cameron PA, Rainer TH. Anaphylaxis presentations to an emergency department in Hong Kong: incidence and predictors of biphasic reactions. *J Emerg Med.* 2005;28(4):381–388.
19. Mullins RJ. Anaphylaxis: risk factors for recurrence. *Clin Exp Allergy.* 2003;33(8):1033–1040.
20. Helbling A, Hurni T, Mueller UR, Pichler WJ. Incidence of anaphylaxis with circulatory symptoms: a study over a 3-year period comprising 940,000 inhabitants of the Swiss Canton Bern. *Clin Exp Allergy.* 2004;34(2):285–290.
21. Boros CA, Kay D, Gold MS. Parent reported allergy and anaphylaxis in 4173 South Australian children. *J Paediatr Child Health.* 2000;36(1):36–40.
22. Lieberman P, Camargo CA Jr, Bohlke K, et al. Epidemiology of anaphylaxis: findings of the American College of Allergy, Asthma and Immunology Epidemiology of Anaphylaxis Working Group. *Ann Allergy Asthma Immunol.* 2006;97(5):596–602.
23. Yocum MW, Butterfield JH, Klein JS, et al. Epidemiology of anaphylaxis in Olmsted County: a population-based study. *J Allergy Clin Immunol.* 1999;104:452–456.
24. Brown AF, McKinnon D, Chu K. Emergency department anaphylaxis: a review of 142 patients in a single year. *J Allergy Clin Immunol.* 2001;108(5):861–866.
25. Braganza SC, Acworth JP, Mckinnon DR, Peake JE, Brown AF. Paediatric emergency department anaphylaxis: different patterns from adults. *Arch Dis Child.* 2006;91(2):159–163.
26. Mertes PM, Lambert M, Guéant-Rodriguez RM, et al. Perioperative anaphylaxis. *Immunol Allergy Clin North Am.* 2009;29(3):429–451.
27. Van der Klau MM, Goudsmit R, Halie MR, et al. A population based case-cohort study of drug-induced anaphylaxis. *Br J Clin Pharmacol.* 1993; 35:400–408.
28. Johansson SG, Florvaag E, Oman H, et al. National pholcodine consumption and prevalence of IgE-sensitization: a multicentre study. *Allergy.* 2009;65(4):498–502.
29. Bilò MB, Bonifazi F. The natural history and epidemiology of insect venom allergy: clinical implications. *Clin Exp Allergy.* 2009;39(10):1467–1476.
30. Gamboa PM, Cáceres O, Antepara I, et al. Two different profiles of peach allergy in the north of Spain. *Allergy.* 2007;62(4):408–414.

31. Dalal I, Binson I, Reifen R, et al. Food allergy is a matter of geography after all: sesame as a major cause of severe IgE-mediated food allergic reactions among infants and young children in Israel. *Allergy.* 2002;57(4):362–365.
32. Yang JJ, Burchard EG, Choudhry S, et al. Differences in allergic sensitization by self-reported race and genetic ancestry. *J Allergy Clin Immunol.* 2008;122(4):820–827.e9.
33. Mulla ZD, Simon MR. Anaphylaxis in Olmsted County: seasonal pattern and suggestions for epidemiologic analysis. *J Allergy Clin Immunol.* 2009;123(5):1194; author reply 1194–1195.
34. Sheikh A, Alves B. Hospital admissions for acute anaphylaxis: time trend study. *BMJ.* 2000;320(7247):1441.
35. Golden DB, Breisch NL, Hamilton RG, et al. Clinical and entomological factors influence the outcome of sting challenge studies. *J Allergy Clin Immunol.* 2006;117(3):670–675.
36. Hourihane JO, Grimshaw KE, Lewis SA, et al. Does severity of low-dose, double-blind, placebo-controlled food challenges reflect severity of allergic reactions to peanut in the community? *Clin Exp Allergy.* 2005;35(9):1227–1233.
37. Summers CW, Pumphrey RS, Woods CN, McDowell G, Pemberton PW, Arkwright PD. Factors predicting anaphylaxis to peanuts and tree nuts in patients referred to a specialist center. *J Allergy Clin Immunol.* 2008;121(3):632–638.
38. Hermann K, von Tschirschnitz M, Ebner von Eschenbach C, Ring J. Histamine, tryptase, norepinephrine, angiotensinogen, angiotensin-converting enzyme, angiotensin I and II in plasma of patients with hymenoptera venom anaphylaxis. *Int Arch Allergy Immunol.* 1994;104(4):379–384.
39. Finkelman FD, Rothenberg ME, Brandt EB, Morris SC, Strait RT. Molecular mechanisms of anaphylaxis: lessons from studies with murine models. *J Allergy Clin Immunol.* 2005;115:449–457.
40. Ishii S, Kuwaki T, Nagase T, et al. Impaired anaphylactic responses with intact sensitivity to endotoxin in mice lacking a platelet-activating factor receptor. *J Exp Med.* 1998;187:1779–1788.
41. Vadas P, Gold M, Perelman B, et al. Platelet-activating factor, PAF acetylhydrolase, and severe anaphylaxis. *N Engl J Med.* 2008;358(1):28–35.
42. Williams P, Sewell WAC Bunn, Pumphrey R, Read G, Jolles S. Clinical immunology review series: an approach to the use of the immunology laboratory in the diagnosis of clinical allergy. *Clin Exp Immunol.* 2008;153(1):10–18.
43. Simon MR, Mulla ZD. A population-based epidemiologic analysis of deaths from anaphylaxis in Florida. *Allergy.* 2008;63(8):1077–1083.
44. Greenberger PA, Rotskoff BD, Lifschultz B. Fatal anaphylaxis: postmortem findings and associated comorbid diseases. *Ann Allergy Asthma Immunol.* 2007;98(3):252–257.
45. http://www.anaphylaxis.org/content/programs/programs_research_deaths.asp. Accessed February 17, 2010.
46. Moneret-Vautrin DA, Kanny G, Parisot L. First survey from the "Allergy Vigilance Network": life-threatening food allergies in France. *Allerg Immunol.* 2002;34(6):194–198.
47. Moneret-Vautrin DA, Morisset M, Flabbee J, Beaudouin E, Kanny G. Epidemiology of life-threatening and lethal anaphylaxis: a review. *Allergy.* 2005;60(4):443–451.
48. http://www.allergy.org.au/mediareleases/peanut_anaph.htm. Acessed 2008.
49. Foucard T, Malmheden Yman I. A study on severe food reactions in Sweden – is soy protein an underestimated cause of food anaphylaxis? *Allergy.* 1999;54:261–265.
50. Foucard T, Yman IM, Nordvall L. Reduced number of fatal and life-threatening reactions to food. Reporting by the medical profession has resulted in effective measures. *Lakartidningen.* 2005;102(46):3465–3468.
51. Pumphrey RS. Lessons for management of anaphylaxis from a study of fatal reactions. *Clin Exp Allergy.* 2000;30(8):1144–1150.
52. Pumphrey RS. Fatal posture in anaphylactic shock. *J Allergy Clin Immunol.* 2003;112(2):451–452.
53. Boulain T, Achard JM, Teboul JL, Richard C, Perrotin D, Ginies G. Changes in BP induced by passive leg raising predict response to fluid loading in critically ill patients. *Chest.* 2002;121(4):1245–1252.
54. Kounis NG, Zavras GM. Histamine-induced coronary artery spasm: the concept of allergic angina. *Br J Clin Pract.* 1991;45(2):121–128.
55. Ridella M, Bagdure S, Nugent K, Cevik C. Kounis syndrome following beta-lactam antibiotic use: review of literature. *Inflamm Allergy Drug Targets.* 2009;8(1):11–16.
56. Morel O, Jesel L, Morel N, et al. Transient left ventricular dysfunction syndrome during anaphylactic shock Vasospasm, Kounis syndrome or epinephrine-induced stunned myocardium? *Int J Cardiol.* 2009 Nov 13. [Epub ahead of print]
57. Pumphrey RS, Nicholls JM. Epinephrine-resistant food anaphylaxis. *Lancet.* 2000;355(9209):1099.
58. Bonadonna P, Perbellini O, Passalacqua G, et al. Clonal mast cell disorders in patients with systemic reactions to Hymenoptera stings and increased serum tryptase levels. *J Allergy Clin Immunol.* 2009;123(3):680–686.
59. Hermann K, Ring J. The renin-angiotensin system in patients with repeated anaphylactic reactions during hymenoptera venom hyposensitization and sting challenge. *Int Arch Allergy Immunol.* 1997;112(3):251–256.
60. Moneret-Vautrin DA, Latarche C. Drugs as risk factors of food anaphylaxis in adults: a case-control study. *Bull Acad Natl Med.* 2009;193(2):351–362; discussion 362–363. [Article in French].
61. Pumphrey R. Anaphylaxis: can we tell who is at risk of a fatal reaction? *Curr Opin Allergy Clin Immunol.* 2004;4(4):285–290.

62. Ford SA, Kam PC, Baldo BA, Fisher MM. Anaphylactic or anaphylactoid reactions in patients undergoing cardiac surgery. *J Cardiothorac Vasc Anesth.* 2001;15(6):684–688.
63. Heytman M, Rainbird A. Use of alpha-agonists for management of anaphylaxis occurring under anaesthesia: case studies and review. *Anaesthesia.* 2004;59(12):1210–1215.
64. Dewachter P, Mouton-Faivre C, Emala CW. Anaphylaxis and anesthesia: controversies and new insights. *Anesthesiology.* 2009;111(5):1141–1150.
65. Harper NJ, Dixon T, Dugué P, et al. Working Party of the Association of Anaesthetists of Great Britain and Ireland. Suspected anaphylactic reactions associated with anaesthesia. *Anaesthesia.* 2009;64(2):199–211.
66. Pumphrey RS, Gowland MH. Further fatal allergic reactions to food in the United Kingdom, 1999–2006. *J Allergy Clin Immunol.* 2007;119(4):1018–1019.
67. Doig RL. Epinephrin; especially in asthma. *Calif State J Med.* 1905;3(2):54–55.
68. Anderson JF, Schultz WH. The cause of serum anaphylactic shock and some methods of alleviating it. *Proc Soc Exper Biol Med.* 1910;vii:32–36.
69. An Apiarist. Bee-sting anaphylaxis? *BMJ.* 1939;1(4094):1306.
70. Yunginger JW, Sweeney KG, Sturner WQ, et al. Fatal food-induced anaphylaxis. *JAMA.* 1988;260(10): 1450–1452.
71. Sampson HA, Mendelson L, Rosen JP. Fatal and near-fatal anaphylactic reactions to food in children and adolescents. *N Engl J Med.* 1992;327(6):380–384.
72. Simons FE, Chan ES, Gu X, Simons KJ. Epinephrine for the out-of-hospital (first-aid) treatment of anaphylaxis in infants: is the ampule/syringe/needle method practical? *J Allergy Clin Immunol.* 2001;108(6):1040–1044.
73. Lockey SD. A new method of administering aqueous epinephrine: the EpiPen, an automatic syringe. *J Asthma Res.* 1980;17(4):153–155.
74. Simons FE, Gu X, Simons KJ. Epinephrine absorption in adults: intramuscular versus subcutaneous injection. *J Allergy Clin Immunol.* 2001;108(5):871–873.
75. Song TT, Nelson MR, Chang JH, et al. Adequacy of the epinephrine autoinjector needle length in delivering epinephrine to the intramuscular tissues. *Ann Allergy Asthma Immunol.* 2005;94(5):539–542.
76. Pumphrey RSH. When should self-injectible epinephrine be prescribed for food allergy and when should it be used? *Curr Opin Allergy Clin Immunol.* 2008;8(3):254–260.
77. Stecher D, Bulloch B, Sales J, Schaefer C, Keahey L. Epinephrine auto-injectors: is needle length adequate for delivery of epinephrine. intramuscularly? *Pediatrics.* 2009;124(1):65–70.
78. Donato AJ, Lesniewski LA, Delp MD. Ageing and exercise training alter adrenergic vasomotor responses of rat skeletal muscle arterioles. *J Physiol.* 2007;579(Pt 1):115–125.
79. Pumphrey RS, Duddridge M, Norton J. Fatal latex allergy. *J Allergy Clin Immunol.* 2001;107(3):558.
80. Mehr S, Robinson M, Tang M. Doctor – how do I use my EpiPen? *Pediatr Allergy Immunol.* 2007;18(5):448–452. Survey of hospital paediatricians' familiarity with auto-injectors showed few would have given correct advice to their patients.
81. Sicherer SH, Forman JA, Noone SA. Use assessment of self-administered epinephrine among food-allergic children and pediatricians. *Pediatrics.* 2000;105(2):359–362.
82. Pouessel G, Deschildre A, Castelain C, et al. Parental knowledge and use of epinephrine auto-injector for children with food allergy. *Pediatr Allergy Immunol.* 2006;17(3):221–22.
83. Ferreira MB, Alves RR. Are general practitioners alert to anaphylaxis diagnosis and treatment? *Allerg Immunol.* 2006;38(3):83–86.
84. Grouhi M, Alshehri M, Hummel D, Roifman CM. Anaphylaxis and epinephrine auto-injector training: who will teach the teachers? *J Allergy Clin Immunol.* 1999;104(1):190–193.

# Chapter 3
# Pathophysiology and Organ Damage in Anaphylaxis

**Stephen F. Kemp and Richard F. Lockey**

**Abstract** Anaphylaxis is an acute, potentially life-threatening multisystem syndrome resulting from the sudden release of mast cell- and basophil-derived mediators into the systemic circulation. Foods, medications, and insect stings cause most anaphylaxis for which a cause can be identified, but virtually any agent capable of directly or indirectly activating mast cells or basophils can cause it. This syndrome can consist of some or all the following signs and symptoms: diffuse pruritus, erythema, urticaria, and/or angioedema; bronchospasm; laryngeal edema; hypotension; and/or cardiac arrhythmias. Some of the other symptoms that can occur include nausea, vomiting, diarrhea, lightheadedness, headache, feeling of impending doom, and unconsciousness. Regardless of the presenting signs or symptoms, which usually present within 5–30 min following the administration of the offending agent, this reaction can progress to respiratory compromise and cardiovascular collapse resulting in human fatalities. Usually, the more rapid the onset of clinical manifestations, the more likely the anaphylaxis will be life threatening. Immediate and appropriate therapy, especially with epinephrine, is mandatory to reverse the reactions. While most reactions are uniphasic, some can be biphasic or protracted. This chapter discusses the immunopathologic mechanisms and effects of anaphylaxis.

**Keywords** Anaphylaxis • Pathophysiology • Severe allergic reactions • Systemic allergic reactions

## 3.1 Background

Anaphylaxis is an acute, potentially life-threatening multisystem syndrome resulting from the sudden release of mast cell- and basophil-derived mediators into the systemic circulation [1]. It most often results from an allergic reaction to foods, therapeutic agents, and insect stings, but it can be induced through either immunologic or non-immunologic mechanisms by any agent capable of producing a sudden, systemic degranulation of mast cells or basophils [2]. The diagnosis of anaphylaxis rests primarily on probability and pattern recognition. Cause and effect often is confirmed retrospectively in subjects who experience objective signs and symptoms of anaphylaxis after reexposure to the culprit agent. Lifetime personal risk of anaphylaxis is presumed to be 1–3%, with a mortality rate of 1% [2], but the incidence may be increasing [3].

Anaphylaxis consists of some or all of the following signs and symptoms: diffuse pruritus, erythema, urticaria, and/or angioedema; bronchospasm; laryngeal edema; hypotension;

S.F. Kemp (✉)
University of Mississippi Medical Center, Jackson, MS, USA
e-mail: skemp@umc.edu

M.C. Castells (ed.), *Anaphylaxis and Hypersensitivity Reactions*,
DOI 10.1007/978-1-60327-951-2_3, © Springer Science+Business Media, LLC 2011

and/or cardiac arrhythmias. Other symptoms can occur such as nausea, vomiting, diarrhea, lightheadedness, headache, feeling of impending doom, and unconsciousness. Cutaneous manifestations are the most common overall, but these may be delayed or absent in rapidly progressive or fatal anaphylaxis. Anaphylaxis often produces signs and symptoms within 5–30 min, but some reactions may be delayed several hours. Respiratory compromise and cardiovascular collapse cause most human fatalities [2, 4]. The more rapid the onset of clinical manifestations after exposure to an offending stimulus, the more likely the anaphylaxis will be life threatening. An analysis of 214 anaphylaxis fatalities during 1 decade in the UK determined that the interval between eating a culprit food and fatal cardiopulmonary arrest averaged 25–35 min, which was longer than for therapeutic agents (mean, 5 min in-hospital; 10–20 min pre-hospital) or insect stings (10–15 min) [4].

Some authors reserve the term "anaphylaxis" for IgE-dependent events and utilize the term "anaphylactoid" to describe IgE-independent reactions, which are clinically indistinguishable. The World Allergy Organization has proposed replacing this traditional nomenclature with "allergic" or "immunologic" (IgE-mediated and non-IgE-mediated [e.g., IgG- and immune complex complement–mediated]) and "non-immunologic" anaphylaxis [5]. Diagnostic criteria intended to enhance prompt recognition of clinical anaphylaxis have been proposed and are discussed elsewhere [1]. Reactions may be immediate and uniphasic or may be delayed, biphasic, or protracted.

## 3.2 Proposed Immunopathologic Mechanisms

Gell and Coombs classified four types of immunopathologic (hypersensitivity) reactions: (1) immediate (IgE-dependent), (2) cytotoxic (IgG-, IgM-dependent), (3) immune complexes (IgG-, IgM-complex-dependent), and (4) delayed (T-lymphocyte-dependent) [6]. Sell proposed an alternate classification based on seven immunopathologic mechanisms with both protective and destructive functions [7]. These are: (1) immune-mediated inactivation/activation reactions of biologically active molecules, (2) antibody-mediated cytotoxic or cytolytic reactions, (3) immune complex reactions, (4) allergic reactions, (5) T-lymphocyte-mediated cytotoxicity, (6) delayed hypersensitivity, and (7) granulomatous reactions. Mechanism 4, in this classification, encompasses both IgE-dependent and IgE-independent anaphylaxis, but several immunopathologic mechanisms may be active in a given individual. For example, transfusion-related anaphylaxis has cytotoxic features and aggregate anaphylaxis involves immune complex formation (e.g., complexes of parenterally infused immunoglobulin), both of which are IgE-independent and yet cause anaphylaxis. Table 3.1 classifies anaphylaxis by pathophysiologic mechanism.

The pathogenesis of anaphylaxis arguably is fairly obscure and its complexity can adversely impact clinical management. Genetic factors and environmental exposure have important roles, but murine models demonstrate two distinct mechanisms of anaphylaxis that also probably apply to humans. The first, which is the classic, IgE-dependent mechanism, is both IL-4 and IL-4 receptor-dependent. It is characterized by an allergen (antigen) cross-linking allergen-specific IgE bound to Fcε(epsilon)RI receptors (high-affinity IgE receptors) on mast cells and/or basophils, which elicits cellular activation and degranulation if intracellular signaling is sufficiently robust. The subsequent release and fulminant propagation of inflammatory mediators and cytokines produce the smooth muscle contraction and increased vascular contractility associated with clinical anaphylaxis. The second mechanism is IgE-independent; requires proportionately more antigen and antibody than the IgE-dependent pathway; is mediated by IgG, Fcγ(gamma)RIII receptors, and macrophages; and can block IgE-dependent anaphylaxis by an interaction between mast cell Fcε(epsilon)RI and Fcγ(gamma)RIIb receptors. Both mechanisms release platelet-activating factor (PAF), while only the IgE-dependent mechanism releases histamine (Fig. 3.1) [8–10].

**Table 3.1** Pathophysiologic mechanisms of anaphylaxis

| |
|---|
| **IgE-dependent, Immunologic** |
| Foods |
| Therapeutic agents |
| Insect venoms |
| Others |
| **IgE-independent, Immunologic** |
| Disturbance of arachidonic acid metabolism |
|   Nonsteroidal anti-inflammatory drugs |
| Complement activation/activation of kallikrein–kinin contact system |
| Radiocontrast media |
| ACE inhibitors |
|   Protamine (possibly) |
| Others: |
| **Non-immunologic** |
| Nonspecific degranulation of mast cells and basophils |
|   Opioids |
|   Muscle relaxants |
| Physical factors |
|   Exercise |
|   Cold, heat |
| Others: c-kit mutation (D816V) |
| **Idiopathic** |

Multiple additional protein motifs, receptors, channels, and molecular signals act at various levels to modulate anaphylaxis induction, however. These have best been characterized in murine models and include the complex interactions of cell-associated tyrosine kinases, intracellular immunoreceptor tyrosine-based activation motifs (ITAMs), intracellular immunoreceptor tyrosine-based inhibition motifs (ITIMs), Src homology 2-containing tyrosine phosphatases 1 and 2 (SHP1 and SHP2), and Src homology 2-containing inositol phosphatase (SHIP) ([8] provides an overview). Examples of ITIM-associated receptors capable of suppressing mast cell activation are Fcγ(gamma)RIIb, CD300a, platelet-endothelial cell adhesion molecule 1 (PECAM-1), paired immunoglobulin-like receptor B (PIR-B), the c-lectin mast cell function–associated antigen (MAFA), sialic acid-binding immunoglobulin-like lectins (Siglecs), and glycoprotein 49B1 (gp49B1) [8, 11]. PIR-B is a surface receptor expressed on both mast cells and macrophages and appears to regulate basal activation of both cells. Examples of ITIM-independent inhibitory receptors include the mast cell receptor for the glycoprotein CD200, the A2b adenosine receptor, and the transient receptor potential cation channel, subfamily M, member 4 (TRPM4) ion channel [8]. Sphingosine kinases also are reported to be determinants of mast cell responsiveness [12].

Antigen-specific IgG antibody blocks IgE-dependent anaphylaxis in immunized mice without precipitating IgE-independent anaphylaxis when anaphylaxis is induced by low-dose allergen but not when it is induced by high-dose allergen [8]. No IgG-dependent anaphylaxis in humans has been reported, but some anaphylactic reactions have been described for which no specific IgE antibodies or mast cell degranulation (e.g., tryptase elevations) could be detected [13–15]. Some of these cases might reflect immunoglobulin-independent activation of inflammatory cells. However, some investigators have speculated that the culprit mechanism might be the well-characterized IgG/Fcγ(gamma)RIII/macrophage/PAF interaction observed in murine anaphylaxis. Human IgG receptors are capable of activating macrophages to secrete PAF, thus enabling potential Fcγ(gamma)RIII-dependent anaphylaxis [8].

Rare individuals have experienced anaphylaxis after receiving therapeutic preparations of IgG anti-IgE antibodies (omalizumab) [16]. Omalizumab blocks binding of IgE to Fcε(epsilon)RI receptors and does not bind Fcε(epsilon)RI-associated IgE [8, 17]. These anaphylactic events

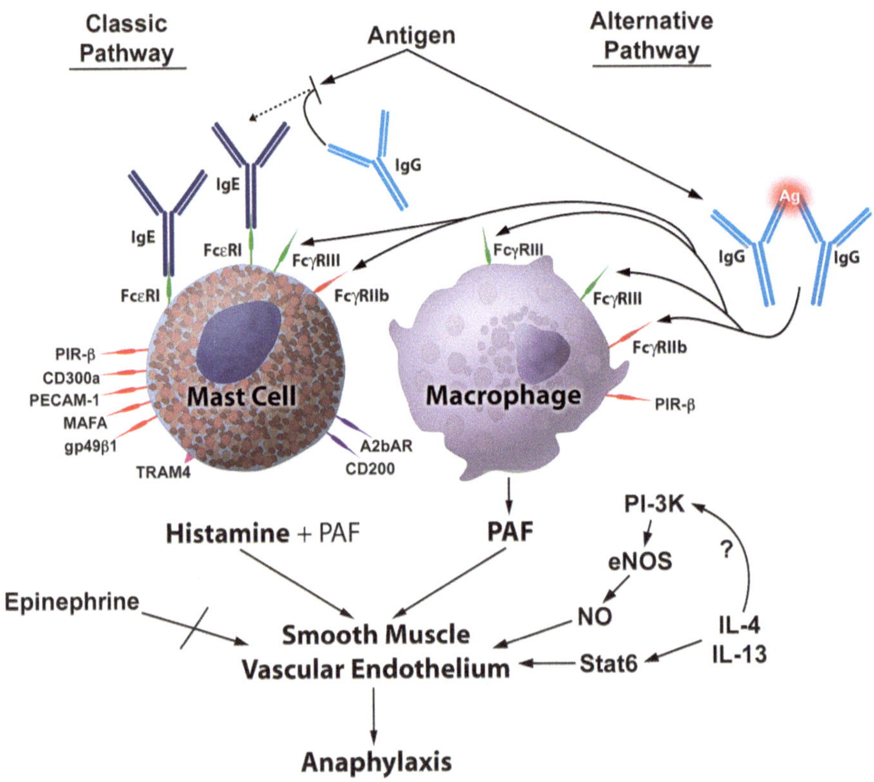


**Fig. 3.1** Mechanisms of anaphylaxis in the mouse. Antigen can cause anaphylaxis in the mouse by (1) cross-linking IgE bound to mast cell Fcε(epsilon)RI, which stimulates histamine and PAF release ("classic pathway"); or (2) binding in large quantities with IgG to form immune complexes that cross-link macrophage Fcγ(gamma)RIII, which stimulates PAF release ("alternative pathway"). Histamine and PAF induce smooth muscle contraction, increased vascular permeability, and other pathophysiologic effects of anaphylaxis. IgG can provide negative feeback on the classic pathway. Nitric oxide, IL-4, and IL-13 can exacerbate anaphylaxis by increasing cellular responsiveness to inflammatory mediators. Epinephrine actions include smooth muscle relaxation and decreased vascular permeability (Modified with permission from [8])

conceivably could be mediated by IgG, with drug-IgG binding to patient IgE [8]. More human data are needed to clarify the causative mechanism.

A mutation of c-kit, a surface membrane tyrosine kinase receptor expressed in all mucosal and connective tissue mast cells, has been associated with anaphylaxis [18] (Table 3.1). Subjects with the D816 V c-kit mutation, present with normal numbers of mast cells in the bone marrow but aberrant expression of CD25 and symptoms of severe anaphylaxis. The entity is described as clonal mast cell activation disorder and screening for this entity should be considered in subjects with severe anaphylactic episodes.

## 3.3 Non-immunologic Anaphylaxis

Non-immunologic anaphylaxis is caused by agents or events that induce sudden, massive mast cell or basophil degranulation in the absence of immunoglobulins. Examples include radiocontrast media, which activate multiple inflammatory pathways including complement and the kallikrein–kinin contact system, and opioids and vancomycin, both of which cause histamine release via direct mast cell degranulation [19].

## 3.4 Chemical Mediators of Anaphylaxis

Biochemical mediators and chemotactic substances are released systemically during anaphylaxis by the degranulation of mast cells and basophils. These include preformed granule-associated substances such as histamine, tryptase, chymase, carboxypeptidase A, and heparin; histamine-releasing factor and other cytokines; and newly generated lipid-derived mediators such as prostaglandin $D_2$, leukotriene $B_4$, PAF, and the cysteinyl leukotrienes, $LTC_4$, $LTD_4$, and $LTE_4$ [2, 19, 20].

The development and severity of anaphylaxis also depend on cellular responsiveness to these mediators. IL-4 and IL-13 are cytokines important in the initial generation of antibody and inflammatory cell responses to anaphylaxis. No comparable human studies have been conducted, but anaphylactic effects in the mouse depend on IL-4Rα(alpha)-dependent IL-4/IL-13 activation of the transcription factor, signal transducer, and activator of transcription 6 (STAT-6). The most rapid, dramatic effect of IL-4 in murine anaphylaxis is a three- to sixfold increase in cellular responsiveness to inflammatory and vasoactive mediators, including histamine, cysteinyl leukotrienes, serotonin, and PAF [8]. PAF causes platelet aggregation and the release of the potent vasoconstrictors serotonin and thromboxane $A_2$ [21]. In murine models, PAF appears to be an important mediator in the development of disseminated intravascular coagulation (DIC) [22].

Rodent models have demonstrated the effectiveness of PAF-receptor antagonists in anaphylaxis [8]. However, the human roles of PAF and PAF acetylhydrolase, the enzyme that inactivates PAF, are becoming increasingly clear. In a prospective study of 41 subjects (age range, 15–74 years) and 23 nonallergic adult controls, serum PAF levels correlated directly and PAF acetylhydrolase levels correlated indirectly with the severity of anaphylaxis [23]. In a companion analysis, PAF acetylhydrolase activity was observed retrospectively to be significantly lower in subjects who experienced fatal peanut-induced anaphylaxis than for five control groups.

Tumor necrosis factor-alpha (TNFα(alpha)), as observed in a murine model of penicillin-induced anaphylaxis, can also play a role in protracted or recurrent events by initiating PAF production. Prolonged mast cell degranulation potentially could cause such events [24]. Thus far, human studies have not reported similar observations.

A mouse model of anaphylaxis indicates that IL-33 can induce antigen-independent systemic anaphylaxis, in a T cell-independent, mast cell-dependent, and ST2 receptor-dependent manner and that IL-33 can directly induce degranulation, eicosanoid, and cytokine production in IgE-sensitized mast cells [25]. The role of IL-33 in human anaphylaxis has not been elucidated, but five atopic subjects who sustained perioperative anaphylaxis had marked IL-33 elevations compared to both atopic and nonatopic controls [25].

Eosinophils may be pro-inflammatory (e.g., release of cytotoxic granule-associated proteins) or anti-inflammatory (e.g., metabolism of vasoactive mediators) [19, 26]. A guinea pig model of anaphylaxis suggests that eosinophils already present in chronically inflamed airways may participate in the acute response to allergen exposure, as well as the role traditionally expected in the late-phase immunologic response [27]. Potential implications for anaphylaxis in humans have not been studied.

### *3.4.1 Histamine and Tryptase*

Histamine activates $H_1$ and $H_2$ receptors. Dose-dependent rhinorrhea, pruritus, bronchospasm, and tachycardia are caused by activation of the $H_1$ receptors, whereas both $H_1$ and $H_2$ receptors mediate flushing, headache, and hypotension [28].

$H_3$ receptors have been implicated in a canine model of anaphylaxis [29] and appear to modulate norepinephrine release from sympathetic nerve fibers in the cardiovascular system. Potential implications for human subjects and anaphylaxis have not been studied. The role of $H_4$ receptors in anaphylaxis, if any, also has not been studied.

Tryptase is a protease that is concentrated selectively and most abundantly in the secretory granules of human mast cells and is released when these cells degranulate. It can activate complement, coagulation pathways, and the kallikrein–kinin contact system with the potential clinical consequences of hypotension, angioedema, clotting, and clot lysis, with the latter variably producing disseminated intravascular coagulation in severe anaphylaxis [4, 19]. Release of ß(beta)-tryptase (mature tryptase) is more specific for activation than α(alpha)-protryptase, which is an inactive monomer. Levels of total tryptase peak 60–90 min after the onset of anaphylaxis and can persist as long as 5 h after the onset of symptoms [19]. Tryptase levels generally correlate with the clinical severity of anaphylaxis [30]. However, an interesting dichotomy may exist in the magnitude of tryptase elevations for those individuals experiencing anaphylaxis after parenteral exposure (e.g., injection, insect sting) versus oral exposure (e.g., food ingestion). In an analysis of anaphylaxis fatalities, the parenterally exposed subjects had higher serum levels of tryptase and lower levels of antigen-specific IgE, whereas those whose demise occurred after oral exposure had low tryptase levels and comparatively high levels of antigen-specific IgE [31]. This difference may be related to the mast cell phenotype the culprit antigen encounters first. Tryptase- and chymase-containing ($MC_{TC}$) mast cells are approximately three times more prevalent in connective tissue than tryptase-containing ($MC_T$) mast cells, whereas the latter cells predominate in pulmonary and intestinal mucosa [31].

Elevations of histamine and tryptase might not correlate clinically. In an emergency department study evaluating subjects who presented with acute allergic reactions, 42 of 97 subjects exhibited increased histamine levels, but only 20 had elevated tryptase levels [32]. Serum histamine levels also correlate with the severity and persistence of cardiopulmonary manifestations but not with the development of urticaria [32, 33].

Possibly because fatal anaphylaxis can occur quickly, many subjects have no distinguishing gross pathologic features at autopsy [34], and postmortem measurements of serum tryptase may be useful in confirming anaphylaxis as the cause of sudden death [31, 35, 36]. However, elevated postmortem tryptase levels have also been reported in fatalities due to other causes, including trauma, heroin injection, and sudden infant death syndrome, all of which can cause mast cell degranulation [19, 37–41]. Thus, postmortem measurement of tryptase might be useful to confirm anaphylaxis fatalities where clinically suspected but it cannot conclusively establish anaphylaxis as cause of death.

### 3.4.2 Arachidonic Acid Metabolites

Arachidonic acid is a phospholipid-derived fatty acid that can be metabolized via the lipoxygenase and cyclooxygenase pathways to generate proinflammatory mediators, such as prostaglandins, leukotrienes, and PAF. Effects of these metabolites include bronchospasm, hypotension, and erythema [19]. Prostaglandin $D_2$ causes vasodilation, increased vasopermeability, and airway smooth muscle bronchoconstriction in various experimental models [42–44]. It is chemotactic for neutrophils and also activates eosinophils [45, 46]. Overproduction of leukotriene $C_4$ enhances mast cell degranulation [19]. Leukotrienes $D_4$ and $E_4$ increase microvascular permeability and both are potent bronchoconstrictors [47–49]. Leukotriene $B_4$ is a chemotactic agent and thus theoretically may contribute to the late phase of biphasic anaphylaxis and to protracted reactions [19].

### 3.4.3 Nitric Oxide in Anaphylaxis

Nitric oxide (NO), a potent autacoid vasodilator, is apparently involved in the complex interaction of regulatory and counter-regulatory mediators in mast cell activation, including anaphylaxis [50, 51].

L-arginine is converted to NO as histamine binds to $H_1$ receptors during phospholipase-C-dependent calcium mobilization. Physiologically, NO participates in the homeostatic control of regional blood pressure and vascular tone. However, its net effects in anaphylaxis appear to be vascular smooth muscle relaxation and enhanced vascular permeability, which are both detrimental in this clinical setting [52]. Increased levels of exhaled nitric oxide have been observed during anaphylaxis [53].

NO may be produced endogenously by inducible nitric oxide synthase (iNOS) or by the constitutively expressed isoforms, endothelial NOS (eNOS) and neuronal NOS (nNOS). eNOS and nNOS presumably produce low amounts of NO for physiologic and/or anti-inflammatory functions, whereas inflammation-associated expression of iNOS and subsequent overproduction of NO and activation of guanylate cyclase have been implicated in the adverse cardiovascular effects of septic shock. It has widely been presumed that this mechanism also applies in anaphylaxis [54].

Cauwels and colleagues, however, suggest that eNOS, rather than iNOS, is a critical mediator of anaphylactic shock experimentally produced by injecting mice with PAF [55]. eNOS-knockout mice survived PAF injection, and soluble guanylate cyclase inhibitors had no effect on the anaphylaxis. Induction of phosphoinositide 3-kinase (PI3K) and protein kinase Akt-mediated phosphorylation were protective. The authors conclude PAF anaphylaxis in mice depends on PI3K/Akt and eNOS-derived NO [55].

### *3.4.4 Other Inflammatory Pathways Are Probably Important*

During episodes of severe anaphylaxis, activation of the complement cascade, the coagulation pathway, and the kallikrein–kinin contact system also occurs. Many of the supporting data are derived from experimental insect sting challenges. Decreases in C4 and C3 and generation of C3a have been observed in anaphylaxis. Evidence for coagulation pathway activation during severe anaphylaxis includes decreases in factor V, factor VIII, and fibrinogen, and fatal disseminated intravascular coagulation in some instances [4, 33]. Of the 196 anaphylaxis fatalities during 10 year in the UK for which sufficient data are available, seven (about 4%) were attributed to DIC [4]. Successful treatment with tranexamic acid has been reported [56]. Decreased high molecular weight kininogen and the formation of factor XIIa-C1 inhibitor and kallikrein-C1 inhibitor complexes indicate contact system activation [33, 57]. Kallikrein activation not only generates bradykinin but also activates factor XII. Factor XII itself can cause clotting and clot lysis via plasmin formation, which itself can activate complement.

In contrast, some mediators may have anti-inflammatory, modulatory effects that limit anaphylaxis. For example, heparin opposes complement activation, modulates tryptase activity, and inhibits clotting, plasmin, and kallikrein [19, 33, 58].

## 3.5 Shock Organs in Anaphylaxis

Organ system involvement varies from species to species and directs the clinical course of anaphylaxis. Factors that determine a specific “shock organ” include variations in the immune response; the location of smooth muscle; and the distribution, rate of degradation, and responsiveness to chemical mediators [59]. In the guinea pig, there is bronchial smooth muscle constriction, which leads to bronchospasm, hypoxemia, and death [60, 61]. The capillary bed is the shock organ for the mouse. Death ensues after severe hypovolemia due to capillary bed dilatation causes fatal tissue hypoxia [62]. Anaphylaxis in rabbits produces fatal pulmonary artery vasoconstriction with right ventricular failure

[61, 63]. The primary shock organ in the dog is the venous system of the liver that contracts and produces severe hepatic congestion [61]. Anaphylaxis in the cat produces acute fatal pulmonary emphysema [64]. In humans, the predominant shock organs are the lung and the heart, and fatalities are divided equally between respiratory arrest and circulatory collapse [4, 65]. Others suggest the spleen may be more important in human anaphylaxis than once was thought [66].

## 3.6 The Heart as Shock Organ in Anaphylaxis

Chemical mediators of anaphylaxis appear to affect the myocardium directly [33, 67]. $H_1$ receptors mediate coronary artery vasoconstriction and increase vascular permeability, whereas $H_2$ receptors increase chronotropy, atrial and ventricular inotropy, and coronary artery vasodilation. The interaction of $H_1$ and $H_2$ receptor stimulation appears to mediate decreased diastolic pressure and increased pulse pressure [68]. PAF also decreases coronary blood flow, delays atrioventricular conduction, and has depressor effects on the heart [69].

Anaphylaxis has been associated clinically with myocardial ischemia and with atrial and ventricular arrhythmias, conduction defects, and repolarization abnormalities [69]. Whether such changes are related to direct mediator effects on the myocardium, to exacerbation of preexisting myocardial insufficiency by the hemodynamic stress of anaphylaxis, to endogenous release of epinephrine from the adrenal medulla in response to stress, or to therapeutically administered epinephrine is unclear [33, 67, 69, 70]. Raper and Fisher describe two previously healthy subjects who developed profound myocardial depression during anaphylaxis [67]. Echocardiography, nuclear imaging, and hemodynamic measurements confirmed the presence of myocardial dysfunction. The anaphylaxis treatment was supplemented with intra-aortic balloon counterpulsation to provide hemodynamic support. Balloon counterpulsation was required for up to 72 h because of persistent myocardial depression, even though other clinical signs of anaphylaxis had resolved. Both subjects recovered with no subsequent evidence of myocardial dysfunction. Thus, the heart can be the primary target of anaphylaxis, even in subjects with no prior cardiovascular disease.

In a retrospective review, the postural history was known for ten individuals who died from anaphylaxis in a nonhospital setting [71]. Four of the 10 fatalities were associated with the assumption of an upright or sitting posture and postmortem findings were consistent with pulseless electrical activity and an "empty heart" attributed to reduced venous return from vasodilation and concomitant volume redistribution.

Increased vascular permeability during anaphylaxis can transfer up to 35% of the intravascular fluid into the extravascular space within 10 min [72]. This shift of effective blood volume causes compensatory release of endogenous catecholamines, endothelins, and angiotensin II [57, 73, 74]. When adequate, these responses may be lifesaving independent of any therapeutic intervention. Some subjects, however, experience abnormal elevations of peripheral vascular resistance (maximal vasoconstriction) yet shock persists due to reduced intravascular volume [75]. Others have decreased systemic vascular resistance, despite elevated levels of endogenous catecholamines [76]. These differences have important clinical implications since the latter scenario may respond favorably to therapeutic doses of vasoconstrictor agents while the former requires large-volume fluid resuscitation and does not respond to vasoconstrictors.

Hypotension can be correlated with elevations of histamine, tryptase, and C3a, but levels of these mediators may not correlate with the presence of flushing, urticaria, or bronchospasm [19]. Angioedema may be related to the appearance of activation products of the contact (kallikrein–kinin) system [57] or to angiotensin converting enzyme levels, which also impact on kinin levels [77].

Levels of enzymes involved in bradykinin metabolism, serum angiotensin converting enzyme (ACE), and aminopeptidase P (APP) were measured in 122 subjects with peanut and tree nut allergy who presented to a regional allergy center with acute allergic reactions after ingestion of these agents [77]. Of these 122, 46 had moderate to severe pharyngeal edema, 36 had moderate to severe bronchospasm, and the remainder lacked these symptoms. Subjects clinically deemed to have severe pharyngeal edema had significantly lower serum ACE levels than those with no pharyngeal edema. Multivariate analysis indicated that subjects with serum ACE concentrations in the lowest quartile were almost ten times more likely to have severe pharyngeal edema than those with higher ACE concentrations. However, subjects with serum ACE levels in the lowest quartile were no more likely than others to have reduced consciousness, bronchospasm, or urticaria. Serum APP levels did not correlate with clinical severity or show any statistical trends. More studies are needed, but these findings suggest a clinical scenario in which some subjects who experience angioedema during anaphylaxis might be more resistant to treatment with epinephrine and second-line therapeutic agents (e.g., antihistamines, corticosteroids) commonly recommended for use after epinephrine.

### 3.6.1 Non-pharmacologic Myocardial Ischemia in Anaphylaxis

Since mast cells accumulate at sites of coronary atherosclerotic plaques, some investigators have suggested that anaphylaxis may promote plaque rupture, thus risking myocardial ischemia [78, 79]. Stimulation of the $H_1$ histamine receptor may also produce coronary artery vasospasm [79–81].

Calcitonin gene-related peptide (CGRP) released during anaphylaxis may help to counteract coronary artery vasoconstriction during anaphylaxis [82, 83]. CGRP, a sensory neurotransmitter widely distributed in cardiovascular tissues, relaxes vascular smooth muscle and has cardioprotective effects in animal models of anaphylaxis [84].

### 3.6.2 Bradycardia During Anaphylaxis

Tachycardia is the rule, but bradycardia may occur during anaphylaxis and thus may not be as useful to distinguish anaphylaxis from a vasodepressor reaction as previously presumed. Relative bradycardia (initial tachycardia followed by a reduction in heart rate despite worsening hypotension) has been reported previously in experimental settings of insect sting anaphylaxis, as well as in trauma patients [33, 57, 85–87].

Bradycardia has also been observed in porcine anaphylaxis induced experimentally by various liposomal preparations. Adenosine and C5a have been implicated [88].

Two distinct phases of physiologic response occur in mammals subjected to hypovolemia. The initial phase is a baroreceptor-mediated sympatho-excitatory response comprised of increased cardiac sympathetic drive and simultaneous withdrawal of resting vagal drive, which together produce tachycardia and peripheral vasoconstriction [86]. When effective blood volume falls by 20–30%, a second phase follows which is characterized by withdrawal of vasoconstrictor drive, relative or absolute bradycardia, increased vasopressin, further catecholamine release as the adrenal axis becomes more active, and hypotension [86, 87]. Atropine administered therapeutically in this hypovolemic scenario reverses the bradycardia but not the hypotension.

Clinical implications of bradycardia in human anaphylaxis and hypovolemic states have not been studied. However, a retrospective analysis of approximately 11,000 trauma patients found that mortality was lower, after adjusting for other mortality factors, in the 29% of hypotensive patients who were bradycardic than for those hypotensive patients with tachycardia [87]. Thus, there may be a compensatory role for bradycardia in these clinical settings of hypotension.

Conduction defects and sympatholytic medications may also produce bradycardia [2]. Excessive venous pooling with decreased venous return (also seen in vasodepressor reactions) may activate tension-sensitive sensory receptors in the infero-posterior portions of the left ventricle, thus resulting in a cardioinhibitory (Bezold–Jarisch) reflex that stimulates the vagus nerve and causes bradycardia [19].

## 3.7 Respiratory Effects of Anaphylaxis

Anaphylaxis may have adverse effects on any part of the respiratory tract. In a compilation of retrospective series of patients with acute nonfatal anaphylaxis, respiratory manifestations were observed in 40–60% of subjects: rhinitis, dyspnea/wheeze, and upper airway angioedema in up to 20%, 50%, and 60%, respectively [19].

Similar observations have been made in cases of fatal anaphylaxis. One report examined 214 anaphylactic fatalities, for which the cause of death could be determined in 196 [4]. Asphyxia was implicated in one-half (98 cases), with pulmonary inflammation in 49, upper airway angioedema in 23, and both upper and lower airway involvement in 26. Fatal respiratory arrest during anaphylaxis occurred almost exclusively in those with preexisting asthma. Another postmortem analysis of 23 unselected cases of fatal anaphylaxis determined that 16 of 20 "immediate" deaths (deaths occurring within 1 h of symptom onset) were due to upper airway edema [65].

## 3.8 Autopsy Findings in Fatal Anaphylaxis

Victims of fatal anaphylaxis often show no distinguishing gross pathologic features at autopsy, possibly because death can occur so rapidly. A retrospective review of 56 cases of fatal anaphylaxis for which autopsy information was available found that death occurred within 1 h for 39 cases [34]. This is consistent with clinical observations that patients whose shock develops rapidly may essentially lack other signs or symptoms. When present however, findings include upper airway edema and petechial hemorrhages in airway mucosa, mucus plugging and hyperinflation of the lungs, and cerebral edema.

## 3.9 Anaerobic Metabolism Complicates Anaphylaxis

Peripheral blood flow is decreased during shock to preserve perfusion of the brain, heart, and kidneys. In septic shock, the paradigm of distributive shock, hypotension results from decreased systemic vascular resistance, and anaerobic metabolism persists in skeletal muscle, despite increased partial pressure of oxygen. This impairment in cellular respiration has been attributed to an unregulated inflammatory process called "cytopathic hypoxia" [89].

Preliminary evidence suggests that anaerobic metabolism also occurs within peripheral tissues during anaphylaxis. One study compared rats with ovalbumin-induced anaphylaxis to a parallel group with severe, nicardipine-induced hypotension [90]. The time course and magnitude of hypotension were similar, and both groups experienced decreased perfusion of skeletal muscle. There were metabolic differences, however. The anaphylactic group showed greater sympatho-excitatory response, with higher plasma catecholamine levels beginning at 20 min and maintained throughout the 60-min protocol. Plasma epinephrine increased 15-fold and norepinephrine increased 10-fold over baseline values in the anaphylactic group. Skeletal muscle blood flow was decreased in both nicardipine- and anaphylaxis-induced hypotensive rats initially. This was followed by a further decrease in the anaphylaxis group that began at 20 min and persisted throughout the observation period. A higher gradient between plasma and interstitial epinephrine reflected more impairment of skeletal muscle blood flow in the anaphylactic animals, possibly due to greater vasoconstriction. The anaphylactic group experienced a larger, more rapid increase in interstitial lactate, and corresponding decrease in interstitial pyruvate, indicating depletion of cellular energy stores. The latter finding was not present in rats with nicardipine-induced hypotension. These findings, combined with decreased perfusion, may partly explain why end-organ injury and irreversible shock in anaphylaxis can develop so quickly [90].

## 3.10 Conclusion

Anaphylaxis involves numerous, complex, immunopathologic mechanisms and interactions. Well-characterized animal models clearly would facilitate a better understanding of the pathophysiologic mechanisms of anaphylaxis and might ultimately assist in diagnosis and treatment, particularly of anaphylactic shock.

## References

1. Sampson HA, Muñoz-Furlong A, Campbell RL, et al. Second symposium on the definition and management of anaphylaxis: summary report. *J Allergy Clin Immunol* 2006;117:391–397.
2. Kemp SF, Lockey RF. Anaphylaxis: a review of causes and mechanisms. *J Allergy Clin Immunol* 2002;110:341–348.
3. Simons FER, Sampson HA. Anaphylaxis epidemic: fact or fiction? *J Allergy Clin Immunol* 2008;122:1166–1168.
4. Pumphrey, RS. Fatal anaphylaxis in the UK, 1992–2001. *Novartis Found Symp* 2004;257:116–128.
5. Johansson SGO, Bieber T, Dahl R, et al. Revised nomenclature for allergy for global use: Report of the Nomenclature Review Committee of the World Allergy Organization, October 2003. *J Allergy Clin Immunol* 2004;113:832–836.
6. Coombs RRA, Gell PGH. Classification of allergic reactions responsible for clinical hypersensitivity and disease. In: Gell PGH, Coombs RRA, Lachmann PJ, eds. *Clinical Aspects of Immunology*, 3rd ed. Oxford, England: Blackwell; 1975:761–781.
7. Sell S. Immunopathology. In: Rich RR, Fleisher TA, Schwartz BD, et al., eds. Clinical Immunology: Principles and Practice. St. Louis, Mo.: Mosby; 1996:449–477.
8. Finkelman FD. Anaphylaxis: lessons from mouse models. *J Allergy Clin Immunol* 2007;120:506–515.
9. Strait RT, Morris SC, Finkelman FD. IgG blocking antibodies inhibit IgE-mediated anaphylaxis in vivo through both antigen interruption and Fcγ(gamma)RIIb cross-linking. *J Clin Invest* 2006;116:833–841.
10. Shibamoto T, Liu W, Cui S, et al. PAF, rather than histamine, participates in mouse anaphylactic hypotension. *Pharmacology* 2008;82:114–120.
11. Yokoi H, Myers A, Matsumoto K, et al. Alteration and acquisition of Siglecs during in vitro maturation of CD34+ progenitors into human mast cells. *Allergy* 2006;61:769–776.
12. Olivera A, Mizugishi K, Tikhonova A, et al. The sphingosine kinase-sphingosine-1-phosphate axis is a determinant of mast cell function and anaphylaxis. *Immunity* 2007;26:287–297.
13. Cheifetz A, Smedley M, Martin S, et al. The incidence and management of infusion reactions to infliximab: a large center experience. *Am J Gastroenterol* 2003;98:1315–1324.
14. Stallmach A, Giese T, Schmidt C, et al. Severe anaphylactic reaction to infliximab: successful treatment with adalimumab—report of a case. *Eur J Gastroenterol Hepatol* 2004;16:627–630.
15. Hod EA, Sokol SA, Zimring JC, Spitalnik SL. Hypothesis: hemolytic transfusion reactions represent an alternative type of anaphylaxis. *Int J Clin Exp Pathol* 2009;2:71–82.
16. Cox L, Platts-Mills TAE, Finegold I, et al. American academy of allergy, asthma & immunology/American college of allergy, asthma and immunology joint task force report on omalizumab-associated anaphylaxis. *J Allergy Clin Immunol* 2007;120:1373–1377.

17. Dreyfus DH, Randolph CC. Characterization of an anaphylactoid reaction to omalizumab. *Ann Allergy Asthma Immunol* 2006;96:624–627.
18. Akin C, Scott LM, Kocabas CN, et al. Demonstration of an aberrant mast-cell population with clonal markers in a subset of patients with "idiopathic" anaphylaxis. *Blood* 2007;110:2331–2333.
19. Lieberman P. Anaphylaxis and anaphylactoid reactions. In: Adkinson NF Jr, Yunginger JW, Busse WW, et al., eds. *Middleton's Allergy: Principles and Practice*, 6th ed. St. Louis, Mo.: Mosby Year Book; 2003:1497–1522.
20. Ono E, Taniguchi M, Mita H, et al. Increased production of cysteinyl leukotrienes and prostaglandin D2 during human anaphylaxis. *Clin Exp Allergy* 2009;39:72–80.
21. Kinn JW, Bache RJ. Effect of platelet activation on coronary collateral blood flow. *Circulation* 1998;98:1431–1437.
22. Choi IH, Ha TY, Lee DG, et al. Occurrence of disseminated intravascular coagulation (DIC) in active systemic anaphylaxis: role of platelet-activating factor. *Clin Exp Immunol* 1995;100:390–394.
23. Vadas P, Gold M, Perelman B, Liss GM, Lack G, Blyth T, et al. Platelet-activating factor, PAF acetylhydrolase, and severe anaphylaxis. *N Engl J Med* 2008;358:28–35.
24. Lieberman P. Biphasic anaphylactic reactions. *Ann Allergy Asthma Immunol* 2005;95:217–228.
25. Pushparaj PN, Tay HK, H'ng SC, et al. The cytokine interleukin-33 mediates anaphylactic shock. *Proc Natl Acad Sci USA* 2009;106:9773–9778.
26. Goetzl EJ, Wasserman SI, Austin KF. Eosinophil polymorphonuclear leukocyte function in immediate hypersensitivity. *Arch Pathol* 1975;99:1–4.
27. Erjefält JS, Korsgren M, Malm-Erjefält M, et al. Acute allergic responses induce a prompt luminal entry of airway tissue eosinophils. *Am J Respir Cell Mol Biol* 2003;29:439–448.
28. Kaliner M, Sigler R, Summers R, Shelhamer JH. Effects of infused histamine: analysis of the effects of H-1 and H-2 receptor antagonists on cardiovascular and pulmonary responses. *J Allergy Clin Immunol* 1981;68:365–371.
29. Chrusch C, Sharma S, Unruh H, et al. Histamine H3 receptor blockade improves cardiac function in canine anaphylaxis. *Am J Respir Crit Care Med* 1999;160:142–149.
30. Schwartz LB. Effector cells of anaphylaxis: mast cells and basophils. *Novartis Found Symp* 2004;257:65–74.
31. Yunginger JW, Nelson DR, Squillace DL, et al. Laboratory investigations of death due to anaphylaxis. *J Forensic Sci* 1991;36:857–865.
32. Lin RY, Schwartz LB, Curry A, et al. Histamine and tryptase levels in patients with acute allergic reactions: an emergency department-based study. *J Allergy Clin Immunol* 2000;106:65–71.
33. Smith PL, Kagey-Sobotka A, Bleecker ER, et al. Physiologic manifestations of human anaphylaxis. *J Clin Invest* 1980;66:1072–1080.
34. Pumphrey RS, Roberts IS. Postmortem findings after fatal anaphylactic reactions. *J Clin Pathol* 2000;53:273–276.
35. Ansari MQ, Zamora JL, Lipscomb MF. Postmortem diagnosis of acute anaphylaxis by serum tryptase analysis. A case report. *Am J Clin Pathol* 1993;99:101–103
36. Schwartz HJ, Yunginger JW, Schwartz LB. Is unrecognized anaphylaxis a cause of sudden unexpected death? *Clin Exp Allergy* 1995;25:866–870.
37. Platt MS, Yunginger JW, Sekula-Perlman A, et al. Involvement of mast cells in sudden infant death syndrome. *J Allergy Clin Immunol* 1994;94:250–256.
38. Randall B, Butts J, Halsey JF. Elevated postmortem tryptase in the absence of anaphylaxis. *J Forensic Sci* 1995;40:208–211.
39. Edston E, van Hage-Hamsten M. β(beta)-Tryptase measurements post-mortem in anaphylactic deaths and in controls. *Forensic Sci Int* 1998;93:135–142.
40. Edston E, Gidlund E, Wickman M, et al. Increased mast cell tryptase in sudden infant death—anaphylaxis, hypoxemia or artifact? *Clin Exp Allergy* 1999;29:1648–1654.
41. Edston E, Eriksson O, van Hage M. Mast cell tryptase in postmortem serum—reference values and confounders. *Int J Legal Med* 2007;121:275–280.
42. Flower RJ, Harvey EA, Kingston WP. Inflammatory effects of prostaglandin D2 in rat and human skin. *Br J Pharmacol* 1976;56:229–233.
43. Hardy CC, Robinson C, Tattersfield AE, Holgate ST. The bronchoconstrictor effect of inhaled prostaglandin D2 in normal and asthmatic men. *N Engl J Med* 1984;311:209–213.
44. Pugliese G, Spokas EG, Marcinkiewicz E, Wong PY. Hepatic transformation of prostaglandin D2 to a new prostanoid, 9 alpha,11 beta-prostaglandin F2, that inhibits platelet aggregation and constricts blood vessels. *J Biol Chem* 1985;260:14621–14625.
45. Goetzl EJ. Oxygenation products of arachidonic acid as mediators of hypersensitivity and inflammation. *Med Clin* NA 1981; 65:809–828.
46. Raible DG, Schulman ES, DiMuzio J, et al. Mast cell mediators prostaglandin-D2 and histamine activate human eosinophils. *J Immunol* 1992;148:3536–3542.

47. Juhlin L, Hammarström S. Effects of intradermally injected leukotriene C4 and histamine in patients with urticaria, psoriasis and atopic dermatitis. *Br J Dermatol* 1982;107 Suppl 23:106–110.
48. Arm JP, Lee TH. Sulphidopeptide leukotrienes in asthma. *Clin Sci* 1993;84:501–510.
49. Austen KF. The Paul Kallós Memorial Lecture. From slow reacting substance of anaphylaxis to leukotriene C4 synthase. *Int Arch Allergy Immunol* 1995;107:19–24.
50. Palmer RMJ, Ferrige AG, Moncada S. Nitric oxide release accounts for the biological activity of endothelium derived relaxing factor. *Nature* 1987;327:524–526.
51. Coleman JW. Nitric oxide: a regulator of mast cell activation and mast cell-mediated inflammation. *Clin Exp Immunol* 2002;129:4–10.
52. Mitsuhata H, Shimizu R, Yokoyama MM. Role of nitric oxide in anaphylactic shock. *J Clin Immunol* 1995;15:277–283.
53. Rolla G, Nebiolo F, Guida G, et al. Level of exhaled nitric oxide during human anaphylaxis. *Ann Allergy Asthma Immunol* 2006;97:264–265.
54. Lowenstein CJ, Michel T. What's in a name? eNOS and anaphylactic shock. *J Clin Invest* 2006;116:2075–2078.
55. Cauwels A, Janssen B, Buys E, et al. Anaphylactic shock depends on PI3K and eNOS-derived NO. *J Clin Invest* 2006;116:2244–2251.
56. De Souza RL, Short T, Warman GR, et al. Anaphylaxis with associated fibrinolysis, reversed with tranexamic acid and demonstrated by thrombelastography. *Anaesth Intensive Care* 2004;32:580–587.
57. van der Linden P-WG, Struyvenberg A, Kraaijenhagen RJ, et al. Anaphylactic shock after insect-sting challenge in 138 persons with a previous insect-sting reaction. *Ann Intern Med* 1993;118:161–168.
58. Kaplan AP, Joseph K, Silverberg M. Pathways for bradykinin formation and inflammatory disease. *J Allergy Clin Immunol* 2002;109:195–209.
59. James LP Jr, Austen KF. Fatal and systemic anaphylaxis in man. *N Engl J Med* 1964;270:597–603.
60. Warren S, Dixon FJ. Antigen tracer studies and histologic observations in anaphylactic shock in the guinea pig. Part 1. *Amer J Med Sci* 1948;216:136–145.
61. Lockey RF, Bukantz SC. Allergic emergencies. *Med Clin North Am* 1974;58:147–156.
62. Munoz J, Bergman RK. Mechanism of anaphylactic death in the mouse. *Nature* 1965;205:199–200.
63. Coca AF. The mechanism of the anaphylaxis reaction in the rabbit. *J Immunol* 1919;4:219–231.
64. McCusker HB, Aitken ID. Anaphylaxis in the cat. *J Pathol Bacteriol* 1966;91:282–285.
65. Greenberger PA, Rotskoff BD, Lifschultz B. Fatal anaphylaxis: postmortem findings and associated comorbid diseases. *Ann Allergy Asthma Immunol* 2007;98:252–257.
66. Trani N, Bonetti LR, Gualandri G, Barbolini G. Immediate anaphylactic death following antibiotics injection: splenic eosinophilia easily revealed by pagoda red stain. *Forensic Sci Int* 2008;181:21–25.
67. Raper RF, Fisher MM. Profound reversible myocardial depression after anaphylaxis. *Lancet* 1988;1:386–388.
68. Bristow MR, Ginsburg R, Harrison DC. Histamine and the human heart: the other receptor system. *Am J Cardiol* 1982;49:249–251.
69. Marone G, Bova M, Detoraki A, et al. The human heart as a shock organ in anaphylaxis. *Novartis Found Symp* 2004;257:133–149.
70. Wittstein IS, Thiemann DR, Lima JAC, et al. Neurohumoral features of myocardial stunning due to sudden emotional stress. *N Engl J Med* 2005;352:539–548.
71. Pumphrey RS. Fatal posture in anaphylactic shock. *J Allergy Clin Immunol* 2003;112: 451–452.
72. Fisher MM. Clinical observations on the pathophysiology and treatment of anaphylactic cardiovascular collapse. *Anaesth Intensive Care* 1986;14:17–21.
73. Hermann K, Rittweger R, Ring J. Urinary excretion of angiotensin I, II, arginine vasopressin and oxytocin in patients with anaphylactoid reactions. *Clin Exp Allergy* 1992;22:845–853.
74. von Tschirschnitz M, von Eschenbach CE, Hermann K, Ring J. Plasma angiotensin II in patients with Hymenoptera venom allergy during hyposensitization [abstract]. *J Allergy Clin Immunol* 1993;91:283.
75. Hanashiro PK, Weil MH. Anaphylactic shock in man: report of two cases with detailed hemodynamics and metabolic studies. *Arch Intern Med* 1967;119:129–140.
76. Fahmy NR. Hemodynamics, plasma histamine and catecholamine concentrations during an anaphylactoid reaction to morphine. *Anesthesiology* 1981;55:329–331.
77. Summers CW, Pumphrey RS, Woods WN, et al. Factors predicting anaphylaxis to peanuts and tree nuts in patients referred to a specialist center. *J Allergy Clin Immunol* 2008;121:632–638.
78. Kovanen PT, Kaartinen M, Paavonen T. Infiltrates of activated mast cells at the site of coronary atheromatous erosion or rupture in myocardial infarction. *Circulation* 1995;92:1084–1088.
79. Kounis NG. Kounis syndrome (allergic angina and allergic myocardial infarction): a natural paradigm? *Int J Cardiol* 2006;110:7–14.
80. Abela GS, Picon PD, Friedl SE, et al. Triggering of plaque disruption and arterial thrombosis in an atherosclerotic rabbit model. *Circulation* 1995;91:776–784.

81. Steffel J, Akhmedov A, Greutert H, et al. Histamine induces tissue factor expression: implications for acute coronary syndromes. *Circulation* 2005;112:341–349.
82. Rubin LE, Levi R. Protective role of bradykinin in cardiac anaphylaxis: coronary-vasodilating and antiarrhythmic activities mediated by autocrine/paracrine mechanisms. *Circ Res*1995;76:434–440.
83. Schuligoi R, Amann R, Donnerer J, Peskar BA. Release of calcitonin gene-related peptide in cardiac anaphylaxis. *N-S Arch Pharmacol* 1997;355:224–229.
84. Rang WQ, Du YH, Hu CP, et al. Protective effects of calcitonin gene-related peptide-mediated evodiamine on guinea-pig cardiac anaphylaxis. *N-S Arch Pharmacol* 2003;367:306–311.
85. Brown SGA, Blackman KE, Stenlake V, Heddle RJ. Insect sting anaphylaxis: prospective evaluation of treatment with intravenous adrenaline and volume resuscitation. *Emerg Med J* 2004;21:149–154.
86. Schadt JC, Ludbrook J. Hemodynamic and neurohumoral responses to acute hypovolemia in conscious mammals. *Am J Physiol* 1991;260:H305–318.
87. Demetriades D, Chan LS, Bhasin P, et al. Relative bradycardia in patients with traumatic hypotension. *J Trauma* 1998;45:534–539.
88. Szebeni J, Baranyi L, Sávay S, et al. Complement activation-related cardiac anaphylaxis in pigs: role of C5a anaphylatoxin and adenosine in liposome-induced abnormalities in ECG and heart function. *Am J Physiol Heart Circ Physiol* 2006;290:H1050–1058.
89. Fink MP. Bench-to-bedside review: cytopathic hypoxia. *Crit Care* 2002;6:491–499.
90. Dewachter P, Jouan-Hureaux V, Franck P, et al. Anaphylactic shock: a form of distributive shock without inhibition of oxygen consumption. *Anesthesiology* 2005;103:40–49.

# Chapter 4
# Mast Cells: Effector Cells of Anaphylaxis

**Mindy Tsai and Stephen J. Galli**

**Abstract** Mast cells are derived from hematopoietic progenitors, which complete their maturation in peripheral tissues. Mast cells are particularly abundant in tissues exposed to the environment, such as the skin, airways, and gastrointestinal tract. Mast cells can be activated to secrete a wide spectrum of mediators, such as histamine and other stored mediators; lipid mediators such as cysteinyl leukotrienes and prostaglandins; and many cytokines, chemokines, and growth factors. IgE-dependent activation of mast cells and basophils and the rapid release of mediators by these cells represent the primary effector mechanisms responsible for the acute manifestations of allergen-induced anaphylaxis in humans. This chapter reviews the basic biology of mast cells, and describes methods for characterizing the functions of mast cells in vivo. We will particularly emphasize the results of studies designed to assess the importance of mast cells in mouse models of active and passive systemic anaphylaxis, and will briefly describe some approaches that are being used to therapeutically target IgE-dependent activation of mast cells.

**Keywords** Antigen • Basophils • c-Kit • Degranulation • Histamine • Mast cells • Mast-cell-deficient mice • IgE • $IgG_1$ • Passive cutaneous anaphylaxis • Platelet-activating factor • Sphingosine-1-phosphate • Stem cell factor

## 4.1 Introduction

Several lines of evidence indicate that IgE-dependent activation of mast cells and basophils and the rapid release of mediators from these effector cells represent the main underlying mechanisms that cause allergen-induced anaphylaxis in humans [1–4]. IgE-dependent activation of mast cells also is critical for many examples of allergen-induced anaphylaxis in mice, particularly those elicited by at low levels of allergen challenge [2, 5]. Studies in mice show that systemic anaphylaxis also can be induced by immune complexes of $IgG_1$ and allergen, and that mast cells have a less important role in such responses than in those involving IgE [5–8]. The extent to which IgG may contribute to the development of systemic anaphylactic reactions in humans is not clear [3, 9, 10].

In humans, these potentially catastrophic systemic allergic reactions are triggered by exposure to otherwise harmless environmental substances, such as peanuts, penicillin, or rubber latex, as well as to venoms of hymenoptera, reptiles, or other animals. In susceptible subjects who have been sensitized

S.J. Galli (✉)
Professor of Pathology and of Microbiology and Immunology Department of Pathology, Stanford University School of Medicine, Stanford, CA, USA
e-mail: sgalli@stanford.edu

M.C. Castells (ed.), *Anaphylaxis and Hypersensitivity Reactions*,
DOI 10.1007/978-1-60327-951-2_4, © Springer Science+Business Media, LLC 2011

to a particular allergen and have developed allergen-specific IgE, reexposure to even minute amounts of that specific allergen results in IgE-dependent aggregation of Fcε(epsilon)RI on the surface of mast cells (and basophils), which in turn initiates intracellular signaling cascades that culminate in mast cell and basophil degranulation with immediate secretion of cytoplasmic granule-associated preformed mediators, for example, vasoactive amines (in humans, histamine), neutral proteases, and proteoglycans, as well as certain cytokines including TNF and VEGF-A. In addition, such activated mast cells and basophils release pro-inflammatory lipid mediators that are synthesized de novo, for example, prostaglandins, leukotrienes, and platelet-activating factor (PAF), and undergo enhanced transcription, translation, and secretion of many growth factors, cytokines, and chemokines [11]. It is likely that many of these mast cell (and/or basophil)-derived mediators contribute to the pathophysiologic manifestation of anaphylaxis; moreover, one of the cytoplasmic granule-associated stored mediators, tryptase, is a well established biomarker for the diagnosis of anaphylaxis in humans [12–14].

This chapter focuses on the effector functions of mast cells in anaphylaxis and particularly review findings derived from studies of mouse models of active and passive anaphylaxis, which were designed to assess the importance of mast cells in the elicitation and progression of local and systemic anaphylactic reactions.

The biochemical mechanisms of mast-cell activation in anaphylaxis have been reviewed recently [15, 16] (see Chap. 20). Like mast cells, basophils also express Fcε(epsilon)RI and secrete histamine upon activation, but basophils are developmentally distinct from mast cells. Several lines of evidence indicate that mast cells and basophils can perform some distinct and some overlapping functions in anaphylaxis. The effector functions of basophils and their mechanisms of activation in anaphylaxis will not be discussed here (see Chap. 5).

## 4.2 The Basic Biology of Mast Cells

Mast cells are widely distributed throughout the vascularized tissues of humans, mice, and other vertebrates. Relatively high numbers of mast cells occur near body surfaces including the skin, airways, and gastrointestinal tract, which are exposed to the environment and where pathogens, allergens, and other environmental agents are frequently encountered [11, 17–19]. Accordingly, mast cells, together with dendritic cells, represent one of the first cell types of the immune system to interact with environmental antigens/allergens, invading pathogens, or external toxins.

Mast cells are derived from hematopoietic stem cells. Unlike granulocytes, mature mast cells do not ordinarily circulate in the blood; instead, circulating mast-cell precursors migrate to the peripheral tissues or (particularly in murine rodents) serosal cavities where they complete their differentiation and maturation and take up residence [11, 17–19]. Mast cells can be long-lived cells that can reenter the cell cycle and proliferate following appropriate stimulation [11–20]. Increased recruitment and/or retention of mast-cell progenitors, followed by their local maturation, also can contribute to the expansion of mast-cell populations in the tissues [11, 17–19, 21]. Studies in mice have established that striking increases in the number of mast cells, as well as local changes in their tissue distribution and/or phenotypic characteristics, can occur during T helper 2 (Th2)-cell-associated responses (e.g., as induced by certain parasites) and that increases in numbers of mast cells also can occur in settings of persistent inflammation and/or tissue remodeling [11, 17–19, 21]. The main survival and developmental factor for mast cells is stem cell factor (SCF, also known as Kit ligand), but many growth factors, cytokines, and chemokines can influence the number and phenotype of mast cells, including interleukin-3 (IL-3), which is of particular importance in mice, Th2-cell-associated cytokines (such as IL-4 and IL-9) and transforming growth factor-β(beta)1 (TGFβ(beta)1), an example of a cytokine that can, in some circumstances, negatively influence mast-cell proliferation or survival [11, 17–19, 21–23].

T cell-derived products may also influence mast-cell populations in humans in vivo. HIV infected patients ($n=3$) or patients with combined immunodeficiency disorders (two patients with severe combined immunodeficiency and one with Omenn's syndrome) exhibited markedly decreased numbers of tryptase-containing mast cells ($MC_T$) in the mucosa of the gastrointestinal tract but no significant differences from normal subjects in the smaller numbers of tryptase and chymase-containing mast cells ($MC_{TC}$) at that site [24]. The reason(s) for such mast-cell depletion in such patients is not yet clear but may reflect impaired T cell-dependent effects on mast-cell populations. In the case of the HIV-infected subjects, it is possible that infection of mast cells with the virus also may have contributed to depletion of $MC_T$ in the gastrointestinal mucosa [25–27].

Various stimuli, in addition to IgE and specific antigen, can activate mast cells to release a wide variety of biologically active products, many of which can potentially mediate pro-inflammatory, anti-inflammatory, and/or immunosuppressive functions and can influence processes of tissue remodeling [11, 21, 28–32]. Furthermore, mast cells can participate in multiple cycles of activation for mediator release and can be differentially activated to release distinct patterns of mediators or cytokines, depending on the type and strength of the activating stimuli [11, 23, 33–36]. The strength and nature of the responsiveness of mast cells to various activating stimuli can be influenced by genetic and microenvironmental factors that affect the expression pattern or functional properties of the surface receptors or signaling molecules that contribute to such responses [11, 32, 33].

The regulation of mast-cell survival and proliferation and the modulation of important phenotypic characteristics of mast cells – including their susceptibility to activation by various stimuli during innate or adaptive immune responses, their ability to store and/or produce various secreted products, and the magnitude and nature of the secretory response of mast cells to specific activation stimuli – can be finely controlled or "tuned" [11]. Therefore, it seems reasonable to hypothesize that, in some settings, mast cells can both enhance and later help to limit certain innate and adaptive immune responses [21, 32].

## 4.3 Approaches to Assess Mast-Cell Functions

Mast-cell function can be studied in vitro using freshly isolated cells from mouse or human tissues (however, such cells usually are available only in limited numbers), or using cultured cells that have been derived in vitro from various sources of hematopoietic tissues (such as bone marrow, peripheral blood, fetal liver), or fetal skin or from embryonic stem cells. Studies using such cells have provided valuable insights into mechanisms by which mast cells might influence anaphylaxis and many other biological responses. Nevertheless, it is exceedingly difficult (and probably impossible) to recapitulate fully in vitro those conditions that are experienced by mast cells in vivo. Thus, to understand the contribution of mast cells in health and disease, we and other investigators have attempted to analyze mast-cell function using experimental mouse models. For example, the roles of mast-cell-associated products can be assessed by studying knockout/transgenic mice in which that product has been deleted or modified by genetic engineering. If a product is selectively expressed by mast cells, and if its deletion/modification does not significantly influence the expression of other mast-cell products, then it is possible to draw conclusions about the role of that mast-cell product in vivo. This approach has been used to analyze functions of several mast-cell-restricted proteases, including mast-cell protease-1 (MCPT1) [37–39], MCPT4 [40, 41], MCPT5 [42], MCPT6 [43–45], MCPT7 [45], and mast-cell carboxypeptidase A3 (CPA3; also known as MC-CPA) [46, 47]. In addition to providing information about the functions of such mast-cell-associated proteases in vivo in various disease models, mice with deficiencies in mast-cell-specific proteases have been used to analyze to what extent the absence of these proteases or their enzymatic activity influences other aspects of mast-cell phenotype, such as the content of other stored mediators (e.g., deficiencies of mast-cell MC-CPA result in reduced expression of MCPT-5 [46] and MC-CPA is absent in MCPT-$5^{-/-}$ mast cells [42], and disruption of the MCPT1 gene in the mouse results in changes in ultrastructural morphology and histochemical staining characteristics of mucosal mast-cells granules [37]).

Models employing genetically mast-cell-deficient mice, such as WBB6F$_1$-*Kit*$^{W/W-v}$ or C57BL/6-*Kit*$^{W-sh/W-sh}$ mice, represent a popular approach to assess the in vivo relevance and biological importance of mast-cell functions that have been proposed based on in vitro observations as well as to quantify the contributions of mast cells to the expression of particular biological responses in vivo. These mice virtually lack tissue mast cells [48–52] due to their defects in the structure or cell expression of the SCF receptor, the c-Kit tyrosine kinase receptor. WBB6F$_1$-*Kit*$^{W/W-v}$ mice have loss-of-function mutations in the c-*Kit* coding sequence [53], whereas C57BL/6-*Kit*$^{W-sh/W-sh}$ mice have an inversion mutation affecting the transcriptional regulatory elements upstream of the Kit transcription start site [54–57]. In addition to their profound deficiency in tissue mast cells, these types of genetically mast-cell-deficient mice exhibit a constellation of other phenotypic abnormalities affecting cell lineages, which, like mast cells, require c-Kit function for aspects of their development, survival, and/or function, or, in the case of C57BL/6-*Kit*$^{W-sh/W-sh}$ mice, reflect other consequences of the inversion mutation [29, 31, 51, 57].

However, the mast-cell deficiency of these mice can be selectively "repaired" by the adoptive transfer of: (1) genetically compatible, purified, or in vitro-derived mast cells from congenic wild-type mice or various transgenic or mutant mice [51, 52]; (2) mast cells derived in vitro from mouse embryonic stem cells [58]; or (3) mast cells that have been transduced with short hairpin RNA to decrease the expression of proteins of interest [59]. These "mast-cell knock-in mice" can then be used to assess the extent to which differences in the biological responses of c-*Kit* mutant mice compared with wild-type mice are due to the lack of mast cells, as opposed to other phenotypic abnormalities, in the c-*Kit* mutant animals.

As noted above, c-*Kit* mutant mice have Kit-related phenotypic abnormalities that affect lineages other than mast cells, but these abnormalities vary depending on the mutations affecting c-Kit structure or cell-specific expression [29, 31, 51, 57]. In general, C57BL/6-*Kit*$^{W-sh/W-sh}$ mice have fewer or milder phenotypic abnormalities than those of WBB6F$_1$-*Kit*$^{W/W-v}$ mice. Moreover, C57BL/6-*Kit*$^{W-sh/W-sh}$ mice are both fertile and have the well-characterized C57BL/6 background. For these reasons, C57BL/6-*Kit*$^{W-sh/W-sh}$ mice are becoming increasingly popular for studies to elucidate the roles of mast cells in vivo. However, it is important to consider that the different genetic backgrounds of WBB6F$_1$-*Kit*$^{W/W-v}$ and C57BL/6-*Kit*$^{W-sh/W-sh}$ mice, as well as the effects of the different mutations in these mice on cell lineages other than mast cells, may influence the results of experiments employing such mice to investigate mast-cell function.

Transgenic mice expressing Cre recombinase under the control of "mast-cell-specific" promoters recently have been generated [60–62]. Such "mast-cell cre mice" are being crossed with other transgenic mice in which the genes of interest are "floxed" in attempts to reduce the expression of specific gene products only (or, at least, predominantly) in the mast-cell lineage. Such approaches may prove to be useful in attempts to analyze to what extent mast cells represent important sources of products (including those with potential effector and/or immunomodulatory functions) that can also be derived from other cell types. "Mast-cell cre" mice could also be mated to other transgenic mice in which important mast-cell survival factors are floxed in order to ablate mast cells selectively. This approach has the promise of permitting the generation of "improved" mast-cell-deficient mouse models that are independent of c-*Kit* mutations. However, time will tell whether various "mast-cell cre" mice achieve truly mast-cell-specific expression of Cre recombinase activity, or can be used to ablate all mast-cell populations without affecting other cell lineages.

## 4.4 Mouse Models of Anaphylaxis

Mouse models of passive anaphylaxis can be elicited locally or systemically by challenging the mice with anti-mouse IgE, or by antigen challenge in mice that have received injections of antigen-specific IgE or $IgG_1$ antibodies. Local or systemic *active* anaphylaxis can be induced by first sensitizing the mice with an antigen to elicit production of antigen-specific IgE and/or $IgG_1$ antibodies, and later challenging the mice with that specific antigen. Studies in mouse models of anaphylaxis have revealed at least two distinct mechanisms for the induction of active systemic anaphylaxis in the mouse [5]. The so-called "classic pathway" (Fig. 4.1) is mediated by cross-linking of IgE receptors (Fcε(epsilon)RI) by binding of allergen to Fcε(epsilon)RI-associated IgE on the mast-cell surface. In mice, current pharmacological evidence indicates that the mediators responsible for this anaphylaxis pathway are primarily histamine and, to a lesser extent, platelet-activating factor (PAF) [5, 7, 8]. It is widely thought that most if not all allergen-induced anaphylactic reactions in humans can be attributed to this classic, IgE-dependent pathway [9, 10]. In humans, IgE-dependent activation of basophils is also thought to contribute to the pathology of IgE-dependent anaphylaxis [3, 4, 9]. Mouse basophils also express Fcε(epsilon)RI [19, 63, 64], but the role of basophils in the "classic" IgE-dependent pathway of anaphylaxis in the mouse is not yet clear (vide infra) (Fig. 4.1).

An alternative pathway for eliciting systemic anaphylaxis in the mouse is thought to involve Fcγ(gamma)RIII, IgG, and PAF [5–7] (Fig. 4.1). Mast cells appear not to have a critical role in such models (although, as discussed below, mast cells may contribute to certain features of these responses) [5–8]. Instead, there is evidence that both macrophages [5, 7] and basophils [8] can contribute significantly to such models, with the relative importance of one or the other cell perhaps depending on the experimental model system analyzed [65]. The involvement of this alternative pathway in human anaphylaxis is less clear, although anaphylaxis has been described in some patients in the absence of evidence of mast-cell degranulation or detectable antigen-specific IgE antibodies [5]. Moreover, some clinical observations have suggested a possible role for IgG-mediated mechanisms in human anaphylaxis [66–69]. In mice, the alternative pathway is thought to require larger amounts of allergen and higher concentrations of IgG antibodies, whereas the classical pathway can be triggered by very small amounts of antigen and IgE [5, 7, 8]. For example, robust IgE/mast-cell-dependent anaphylactic reactions can even be elicited in mice in the absence of measureable serum IgE [70].

We think it is likely that the relative importance of the IgE- versus IgG-dependent pathways of anaphylaxis in mouse models of active systemic anaphylaxis, as well as the extent to which such models depend on mast cells, basophils, or macrophages (or other cell types), will depend on the characteristics of the anaphylactic models tested, including the amount and type of allergen, the protocols used to elicit the responses, and perhaps the strain background of the mice.

As described below, various mouse models of active or passive local or systemic anaphylaxis have been studied using genetically mast-cell-deficient mice (including WCB6F$_1$-*Kitl*$^{Sl/Sl-d}$, WBB6F$_1$-*Kit*$^{W/W-v}$, or C57BL/6-*Kit*$^{W-sh/W-sh}$ mice), the corresponding wild-type mice, and, in some cases, mast-cell knock-in mice. Such approaches have permitted investigators to analyze the role of mast cells in examples of $IgG_1$- or IgE-dependent local or systemic anaphylactic reactions in the mouse.

## 4.5 IgE-Dependent Passive Systemic Anaphylaxis

The central role of mast cells in the development of IgE-mediated systemic anaphylaxis was demonstrated in studies employing intravenous infusion or intraperitoneal injection of anti-mouse IgE [7, 71–73], or antigen challenge in mice that had previously received antigen-specific IgE

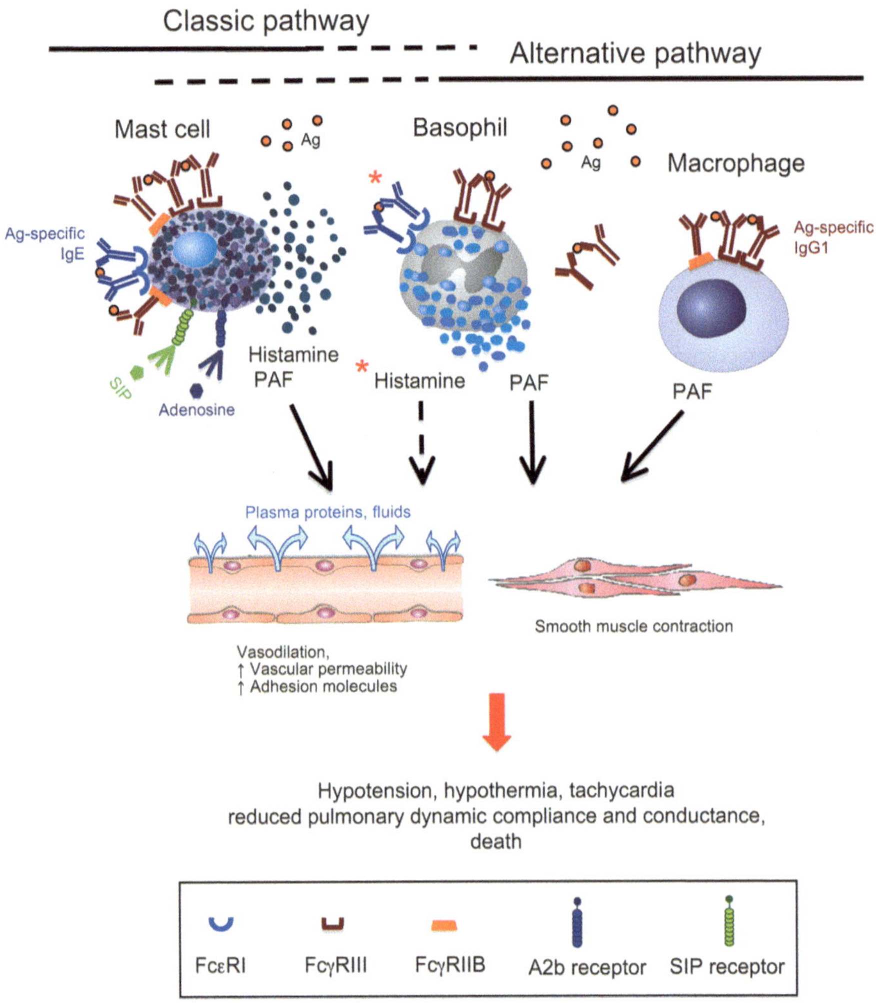


**Fig. 4.1** Effector mechanisms in mouse models of systemic anaphylaxis. Mouse models of systemic anaphylaxis can be elicited by antigen challenge in mice that have been sensitized with that specific antigen (active anaphylaxis) or with antigen-specific $IgG_1$ or IgE (passive anaphylaxis). Depending on the experimental models, these reactions are mediated by classic and/or alternative anaphylactic pathways. *Classic Pathway:* Mast cells are the primary effector cells involved in the classic anaphylactic pathway and induce pathophysiological changes by releasing histamine, PAF (in the mouse, it appears that mast-cell-derived histamine is more important than mast-cell-derived PAF in this setting), and other mediators upon aggregation of their high-affinity IgE receptors (Fcε(epsilon)RI) with antigen and antigen-specific IgE. IgE-dependent mast-cell degranulation can be enhanced by S1P, but inhibited by adenosine binding to A2b receptor (other factors also can enhance or suppress the mast cells' response). The IgE/Fcε(epsilon)RI/basophil pathway (marked * in the figure) reflects expression of the high-affinity IgE receptor mouse basophils, and increased levels of IgE can increase surface expression of Fcε(epsilon)RI in mouse and human basophils and enhance IgE-dependent function in (human) basophils, as well as in mouse or human mast cells. Histamine derived from basophils stimulated with IgE and antigen is thought to contribute to systemic anaphylaxis in humans, but the role of the IgE/Fcε(epsilon)RI/basophil/histamine (or PAF) axis in mouse models of systemic anaphylaxis is not yet clear. *Alternative Pathway:* The alternative pathway is induced by the release of PAF from macrophages and/or basophils activated by the binding of antigen-$IgG_1$ immune complexes to the low-affinity IgG receptor, Fcγ(gamma)RIII. In either pathway, potent chemical mediators produced by these effector cells stimulate endothelial cells and smooth muscle cells, resulting in reductions in blood pressure and body temperature, tachycardia, pulmonary dysfunction, and mortality. Although mast cells are not required in the Fcγ(gamma)RIII/$IgG_1$ pathway, there is evidence that they can amplify certain features of the responses. Both classic and alternative pathways can be modulated by the expression of inhibitory receptors, such as Fcγ(gamma)RIIB, which can diminish signaling via Fcε(epsilon)RI and Fcγ(gamma) RIII receptors. Either IgG (shown) or IgE (albeit at low affinity, see text) can mediate inhibition of mast-cell responses via Fcγ(gamma)RIIB in some model systems. This figure is modified after one from [5]

[6, 74–78]. In wild-type mice, such treatments induced extensive mast-cell degranulation [71, 72, 74], release of mast-cell-associated mediators [7, 77, 78] (MCPT-1, histamine, PAF), reductions in body temperature [7, 75], significant reductions in pulmonary dynamic compliance and conductance [71, 73, 74], and, in some protocols, significant mortality [7, 71–74]. By contrast, identically challenged mast-cell-deficient WBB6F$_1$-*Kit*$^{W/W-v}$ or WCB6F$_1$-*Kitl*$^{Sl/Sl-d}$ mice exhibited little or no alterations in body temperature [7], cardiopulmonary function, or mortality [6, 7, 71, 72, 74] (Table 4.1). Studies in WBB6F$_1$-*Kit*$^{W/W-v}$ mast-cell knock-in mice also showed that IgE-mediated activation of mast cells can enhance airway responsiveness to cholinergic stimulation [73]. Pretreatment with the H1 antihistamine triprolidine and, to a lesser extent, with the PAF antagonist CV 6209, significantly inhibited anti-IgE-induced hypothermia in wild-type mice, indicating the involvement of both histamine and PAF in this feature of the model [7]. Mouse basophils, like mouse mast cells, make histamine [79, 80], but the role of basophil-derived histamine in IgE-dependent models of anaphylaxis in mice is not clear.

Notably, even though mast cells are thought to be the most critical effector cells in IgE-dependent systemic anaphylaxis, mast-cell hyperplasia induced by the chronic treatment of wild-type mice with stem cell factor (SCF), the c-Kit ligand, and the major regulator of mast-cell survival and development [18, 19, 53] did not enhance the severity of IgE-induced systemic anaphylaxis [74]. This interesting result may have reflected the phenotypic and functional changes that were induced in mast cells by such SCF treatment. Whatever the explanation for the findings in that study, they illustrate that the intensity of IgE- and mast-cell-dependent biological responses does not necessarily correlate solely with the numbers of mast cells in the affected tissues.

In contrast to the results in mice, which develop marked increases in mast cell populations in response to treatment with SCF, human subjects with mastocytosis are susceptible to the development of very severe anaphylaxis, whether in response to allergens such as insect venoms [81–83] or based on as yet unknown "idiopathic" mechanisms [81, 84]. In some of these patients, gain-of-function

**Table 4.1** Evidence for roles of mast cells in mouse models of passive systemic anaphylaxis derived from studies using genetically mast-cell-deficient mice

| Model | Findings in genetically mast-cell-deficient mice versus the corresponding wild-type (+/+) mice |
|---|---|
| IgE-mediated passive anaphylaxis (elicited by anti-IgE or antigen-specific-IgE + antigen) | Significant mast-cell degranulation, elevation of heart rate, reductions in pulmonary dynamic compliance ($C_{dyn}$) and conductance ($G_L$), a drop in body temperature, and some mortality were observed in +/+ mice, but not in mast-cell-deficient WBB6F$_1$-*Kit*$^{W/W-v}$ [6, 7, 71, 72, 75] or WCB6F$_1$-*Kitl*$^{Sl/Sl-d}$ mice [71, 74]. |
| IgG$_1$-mediated passive anaphylaxis (elicited by antigen-specific IgG$_1$+ antigen) | Compared to +/+ mice, mast-cell-deficient WBB6F$_1$-*Kit*$^{W/W-v}$ mice developed tachycardia more slowly, exhibited smaller declines in pulmonary dynamic compliance ($C_{dyn}$) and conductance ($G_L$), and had reduced mortality [6], but WBB6F$_1$-*Kit*$^{W/W-v}$ and +/+ mice developed similar levels of hypothermia [75] elicited by antigen and DNP-specific IgG$_1$. C57BL/6-*Kit*$^{W-sh/W-sh}$ developed reduced hypothermia compared to +/+ mice in a model of passive anaphylaxis elicited by penicillin V-specific IgG$_1$ [8]. |
| Fcγ(gamma)RIII-mediated anaphylaxis (elicited by anti-Fcγ(gamma)RII/RIII [2.4G2] antibody) | Naïve WBB6F$_1$-*Kit*$^{W/W-v}$ mice developed less hypothermia than +/+ mice after IV administration of 2.4G2 (100 μg/mouse) [75]. By contrast, mast-cell-deficient WBB6F$_1$-*Kit*$^{W/W-v}$ mice that had been primed with goat anti-mouse IgD exhibited an enhanced drop in body temperature compared to +/+ mice following IV administration of 2.4G2 (100 μg/mouse) [7]. |

mutations of c-*Kit* may render the mast cells more susceptible to SCF and/or other stimuli which can trigger the release of mast-cell mediators [15, 83, 85] (see Chap. 16).

In addition to the effects of such c-Kit-related or other intrinsic differences in the susceptibility of mast cells to stimuli of activation, or in the nature of their responses to such stimuli, it appears that the activation of mast cells in IgE-dependent systemic reactions can be substantially modulated by inflammatory mediators produced by mast cells or other cell types. Sphingosine-1-phosphate (S1P), a plasma-membrane sphingolipid-derived mediator involved in immune-cell trafficking which can be produced by mast cells and other cell types [86, 87], is an example of such a mediator. A strong correlation has been identified between serum S1P and plasma histamine concentrations in a mouse model of IgE-mediated passive systemic anaphylaxis, suggesting a role for SIP in regulating mast-cell degranulation in this setting in vivo [77]. Although mast-cell responsiveness to Fcε(epsilon)RI aggregation can be enhanced by SIP from intracellular and extracellular sources, studies using sphingosine kinase-1 (Sphk1)-, Sphk2-, or Sphk1,2-deficient mice showed that SIP derived from cells other than mast cells probably represents the main source of SIP in this model of anaphylaxis, and that SphK2 was required for mouse mast-cell S1P production and Fcε(epsilon) RI-dependent degranulation [77]. Evidence has been reported from work with in vitro-derived human mast cells indicating that, in contrast to mouse mast cells, S1P can potently induce degranulation of human mast cells [88]. Moreover, based on using siRNA to downregulate the products, SphK1, rather than SphK2, markedly enhanced IgE- and antigen-induced human mast-cell degranulation and migration in vitro, but that both SphK1 and SphK2 contributed to human mast-cell cytokine secretion [88]. Thus, while there is strong evidence that S1P represents a potentially important enhancer of mast-cell activation in response to IgE and specific antigen in both mice and humans, there may be important differences between these species in the details of how S1P is produced by mast cells, as well as in the effects of S1P on mast-cell function.

The importance of Fcε(epsilon)RI in mediating the "classic" IgE- and mast-cell-dependent anaphylaxis pathway has been shown using mice deficient in the expression of Fcε(epsilon)RI α(alpha) chain, the IgE-binding component of the IgE receptor complex [6, 7, 75]. Miyajima et al. [6] showed that Fcε(epsilon)RI α(alpha) chain −/− mice did not develop significant mast-cell degranulation or cardiopulmonary changes, nor did these mice exhibit significant mortality, during attempts to elicit IgE-dependent passive systemic anaphylaxis. Nevertheless, in vivo studies conducted in mice deficient in expression of Fcγ(gamma)RIIB or Fcγ(gamma)RIII receptors suggest that the intensity of IgE-dependent passive systemic anaphylaxis can be modulated by the expression of Fc receptors for IgG. Fcγ(gamma)RIIB$^{-/-}$ and Fcγ(gamma)RIII$^{-/-}$ mice can exhibit augmented and attenuated IgE-dependent systemic anaphylaxis responses, respectively, which is thought to reflect the consequences of low affinity binding of IgE or IgE immune complexes to Fcγ(gamma)RIIB or Fcγ(gamma)RIII [89, 90]. These findings indicate that at least some IgE-mediated responses in mice reflect effects attributable to low-affinity interactions of IgE with Fcγ(gamma)RIII and Fcγ(gamma) RII receptors (which can be expressed on mast cells and other cell types), as well as the more widely recognized effects of the high-affinity binding of IgE to Fcε(epsilon)RI.

Recently, basophils were shown to play a pivotal role in $IgG_1$-mediated anaphylaxis in mice that had been passively sensitized with penicillin V-specific $IgG_1$ monoclonal antibody, and then challenged with an intravenous infusion of PenV-conjugated bovine-serum albumin [8]. In this mouse model of "penicillin shock," antibody-dependent depletion of basophils substantially suppressed the $IgG_1$-, but not IgE-, mediated anaphylactic reactions. By contrast, mast-cell-deficient C57BL/6-$Kit^{W-sh/W-sh}$ mice developed significant reductions in body temperature in response to PenV-$IgG_1$/PenV-BSA treatment, albeit slightly less severe than that in the wild-type mice [8]. This observation is in accord with the results of previous reports in which treatment with anti-DNP-$IgG_1$ followed by challenge with DNP-HSA-induced passive systemic anaphylaxis in genetically mast-cell-deficient $Kit^{W/W-v}$ mice [6, 75].

## 4.6 IgE- or $IgG_1$-Dependent Passive Local Anaphylaxis

Other studies using "mast-cell knock-in mice" have revealed the essential roles of mast cells in several acute and late phase features of the IgE-dependent responses that were elicited locally after the passive transfer of the antibody into the skin [91–93] or gastrointestinal tract [94, 95]. These mast-cell-dependent changes included acute swelling of the skin [91, 92], local extravasation of fibrinogen, and deposition of cross-linked fibrin in the dermis [91], the recruitment of leukocytes during the "late phase" of the response in the skin or stomach wall [92, 94], the enhancement of levels of type 1 collagen mRNA in fibroblasts at the site of the skin reaction [93], and the promotion of histamine-dependent migration of Langerhans cells to lymph nodes draining the skin [96]. Some of these studies also provided evidence that the recruitment of circulating inflammatory cells, including neutrophils and monocytes, to sites of acute IgE- and mast-cell-dependent responses in the skin or stomach is promoted by TNF [92, 95].

Although passive cutaneous anaphylaxis (PCA) is most often elicited using IgE, it can also be induced in mice injected with a subset of $IgG_1$ antibodies called "anaphylactic $IgG_1$" antibodies [97]. Mouse mast cells express the low-affinity receptor (Fcγ(gamma)RIII) for $IgG_1$ and can be activated by antigen/$IgG_1$ complexes [98]. Unlike $IgG_1$-dependent systemic anaphylaxis, which can be elicited in mice which lack mast cells [6, 8, 75], $IgG_1$-mediated PCA reactions appear to require the presence of dermal mast cells [99], as well as the expression of Fcγ(gamma)RIII [97, 100]. It is interesting that mast cells are critical for the expression of $IgG_1$-dependent PCA reactions but not for $IgG_1$-dependent passive systemic anaphylaxis. At least in part, this may reflect the more ready accessibility of $IgG_1$-antigen immune complex to target mast cells in the skin during PCA protocols, as well as the relative paucity of alternative potential effector cells (e.g., basophils and various monocyte/macrophage populations) at that site as opposed to when sensitization and challenge occurs via the systemic route.

Although the presence of dermal mast cells is required for the expression of IgE- or $IgG_1$-dependent PCA responses, the features of such responses may be influenced by products of mast cells that have autocrine or paracrine effects on mast cells, thus "tuning" the features of the mast cells' response. For example, osteopontin (a mediator implicated in bone remodeling and immune responses) can be produced by mouse mast cells as well as other cell types and can enhance IgE-dependent mast-cell degranulation in vitro, and mice which genetically lack osteopontin exhibit IgE- and mast-cell-dependent PCA reactions which are significantly reduced compared to those in the corresponding wild-type mice [101]. Mast-cell- and IgE-mediated cutaneous anaphylaxis reactions also can be critically regulated by intracellular proteins that regulate calcium influx upon Fcε(epsilon)RI aggregation in mast cells (TRPM4, STIM1, CRACM1 [also known as Orai1], etc.) (see Chapter 7), as well as by the expression of activating or inhibitory receptors on the cell surface. For example, Fcε(epsilon)RI α(alpha) chain-deficient mice are resistant to IgE-dependent PCA [102], but deletion of the ITIM-containing LILRB4 (formerly designated gp49B1) receptors [103] in mice results in increased tissue swelling and mast-cell degranulation at sites of IgE-mediated PCA reactions [104]. The mast-cell-expressed chemerin-binding mCCRL2 receptor also appears to enhance the tissue swelling and leukocyte infiltrates associated with IgE-dependent PCA reactions in mice [105]. CysLT(1)R, a receptor for cysteinyl leukotrienes (cysLTs), also can enhance IgE-dependent PCA reactions, as shown by reduced plasma protein extravasation at sites of such reactions in CysLT(1)R-deficient mice [106]. By contrast, the expression of A2b adenosine receptors on mast cells can limit the magnitude of IgE-mediated passive systemic anaphylaxis, as well as local cutaneous anaphylaxis responses [76].

## 4.7 Active Systemic or Local Anaphylaxis

Active anaphylaxis can be induced locally or systemically by the administration of certain protein antigens or haptens to mice that have been previously sensitized with the same or closely related agents. The adaptive immune responses elicited by active antigen sensitization are usually associated with production of antigen-specific IgE, as well as $IgG_1$ [6, 7, 72, 75]. While mice lacking the FcRγ(gamma) chain common to Fcε(epsilon)RI and Fcγ(gamma)RI/III cannot express active anaphylaxis induced by ovalbumin [6] or DNP-KLH administration [75], active anaphylaxis can be readily elicited in Fcε(epsilon)RI α(alpha) chain –/– mice [7, 75] or in genetically mast-cell-deficient mice [6, 7, 72, 107–110].

Such work shows that mast cells are not essential for the development of hypotension, hypothermia, death, or some of the cardiopulmonary changes associated with certain models of active anaphylaxis [6, 7, 72, 75, 110] (Table 4.2). However, in some models, individual features of the responses can differ significantly from those of the corresponding reactions which are elicited in mice in which the IgE/Fcε(epsilon)RI/mast-cell pathway is intact. For example, studies using $WBB6F_1$-$Kit^{W/W-v}$ mice that had been repaired of their mast-cell deficiency (nonselectively) by bone marrow transplantation have suggested that mast cells (or perhaps other bone marrow-derived cells that differ between $Kit^{W/W-v}$ mice and wild-type mice) can contribute to tachycardia in one model of fatal active anaphylaxis [110]. Moreover, although $IgG_1$-dependent systemic anaphylaxis can be elicited in the absence of mast cells, mast-cell-deficient $WBB6F_1$-$Kit^{W/W-v}$ mice developed delayed and less-striking increases in heart rate, much smaller reductions in airway function, and lower mortality (1 death/6 $Kit^{W/W-v}$ mice versus 5 deaths/6 +/+ mice, $p=0.08$) than did the corresponding wild-type mice [6]. However, the extent to which these differences reflected the mast-cell deficiency of the $WBB6F_1$-$Kit^{W/W-v}$ mice, as opposed to other consequences of their mutations, has not yet been established.

In a model of ovalbumin-induced active anaphylaxis using a protocol in which both IgE and $IgG_1$ antibodies are elicited, Fcε(epsilon)RI α(alpha) chain –/– mice and the corresponding wild-type mice exhibited similar levels of extensive degranulation of peribronchial and dermal mast cells, and similarly high mortality rates [6]. However, the Fcε(epsilon)RI α(alpha) chain –/– mice, in

**Table 4.2** Evidence for roles of mast cells in mouse models of active systemic anaphylaxis derived from studies using genetically mast-cell-deficient mice

| Feature(s) of the response | Findings in genetically mast-cell-deficient mice versus the corresponding wild-type (+/+) mice |
|---|---|
| Death | Mast-cell-deficient $WBB6F_1$-$Kit^{W/W-v}$ [7, 72, 107–110] or $WCB6F_1$-$Kitl^{Sl/Sl-d}$ mice [109, 110] mice exhibited similar mortality rates associated with systemic anaphylaxis to OVA [6, 108, 109], BSA [107], bovine γ(gamma)-globulin [110], or goat anti-mouse IgD [7, 72]. |
| Body temperature | Mast-cell-deficient WBB6F1-$Kit^{W/W-v}$ and +/+ mice exhibited similar drops in body temperature associated with systemic anaphylaxis to goat anti-mouse IgD [7]. |
| Pulmonary function | $WBB6F_1$-$Kit^{W/W-v}$ mice exhibited reductions in pulmonary dynamic compliance ($C_{dyn}$) and conductance ($G_L$), which were similar to those observed in +/+ mice [72, 110]. In a model of active anaphylaxis to OVA [6], $WBB6F_1$-$Kit^{W/W-v}$ mice developed declines in $G_L$ and $C_{dyn}$, which were slower and more modest than those in the +/+ mice. |
| Heart rate and blood pressure | Mast-cell-deficient $WBB6F_1$-$Kit^{W/W-v}$ mice exhibited a much smaller increase in heart rate (HR) [6, 110], or no significant increase in HR [110], during systemic anaphylaxis to OVA [6] or bovine γ(gamma)-globulin [110]. However, in bovine γ(gamma)-globulin-induced systemic anaphylaxis, $WBB6F_1$-$Kit^{W/W-v}$ mice exhibited a more rapid and profound drop in blood pressure, than did +/+ mice [110]. |

comparison to the corresponding wild-type mice, exhibited slightly more prolonged tachycardia and more prolonged or substantial reductions in lung conductance and dynamic compliance, respectively, in this model of active anaphylaxis [6]. Similarly, in a model of $IgG_1$-dependent passive systemic anaphylaxis, which was associated with little or no morphological evidence of mast-cell degranulation, the responses in Fcε(epsilon)RI α(alpha) chain –/– mice were associated with levels of tachycardia and early reductions in lung conductance, which were significantly greater than those in wild-type mice [6]. These findings may have reflected increased signaling via Fcγ(gamma)RIII in Fcε(epsilon)RI α(alpha) chain –/– mice, due to increased availability of the FcRγ(gamma) chain for incorporation into Fcγ(gamma)RIII since, in the absence of the Fcε(epsilon)RI α(alpha)chain, none of the FcRγ(gamma) chain is used for assembly of the Fcε(epsilon)RI [75]. Alternatively, it is possible that mast-cell activation via Fcε(epsilon)RI can actually serve to limit the intensity of some of the features of active anaphylaxis in which the $IgG_1$/Fcγ(gamma)RIII pathway has an important role.

The $IgG_1$-dependent components of systemic anaphylactic reactions in actively immunized mice probably involve the participation of many cell types, including macrophages [7], basophils [52] and other granulocytes [8, 111], and platelets [112], as well as mast cells [6, 98]. For example, in an active model of systemic anaphylaxis induced by goat anti-mouse IgD antibody (goat IgG), it has been reported that macrophages, rather than mast cells, contribute importantly to the expression of $IgG_1$-dependent responses [7]. Platelet-activating factor (PAF) appears to be an important mediator for this mast-cell-independent anaphylaxis pathway. In other models of $IgG_1$-dependent passive anaphylaxis, basophils appear to be more important than macrophages as a source of PAF [8].

Two groups have challenged $WBB6F_1$-$Kit^{W/W-v}$ mice and the corresponding +/+ wild-type mice with the anti-Fcγ(gamma)RII/III antibody, 2.4G2 (100 μg/mouse), to elicit Fcγ(gamma)RIII-dependent responses (Table 4.1). Naïve $WBB6F_1$-$Kit^{W/W-v}$ mice developed significantly *less* hypothermia than +/+ mice after IV administration of 2.4G2 [75]. By contrast, mast-cell-deficient $WBB6F_1$-$Kit^{W/W-v}$ mice that had been primed with goat anti-mouse IgD exhibited an *enhanced* drop in body temperature compared to +/+ mice following IV administration of 2.4G2 [7]. While the reason for the difference in the results obtained in the two models tested has not yet been identified, it is possible that the contribution of mast cells to this response may depend on factors which alter either the levels of FcRγ(gamma)III on the mast-cell surface and/or the cells' functional response to activation via that receptor. Alternatively, naïve versus goat anti-mouse IgD-primed $WBB6F_1$-$Kit^{W/W-v}$ mice may differ from the corresponding +/+ mice in the contribution of other cell types which are affected by the $Kit^{W/W-v}$ mutations.

In summary, studies in wild-type mice, mast-cell-deficient mice, and mice deficient in either the α(alpha) chain of the Fcε(epsilon)RI or the γ(gamma) chain common to Fcε(epsilon)RI and Fcγ(gamma)RIII indicate that both IgE and $IgG_1$ antibodies can contribute to active systemic anaphylaxis in the mouse. The IgE-dependent component of such responses appears to be largely mast-cell-dependent. By contrast, studies in mast-cell-deficient mice and other lines of evidence suggest that mast cells can contribute to the intensity or kinetics of some of the features of $IgG_1$-dependent systemic anaphylaxis, but their role in the $IgG_1$-depedent components of active anaphylaxis is less important than their contributions to the IgE-dependent components of the response.

Another mouse model of active anaphylaxis has been reported to involve IgE but not mast cells [113]. In this model of active fatal anaphylaxis induced by penicillin V (Pen V), Pen V challenge elicited a biphasic response that was correlated with early and late phase production of PAF [114]. Studies in $Kit^{W/W-v}$ mice indicated that mast cells were not required for the expression of either the immediate or late phase responses induced by Pen V in this model [114]. While evidence was presented to indicate that the response to Pen V was dependent on IgE rather than $IgG_1$ antibodies [115], it would be of interest to attempt to elicit such Pen V-induced active anaphylaxis in IgE- deficient mice, as this might provide additional evidence that this is an entirely IgE-dependent model system. Although the cells responsible for this model of Pen V-induced active anaphylaxis have not been identified, the work of Hajime Karasuyama et al. on another model of PenV-induced anaphylaxis

[8] indicates that basophils represent one candidate. The finding that NK cells can be activated by antigen and IgE, via the binding of IgE to Fcγ(gamma)RIII receptors [116], raises the possibility that NK cells, in addition to mast cells and basophils, might contribute to some IgE-dependent immune responses.

## 4.8 Mast Cells in Peanut Allergy

Peanut allergy is the most common cause of food-induced fatal anaphylaxis [117, 118] (see Chap. 21). In humans with severe peanut allergy, subcutaneous injections of the anti-IgE antibody TNX-901 permits the subjects to tolerate significantly higher amounts of orally administered peanut protein before experiencing an allergic response [119]. These data are consistent with a role for IgE-induced activation of mast cells, basophils, and possibly other cell types which can interact with IgE, in this setting. However, in many cases of peanut-induced anaphylaxis in humans, analyses of blood specimens have not demonstrated elevated levels of tryptase [120]. Whether these findings reflect a lack of an important role for mast cells in the pathology in such patients is not yet clear. For example, the data are also compatible with the interpretation that mast cells contribute to anaphylaxis in this setting, but do so in a way that results in little or no, and/or a delayed, release of tryptase into the circulation.

A few studies have used mouse models in an attempt to evaluate the contribution of mast cells to peanut allergy. In one model, systemic anaphylactic responses were elicited by intraperitoneal injection of crude peanut extract given 2 weeks after 4 weekly oral administrations of peanut proteins in the presence of cholera toxin. Peanut hypersensitivity was induced in wild-type mice, which exhibited elevated levels of plasma histamine and leukotrienes, as well as a reduction in body temperature. By contrast, mast-cell-deficient $Kit^{W/W-v}$ mice were resistant to peanut-induced systemic anaphylaxis. Fcε(epsilon)RI α(alpha) chain –/– mice exhibited anaphylactic responses with reduced severity in this mouse model of peanut allergy, implicating IgE in the response [121]. While these findings suggest an important contribution of mast cells, as well as IgE and Fcε(epsilon) RI, in the effector mechanism in peanut allergy in this model, the extent of the contribution of mast cells has not yet been confirmed by analyzing mast-cell-engrafted $Kit^{W/W-v}$ mice [121].

In another study, injection of BALB/c and C57BL/6 mice with peanut or tree nut extracts, in conjunction with a β(beta)-adrenergic receptor antagonist and long-acting IL-4, induced complement activation and an antibody-independent, innate immune response-dependent anaphylactoid reaction that, based on pharmacological evidence, involved PAF and histamine [122]. Studies in mice injected with an anti-c-Kit antibody to deplete mast cells, or in mice treated with cromolyn to interfere with mast-cell degranulation, indicated that mast cells were not essential for the occurrence of these peanut/tree nut-induced anaphylactoid reactions. It is not clear whether antibody-independent complement activation occurs during or, if so, represents an important feature of, anaphylactic reactions to peanuts in humans. However, complement activation has been reported during severe cases of allergen-induced anaphylaxis in humans [123, 124], and it is possible that both IgE and specific antigen and complement-derived anaphylatoxins can contribute to high levels of mast-cell activation and mediator release during some cases of anaphylaxis.

## 4.9 Mast Cells in Intestinal Anaphylaxis

The role of mast cells in the expression of intestinal anaphylaxis has been investigated using mast-cell-deficient mice, in wild-type mice treated with anti-c-Kit antibody (ACK2) to deplete mast cells, and in wild-type mice treated with cromolyn sodium to "stabilize" mast cells. Studies in mast-cell-deficient mice that had been repaired of their mast-cell deficiency nonselectively by the transfer of wild-type bone marrow cells provided evidence that mast cells can promote the enhanced secretion of ions (primarily $Cl^-$) by the small intestine during active intestinal hypersensitivity [108]. This work suggested that mast cells contribute significantly to this response in part by influencing the function of intestinal nerves [125]. In another study, exposure of OVA/alum-sensitized wild-type mice to repeated administrations of intragastric OVA induced a dose-dependent acute diarrhea associated with increased intestinal permeability, eosinophilia, increased numbers of gut mast cells, and marked degranulation of intestinal mucosal mast cells. This model of intestinal anaphylaxis appears to be mediated via the mast-cell/Fcε(epsilon)RI/IgE-dependent pathway, since such allergic diarrhea could not be elicited or was markedly attenuated in wild-type mice treated with anti-c-Kit antibody (ACK2) or anti-IgE antibody (EM-95), or in Fcε(epsilon)RI α(alpha) chain-deficient mice [126]. Based on pharmacological evidence, it appears that the important mediators in this model of allergic diarrhea are serotonin, platelet-activating factor (PAF) [126] and IL-9 [127], a cytokine which can enhance the growth, recruitment, and effector function of mast cells [128].

## 4.10 Roles of Mast Cells in Other Immune or Nonimmune Mechanisms of Anaphylaxis

An immunologically specific pathway that can produce a mast-cell-dependent immediate hypersensitivity-like reaction independently of IgE or $IgG_1$ antibodies has been reported by Redegeld et al., who have provided evidence that transfer of Ig light chains, which are free of intact immunoglobulins, can transfer antigen-specific reactivity into naïve mice [129, 130]. Local challenge of the sensitized mice with the specific antigen can induce mast-cell degranulation, vascular leakage, and edema in the skin, as well as acute bronchoconstriction, in wild-type mice but not in mast-cell-deficient mice [129, 130]. Intriguingly, the mechanism(s) by which light chains can have these effects on mast cells, and, specifically, the receptor(s) through which such Ig light chains can signal mast cells and perhaps other effector cells to exhibit cellular functions, have not yet been defined. Nevertheless, these studies point to yet another mast-cell-dependent pathway with the potential to contribute to immediate hypersensitivity responses. The extent to which such a mechanism might contribute to antigen-specific immune responses in humans remains to be determined.

In humans, signs and symptoms of anaphylaxis that are similar to those elicited by IgE and allergens can also develop by other immunological or non-immunological mechanisms. Such IgE-independent immunological mechanisms include those elicited by immune complexes, activation of the complement or coagulation systems, or activation of T cells or platelets [10]. Non-immunologic mechanisms include those initiated by exercise, by exposure to cold air or water, X-ray materials, or certain medications, or by "idiopathic" mechanisms, which remain to be elucidated. In some individuals, anaphylactic reactions can be induced upon initial exposure to agents (such as drugs, antigens, or radiocontrast materials) without prior sensitization [3, 9, 10]. The involvement of mast cells in such IgE-independent anaphylactic reactions (which used to be called "anaphylactoid" reactions [131]) is less understood than is the role of mast cells in IgE-dependent anaphylaxis. Given the functional versatility and the wide spectrum of stimuli that can activate mast cells, it is possible that these reactions can be aggravated by the direct release of mediators from mast cells. For example, complement activation and generation of anaphylatoxins (C3a and C5a) can occur during immune complex- and complement-mediated activation of anaphylaxis in humans (which can occur, e.g., following the administration of blood components), or can occur during cases of presumably IgE-dependent severe anaphylaxis induced by agents such as hymenoptera venom [123, 124, 132], penicillin derivatives [133], or peanut extracts [122]. Anaphylatoxins have potent activities in stimulating vascular permeability and smooth muscle contraction and can directly induce mast cells to release potent anaphylactic mediators [134], resulting in hypotension, respiratory distress, and other signs and symptoms in anaphylaxis.

Although the clinical diagnosis and current approaches for the acute treatment of anaphylaxis do not depend on which of the many different potential effector mechanisms initially triggered the disorder, a better understanding of the effector mechanisms leading to mast-cell activation in anaphylaxis may offer novel targets for therapeutic intervention and may also provide valuable information for long-term risk reduction [3, 9, 10].

## 4.11 Manipulation of Mast-Cell Effector Function

The treatment of anaphylaxis includes systemic administration of epinephrine (which counteracts the effects of mast-cell-derived and other mediators on critical end organs) and antihistamines (which block actions of histamine derived from mast cells, basophils, and perhaps, to a lesser extent, other sources) [3, 9, 10]. However, additional approaches, such as those targeting the IgE-dependent activation of mast cells, are under investigation. As noted above, treatment with the anti-IgE antibody TNX-901 increased the tolerance of peanut allergic patients to peanut antigen [119]. The anti-IgE antibody omalizumab also has been used successfully for the treatment of one patient with a severe case of apparently "idiopathic" cold-induced urticaria, strongly suggesting some role for IgE in that patient's disorder [135].

Administration of anti-IgE reduces free IgE in the serum and tissues, results in reduction in the numbers of IgE receptors on mast cells and basophils, and may have other beneficial effects as well. The reduction in numbers of Fcε(epsilon)RI expressed by mast cells following anti-IgE therapy (as assessed by immunohistochemistry) is associated with a substantially reduced acute wheal response, as well as, in two-thirds of the subjects, a reduction in the size of the subsequent late phase reaction upon intradermal challenge with antigen, presumably reflecting reduced IgE-dependent activation of dermal mast cells [136, 137]. In addition to stabilizing expression of Fcε(epsilon)RI on the mast-cell surface, the binding of certain preparations of monomeric IgE can also promote the survival of human [138] and mouse [139–142] mast cells. However, we are not aware of reports documenting any changes in levels of tissue mast cells in human subject treated with anti-IgE antibodies [137].

Another approach for inhibiting mast-cell degranulation/activation is to use IgE Fc–IgG Fc fusion proteins to co-engage mast-cell Fcε(epsilon)RI with the inhibitory receptor, Fcγ(gamma) RIIB [143–145]. Similarly, bifunctional antibodies that cross-link Fcε(epsilon)RI and other ITIM containing molecules (e.g., CD300a) [146], or agonists which directly target intracellular tyrosine phosphatases [147], can also reduce mast-cell activation. While the potential utility of these approaches is supported based on in vitro studies [143, 145, 148] or tests in experimental animals [143, 145, 148], they so far have not been tested in clinical trials.

In mice, mast-cell IgE-dependent effector function can also be modulated by regulatory T cells (Treg). In a mouse model of IgE-mediated passive systemic anaphylaxis, assessment of histamine levels in the serum showed that mast-cell activation in response to challenge with IgE and specific antigen was significantly increased, relative to values in wild-type mice, either in wild-type mice that had been depleted of Treg in vivo or in OX40-deficient mice [78]. In vitro studies showed that Treg can directly inhibit Fcε(epsilon)RI-dependent mast-cell degranulation (but not mast-cell production of IL-6 or TNF) through cell–cell contact involving interactions between OX40 expressed on Treg and OX40 ligand expressed by mast cells [78]. This study defined a novel, Treg-dependent mechanism which can suppress mast-cell degranulation and which could serve to limit anaphylaxis and perhaps other IgE-dependent responses. However, this elegant and interesting work has been conducted entirely in mice, and its relevance to human anaphylaxis is not yet clear.

Moreover, while mast cell–T cell interactions represent a complex area of study that is beyond the scope of this chapter, in vitro data support the conclusion that both human [149] and mouse [150] mast cells can promote T cell proliferation [149, 150] and cytokine release [150], at least in part in an OX40–OX40L-dependent manner. Taken together with the work of Gri et al. [78], these findings indicate that OX40–OX40L interactions between mast cells and T cells can significantly influence the function of each of the participating cell types.

Rapid desensitization can provide temporary protection from IgE-associated anaphylaxis or from anaphylactic reactions induced independently of IgE by aspirin or nonsteroidal anti-inflammatory drugs [151]. Rapid desensitization is achieved by administrating small doses of the offending agent over a short period of time, in a setting in which appropriate resuscitation can be performed should the anaphylactic reaction occur [151].

This approach can be used successfully in patients who are highly allergic to drugs, humanized monoclonal antibodies, or other proteins (e.g., insulin) [151]. While there are many studies focused on the effects of desensitization and other immunotherapy protocols on basophils [152–157], some in vitro studies have suggested that mast cells [151, 154–161] also represent potentially important cellular targets of such desensitization protocols [151]. For example, purified human skin mast cells [154, 260], rat peritoneal mast cells [159], and mouse bone marrow derived cultured mast cells [158, 161] can be "desensitized" by repeated exposure to gradually increasing amounts of anti-IgE or suboptimal doses of antigens, an in vitro protocol which mimics protocols of rapid desensitization in vivo. While the mechanisms that account for the unresponsiveness exhibited by such mast cells remain to be fully defined, some intracellular signaling molecules and transcription factors already have been implicated. Incubation with low concentrations of antigens leads to a reduction in Syk protein expression in human skin mast cells and peripheral blood basophils [154]. Furthermore, bone marrow-derived cultured mast cells from wild-type mice but not STAT6-deficient mice could be rendered unresponsive to IgE- and antigen-dependent activation by incubation with suboptimal doses of antigen in the presence of calcium [161].

## 4.12 Conclusions

Experiments employing mutant mice that lack mast cells or other critical signaling components in IgE and/or $IgG_1$ antibody-dependent pathways have been useful in defining the importance of mast cells, and various mast-cell activation mechanisms, in local or systemic models of active or passive anaphylaxis in mice. Such studies show that mast cells have a critically important role in anaphylactic reactions that involve IgE. Indeed, in most of the models of passive local or systemic anaphylaxis tested, little or no responsiveness to challenge with IgE and specific antigen can be detected in the absence of mast cells by any of the forms of assessment utilized to date. While evidence has been reported that some IgE-dependent systemic responses to certain penicillin-related antigens may be elicited in mice which lack mast cells [113, 114], this conclusion has been questioned by others [5, 8] and the IgE dependence of this model of anaphylaxis needs additional study.

In contrast to the critical role of mast cells in IgE-dependent responses, work conducted in mast-cell-deficient mice clearly indicates that mast cells are not required for the development of various models of active or $IgG_1$-mediated passive systemic anaphylaxis. However, evidence derived from comparisons of such responses in mast cell-deficient WB$B6F_1$-$Kit^{W/W-v}$ mice versus the corresponding wild-type mice suggests that mast cells can amplify the rate of development or magnitude of some features of these reactions, including (in the case of $IgG_1$-dependent passive systemic anaphylaxis) the associated mortality [6]. Moreover, in contrast to $IgG_1$-dependent passive systemic anaphylactic responses, which clearly can occur in the absence of mast cells, dermal mast cells appear to be required for expression of $IgG_1$-dependent passive cutaneous anaphylaxis reactions.

While the importance of mast cells in anaphylaxis (especially IgE-dependent anaphylaxis) is clear, we are just beginning to understand how the roles of mast cells in IgE-dependent and other models of anaphylaxis can be influenced by factors that can modulate mast-cell function in these settings. Such factors include ligands of receptors that are expressed by mast cells and that can enhance or suppress mast-cell activation or mediator release, products of mast cells or other cell types that can promote or inhibit mast-cell function, direct interactions between mast cells and other cells with immunoregulatory function, and the effects of "desensitization" protocols, which render mast cells less responsive to the offending allergen. These are important areas of current research, and ones which, with luck, may reveal additional options for the management, diagnosis, and treatment of these devastating disorders.

## References

1. Bochner BS, Lichtenstein LM. Anaphylaxis. *N Engl J Med.* 1991;324:1785–1790.
2. Galli SJ. Pathogenesis and management of anaphylaxis: current status and future challenges. *J Allergy Clin Immunol.* 2005;115:571–574.
3. Sampson HA, Munoz-Furlong A, Bock SA, et al. Symposium on the definition and management of anaphylaxis: summary report. *J Allergy Clin Immunol.* 2005;115:584–591.
4. Simons FE. 9. Anaphylaxis. *J Allergy Clin Immunol.* 2008;121:S402–407; quiz S420.
5. Finkelman FD. Anaphylaxis: lessons from mouse models. *J Allergy Clin Immunol.* 2007;120:506–515; quiz 516–507.
6. Miyajima I, Dombrowicz D, Martin TR, Ravetch JV, Kinet JP, Galli SJ. Systemic anaphylaxis in the mouse can be mediated largely through IgG1 and Fc gammaRIII. Assessment of the cardiopulmonary changes, mast cell degranulation, and death associated with active or IgE- or $IgG_1$-dependent passive anaphylaxis. *J Clin Invest.* 1997;99:901–914.
7. Strait RT, Morris SC, Yang M, Qu XW, Finkelman FD. Pathways of anaphylaxis in the mouse. *J Allergy Clin Immunol.* 2002;109:658–668.
8. Tsujimura Y, Obata K, Mukai K, et al. Basophils play a pivotal role in immunoglobulin-G-mediated but not immunoglobulin-E-mediated systemic anaphylaxis. *Immunity.* 2008;28:581–589.
9. Sampson HA, Munoz-Furlong A, Campbell RL, et al. Second symposium on the definition and management of anaphylaxis: summary report – Second National Institute of Allergy and Infectious Disease/Food Allergy and Anaphylaxis Network symposium. *J Allergy Clin Immunol.* 2006;117:391–397.
10. Simons FE, Frew AJ, Ansotegui IJ, et al. Risk assessment in anaphylaxis: current and future approaches. *J Allergy Clin Immunol.* 2007;120:S2–24.
11. Galli SJ, Kalesnikoff J, Grimbaldeston MA, Piliponsky AM, Williams CM, Tsai M. Mast cells as "tunable" effector and immunoregulatory cells: recent advances. *Annu Rev Immunol.* 2005;23:749–786.
12. Brown SG, Blackman KE, Heddle RJ. Can serum mast cell tryptase help diagnose anaphylaxis? Emerg Med Australas. 2004;16:120–124.
13. Levy JH. Biomarkers in the diagnosis of anaphylaxis: making nature disclose her mysteries. Clin Exp Allergy. 2009;39:5–7.
14. Ono E, Taniguchi M, Mita H, et al. Increased production of cysteinyl leukotrienes and prostaglandin D2 during human anaphylaxis. Clin Exp Allergy. 2009;39:72–80.
15. Peavy RD, Metcalfe DD. Understanding the mechanisms of anaphylaxis. Curr Opin Allergy Clin Immunol. 2008;8:310–315.
16. Kalesnikoff J, Galli SJ. Anaphylaxis: mechanisms of mast cell activation. *Chem Immunol Allergy.* 2010;95: 45–66.
17. Kitamura Y. Heterogeneity of mast cells and phenotypic change between subpopulations. Annu Rev Immunol. 1989;7:59–76.
18. Metcalfe DD, Baram D, Mekori YA. Mast cells. Physiol Rev. 1997;77:1033–1079.
19. Kawakami T, Galli SJ. Regulation of mast-cell and basophil function and survival by IgE. Nat Rev Immunol. 2002;2:773–786.
20. Tsai M, Shih LS, Newlands GF, et al. The rat c-*kit* ligand, stem cell factor, induces the development of connective tissue-type and mucosal mast cells in vivo. Analysis by anatomical distribution, histochemistry, and protease phenotype. J Exp Med. 1991;174:125–131.
21. Galli SJ, Grimbaldeston M, Tsai M. Immunomodulatory mast cells: negative, as well as positive, regulators of immunity. Nat Rev Immunol. 2008;8:478–486.

22. Miller HR, Wright SH, Knight PA, Thornton EM. A novel function for transforming growth factor-beta1: upregulation of the expression and the IgE-independent extracellular release of a mucosal mast cell granule-specific beta-chymase, mouse mast cell protease-1. Blood. 1999;93:3473–3486.
23. Ryan JJ, Kashyap M, Bailey D, et al. Mast cell homeostasis: a fundamental aspect of allergic disease. Crit Rev Immunol. 2007;27:15–32.
24. Irani AM, Craig SS, DeBlois G, Elson CO, Schechter NM, Schwartz LB. Deficiency of the tryptase-positive, chymase-negative mast cell type in gastrointestinal mucosa of patients with defective T lymphocyte function. J Immunol. 1987;138:4381–4386.
25. Bannert N, Farzan M, Friend DS, et al. Human mast cell progenitors can be infected by macrophagetropic human immunodeficiency virus type 1 and retain virus with maturation in vitro. J Virol. 2001;75:10808–10814.
26. Li Y, Li L, Wadley R, et al. Mast cells/basophils in the peripheral blood of allergic individuals who are HIV-1 susceptible due to their surface expression of CD4 and the chemokine receptors CCR3, CCR5, and CXCR4. Blood. 2001;97:3484–3490.
27. Sundstrom JB, Ellis JE, Hair GA, et al. Human tissue mast cells are an inducible reservoir of persistent HIV infection. Blood. 2007;109:5293–5300.
28. Mekori YA, Metcalfe DD. Mast cells in innate immunity. Immunol Rev. 2000;173:131–140.
29. Grimbaldeston MA, Metz M, Yu M, Tsai M, Galli SJ. Effector and potential immunoregulatory roles of mast cells in IgE-associated acquired immune responses. Curr Opin Immunol. 2006;18:751–760.
30. Dawicki W, Marshall JS. New and emerging roles for mast cells in host defence. Curr Opin Immunol. 2007;19:31–38.
31. Metz M, Grimbaldeston MA, Nakae S, Piliponsky AM, Tsai M, Galli SJ. Mast cells in the promotion and limitation of chronic inflammation. Immunol Rev. 2007;217:304–328.
32. Kalesnikoff J, Galli SJ. New developments in mast cell biology. Nat Immunol. 2008;9:1215–1223.
33. Blank U, Rivera J. The ins and outs of IgE-dependent mast-cell exocytosis. Trends Immunol. 2004;25:266–273.
34. Galli SJ, Nakae S, Tsai M. Mast cells in the development of adaptive immune responses. Nat Immunol. 2005;6:135–42.
35. Sayed BA, Brown MA. Mast cells as modulators of T-cell responses. Immunol Rev. 2007;217:53–64.
36. Theoharides TC, Kempuraj D, Tagen M, Conti P, Kalogeromitros D. Differential release of mast cell mediators and the pathogenesis of inflammation. Immunol Rev. 2007;217:65–78.
37. Wastling JM, Knight P, Ure J, et al. Histochemical and ultrastructural modification of mucosal mast cell granules in parasitized mice lacking the beta-chymase, mouse mast cell protease-1. Am J Pathol. 1998;153:491–504.
38. Knight PA, Wright SH, Lawrence CE, Paterson YY, Miller HR. Delayed expulsion of the nematode Trichinella spiralis in mice lacking the mucosal mast cell-specific granule chymase, mouse mast cell protease-1. J. Exp. Med. 2000;192:1849–1856.
39. Lawrence CE, Paterson YY, Wright SH, Knight PA, Miller HR. Mouse mast cell protease-1 is required for the enteropathy induced by gastrointestinal helminth infection in the mouse. Gastroenterology. 2004;127:155–165.
40. Tchougounova E, Pejler G, Abrink M. The chymase, mouse mast cell protease 4, constitutes the major chymotrypsin-like activity in peritoneum and ear tissue. A role for mouse mast cell protease 4 in thrombin regulation and fibronectin turnover. J Exp Med. 2003;198:423–431.
41. Magnusson SE, Pejler G, Kleinau S, Abrink M. Mast cell chymase contributes to the antibody response and the severity of autoimmune arthritis. FASEB J. 2009;23:875–882.
42. Abonia JP, Friend DS, Austen WG Jr, et al. Mast cell protease 5 mediates ischemia-reperfusion injury of mouse skeletal muscle. J Immunol. 2005;174:7285–7291.
43. Thakurdas SM, Melicoff E, Sansores-Garcia L, et al. The mast cell-restricted tryptase mMCP-6 has a critical immunoprotective role in bacterial infections. J Biol Chem. 2007;282:20809–20815.
44. Shin K, Watts GF, Oettgen HC, et al. Mouse mast cell tryptase mMCP-6 is a critical link between adaptive and innate immunity in the chronic phase of *Trichinella spiralis* infection. J Immunol. 2008;180:4885–4891.
45. McNeil HP, Shin K, Campbell IK, et al. The mouse mast cell-restricted tetramer-forming tryptases mouse mast cell protease 6 and mouse mast cell protease 7 are critical mediators in inflammatory arthritis. Arthritis Rheum. 2008;58:2338–2346.
46. Feyerabend TB, Hausser H, Tietz A, et al. Loss of histochemical identity in mast cells lacking carboxypeptidase A. Mol Cell Biol. 2005;25:6199–6210.
47. Schneider LA, Schlenner SM, Feyerabend TB, Wunderlin M, Rodewald HR. Molecular mechanism of mast cell mediated innate defense against endothelin and snake venom sarafotoxin. J Exp Med. 2007;204:2629–2639.
48. Kitamura Y, Go S, Hatanaka K. Decrease of mast cells in *W/W^v^* mice and their increase by bone marrow transplantation. Blood. 1978;52:447–452.

49. Lyon MF, Glenister PH. A new allele sash ($W^{sh}$) at the *W*-locus and a spontaneous recessive lethal in mice. Genet Res. 1982;39:315–322.
50. Nakano T, Sonoda T, Hayashi C, et al. Fate of bone marrow-derived cultured mast cells after intracutaneous, intraperitoneal, and intravenous transfer into genetically mast cell-deficient $W/W^{v}$ mice. Evidence that cultured mast cells can give rise to both connective tissue type and mucosal mast cells. J Exp Med. 1985;162:1025–1043.
51. Grimbaldeston MA, Chen CC, Piliponsky AM, Tsai M, Tam SY, Galli SJ. Mast cell-deficient *W-sash* c-*kit* mutant $Kit^{W-sh/W-sh}$ mice as a model for investigating mast cell biology in vivo. Am J Pathol. 2005;167:835–848.
52. Wolters PJ, Mallen-St Clair J, Lewis CC, et al. Tissue-selective mast cell reconstitution and differential lung gene expression in mast cell-deficient $Kit^{W-sh}/Kit^{W-sh}$ sash mice. Clin Exp Allergy. 2005;35:82–88.
53. Galli SJ, Zsebo KM, Geissler EN. The kit ligand, stem cell factor. Adv Immunol. 1994;55:1–96.
54. Duttlinger R, Manova K, Chu TY, et al. *W-sash* affects positive and negative elements controlling c-*kit* expression: ectopic c-*kit* expression at sites of kit-ligand expression affects melanogenesis. Development. 1993;118:705–717.
55. Nagle DL, Kozak CA, Mano H, Chapman VM, Bucan M. Physical mapping of the *Tec* and *Gabrb1* loci reveals that the $W^{sh}$ mutation on mouse chromosome 5 is associated with an inversion. Hum Mol Genet. 1995;4:2073–2079.
56. Berrozpe G, Timokhina I, Yukl S, et al. The $W^{sh}$, $W^{57}$, and *Ph Kit* expression mutations define tissue-specific control elements located between -23 and -154 kb upstream of *Kit*. Blood. 1999;94:2658–2666.
57. Nigrovic PA, Gray DH, Jones T, et al. Genetic inversion in mast cell-deficient ($W^{sh}$) mice interrupts *corin* and manifests as hematopoietic and cardiac aberrancy. Am J Pathol. 2008;173:1693–1701.
58. Tsai M, Wedemeyer J, Ganiatsas S, Tam SY, Zon LI, Galli SJ. In vivo immunological function of mast cells derived from embryonic stem cells: an approach for the rapid analysis of even embryonic lethal mutations in adult mice in vivo. Proc Natl Acad Sci USA. 2000;97:9186–9190.
59. Metz M, Piliponsky AM, Chen CC, et al. Mast cells can enhance resistance to snake and honeybee venoms. Science. 2006;313:526–530.
60. Scholten J, Hartmann K, Gerbaulet A, et al. Mast cell-specific Cre/loxP-mediated recombination in vivo. Transgenic Res. 2008;17:307–315.
61. Musch W, Wege AK, Mannel DN, Hehlgans T. Generation and characterization of alpha-chymase-Cre transgenic mice. Genesis. 2008;46:163–166.
62. Feyerabend TB, Terszowski G, Tietz A, et al. Deletion of Notch1 converts pro-T cells to dendritic cells and promotes thymic B cells by cell-extrinsic and cell-intrinsic mechanisms. Immunity. 2009;30:67–79.
63. Lantz CS, Yamaguchi M, Oettgen HC, et al. IgE regulates mouse basophil Fc epsilon RI expression in vivo. J Immunol. 1997;158:2517–2521.
64. Sullivan BM, Locksley RM. Basophils: a nonredundant contributor to host immunity. Immunity. 2009;30:12–20.
65. Galli SJ, Franco CB. Basophils are back! Immunity. 2008;28:495–497.
66. Hedin H, Richter W, Messmer K, Renck H, Ljungstrom KG, Laubenthal H. Incidence, pathomechanism and prevention of dextran-induced anaphylactoid//anaphylactic reactions in man. Dev Biol Stand. 1980;48:179–189.
67. Bergamaschini L, Mannucci PM, Federici AB, Coppola R, Guzzoni S, Agostoni A. Posttransfusion anaphylactic reactions in a patient with severe von Willebrand disease: role of complement and alloantibodies to von Willebrand factor. J Lab Clin Med. 1995;125:348–355.
68. Cheifetz A, Smedley M, Martin S, et al. The incidence and management of infusion reactions to infliximab: a large center experience. Am J Gastroenterol. 2003;98:1315–1324.
69. Umeda Y, Fukumoto Y, Miyauchi T, et al. Anaphylactic shock related to aprotinin induced by anti-aprotinin immunoglobulin G antibody alone; report of a case. Kyobu Geka. 2007;60:69–71.
70. Fish SC, Donaldson DD, Goldman SJ, Williams CM, Kasaian MT. IgE generation and mast cell effector function in mice deficient in IL-4 and IL-13. J Immunol. 2005;174:7716–7724.
71. Martin TR, Galli SJ, Katona IM, Drazen JM. Role of mast cells in anaphylaxis. Evidence for the importance of mast cells in the cardiopulmonary alterations and death induced by anti-IgE in mice. J Clin Invest. 1989;83:1375–1383.
72. Takeishi T, Martin TR, Katona IM, Finkelman FD, Galli SJ. Differences in the expression of the cardiopulmonary alterations associated with anti-immunoglobulin E-induced or active anaphylaxis in mast cell-deficient and normal mice. Mast cells are not required for the cardiopulmonary changes associated with certain fatal anaphylactic responses. J Clin Invest. 1991;88:598–608.
73. Martin TR, Takeishi T, Katz HR, Austen KF, Drazen JM, Galli SJ. Mast cell activation enhances airway responsiveness to methacholine in the mouse. J Clin Invest. 1993;91:1176–1182.
74. Ando A, Martin TR, Galli SJ. Effects of chronic treatment with the c-*kit* ligand, stem cell factor, on immunoglobulin E-dependent anaphylaxis in mice. Genetically mast cell-deficient $Sl/Sl^{d}$ mice acquire anaphylactic

responsiveness, but the congenic normal mice do not exhibit augmented responses. J Clin Invest. 1993;92:1639–1649.
75. Dombrowicz D, Flamand V, Miyajima I, Ravetch JV, Galli SJ, Kinet JP. Absence of Fc epsilonRI alpha chain results in upregulation of Fc gammaRIII-dependent mast cell degranulation and anaphylaxis. Evidence of competition between Fc epsilonRI and Fc gammaRIII for limiting amounts of FcR beta and gamma chains. J Clin Invest. 1997;99:915–925.
76. Hua X, Kovarova M, Chason KD, Nguyen M, Koller BH, Tilley SL. Enhanced mast cell activation in mice deficient in the A2b adenosine receptor. J Exp Med. 2007;204:117–128.
77. Olivera A, Mizugishi K, Tikhonova A, et al. The sphingosine kinase-sphingosine-1-phosphate axis is a determinant of mast cell function and anaphylaxis. Immunity. 2007;26:287–297.
78. Gri G, Piconese S, Frossi B, et al. CD4+CD25+ regulatory T cells suppress mast cell degranulation and allergic responses through OX40-OX40L interaction. Immunity. 2008;29:771–781.
79. Charles N, Watford WT, Ramos HL, et al. Lyn kinase controls basophil GATA-3 transcription factor expression and induction of Th2 cell differentiation. Immunity. 2009;30:533–543.
80. Schneider E, Petit-Bertron AF, Bricard R, et al. IL-33 activates unprimed murine basophils directly in vitro and induces their in vivo expansion indirectly by promoting hematopoietic growth factor production. J Immunol. 2009;183:3591–3597.
81. Brockow K, Jofer C, Behrendt H, Ring J. Anaphylaxis in patients with mastocytosis: a study on history, clinical features and risk factors in 120 patients. Allergy. 2008;63:226–232.
82. Bonadonna P, Perbellini O, Passalacqua G, et al. Clonal mast cell disorders in patients with systemic reactions to Hymenoptera stings and increased serum tryptase levels. J Allergy Clin Immunol. 2009;123: 680–686.
83. Metcalfe DD, Schwartz LB. Assessing anaphylactic risk? Consider mast cell clonality. J Allergy Clin Immunol. 2009;123:687–688.
84. Ring J, Darsow U. Idiopathic anaphylaxis. Curr Allergy Asthma Rep. 2002;2:40–45.
85. Iwaki S, Spicka J, Tkaczyk C, et al. Kit- and Fc epsilonRI-induced differential phosphorylation of the transmembrane adaptor molecule NTAL/LAB/LAT2 allows flexibility in its scaffolding function in mast cells. Cell Signal. 2008;20:195–205.
86. Rivera J, Proia RL, Olivera A. The alliance of sphingosine-1-phosphate and its receptors in immunity. Nat Rev Immunol. 2008;8:753–763.
87. Ryan JJ, Spiegel S. The role of sphingosine-1-phosphate and its receptors in asthma. Drug News Perspect. 2008;21:89–96.
88. Oskeritzian CA, Alvarez SE, Hait NC, Price MM, Milstien S, Spiegel S. Distinct roles of sphingosine kinases 1 and 2 in human mast-cell functions. Blood. 2008;111:4193–4200.
89. Takizawa F, Adamczewski M, Kinet JP. Identification of the low affinity receptor for immunoglobulin E on mouse mast cells and macrophages as Fc gamma RII and Fc gamma RIII. J Exp Med. 1992;176:469–475.
90. Ujike A, Ishikawa Y, Ono M, et al. Modulation of immunoglobulin (Ig)E-mediated systemic anaphylaxis by low-affinity Fc receptors for IgG. J Exp Med. 1999;189:1573–1579.
91. Wershil BK, Mekori YA, Murakami T, Galli SJ. $^{125}$I-fibrin deposition in IgE-dependent immediate hypersensitivity reactions in mouse skin. Demonstration of the role of mast cells using genetically mast cell-deficient mice locally reconstituted with cultured mast cells. J Immunol. 1987;139:2605–2614.
92. Wershil BK, Wang ZS, Gordon JR, Galli SJ. Recruitment of neutrophils during IgE-dependent cutaneous late phase reactions in the mouse is mast cell-dependent. Partial inhibition of the reaction with antiserum against tumor necrosis factor-alpha. J Clin Invest. 1991;87:446–453.
93. Gordon JR, Galli SJ. Promotion of mouse fibroblast collagen gene expression by mast cells stimulated via the Fc epsilon RI. Role for mast cell-derived transforming growth factor beta and tumor necrosis factor alpha. J Exp Med. 1994;180:2027–2037.
94. Wershil BK, Furuta GT, Wang ZS, Galli SJ. Mast cell-dependent neutrophil and mononuclear cell recruitment in immunoglobulin E-induced gastric reactions in mice. Gastroenterology. 1996;110:1482–1490.
95. Furuta GT, Schmidt-Choudhury A, Wang MY, et al. Mast cell-dependent tumor necrosis factor alpha production participates in allergic gastric inflammation in mice. Gastroenterology. 1997;113:1560–1569.
96. Jawdat DM, Albert EJ, Rowden G, Haidl ID, Marshall JS. IgE-mediated mast cell activation induces Langerhans cell migration in vivo. J Immunol. 2004;173:5275–5282.
97. Silva SR, Casabuono A, Jacysyn JF, et al. Sialic acid residues are essential for the anaphylactic activity of murine IgG1 antibodies. J Immunol. 2008;181:8308–8314.
98. Latour S, Bonnerot C, Fridman WH, Daeron M. Induction of tumor necrosis factor-alpha production by mast cells via Fc gamma R. Role of the Fc gamma RIII gamma subunit. J Immunol. 1992;149:2155–2162.
99. Arimura A, Nagata M, Takeuchi M, Watanabe A, Nakamura K, Harada M. Active and passive cutaneous anaphylaxis in WBB6F1 mouse, a mast cell-deficient strain. Immunol Invest. 1990;19:227–233.
100. Hazenbos WL, Gessner JE, Hofhuis FM, et al. Impaired IgG-dependent anaphylaxis and Arthus reaction in Fc gamma RIII (CD16) deficient mice. Immunity. 1996;5:181–188.

101. Nagasaka A, Matsue H, Matsushima H, et al. Osteopontin is produced by mast cells and affects IgE-mediated degranulation and migration of mast cells. Eur J Immunol. 2008;38:489–499.
102. Dombrowicz D, Flamand V, Brigman KK, Koller BH, Kinet JP. Abolition of anaphylaxis by targeted disruption of the high affinity immunoglobulin E receptor alpha chain gene. Cell. 1993;75:969–976.
103. Katz HR. Inhibition of pathologic inflammation by leukocyte Ig-like receptor B4 and related inhibitory receptors. Immunol Rev. 2007;217:222–230.
104. Daheshia M, Friend DS, Grusby MJ, Austen KF, Katz HR. Increased severity of local and systemic anaphylactic reactions in gp49B1-deficient mice. J Exp Med. 2001;194:227–234.
105. Zabel BA, Nakae S, Zuniga L, et al. Mast cell-expressed orphan receptor CCRL2 binds chemerin and is required for optimal induction of IgE-mediated passive cutaneous anaphylaxis. J Exp Med. 2008;205:2207–2220.
106. Maekawa A, Austen KF, Kanaoka Y. Targeted gene disruption reveals the role of cysteinyl leukotriene 1 receptor in the enhanced vascular permeability of mice undergoing acute inflammatory responses. J Biol Chem. 2002;277:20820–20824.
107. Jacoby W, Cammarata PV, Findlay S, Pincus SH. Anaphylaxis in mast cell-deficient mice. J Invest Dermatol. 1984;83:302–304.
108. Ha TY, Reed ND, Crowle PK. Immune response potential of mast cell-deficient *W/W^v^* mice. Int Arch Allergy Appl Immunol. 1986;80:85–94.
109. Ha TY, Reed ND. Systemic anaphylaxis in mast-cell-deficient mice of $W/W^v$ and $Sl/Sl^d$ genotypes. Exp Cell Biol. 1987;55:63–68.
110. Martin TR, Ando A, Takeishi T, Katona IM, Drazen JM, Galli SJ. Mast cells contribute to the changes in heart rate, but not hypotension or death, associated with active anaphylaxis in mice. J Immunol. 1993;151:367–376.
111. Kimura S, Nagata M, Takeuchi M, Takano K, Harada M. Anti-granulocyte antibody suppression of active and passive anaphylactic shock in WBB6F1-$W/W^v$ mice. Cell Mol Life Sci. 1997;53:663–666.
112. Cara DC, Ebbert KV, McCafferty DM. Mast cell-independent mechanisms of immediate hypersensitivity: a role for platelets. J Immunol. 2004;172:4964–4971.
113. Choi IH, Shin YM, Park JS, et al. Immunoglobulin E-dependent active fatal anaphylaxis in mast cell-deficient mice. J Exp Med. 1998;188:1587–1592.
114. Choi IW, Kim YS, Kim DK, et al. Platelet-activating factor-mediated NF-kappaB dependency of a late anaphylactic reaction. J Exp Med. 2003;198:145–151.
115. Park JS, Choi IH, Lee DG, et al. Anti-IL-4 monoclonal antibody prevents antibiotics-induced active fatal anaphylaxis. J Immunol. 1997;158:5002–5006.
116. Arase N, Arase H, Hirano S, Yokosuka T, Sakurai D, Saito T. IgE-mediated activation of NK cells through Fc gamma RIII. J Immunol. 2003;170:3054–3058.
117. Bock SA, Munoz-Furlong A, Sampson HA. Fatalities due to anaphylactic reactions to foods. J Allergy Clin Immunol. 2001;107:191–193.
118. Sicherer SH, Sampson HA. Food allergy: recent advances in pathophysiology and treatment. Annu Rev Med. 2009;60:261–277.
119. Leung DY, Sampson HA, Yunginger JW, et al. Effect of anti-IgE therapy in patients with peanut allergy. N Engl J Med. 2003;348:986–993.
120. Sampson HA, Mendelson L, Rosen JP. Fatal and near-fatal anaphylactic reactions to food in children and adolescents. N Engl J Med. 1992;327:380–384.
121. Sun J, Arias K, Alvarez D, et al. Impact of CD40 ligand, B cells, and mast cells in peanut-induced anaphylactic responses. J Immunol. 2007;179:6696–6703.
122. Khodoun M, Strait R, Orekov T, et al. Peanuts can contribute to anaphylactic shock by activating complement. J Allergy Clin Immunol. 2009;123:342–351.
123. Smith PL, Kagey-Sobotka A, Bleecker ER, et al. Physiologic manifestations of human anaphylaxis. J Clin Invest. 1980;66:1072–1080.
124. van der Linden PW, Hack CE, Kerckhaert JA, Struyvenberg A, van der Zwan JC. Preliminary report: complement activation in wasp-sting anaphylaxis. Lancet. 1990;336:904–906.
125. Perdue MH, Masson S, Wershil BK, Galli SJ. Role of mast cells in ion transport abnormalities associated with intestinal anaphylaxis. Correction of the diminished secretory response in genetically mast cell-deficient $W/W^v$ mice by bone marrow transplantation. J Clin Invest. 1991;87:687–693.
126. Brandt EB, Strait RT, Hershko D, et al. Mast cells are required for experimental oral allergen-induced diarrhea. J Clin Invest. 2003;112:1666–1677.
127. Forbes EE, Groschwitz K, Abonia JP, et al. IL-9- and mast cell-mediated intestinal permeability predisposes to oral antigen hypersensitivity. J Exp Med. 2008;205:897–913.
128. Hauber HP, Bergeron C, Hamid Q. IL-9 in allergic inflammation. Int Arch Allergy Immunol. 2004;134:79–87.

129. Redegeld FA, van der Heijden MW, Kool M, et al. Immunoglobulin-free light chains elicit immediate hypersensitivity-like responses. Nat Med. 2002;8:694–701.
130. Kraneveld AD, Kool M, van Houwelingen AH, et al. Elicitation of allergic asthma by immunoglobulin free light chains. Proc Natl Acad Sci USA. 2005;102:1578–1583.
131. Johansson SG, Bieber T, Dahl R, et al. Revised nomenclature for allergy for global use: Report of the Nomenclature Review Committee of the World Allergy Organization, October 2003. J Allergy Clin Immunol. 2004;113:832–836.
132. De Carolis C, Perricone R, De Sanctis G, Fontana L. Complement activation by Hymenoptera venom allergenic extracts. J Allergy Clin Immunol. 1982;70:219–220.
133. von Zabern I, Przyklenk H, Nolte R, Vogt W. Effect of different penicillin derivatives on complement components in human serum. Int Arch Allergy Appl Immunol. 1984;75:164–172.
134. Erdei A, Andrasfalvy M, Peterfy H, Toth G, Pecht I. Regulation of mast cell activation by complement-derived peptides. Immunol Lett. 2004;92:39–42.
135. Boyce JA. Successful treatment of cold-induced urticaria/anaphylaxis with anti-IgE. J Allergy Clin Immunol. 2006;117:1415–1418.
136. MacGlashan DW Jr, Bochner BS, Adelman DC, et al. Down-regulation of Fc(epsilon)RI expression on human basophils during in vivo treatment of atopic patients with anti-IgE antibody. J Immunol. 1997;158:1438–1445.
137. Beck LA, Marcotte GV, MacGlashan D, Togias A, Saini S. Omalizumab-induced reductions in mast cell Fce psilon RI expression and function. J Allergy Clin Immunol. 2004;114:527–530.
138. Matsuda K, Piliponky AM, Nakae S, Kawakami T, Tsai M, Galli SJ. IgE enhances human mast cell survival and chemokine production: IL-4 augments the secretory response. J Allergy Clin Immunol. 2005;116:1357–1363.
139. Asai K, Kitaura J, Kawakami Y, et al. Regulation of mast cell survival by IgE. Immunity. 2001;14:791–800.
140. Kalesnikoff J, Huber M, Lam V, et al. Monomeric IgE stimulates signaling pathways in mast cells that lead to cytokine production and cell survival. Immunity. 2001;14:801–811.
141. Kitaura J, Song J, Tsai M, et al. Evidence that IgE molecules mediate a spectrum of effects on mast cell survival and activation via aggregation of the FcepsilonRI. Proc Natl Acad Sci USA. 2003;100:12911–12916.
142. Kohno M, Yamasaki S, Tybulewicz VL, Saito T. Rapid and large amount of autocrine IL-3 production is responsible for mast cell survival by IgE in the absence of antigen. Blood. 2005;105:2059–2065.
143. Zhu D, Kepley CL, Zhang K, Terada T, Yamada T, Saxon A. A chimeric human-cat fusion protein blocks cat-induced allergy. Nat Med. 2005;11:446–449.
144. Kalesnikoff J, Galli SJ. Nipping cat allergy with fusion proteins. Nat Med. 2005;11:381–382.
145. Mertsching E, Bafetti L, Hess H, et al. A mouse Fcgamma-Fcepsilon protein that inhibits mast cells through activation of FcgammaRIIB, SH2 domain-containing inositol phosphatase 1, and SH2 domain-containing protein tyrosine phosphatases. J Allergy Clin Immunol. 2008;121:441–447 e445.
146. Bachelet I, Munitz A, Levi-Schaffer F. Abrogation of allergic reactions by a bispecific antibody fragment linking IgE to CD300a. J Allergy Clin Immunol. 2006;117:1314–1320.
147. Ong CJ, Ming-Lum A, Nodwell M, et al. Small-molecule agonists of SHIP1 inhibit the phosphoinositide 3-kinase pathway in hematopoietic cells. Blood. 2007;110:1942–1949.
148. Zhang K, Kepley CL, Terada T, Zhu D, Perez H, Saxon A. Inhibition of allergen-specific IgE reactivity by a human Ig Fcgamma-Fcepsilon bifunctional fusion protein. J Allergy Clin Immunol. 2004;114:321–327.
149. Kashiwakura J, Yokoi H, Saito H, Okayama Y. T cell proliferation by direct cross-talk between OX40 ligand on human mast cells and OX40 on human T cells: comparison of gene expression profiles between human tonsillar and lung-cultured mast cells. J Immunol. 2004;173:5247–5257.
150. Nakae S, Suto H, Iikura M, et al. Mast cells enhance T cell activation: importance of mast cell costimulatory molecules and secreted TNF. J Immunol. 2006;176:2238–2248.
151. Castells M. Desensitization for drug allergy. Curr Opin Allergy Clin Immunol. 2006;6:476–481.
152. MacGlashan D Jr, Lavens-Phillips S, Katsushi M. IgE-mediated desensitization in human basophils and mast cells. Front Biosci. 1998;3:d746–756.
153. MacGlashan D Jr. Desensitization of IgE-mediated IL-4 release from human basophils. J Leukoc Biol. 1998;63:59–67.
154. Kepley CL. Antigen-induced reduction in mast cell and basophil functional responses due to reduced Syk protein levels. Int Arch Allergy Immunol. 2005;138:29–39.
155. Plewako H, Wosinska K, Arvidsson M, et al. Basophil interleukin 4 and interleukin 13 production is suppressed during the early phase of rush immunotherapy. Int Arch Allergy Immunol. 2006;141:346–353.
156. Nagao M, Hiraguchi Y, Hosoki K, et al. Allergen-induced basophil CD203c expression as a biomarker for rush immunotherapy in patients with Japanese cedar pollinosis. Int Arch Allergy Immunol. 2008;146 Suppl 1:47–53.
157. MacGlashan D Jr, Vilarino N. Polymerization of actin does not regulate desensitization in human basophils. J Leukoc Biol. 2009;85:627–637.

158. Ishizaka T, Sterk AR, Daeron M, Becker EL, Ishizaka K. Biochemical analysis of desensitization of mouse mast cells. J Immunol. 1985;135:492–501.
159. Shalit M, Levi-Schaffer F. Challenge of mast cells with increasing amounts of antigen induces desensitization. Clin Exp Allergy. 1995;25:896–902.
160. Rubinchik E, Shalit M, Levi-Schaffer F. Responsiveness of human skin mast cells to repeated activation: an in vitro study. Allergy. 1998;53:14–19.
161. Morales AR, Shah N, Castells M. Antigen-IgE desensitization in signal transducer and activator of transcription 6-deficient mast cells by suboptimal doses of antigen. Ann Allergy Asthma Immunol. 2005;94:575–580.

# Chapter 5
# Basophils in Anaphylaxis

**David E. Sloane and Donald MacGlashan**

**Abstract** Human basophils are the least common (and arguably the least well understood) peripheral blood leukocyte. Their roles in normal physiology and homeostasis are unknown, but their ability to bind IgE, to release histamine, leukotrienes, and other mediators, and to move into extravascular tissues suggest that they may participate in allergic reactions, including anaphylaxis. Although basophils share many salient features with mast cells, it is now widely accepted that these are two distinct cell types. Recent evidence from murine models of anaphylaxis indicates a role for basophils in some situations, but if (and, if so, how) basophils contribute to anaphylaxis in humans is as yet undetermined.

**Keywords** Anaphylaxis • Basophil • FcεRI • IgE receptor • Murine model • Platelet-activating factor • Signal transduction

## 5.1 Introduction

Recent attention has focused on the potential immunoregulatory functions of basophils. But this cell, originally identified by the appearance and staining qualities of its characteristic granules, was first hypothesized to be an effector cell of allergic reactions, based on the identification of substances known to be produced by the basophil (most famously, histamine) in tissues affected by allergic inflammation. This putative role in allergy was reinforced by the discovery that basophils are able to generate *de novo* prodigious amounts of selected lipid mediators rapidly after activation. Indeed, the presence of elevated concentrations of extracellular histamine and leukotrienes such as leukotriene $C_4$ ($LTC_4$) along with the infiltration of a tissue by peripheral blood basophils and eosinophils, and the degranulation of resident mast cells may fairly be said to *define* allergic inflammation. What is currently at issue is the relationship among basophils, mast cells, and eosinophils in initiating, maintaining, and resolving the stereotyped immune system activity conventionally called "allergic," as well as the molecular details of how each of these three cell types makes its contribution. Thus, although basophils produce and release substances such as histamine, lipid mediators, and interleukin (IL) 4 – substances that recapitulate the signs and symptoms of allergic reactions such as anaphylaxis – it is not yet clear that basophils are involved in the pathobiology of anaphylaxis.

Resolving questions about the roles of mast cells and basophils is confounded by the similarity between basophils and mast cells. While these two cells are certainly distinct in anatomic distribution,

D.E. Sloane (✉)
Rheumatology, Immunology, and Allergy Brigham and Women's Hospital Smith Building
1 Jimmy Fund Way Room 636, Boston, MA, 02115
e-mail: dsloane@partners.org

M.C. Castells (ed.), *Anaphylaxis and Hypersensitivity Reactions*,
DOI 10.1007/978-1-60327-951-2_5, © Springer Science+Business Media, LLC 2011

life span, and morphology, they resemble each other closely enough in their cell surface receptors and the mediators they release upon activation to make a precise determination of their relative contributions to human anaphylaxis an elusive goal.

This chapter briefly reviews the basic biology of the basophil, with emphasis on the biology of interleukin (IL)-3 and what is known of basophil signal transduction. As will be readily appreciated, despite impressive recent progress and assiduous study, what is known about the basophil in the broad immunologic schema is meager compared to the questions that remain about the basic biology of this rarest of granulocytes, its roles in healthy homeostasis, and its activity in disease. Wherever possible, this chapter relies upon studies of human basophils. However, data from murine models of signal transduction and anaphylaxis are cited where they are hoped to be germane to an accurate understanding of human basophil physiology in general and to the part played by this cell in human anaphylaxis specifically. But, as both basophils and anaphylaxis differ significantly between these two species, comparisons require caution.

## 5.2 Review of Basophil Biology

### *5.2.1 Ontogeny*

Like other granulocytes (neutrophils and eosinophils), basophils are believed to originate in the bone marrow and to derive from hematopoietic stem cells that differentiate down the common myeloid progenitor (CMP) pathway, a $CD34^+$ cell that may give rise to any nonlymphoid leukocyte [1]. Developmental relationships among basophils, mast cells, and eosinophils are not entirely clear. Data from murine studies suggest that basophils are more closely related to mast cells than to eosinophils [2], as a common basophil–mast cell precursor has been isolated. However, other data suggest that human basophils may be related more closely to eosinophils than mast cells [3–5]. Current thinking holds that basophils are "fully matured" when they exit the bone marrow into the peripheral circulation, whereas mast cells do not mature until they exit the circulation, entering tissues such as the skin, lung, and gut. This view is based on the observation that basophils can be identified in peripheral blood, isolated, and made to function (e.g., degranulate, generate lipid mediators, and release cytokines), whereas the same cannot yet be said of mast cells, whose blood-borne precursors so far defy easy identification and isolation. However, basophils are also able to exit the circulation and enter tissues, where they may undergo significant biochemical alterations. Others have raised the possibility that some human peripheral blood mononuclear cells with metachromatic granules and expressing low levels of the c-kit receptor on their surface are mast cell precursors rather than basophils [6].

### *5.2.2 Morphology and Biochemistry*

Basophils typically have a bilobed nucleus, but their salient feature is their numerous metachromatic granules. Mast cells possess a greater number of granules with similar staining characteristics, and generally have a single bean-shaped nucleus. Mast cells are heterogeneous, with $MC_T$ distributed at mucosal surfaces and possessing "scroll-rich" granules containing tryptase as the dominant protease, while $MC_{TC}$ are located in the skin and submucosae and having "scroll-poor" granules with the proteases carboxypeptidase, cathepsin-G, and chymase as well as tryptase [7]. Basophils, in contrast, are generally believed to be homogeneous, as no definitive data indicate distinct basophil subtypes.

The histamine content of a basophil is 0.5–1.5 pg/cell, considerably less than the 3–4 pg/cell found in mast cells [8]. Basophils and mast cells also differ in their capacity for lipid mediator generation. While they share the capacity to synthesize $LTC_4$, it seems that mast cells alone are able to make prostaglandin $D_2$ ($PGD_2$), as basophils do not express the enzyme $PGD_2$ synthase. Platelet-activating factor (PAF), a mediator that may play an important role in anaphylaxis (see below), is synthesized by human basophils, but the dominant form of this lipid mediator is the so-called acyl-PAF, which does not appear to be physiologically active [9]. However, studies of anaphylaxis in mice have suggested a role for PAF generated by basophils. Basophils contain small amounts of tryptase, typically on the order of 0.05 pg per cell, which is estimated to be 0.4% that of mast cells [10].

### 5.2.3 Life Span

Basophils isolated from peripheral blood survive in culture with a half-life ($t_{½}$) of approximately 24 h. Supplementation with the cytokine IL-3 extends this to a $t_{½}$ of 3 days (see below). This is in apparent contrast to mast cells, which live for months to years in peripheral tissues. It has been estimated that bone marrow cells that can be considered maturing basophils may live for 3–6 days before leaving the marrow where their circulation time is very brief (ca. 12 h) before migrating to tissues.

### 5.2.4 Extravasation

Basophils express a number of chemokine receptors [11] and the molecule VLA-4 (CD49d/CD29), allowing them to respond to a broad array of chemotactic agents and to leave the circulation and enter sites of inflammation where the vessel endothelium has upregulated VCAM-1. Increased number of basophils have been observed in the airways of atopic asthmatics after allergen challenge [12], in the lungs of patients with fatal asthma [13], and in late phase allergic reactions in skin [14]. The survival of basophils in the tissues is not known, but if studies of eosinophils are a guide, the life span may be dependent on the local cytokine environment in the tissue.

### 5.2.5 Activation

The best characterized activating molecule expressed on the surface of basophils is the high affinity receptor for IgE, FcεRI [15]. Indeed, it is the constitutive expression of the $\alpha\beta\gamma_2$ form of Fcε(epsilon)RI and the histamine-containing metachromatic granules that are the most striking similarities between basophils and mast cells. Unlike other Ig receptors, Fcε(epsilon)RI binds its IgE before the antibody binds antigen, arming the basophil to respond to contact with a polyvalent antigen molecule that cross-links allergen-specific IgE. If a sufficient number of Fcε(epsilon)RI receptors are cross-linked, the basophil rapidly (within minutes) degranulates and generates lipid mediators, and later (hours) produces newly synthesized cytokines such as IL-4. However, basophils possess a variety of other activating and inhibitor receptors, allowing them to respond to stimuli by IgE-independent mechanisms as well [16]. Among these other activating receptors, murine basophils express CD16A, the Fcγ(gamma)RIIIA receptor for the constant region of IgG, which allows basophils from this species to respond with mediator generation to the presence of IgG-antigen complexes. This is hypothesized to be an important mechanism by which basophils may contribute to anaphylaxis in mice. Human basophils, however, do not express Fcγ(gamma)RIIIA. Although it has been reported that these cells do express Fcγ(gamma)RIIIB (CD16B), the level of expression is one to three log-fold lower than that of human neutrophils, and cross-linking of this receptor (which does not associate with the common γ(gamma) chain, see below) does not seem to elicit basophil degranulation [17]. Thus, it is presently unclear whether human basophils activate in response to IgG-antigen complexes. Indeed, while these cells may express low levels of Fcγ(gamma)RIIA (CD32A), an activating receptor for IgG, they clearly express functional Fcγ(gamma)RIIB (CD32B), an inhibitory IgG receptor [18]. Of these two IgG receptors, the latter seems to be dominant, as co-ligation to Fcε(epsilon)RI dramatically attenuates basophil activation signals and degranulation [19]. In clinical situations of allergen exposure and sensitization, where patients may respond immunologically by producing both IgE and IgG, this may actually prevent basophil activation to antigen. Human basophils, unlike their murine counterparts, do express other activating receptors, such as LILRA-2 (previously known as LIR-7), cross-linking of which induces mediator release [20, 21]. As the natural ligands for LILRA-2 are currently unidentified, however, whether this receptor allows basophils to participate in anaphylaxis is unknown.

As detailed below, it is the common γ(gamma) chain shared by Fcε(epsilon)RI and Fcγ(gamma) RIIIA (as well as other activating Fc receptors) that, by phosphorylation of the immunoreceptor tyrosine-base activation motifs (ITAMs) in its cytoplasmic tail, allows extracellular events such as the cross-linking of Fcε(epsilon)RI-bound IgE to initiate intracellular biochemical changes. These intracellular signaling events culminate in the release of inflammatory mediators from three basophil "compartments": the granules containing preformed mediators such as histamine, the lipid mediator pathways leading to $LTC_4$ and PAF generation, and the protein synthetic pathways eventuating in the production of cytokines such as IL-4 (Fig. 5.1).

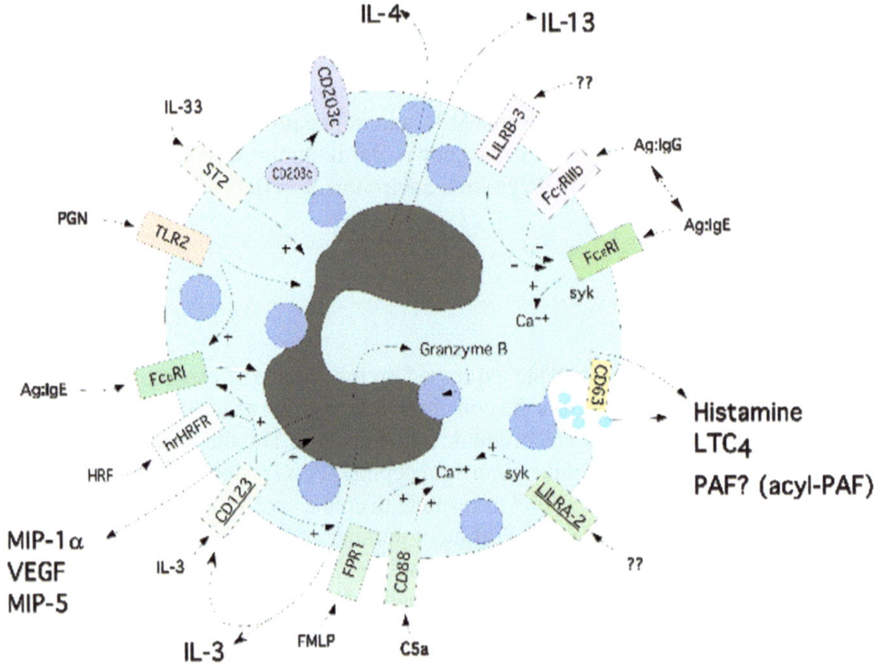


**Fig. 5.1** Receptors and mediators associated with human basophils. Selected interactions are indicated by *arrows*. HRF = histamine releasing factor; TLR = toll-like receptors; $LTC_4$ = leukotriene $C_4$; PAF = platelet-activating factor; VEGF = vascular endothelial growth factor; IL4, IL13, or IL3 = interleukin-4 or -13 or -3; MIP-1a = CCL3; MIP-5 = CCL15; Ag = antigen

## 5.2.6 *Signal Transduction: Fcε(epsilon)RI-Mediated Signal Transduction in Human Basophils*

### 5.2.6.1 Lyn Kinase and Syk Kinase

The IgE receptor has no known intrinsic enzymatic activity. It likely signals by means of kinases recruited when specific antigens binding to specific IgE antibodies occupying the receptor lead to receptor aggregation. This three-subunit (α(alpha)β(beta)γ(gamma)$_2$) receptor requires aggregation to generate the signaling steps that lead to mediator release. The current model proposes that a src-family kinase, probably lyn, is closely associated with the receptor and is only capable of phosphorylating a different receptor to which it is not directly associated [22]. Phosphorylation of the beta subunit by an adjacent lyn kinase, allows lyn to bind with much higher affinity, enhancing further phosphorylation of the gamma subunit. Phosphorylation of the gamma subunit allows the ZAP-70 family kinase, syk, to bind and become more active, initiating many of the steps that lead to mediator release. These details come from studies of rodent cell lines [23–31]. While only rudimentary information is known about the reaction in human cells, the general characteristics appear the same. Phosphorylation of the gamma subunit has been demonstrated [32], changes in the phosphorylation of lyn have been noted [32], and syk is an obligate participant in the early signaling reaction [33].

### 5.2.6.2 Fyn Kinase

In rodent mast cells, it is now well established that the src-family kinase fyn is also an initiator of a parallel set of pathways, some of which counter-regulate lyn [34]. Since these particular src-family kinases have one inhibitory and one activating tyrosine phosphorylation sites, it is possible to observe these enzymes switching between inactive and active states, by monitoring the phosphorylation of these tyrosines. Such changes can be observed in lyn during activation of human basophils but thus far, no changes in fyn, which is clearly present, have been observed [32]. Further study will be needed to know if these results imply an inactivity for fyn in the basophil reaction.

One of the characteristics of peripheral blood human basophils that distinguishes this cell from its rodent mast cell counterparts [35] is that the receptor is not lost from the cell surface minutes to hours following aggregation [36, 37]. This canonical means of downregulating the receptor response does occur in human cells, but on a timescale of many hours and days. A second difference between human and rodent basophils is the ability of rodent monomeric IgE to initiate many of the classical elements of the aggregation reaction [38–40]. Murine monomeric IgE has been shown to initiate signaling, but it is an attribute only of certain IgE antibodies [39]. Aggregation is likely required since monovalent antigen inhibits signaling, but the nature of the aggregation is unclear. Examples of this behavior of IgE on human cells are unusual [40, 41].

### 5.2.6.3 Phosphatidyl Inositol 3′ Kinase (PI3K)

Other characterized early signaling steps in human basophils include the activation of phosphatidyl inositol 3′ kinase (PI3K) [41]. This enzyme is recruited to the plasma membrane by phosphorylation of its regulatory subunit by syk (or possibly an early syk-dependent tyrosine kinase) [42, 43]. The activities of PI3K are required for secretion; relatively selective inhibitors of PI3K completely ablate the secretion of all known mediators. This enzyme may play multiple roles, but a primary task for PI3K is to phosphorylate plasma membrane phosphatidyl inositol. The phosphatidylinositol 3,4,5 phosphate acts as a ligand for proteins that possess PH domains, recruiting these proteins to the cell membrane. Several important proteins that are thus recruited, including btk [44] and PLCγ(gamma)1/γ(gamma)2. In rodent mast cells, the recruitment of PLCγ(gamma)1/γ(gamma)2 to the membrane and its activity are considered critical to the IgE-mediated reaction [45, 46] and inhibition of the PI3K that generates the PIP3 needed for PLCγ(gamma)1/γ(gamma)2 recruitment markedly inhibits the cytosolic calcium response. In human basophils, however, this effect is considerably blunted. Very high concentrations of the PI3K inhibitor, LY294002, only partially inhibit the calcium response [47]. These results suggest that there are significant differences in the sequencing of steps in human basophils compared to those operative in rodent mast cells.

#### 5.2.6.4 SH-2-Containing 5′ Inositol Phosphatase-1 (SHIP-1)

A downregulatory reaction that has been studied in some detail in rodent mast cells is the recruitment of the 5′ inositol phosphatase, SHIP-1 [48, 49]. Knocking out this enzyme results in an exaggerated response to IgE-mediated stimulation of mast cells [50]. SHIP-1 is also recruited and phosphorylated in human basophils [32]. Its phosphorylation kinetics suggest that its participation is transitory, but it shows a kinetic profile of somewhat longer duration than signaling elements that lie downstream of the generation of PIP3 by PI3K. It has been suggested that its heightened phosphorylation on the supraoptimal side of the anti-IgE Ab dose–response curve may contribute to the blunted histamine release on this side of the dose–response curve [51].

#### 5.2.6.5 MAP Kinase Pathway

In all mast cells and basophils studied to date, the activation of the MAPK family of enzymes is common. In human basophils, the pathway that leads to the ERK phosphorylation is critical for the activation of cPLA2 and therefore the generation of $LTC_4$ [52]. The pathway does not regulate histamine or IL-4 secretion. However, the top of this pathway is the GTP-binding protein p21ras. This small GTP-binding protein is intimately linked to PI3K in basophils, as inhibition of PI3K prevents the activation of p21ras [47]. This appears to be unique to basophils, and is not found in human or rodent mast cells. The significance is not clear, but downregulatory elements like SHIP1 might be expected to have a direct influence on the duration of activity of this pathway if the linkage to PI3K is related to its generation of PIP3.

#### 5.2.6.6 Dynamics and Variability of Syk Expression

As in mast cells, the activities of syk are critical for the IgE-mediated reaction in basophils. But surprisingly, expression of this critical enzyme appears highly restricted [52]. The typical basophil expresses 150,000 IgE receptors but only expresses 25,000 syk molecules [53]. In contrast, there are typically 100,000 lyn molecules. If all receptors were aggregated (as is expected if the stimulus is anti-IgE antibody), then syk levels may be rate limiting. Other leukocytes express 10–30 times more syk than basophils [54]. In addition, CD34 progenitors express 10–12-fold more syk. Between the CD34+ progenitor stage and the subsequently developed peripheral blood basophil, syk expression is greatly diminished. In addition, there is a broad range of syk expression among individuals. In some, syk expression is essentially absent, and their basophils do not respond to IgE-mediated stimulation, although they express typical IgE receptor densities [55]. In the general population, the expression of syk in basophils is an accurate predictor of how well their basophils will respond to IgE-mediated stimulation [53]. In a survey of 20 signaling elements, only syk expression showed a coefficient of variation as broad as anti-IgE-mediated histamine release, and only syk expression was correlated with maximal histamine release [56]. There is no correlation between syk expression in basophils and syk expression in any other type of leukocyte [54, 57], suggesting that the regulation of syk expression in basophils is a unique process. Since syk expression determines the basophil's response to IgE-mediated stimulation and the magnitude of the basophil response has a relationship to the expression of allergic asthma (and possibly to atopy in general) [58–60], there may be an important relationship between regulation of syk expression and asthma.

#### 5.2.6.7 Regulation of Syk Expression

A second characteristic of syk expression may be germane to the process of clinical desensitization. IgE-mediated activation leads to a loss of syk that takes place over the course of 4–12 h [61]. An intriguing feature of this aggregated receptor-mediated loss is that it appears integrative. Levels of stimulation too weak to induce significant histamine release nevertheless induce some loss of syk. Prolonged weak stimulation effectively diminishes expression of syk. In a survey of 25 signaling elements known to participate in IgE-mediated signaling in human basophils, only three were downregulated [53]. In addition to the loss of syk expression (70% loss) after 18 h of stimulation, there was modest loss of Fcε(epsilon)RIα(alpha) (30%) and an even more modest loss of lyn (15%). The integrative nature of the loss of syk is consistent with the outcome of clinical desensitization, namely a loss in the individual's ability to respond to antigenic challenge after a prolonged and progressively escalating exposure to antigen. But the loss of syk is an event that alters responsiveness to all antigenic stimulation, while a hallmark of clinical desensitization is its antigenic specificity.

The highly variable suppression of syk, and its low levels of expression that are unique to basophils (among the granulocytes), raises questions about the source of the variation. Recent studies of culture-derived basophils have shown that CD34 progenitors express 11-fold more syk than a peripheral blood basophil. Basophils derived from these CD34 progenitors, following 21 days of culture in IL-3, also express 11-fold more syk than peripheral blood basophils. Exposing the culture to a pre-aggregated IgE–anti-IgE mixture for the entire 21-day culture downregulates syk expression to levels observed in peripheral blood basophils. Despite the decrease in syk expression, the cells label normally with alcian blue, contain normal levels of histamine, and express cell surface Fcε(epsilon)RI at levels equivalent to cells not treated this way [54]. Whether or not these studies accurately reflect the events occurring in vivo, the results do demonstrate that it is possible to induce syk downregulation by a constitutively present aggregation of Fcε(epsilon)RI and still generate a basophil with normal characteristics.

#### 5.2.6.8 Variability of SHIP-1 Expression

Although syk expression was found to correlate with maximum histamine release induced by anti-IgE antibody, the correlation could be marginally improved by including in the regression relationship the expression level of SHIP-1 [53]. As noted above, this signaling element is considered downregulatory, so that increased expression would be expected to suppress histamine release or cellular sensitivity. This is true, although only weakly so. Indeed, the distribution of SHIP-1 expression in the general population is quite narrow. But there is a subpopulation of subjects whose basophils are uniquely sensitive to the secretagogue histamine-releasing factor (HRF, or TCTP) [62–64], and these individuals show a depressed levels of SHIP-1 expression in their basophils, approximately fivefold below the typical level. At the opposite end of the spectrum, there is a subset of patients with chronic urticaria that have basophils nearly unresponsive to IgE-mediated stimulation, despite having normal levels of syk expression. Basophils from these patients express higher levels of SHIP-1 [65, 66]. Therefore, there are two special cases in humans where the expression level of SHIP-1 appears to have a marked influence on basophil function in a manner consistent with observations in SHIP-1 knockout mice.

#### 5.2.6.9 Nuclear Factor of Activated T Cells (NFAT)

In rodent mast cell models, there has been some study of later signaling events. Some of the steps of granule fusion have been explored, and a couple of pathways leading to cytokine release have been studied. Studies of these pathways in human basophils have been limited to one study of NFAT expression. NFAT is a nuclear transcription factor that is heavily phosphorylated in the cytoplasm of resting cells. It is activated by dephosphorylation, a process that is mediated by the phosphatase calcineurin that is, in turn, activated by elevations of cytosolic calcium modulating the binding of calmodulin to calcineurin. Since the signals that lead to elevations in cytosolic calcium are well understood in mast cells, the NFAT pathway is well defined. NFAT2 is not commonly expressed in leukocytes, but in human basophils NFAT2 appears to mediate IgE-induced signaling for IL-4 secretion [67].

### 5.2.7 *Effects of IL-3*

Regulation of human basophil function occurs by many pathways, but the influence of IL-3 is both broad spectrum and marked, and operates at all stages of basophil development. In terms of development, in mice, IL-3 appears to alter the frequency of basophil progenitors [68]. In cultures of human CD34+ progenitors, the chronic presence of IL-3 leads to cells with many characteristics of peripheral blood basophils [69], shifting development away from a mast cell or eosinophil pathway.

#### 5.2.7.1 Effects on Basophil Mediator Secretion

In peripheral blood basophils, exposure to IL-3 has a multiplicity of effects that occur on various timescales. There is an immediate effect, taking place with 2–5 min, that is independent of gene transcription or translation [70, 71], with enhancement of mediator release in response to other stimuli. These changes occur because IL-3-mediated signaling shares components with other activating receptors [72, 73]. For example, IL-3 induces a transient activation of the p21ras->Erk pathway [72, 73]. As noted above, activation of this pathway is required for the secretion of $LTC_4$ from basophils. Through this pathway, IL-3 causes a transitory (lasting about 1 h) phosphorylation of cytosolic PLA2, one of two known conditions necessary for this enzyme to be optimally active. The second condition is an elevation in cytosolic calcium. Therefore, any stimulus that leads to an elevation of cytosolic calcium immediately induces $LTC_4$ release [71]. This is most apparent with the anaphylatoxin C5a, which alone only weakly induces $LTC_4$ release, despite initiating a very brisk release of histamine. The activation of cPLA2 following C5a lags behind the very transient increase in cytosolic calcium that follows exposure to C5a. A short pretreatment with IL-3 provides a preexisting phosphorylation of cPLA2, so that when C5a induces an influx of calcium, robust $LTC_4$ release quickly follows. Other secretagogues are influenced by IL-3 in a similar way. The transient activation of the Erk pathway that follows IL-3 is accomplished by a process that is not yet identified [73]. It appears that there is an unidentified phosphatase whose activity is curtailed by IL-3 incubation so that phosphorylation of Erk is prolonged. This suppression of a downregulatory event also alters the activation profile of secretagogues. With respect to IgE-mediated release, there are no clearly induced changes in the patterns of signaling. The effects may be downstream of the early events.

Within the time frame of 8–24 h, IL-3 causes additional phenotypic changes in basophils. One notable effect is to alter the cytosolic calcium response initiated by a stimulus [71]. The basis for the change in calcium handling by the cell is unknown for human basophils. It is speculated that an influx pathway is added to the mix of store-operated calcium channels that lead to a sustained elevation of cytosolic calcium. Again, the response to C5a exemplifies this effect most clearly. As noted above, without IL-3, C5a induces a very transient elevation in cytosolic calcium; essentially no influx phase follows the stimulation (even though one might expect that with the very strong discharging of internal stores that follow C5a, it would be possible to observe influx). Following 18–24 h of IL-3 exposure, C5a induces a strong influx component to the calcium response. This change also allows C5a to induce $LTC_4$ release, though in this instance the mechanism differs from the effects after a short exposure to IL-3. The cytosolic calcium responses induced by other secretagogues, including those that are IgE-mediated, are similarly augmented by longer term IL-3 exposure.

#### 5.2.7.2 Effects on Basophil Survival

The effects at 8–24 h are sensitive to transcription and translation inhibitors. Indeed, the number of changes induced by IL-3 in this time frame is extensive. In microarray studies, nearly 500 genes change at least fourfold (in either direction) and the changes in approximately 200 genes exceed the Bonferroni-corrected *p*-value needed for significance (unpublished data). Like all polymorphonuclear leukocytes, the basophil does not survive well in culture despite supplementation with cytokines. IL-3 is a better cytokine than IL-5, GM-CSF, or NGF for protecting the cell from apoptosis [72]. Indeed, these other cytokines, which have weak, transitory effects on basophil function, provide poor protection from apoptosis. Recent studies have shown that IL-3 induces the enhanced presence of PIM-1 [74]. This protein is critical in the survival pathways of leukocytes. Basophils tend to express more PIM-1 before IL-3 treatment, which may explain why they survive somewhat better in culture than eosinophils or neutrophils. IL-3 induces a 5–10-fold change in PIM-1, which blunts many of apoptotic pathways (increased caspase-9 induction, for example).

There is a third phase to the IL-3 effect on basophils. This is most apparent when considering the basophil phenotype called the "non-releaser." While secreting normally in response to seven transmembrane receptor secretagogues like fMLP or C5a, these cells respond poorly or not at all to stimulation with antigen or anti-IgE antibody [55]. As noted above, such cells do not express syk appreciably. How this occurs is still under investigation, but treating these cells for 3 days with IL-3 partially reverses the deficiency in syk expression [53, 75] and results in a cell that responds better to stimulation with anti-IgE Ab [76]. The effect is not apparent after only 24 h. Syk is not the only early signaling element whose expression is modified; at least five other proteins critical for signaling or downregulation are enhanced [53]. For example, the expression of SHIP-1 is enhanced, considerably more so than that of syk. Basophils undergo complex phenotypic changes in response to prolonged exposure to IL-3, resulting in greater responsiveness to all forms of stimulation.

## 5.3 Evidence of Basophil Involvement in Anaphylaxis

The belief that basophils play a role in anaphylaxis is based primarily on the observation that basophils are capable of generating and releasing significant concentrations of chemical substances that not only are present in patients with anaphylaxis, but when infused into human test subjects or experimental animals induce symptoms and signs that resemble the clinical picture of this allergic diathesis. Such observations constitute circumstantial evidence at best, as mast cells are also able to produce such mediators. The attractive hypothesis that basophils are nevertheless involved in anaphylaxis is supported by their expression of receptors that allow basophils to respond with mediator release to stimuli such as allergens that are recognized triggers of anaphylaxis. Although the evidence is circumstantial, the infiltration of basophils into the tissues of organs whose physiologic functions are commonly affected in anaphylaxis further buttresses the argument that these cells participate in these reactions.

### *5.3.1 Basophil Mediators*

#### 5.3.1.1 Histamine

Although basophils contain, on average, only 25–33% of the histamine possessed by mast cells [8, 15], the rapid aggregate release of this preformed mediator by the degranulation of many basophils activated nearly simultaneously may result in significantly elevated concentrations of this vasoactive amine. Histamine has been shown to reproduce the symptoms and signs of anaphylaxis in humans [77], including flushing, headache, and tachycardia. The inhibition of the histamine H1 receptor can attenuate these changes [78]. Importantly, mast cells and basophils are the only human cells known to produce significant amounts of histamine, in contrast to other mammals, such as rabbits, whose platelets also contain and release histamine.

#### 5.3.1.2 Leukotriene $C_4$

Like histamine, $LTC_4$ is released in significant amounts by activated basophils with a kinetic profile almost as rapid as that of histamine [79]. Once released from basophils in physiologic contexts such as peripheral blood (as opposed to in vitro experiments with highly purified basophils), $LTC_4$ is rapidly metabolized to $LTD_4$ and $LTC_4$, which are also biologically active. In the upper airway, these mediators cause rhinitis, a common clinical feature of some patients with anaphylaxis. $LTC_4$ is a potent bronchoconstrictor that may contribute to the asthma symptoms that often attends anaphylaxis, such as dyspnea, wheezing, coughing, and chest tightness, as well as the reversible airflow obstruction correlated with these symptoms. In skin, $LTC_4$ causes vasodilation and augmentation of transendothelial fluid flux that manifests as a wheal and flare reaction reminiscent of the urticaria and flushing seen in many patients with anaphylaxis [80].

#### 5.3.1.3 Platelet-Activating Factor

Platelet-activating factor (PAF) is a lipid autocoid that contributes to inflammation at least in part by binding to a specific cell surface receptor [81]. Its actions in some contexts may be predominantly via a juxtracrine mechanism, in which PAF expressed on the surface of endothelial cells and leukocytes influences the movement and activation state of neighboring cells. In addition, PAF may bind to intracellular receptors in target cells. In such cases, the determination of "free" extracellular PAF may not be a reliable indicator of PAF activity [81]. However, PAF production and release by basophils in response to both physiologic and non-physiologic stimuli (including anti-IgE) has been demonstrated in vitro, though at concentrations one to two log-fold lower than that of $LTC_4$ [9]. The relevance of PAF to human anaphylaxis was recently investigated in a study of patients with fatal peanut anaphylaxis [82], in which serum concentrations of PAF were directly correlated with the severity of anaphylaxis while the activity of PAF acetylhydrolase, an enzyme that regulates PAF activity by degrading the autocoid, was inversely correlated. This study fuels speculation for the involvement of basophils in some forms of anaphylaxis as elevations in mast cell tryptase are generally absent in food-induced anaphylaxis, suggesting that some non-mast cell is at work in this context. Whether food antigens activate basophils by means of IgE-dependent or IgE-independent mechanisms, leading to the production and release of PAF to bring about anaphylaxis in the absence of significant tryptase release, however, remains a speculation, as experimental support from human studies is so far lacking.

#### 5.3.1.4 IL-4

Human and murine basophils produce significant amounts of IL-4 in response to physiologic stimuli such as cross-linking of IgE and LILRA-2 [20, 83]. This suggests an immunoregulatory role for basophils, and experiments in mice have demonstrated their participation in primary and secondary adaptive immune responses [84]. In a murine model of fatal anaphylaxis, blockade of IL-4 during the sensitization phase of both wild-type and mast cell deficient ($W/W^V$) animals prevented the generation of antigen-specific IgE and fatal anaphylaxis, but it is not clear that the source of this IL-4 was the basophil [85]. Human basophils are also potent sources of IL-13 [86], a number of chemokines, and vascular endothelial growth factor, but as these proteins require many hours for their secretion, their precise roles in mediating anaphylaxis (either acute or "late phase" secondary reactions) are not clear.

### *5.3.2 Basophil Receptors*

Fcε(epsilon)RI allows basophil activation in response to small amounts of allergen, and such activation leads to the release of histamine, lipid mediators, and IL-4, all of which have been shown (either in humans or in model animals such as guinea pigs and mice) either to effect physiologic changes consistent with anaphylaxis or to exacerbate anaphylaxis. In addition, Fcγ(gamma)RIIIA allows murine basophil activation in response to antigen-IgG complexes, which typically form in the presence of higher concentrations of antigen than those that activate the IgE-Fcε(epsilon)RI system. As noted above, however, human basophils do not express this receptor, and the expression and function of Fcγ(gamma)RIIIB on these cells are dubious and unclear.

### *5.3.3 Location of Basophils*

#### 5.3.3.1 Circulation in Peripheral Blood

Many of the most severe cases of anaphylaxis and those with the most rapid progression of symptoms occur with the intravenous administration of medications or other agents to which the patient is allergic. Since mature mast cells are not normally present in the peripheral circulation, whereas competent basophils are typically found in the circulation, basophils would be the first cell whose activation would be sufficient for causing anaphylaxis to encounter the intravenous antigen.

#### 5.3.3.2 Migration into Tissues Involved in Allergic Reactions

As noted above, the expression of an array of chemokine receptors renders basophils sensitive to a variety of molecules capable of inducing their migration from the circulation into tissues. These receptors include (but are not limited to) CCR2, CCR3, and CXCR4 [15], and one or more of them may attract basophils to anatomic locations involved in anaphylaxis. Basophils have been found to be recruited to the nasal mucosa after allergen challenge [87], in the airways of patients with severe and fatal asthma [13, 88], and in allergen challenged skin [14]. While basophils infiltrating these tissues have been shown to release granule and lipid mediators as well as cytokines [89], their entry and activation likely occur on a timescale more consistent with the "late phase" of an allergic reaction [90, 91]. This argues against a role for basophils in the rapid and acute anaphylactic reaction to inhaled or intradermally encountered allergens (as in reactions to the stings of Hymenoptera), but would be consistent with a contribution by the basophil to the recurrent or delayed symptoms seen hours later in up to one-third of patients with anaphylaxis. The infiltration of the alimentary tract by basophils has been less well studied, making it difficult to do more than hypothesize about the involvement of basophils in food-induced anaphylaxis. However, the absence of mast cell tryptase in this setting, in stark contrast to other forms of anaphylaxis, in which an elevation in the serum tryptase is a clinically reliable marker for mast cell activation and helps establish the diagnosis, leads some to argue that basophils may be the dominant cell involved in food-induced anaphylaxis [7].

## 5.4 Evidence for Basophil Activity in Human Anaphylaxis

Although a belief that basophils are directly involved in human anaphylaxis is widespread, it is supported by little direct evidence. This is unsurprising, given the difficulty of studying the function of a rare and short-lived peripheral blood cell in an acute and transient life-threatening condition. A negative piece of circumstantial evidence of basophil involvement in anaphylaxis comes from a comparison of the best-known states of basophilia (which occurs in rare oncologic conditions such as the accelerated phase of chronic myelogenous leukemia [CML]) with mastocytosis. In the latter disease, the superabundance of mast cells is clearly associated with an increased risk of anaphylaxis, often associated with the stings of Hymenoptera. Indeed, sting- or opioid-induced anaphylaxis may be the presenting event that unmasks mastocytosis [92]. However, the superfluity of basophils in CML does not seem to be accompanied by a parallel increase in the risk of anaphylaxis, though basophils from such patients have been studied for mediator release [93]. A search of the PubMed database (accessed January 11, 2010) for reports on patients with basophilia and anaphylaxis yielded two cases, both of which were in pediatric patients whose reactions appeared to be the result of basophil degranulation induced by chemotherapy [94, 95]. A ready counterargument to this observation is that the basophils in CML carry the Philadelphia chromosome and are likely to be functionally abnormal.

## 5.5 Evidence for Basophil Activity in Murine Models of Anaphylaxis

Mammalian models of anaphylaxis have historically included dogs and guinea pigs. However, the currently dominant model organism is the mouse, though strain-specific differences may make aggregating all such models misleading. See Table 5.1 for a comparison and contrast of human and

**Table 5.1** Selected activating and inhibitory receptors expressed by human and murine basophils

| Receptor | Activating/inhibitory | Ligand | Human | Mouse |
|---|---|---|---|---|
| Fcε(epsilon)RI | Activating | IgE + antigen | Yes | Yes |
| Fcγ(gamma)RIIB | Inhibitory | IgG + antigen | Yes | Unknown |
| Fcγ(gamma)RIIIA | Activating | IgG + antigen | No | Yes |
| Fcγ(gamma)RIIIB | Unknown | IgG + antigen | Possibly | Unknown |
| LILRA-2 | Activating | Unknown | Yes | No |
| LILRB-3 | Inhibitory | Unknown | Yes | No |
| CD88 | Activating | C5a | Yes | Yes |
| FPR1 | Activating | fMLP | Yes | Yes |

Abbreviations: *Fcγ (gamma)R* = receptor for the Fc portion of IgG; *Fcε(epsilon)RI* = type I receptor for the Fc portion of IgE; *FPR1* = f-Met-Leu-Phe peptide receptor-1; *LILR* = leukocyte immunoglobulin-like receptor. Comparison between human and murine basophils of the expression of basophil surface receptors

murine basophils. In contrast to the situation with humans, in whom identification of the basophil is relatively straightforward but in whom there is a dearth of direct evidence for this cell having a role in anaphylaxis, recent data exploring some murine models of anaphylaxis present a compelling argument for the involvement of basophils.

The utility of murine models in drawing conclusions that will elucidate human anaphylaxis may depend exquisitely on the details of the experimental system [96]. In active anaphylaxis, mice are sensitized to one or more antigens and allowed to form their own antibodies (IgE, IgG) to them. Examples include proteins such as ovalbumin and peanut extract, and the hapten penicillin. Thereafter, the mice are challenged with the antigen either orally or intravenously. Metrics of anaphylaxis include alterations in mouse behavior ("shallow respirations, lethargy, decreased response to tactile stimuli" [97]), changes in physiologic parameters (increased heart rate, decreased pulmonary conductance and dynamic compliance [98], decreased rectal temperature [99]), gross or microscopic pathologic changes (increased vascular permeability as measured by leakage of Evans blue dye, quantification of mast cell degranulation [98]), and death. In passive anaphylaxis, antigen-specific antibodies (IgE, $IgG_1$) are injected into the experimental animal – either systemically (intravenously) or locally (intradermally) – which is thereafter challenged with the relevant antigen (again, either intravenously or intradermally) to effect a response. The chemical properties of the antigen and the genetic background of the mice employed may also be a crucial determinant of the response, both in the sensitization phase and the challenge phase.

Studies supporting a role for basophils have lagged behind those exploring the contributions of mast cells to murine models of anaphylaxis for two reasons: first, because murine basophils have been difficult to identify [100], leading some to question identity of cells called basophils [101] or even to doubt the very existence of this cell type in this species; second, because a mouse with a genetic deficiency in basophil production has not yet been discovered or engineered, in contrast to the $W/W^V$ mouse and other mast cell deficient mice such as the $Kit^{W-sh/W-sh}$ mouse. Recent progress has been made by consensus on the flow cytometric characteristics of murine basophils (defining them as $CD49b^+/IgE^+$ peripheral blood or spleen cells) and by the development of the Ba103 monoclonal antibody that binds to CD200R3 and effectively removes 80–90% of murine basophils [102].

An early study predating these advances suggested that basophils might play an important role in a murine model of anaphylaxis [97]. After sensitization to bovine serum albumin (BSA), wild-type and $W/W^V$ mast cell deficient mice were challenged with tail vein injection of BSA. Despite the greatly reduced number of mast cells, $W/W^V$ mice developed anaphylaxis (generally fatal) and had equal numbers of peripheral blood basophils (identified as Alcian blue staining cells) as their wild-type counterparts, leading the authors to question the absolute hegemony of the mast cell in this model of anaphylaxis. Interestingly, while the control mice had higher concentrations of histamine than the $W/W^V$ mice, the authors were not able to demonstrate significant changes in the histamine concentration before and after challenge with BSA, suggesting that histamine might not be the most important mediator in this model of anaphylaxis.

A seminal study investigating active anaphylaxis in response to ovalbumin+alum+pertussis toxin (OVA) and confirmed by experiments with bovine gamma globulin indicated that anaphylaxis can occur in the absence of IgE [98]. The authors documented the induction of antigen-specific $IgG_1$ production, elevated plasma histamine concentrations, and mast cell degranulation, but did not assess specifically for basophil activation. This study established that IgE-independent mechanisms could bring about anaphylaxis in mice.

Using similar methods, this conclusion was reinforced and clarified when OVA-induced active anaphylaxis was shown to occur in mice genetically lacking the α(alpha) chain of Fcε(epsilon)RI (Fcε(epsilon)RI-α(alpha)$^{-/-}$) [103]. Interestingly, while such mice had more severe disturbances of physiologic variables than their wild-type counterparts, they had significantly less mast cell degranulation in biopsied tissues, suggesting that some other cell was involved. When mice genetically lacking the common γ(gamma) chain (FcR-γ(gamma)$^{-/-}$) employed by Fcε(epsilon)RI and Fcγ(gamma)RIII were challenged, however, none died, suffered changes in heart rate or pulmonary function, or demonstrated mast cell degranulation, whereas anaphylaxis was fatal for all matched wild-type mice and was preceded by heart and lung dysfunction and accompanied by mast cell degranulation. Passive sensitization with murine antibodies of specific isotypes allowed further insights into these results, and demonstrated that $IgG_1$ could cause deadly anaphylaxis in wild-type and Fcε(epsilon)RI-α(alpha)$^{-/-}$ mice, but not in FcR-γ(gamma)$^{-/-}$ mice. Importantly, passive anaphylaxis induced in $IgG_1$ sensitized mice was not accompanied by mast cell activation, again suggesting that some other cell type capable of responding to $IgG_1$+antigen was responsible. However, when the authors used W/W$^V$ mast cell deficient mice in the $IgG_1$ passive anaphylaxis model, antigen challenge induced a significantly less-severe response, indicating that mast cells were likely to be involved importantly, though not exclusively. This study supported the notion that one or more non-mast cells that express receptors using the FcR-γ(gamma) chain (Fcγ(gamma)RI and Fcγ(gamma)RIII) and capable of releasing relevant mediators are activated in these models of anaphylaxis. Candidate cells in mice include macrophages and basophils.

Using the hapten penicillin V (PCN), fatal anaphylaxis was shown to occur in W/W$^V$ mice with the same 100% mortality as mast cell sufficient controls [85]. This model of active anaphylaxis was IgE-dependent, as treatment with anti-IL-4 during the sensitization phase ablated the production of PCN-specific IgE but not PCN-specific $IgG_1$ and was completely protective in terms of fatality. Importantly, mast cell deficient mice died in the absence of significant elevations in plasma histamine concentrations, but with increased plasma concentrations of PAF. A PAF receptor antagonist protected mice from death due to anaphylaxis. Passive IgE-mediated anaphylaxis was milder but occurred in all W/W$^V$ mice. The authors suggested that one or more cells capable of binding IgE and releasing PAF upon activation was responsible for the findings among the mast cell deficient mice, and since IgE-mediated anaphylaxis seems to be absolutely dependent upon functional Fcε(epsilon)RI, they suspected the basophil was that cell.

A recent study provided the clearest evidence for basophil involvement in a murine model of anaphylaxis to date [99]. Using $IgG_1$ to passively sensitize wild-type and mast cell deficient Kit$^{W-sh/W-sh}$ mice to PCN, the authors first showed that intravenous PCN challenge caused a drop in rectal temperature consistent with anaphylaxis. Flow cytometry demonstrated that basophils were the cells that most efficiently captured $IgG_1$+PCN+BSA immune complexes. Depletion of basophils with the Ba103 antibody-protected $IgG_1$ passively sensitized mice (wild type and Kit$^{W-sh/W-sh}$) but not IgE passively sensitized mice to PCN-BSA-induced anaphylaxis, while depletion of macrophages, NK cells, or neutrophils did not. A PAF inhibitor protected mice from this form of anaphylaxis, and PCN-BSA elicited PAF release from the basophil-containing subset of spleen and peritoneal cells. Additional ex vivo experiments with these cells demonstrated that culture supernatants induced contraction in human umbilical vein endothelial cells, an effect also blocked by the PAF inhibitor. Last, this study demonstrated that depletion of basophils with Ba103 rescued Kit$^{W-sh/W-sh}$ but not mast cell sufficient wildtype mice from *active* PCN-induced anaphylaxis. The model that emerges from this study is one in which anaphylaxis may be IgE, mast cell, and histamine dependent in some cases and $IgG_1$, basophil, and PAF dependent in others [104].

## 5.6 Conclusion

The hypothesis that basophils are involved in the pathobiology of anaphylaxis finds supportive evidence in a variety of studies, but the precise contributions of these cells remain unclear. This hypothesis is based on the reasonable and consistent observations that basophils are present in the relevant anatomic locations involved in anaphylaxis, express receptors for IgE that enable them to bind and respond to antigens that elicit anaphylaxis, and that upon activation by such antigens these cells release mediators that can effect symptoms and signs of anaphylaxis. While there are compelling data for basophil involvement in anaphylaxis in some murine models, doubts remain about the relationship between human anaphylaxis and these murine models [96]. Anaphylaxis is likely a syndrome rather than a single disease, and basophils may play a role in some forms but not others. Among the critical issues is whether anaphylaxis in humans exposed to small amounts of allergen (e.g., from an intradermal sting from an insect or the ingestion of a single peanut) is brought about by the same mechanisms as that induced by exposure to a large amount of allergen (as with the intravenous administration of a drug such as penicillin). It may be that in the former situation mast cells are dominant, while in the latter case basophils are more important. Despite significant challenges, newer tools currently in development should provide experimental support for some of these hypotheses, and future studies in humans hopefully will elucidate any contribution of the basophil to these most severe allergic reactions.

## References


1. Falcone FH, Haas H, Gibbs BF. The human basophil: a new appreciation of its role in immune responses. *Blood.* 2000;96(13):4028–4038.
2. Arinobu Y, Iwasaki H, Gurish MF, et al. Developmental checkpoints of the basophil/mast cell lineages in adult murine hematopoiesis. *Proc Natl Acad Sci USA.* 2005;102(50):18105–18110.
3. Boyce JA, Friend D, Matsumoto R, Austen KF, Owen WF. Differentiation in vitro of hybrid eosinophil/basophil granulocytes: autocrine function of an eosinophil developmental intermediate. *J Exp Med.* 1995;182(1):49–57.
4. Denburg JA, Telizyn S, Messner H, et al. Heterogeneity of human peripheral blood eosinophil-type colonies: evidence for a common basophil–eosinophil progenitor. *Blood.* 1985;66(2):312–318.
5. Denburg JA. The origins of basophils and eosinophils in allergic inflammation. *J Allergy Clin Immunol.* 1998;102(5):S74–S76.
6. Li L, Li Y, Reddel SW, et al. Identification of basophilic cells that express mast cell granule proteases in the peripheral blood of asthma, allergy, and drug-reactive patients. *J Immunol.* 1998;161(9):5079–5086.
7. Hsu FI, Boyce JA. Biology of mast cells and their mediators. In: Adkinson NF Jr, Bochner BS, Busse WW, Holgate ST, Lemanske RF Jr, Simons FER, eds. *Middleton's Allergy: Principles and Practice.* Philadelphia: Elsevier, a division of Mosby; 2009: 311–328.
8. Bochner BS, Lichtenstein LM. Anaphylaxis. *N Engl J Med.* 1991;324(25):1785–1790.
9. Lie WJ, Homburg CH, Kuijpers TW, et al. Regulation and kinetics of platelet-activating factor and leukotriene C4 synthesis by activated human basophils. *Clin Exp Allergy.* 2003;33(8):1125–1134.
10. Castells MC, Irani AM, Schwartz LB. Evaluation of human peripheral blood leukocytes for mast cell tryptase. *J Immunol.* 1987;138(7):2184–2189.
11. Marone G, Triggiani M, de Paulis A. Mast cells and basophils: friends as well as foes in bronchial asthma? *Trends Immunol.* 2005;26(1):25–31.
12. Gauvreau GM, Lee JM, Watson RM, Irani AM, Schwartz LB, ÓByrne PM. Increased numbers of both airway basophils and mast cells in sputum after allergen inhalation challenge of atopic asthmatics. *Am J Respir Crit Care Med.* 2000;161(5):1473–1478.
13. Kepley CL, McFeeley PJ, Oliver JM, Lipscomb MF. Immunohistochemical detection of human basophils in postmortem cases of fatal asthma. *Am J Respir Crit Care Med.* 2001;164(6):1053–1058.
14. Macfarlane AJ, Kon OM, Smith SJ, et al. Basophils, eosinophils, and mast cells in atopic and nonatopic asthma and in late-phase allergic reactions in the lung and skin. *J Allergy Clin Immunol.* 2000; 105(1Pt1):99–107.
15. Schroeder JT. Biology of basophils. In: Adkinson NF Jr, Bochner BS, Busse WW, Holgate ST, Lemanske RF Jr, Simons FER, eds. *Middleton's Allergy: Principles and Practice.* Philadelphia: Elsevier, a division of Mosby; 2009: 329–340.

16. Sullivan BM, Locksley RM. Basophils: a nonredundant contributor to host immunity. *Immunity.* 2009; 30(1):12–20.
17. Meknache N, Jonsson F, Laurent J, Guinnepain MT, Daeron M. Human basophils express the glycosylphosphatidylinositol-anchored low-affinity IgG receptor Fcγ(gamma)RIIIB (CD16B). *J Immunol.* 2009; 182(4):2542–2550.
18. Kepley CL, Cambier JC, Morel PA, et al. Negative regulation of Fcε(epsilon)RI signaling by Fcγ(gamma)RII costimulation in human blood basophils. *J Allergy Clin Immunol.* 2000;106(2):337–348.
19. Zhu D, Kepley CL, Zhang M, Zhang K, Saxon A. A novel human immunoglobulin Fcγ(gamma) Fcε(epsilon) bifunctional fusion protein inhibits Fcε(epsilon) RI-mediated degranulation. *Nat Med.* 2002;8(5):518–521.
20. Sloane DE, Tedla N, Awoniyi M, et al. Leukocyte immunoglobulin-like receptors: novel innate receptors for human basophil activation and inhibition. *Blood.* 2004;104(9):2832–2839.
21. MacGlashan DW Jr, Ishmael S, MacDonald SM, Langdon JM, Arm JP, Sloane DE. Induced loss of Syk in human basophils by non-IgE-dependent stimuli. *J Immunol.* 2008;180(6):4208–4217.
22. Pribluda VS, Pribluda C, Metzger H. Transphosphorylation as the mechanism by which the high-affinity receptor for IgE is phosphorylated upon aggregation. *Proc Natl Acad Sci USA.* 1994;91(23):11246–11250.
23. Kent UM, Mao SY, Wofsy C, Goldstein B, Ross S, Metzger H. Dynamics of signal transduction after aggregation of cell-surface receptors: studies on the type I receptor for IgE. *Proc Natl Acad Sci USA.* 1994;91(8):3087–3091.
24. Yamashita T, Mao SY, Metzger H. Aggregation of the high-affinity IgE receptor and enhanced activity of p53/56lyn protein-tyrosine kinase. *Proc Natl Acad Sci USA.* 1994;91(23):11251–11255.
25. Vonakis BM, Chen H, Haleem-Smith H, Metzger H. The unique domain as the site on Lyn kinase for its constitutive association with the high affinity receptor for IgE. *J Biol Chem.* 1997;272:24072–24080.
26. Torigoe C, Goldstein B, Wofsy C, Metzger H. Shuttling of initiating kinase between discrete aggregates of the high affinity receptor for IgE regulates the cellular response. *Proc Natl Acad Sci USA.* 1997;94:1372–1377.
27. Faeder JR, Hlavacek WS, Reischl I, et al. Investigation of early events in Fcε(epsilon) RI-mediated signaling using a detailed mathematical model. *J Immunol.* 2003;170(7):3769–3781.
28. Kihara H, Siraganian RP. Src homology 2 domains of Syk and Lyn bind to tyrosine-phosphorylated subunits of the high affinity IgE receptor. *J Biol Chem.* 1994;269(35):22427–22432.
29. Zhang J, Berenstein EH, Evans RL, Siraganian RP. Transfection of Syk protein tyrosine kinase reconstitutes high affinity IgE receptor-mediated degranulation in a Syk-negative variant of rat basophilic leukemia RBL-2H3 cells. *J Exp Med.* 1996;184(1):71–79.
30. Jouvin MH, Adamczewski M, Numerof R, Letourneur O, Valle A, Kinet JP. Differential control of the tyrosine kinase lyn and syk by the two signaling chains of the high affinity immunoglobulin E receptor. *J Biol Chem.* 1994;269:5918–5925.
31. Scharenberg AM, Lin S, Cuenod B, Yamamura H, Kinet JP. Reconstitution of interactions between tyrosine kinases and the high affinity IgE receptor which are controlled by receptor clustering. *EMBO J.* 1995;14(14):3385–3394.
32. MacGlashan DW Jr, Vilarino N. Nonspecific desensitization, functional memory and the characteristics of SHIP phosphorylation following IgE-mediated stimulation of human basophils. *J Immunol.* 2006;177:1040–1051.
33. Vilarino N, MacGlashan D Jr. Transient transfection of human peripheral blood basophils. *J Immunol Methods.* 2005;296(1–2):11–18.
34. Parravicini V, Gadina M, Kovarova M, et al. Fyn kinase initiates complementary signals required for IgE-dependent mast cell degranulation. *Nat Immunol.* 2002;3(8):741–748.
35. Isersky C, Rivera J, Segal DM, Triche T. The fate of IgE bound to rat basophilic leukemia cells. II. Endocytosis of IgE oligomers and effect on receptor turnover. *J Immunol.* 1983;131(1):388–396.
36. MacGlashan DW Jr, Mogowski M, Lichtenstein LM. Studies of antigen binding on human basophils. II. Continued expression of antigen-specific IgE during antigen-induced desensitization. *J Immunol.* 1983;130(5):2337–2342.
37. MacGlashan DW Jr. Endocytosis, re-cycling and degradation of unoccupied Fcε(epsilon)RI in Human Basophils. *J Leuk Biol.* 2007;82:1003–1010.
38. Kalesnikoff J, Huber M, Lam V, et al. Monomeric IgE stimulates signaling pathways in mast cells that lead to cytokine production and cell survival. *Immunity.* 2001;14(6):801–811.
39. Kawakami T, Kitaura J. Mast cell survival and activation by IgE in the absence of antigen: a consideration of the biologic mechanisms and relevance. *J Immunol.* 2005;175(7):4167–4173.
40. Matsuda K, Piliponsky AM, Iikura M, et al. Monomeric IgE enhances human mast cell chemokine production: IL-4 augments and dexamethasone suppresses the response. *J Allergy Clin Immunol.* 2005;116(6):1357–1363.
41. Xie L, Schroeder JT, Langdon JM, Sora-Scott RS, Kawakami T, MacDonald SM. Human IgE+and IgE- are not equivalent to mouse highly cytokinergic IgE. *J Allergy Clin Immunol.* 2008;121(4):1027–1033.
42. Jiang K, Zhong B, Gilvary DL, et al. Syk regulation of phosphoinositide 3-kinase-dependent NK cell function. *J Immunol.* 2002;168(7):3155–3164.
43. MacGlashan DW Jr, Undem BJ. Inducing an Anergic state in mast cells and basophils without secretion. *J Allergy Clin Immunol.* 2008;121(6):1500–1506.

44. Hata D, Kawakami Y, Inagaki N, et al. Involvement of Bruton's tyrosine kinase in Fcε(epsilon)RI-dependent mast cell degranulation and cytokine production. *J Exp Med.* 1998;187(8):1235–1247.
45. Tkaczyk C, Beaven MA, Brachman SM, Metcalfe DD, Gilfillan AM. The phospholipase C gamma 1-dependent pathway of Fc epsilon RI-mediated mast cell activation is regulated independently of phosphatidylinositol 3-kinase. *J Biol Chem.* 2003;278(48):48474–48484.
46. Manetz TS, Gonzalez-Espinosa C, Arudchandran R, Xirasagar S, Tybulewicz V, Rivera J. Vav1 regulates phospholipase cgamma activation and calcium responses in mast cells. *Mol Cell Biol.* 2001;21(11):3763–774.
47. Miura K, MacGlashan DW Jr. Phosphatidylinositol-3 kinase regulates p21ras activation during IgE-mediated stimulation of human basophils. *Blood.* 2000;96:2199–2205.
48. Kimura T, Sakamoto H, Appella E, Siraganian RP. The negative signaling molecule SH2 domain-containing inositol- polyphosphate 5-phosphatase (SHIP) binds to the tyrosine-phosphorylated beta subunit of the high affinity IgE receptor. *J Biol Chem.* 1997;272(21):13991–13996.
49. Rauh MJ, Kalesnikoff J, Hughes M, Sly L, Lam V, Krystal G. Role of Src homology 2-containing-inositol 5′-phosphatase (SHIP) in mast cells and macrophages. *Biochem Soc Trans.* 2003;31(Pt 1):286–291.
50. Huber M, Helgason CD, Damen JE, Liu L, Humphries RK, Krystal G. The src homology 2-containing inositol phosphatase (SHIP) is the gatekeeper of mast cell degranulation. *Proc Natl Acad Sci USA.* 1998;95(19):11330–11335.
51. Gibbs BF, Rathling A, Zillikens D, Huber M, Haas H. Initial Fcε(epsilon) RI-mediated signal strength plays a key role in regulating basophil signaling and deactivation. *J Allergy Clin Immunol.* 2006;118(5):1060–1067.
52. Miura K, Schroeder JT, Hubbard WC, MacGlashan DW Jr. Extracellular signal-regulated kinases regulate leukotriene C4 generation, but not histamine release or IL-4 production from human basophils. *J Immunol.* 1999;162(7):4198–4206.
53. MacGlashan DW Jr. Relationship between Syk and SHIP expression and secretion from human basophils in the general population. *J Allergy Clin Immunol.* 2007;119:626–633.
54. Ishmael S, MacGlashan DW Jr. Syk expression in peripheral blood leukocytes, CD34+ progenitors and CD34-derived basophils. *J Leukoc Biol.* 2009; 2010;87:291–300.
55. Nguyen KL, Gillis S, MacGlashan DW Jr. A comparative study of releasing and nonreleasing human basophils: nonreleasing basophils lack an early component of the signal transduction pathway that follows IgE cross-linking. *J Allergy Clin Immunol.* 1990;85(6):1020–1029.
56. Ishmael S, MacGlashan D Jr. Early signal protein expression profiles in basophils: a population study. *J Leukoc Biol.* 2009;86(2):313–325.
57. Kepley CL, Youssef L, Andrews RP, Wilson BS, Oliver JM. Syk deficiency in nonreleaser basophils. *J Allergy Clin Immunol.* 1999;104(2Pt1):279–284.
58. Busse WW, Swenson CA, Sharpe G, Koschat M. Enhanced basophil histamine release to concanavalin A in allergic rhinitis. *J Allergy Clin Immunol.* 1986;78:90–97.
59. Gaddy JN, Busse WW. Enhanced IgE-dependent basophil histamine release and airway reactivity in asthma. *Am Rev Respir Dis.* 1986;134(5):969–974.
60. Casolaro V, Spadaro G, Marone G. Human basophil releasability. VI. Changes in basophil releasability in patients with allergic rhinitis or bronchial asthma. *Am Rev Respir Dis.* 1990;142:1108–1111.
61. MacGlashan D, Miura K. Loss of syk kinase during IgE-mediated stimulation of human basophils. *J Allergy Clin Immunol.* 2004;114(6):1317–1324.
62. MacDonald SM, Lichtenstein LM, Proud D, et al. Studies of IgE-dependent histamine releasing factors: heterogeneity of IgE. *J Immunol.* 1987;139(2):506–512.
63. Schroeder JT, Lichtenstein LM, MacDonald SM. An immunoglobulin E-dependent recombinant histamine-releasing factor induces interleukin-4 secretion from human basophils. *J Exp Med.* 1996;183(3):1265–1270.
64. Schroeder JT, Lichtenstein LM, MacDonald SM. Recombinant HRF enhances IgE-dependent IL-4 and IL-13 secretion by human basophils. *J Immunol.* 1997;159:447–452.
65. Baker R, Vasagar K, Ohameje N, et al. Basophil histamine release activity and disease severity in chronic idiopathic urticaria. *Ann Allergy Asthma Immunol.* 2008;100(3):244–249.
66. Eckman JA, Hamilton RG, Gober LM, Sterba PM, Saini SS. Basophil Phenotypes in chronic idiopathic urticaria in relation to disease activity and autoantibodies. *J Invest Dermatol.* 2008;128:1956–1963.
67. Schroeder JT, Miura K, Kim HH, Sin A, Cianferoni A, Casolaro V. Selective expression of nuclear factor of activated T cells 2/c1 in human basophils: evidence for involvement in IgE-mediated IL-4 generation. *J Allergy Clin Immunol.* 2002;109(3):507–513.
68. Ohmori K, Luo Y, Jia Y, et al. IL-3 induces basophil expansion in vivo by directing granulocyte-monocyte progenitors to differentiate into basophil lineage-restricted progenitors in the bone marrow and by increasing the number of basophil/mast cell progenitors in the spleen. *J Immunol.* 2009;182(5):2835–2841.
69. Kepley CL, Pfeiffer JR, Schwartz LB, Wilson BS, Oliver JM. The identification and characterization of umbilical cord blood-derived human basophils. *J Leukoc Biol.* 1998;64(4):474–483.
70. Kurimoto Y, de Weck AL, Dahinden CA. Interleukin 3-dependent mediator release in basophils triggered by C5a. *J Exp Med.* 1989;170(2):467–479.

71. Miura K, MacGlashan DW Jr. Dual phase priming by interleukin-3 for leukotriene C4 generation in human basophils. *J Immunol.* 2000;164:3026–3034.
72. Miura K, Saini SS, Gauvreau G, MacGlashan DW Jr. Differences in functional consequences and signal transduction induced by IL-3, IL-5 and NGF in human basophils. *J Immunol.* 2001;167:2282–2291.
73. Vilarino N, Miura K, MacGlashan DW Jr. Acute IL-3 priming up-regulates the stimulus-induced Raf-1-Mek-Erk cascade independently of IL-3-induced activation of Erk. *J Immunol.* 2005;175(5):3006–3014.
74. Didichenko SA, Spiegl N, Brunner T, Dahinden CA. IL-3 induces a Pim1-dependent antiapoptotic pathway in primary human basophils. *Blood.* 2008;112(10):3949–3958.
75. Kepley CL, Youssef L, Andrews RP, Wilson BS, Oliver JM. Multiple defects in Fcε(epsilon)RI signaling in Syk-deficient nonreleaser basophils and IL-3-induced recovery of Syk expression and secretion. *J Immunol.* 2000;165(10):5913–5920.
76. Yamaguchi M, Hirai K, Ohta K, et al. Culturing in the presence of IL-3 converts anti-IgE nonresponding basophils into responding basophils. *J Allergy Clin Immunol.* 1996;97:1279–1287.
77. Kaliner M, Shelhamer JH, Ottesen EA. Effects of infused histamine: correlation of plasma histamine levels and symptoms. *J Allergy Clin Immunol.* 1982;69(3):283–289.
78. Kaliner M, Sigler R, Summers R, Shelhamer JH. Effects of infused histamine: analysis of the effects of H-1 and H-2 histamine receptor antagonists on cardiovascular and pulmonary responses. *J Allergy Clin Immunol.* 1981;68(5):365–371.
79. MacGlashan DW Jr, Peters SP, Warner J, Lichtenstein LM. Characteristics of human basophil sulfidopeptide leukotriene release: releasability defined as the ability of the basophil to respond to dimeric cross-links. *J Immunol.* 1986;136(6):2231–2239.
80. Peebles RS, Jr., Boyce J.A. Lipid mediators of hypersensitivity and inflammation. In: Adkinson NF Jr, Bochner BS, Busse WW, Holgate ST, Lemanske RF Jr, Simons FER, eds. *Middleton's Allergy: Principles and Practice.* Philadelphia, PA: Elsevier, a division of Mosby; 2009:203–221.
81. Prescott SM, Zimmerman GA, Stafforini DM, McIntyre TM. Platelet-activating factor and related lipid mediators. *Annu Rev Biochem.* 2000;69:419–445.
82. Vadas P, Gold M, Perelman B, et al. Platelet-activating factor, PAF acetylhydrolase, and severe anaphylaxis. *N Engl J Med.* 2008;358(1):28–35.
83. MacGlashan D Jr, White JM, Huang SK, Ono SJ, Schroeder JT, Lichtenstein LM. Secretion of IL-4 from human basophils. The relationship between IL-4 mRNA and protein in resting and stimulated basophils. *J Immunol.* 1994;152(6):3006–3016.
84. Sokol CL, Barton GM, Farr AG, Medzhitov R. A mechanism for the initiation of allergen-induced T helper type 2 responses. *Nat Immunol.* 2008;9(3):310–318.
85. Choi IH, Shin YM, Park JS, et al. Immunoglobulin E-dependent active fatal anaphylaxis in mast cell-deficient mice. *J Exp Med.* 1998;188(9):1587–1592.
86. Ochensberger B, Daepp GC, Rihs S, Dahinden CA. Human blood basophils produce interleukin-13 in response to IgE-receptor-dependent and -independent activation. *Blood.* 1996;88(8):3028–3037.
87. Kleinjan A, McEuen AR, Dijkstra MD, Buckley MG, Walls AF, Fokkens WJ. Basophil and eosinophil accumulation and mast cell degranulation in the nasal mucosa of patients with hay fever after local allergen provocation. *J Allergy Clin Immunol.* 2000;106(4):677–686.
88. Charles TJ, Williams SJ, Seaton A, Bruce C, Taylor WH. Histamines, basophils and eosinophils in severe asthma. *Clin Sci.* 1979;57(1):39–45.
89. Schroeder JT, Lichtenstein LM, Roche EM, Xiao H, Liu MC. IL-4 production by human basophils found in the lung following segmental allergen challenge. *J Allergy Clin Immunol.* 2001;107(2):265–271.
90. Naclerio RM, Proud D, Togias AG, et al. Inflammatory mediators in late antigen-induced rhinitis. *N Engl J Med.* 1985;313(2):65–70.
91. Guo CB, Liu MC, Galli SJ, Bochner BS, Kagey-Sobotka A, Lichtenstein LM. Identification of IgE-bearing cells in the late-phase response to antigen in the lung as basophils. *Am J Respir Cell Mol Biol.* 1994;10(4):384–390.
92. Liberman PL. Anaphylaxis. In: Adkinson NF Jr, Bochner BS, Busse WW, Holgate ST, Lemanske RF Jr, Simons FER, ed. *Middleton's Allergy: Principles and Practice.* 2009; 1027–1049.
93. Lewis RA, Goetzl EJ, Wasserman SI, Valone FH, Rubin RH, Austen KF. The release of four mediators of immediate hypersensitivity from human leukemic basophils. *J Immunol.* 1975;114(1Pt1):87–92.
94. Bernini JC, Timmons CF, Sandler ES. Acute basophilic leukemia in a child. Anaphylactoid reaction and coagulopathy secondary to vincristine-mediated degranulation. *Cancer.* 1995;75(1):110–114.
95. Berkowitz FE, Wehde S, Ngwenya ET, Greeff M, Wadee AA, Rabson AR. Anaphylactic shock due to cytarabine in a leukemic child. *Am J Dis Child.* 1987;141(9):1000–1001.
96. Finkelman FD. Anaphylaxis: lessons from mouse models. *J Allergy Clin Immunol.* 2007;120(3):506–515.
97. Jacoby W, Cammarata PV, Findlay S, Pincus SH. Anaphylaxis in mast cell-deficient mice. *J Invest Dermatol.* 1984;83(4):302–304.

98. Oettgen HC, Martin TR, Wynshaw-Boris A, Deng C, Drazen JM, Leder P. Active anaphylaxis in IgE-deficient mice. *Nature.* 1994;370(6488):367–370.
99. Tsujimura Y, Obata K, Mukai K, et al. Basophils play a pivotal role in immunoglobulin-G-mediated but not immunoglobulin-E-mediated systemic anaphylaxis. *Immunity.* 2008;28(4):581–589.
100. Dvorak AM. The mouse basophil, a rare and rarely recognized granulocyte. *Blood.* 2000;96(4):1616–1617.
101. Lee JJ, McGarry MP. When is a mouse basophil not a basophil? *Blood.* 2007;109(3):859–861.
102. Kojima T, Obata K, Mukai K, et al. Mast cells and basophils are selectively activated in vitro and in vivo through CD200R3 in an IgE-independent manner. *J Immunol.* 2007;179(10):7093–7100.
103. Miyajima I, Dombrowicz D, Martin TR, Ravetch JV, Kinet JP, Galli SJ. Systemic anaphylaxis in the mouse can be mediated largely through IgG1 and Fcγ(gamma)RIII. Assessment of the cardiopulmonary changes, mast cell degranulation, and death associated with active or IgE- or IgG1-dependent passive anaphylaxis. *J Clin Invest.* 1997;99(5):901–914.
104. Galli SJ, Franco CB. Basophils are back! *Immunity.* 2008;28(4):495–497.

# Chapter 6
# Protease Mediators of Anaphylaxis

**George H. Caughey**

**Abstract** This chapter reviews the history of studies of mast cell and basophil protease biology and attempts to synthesize current concepts bearing upon their likely contributions to anaphylaxis, focusing on enzymes in the histamine-rich intracellular granules in humans and rodents. As a class, peptidases and proteases are the major proteins of mast cell secretory granules, but seem to be less abundant in basophil granules. The peptidases are secreted with histamine during anaphylactic degranulation. Typically, they are cationic proteins that are packaged in the granule with polyanionic heparin and chondroitin sulfate proteoglycans, and are released in association with them. The peptidases, which differ widely in mechanistic class and substrate specificity, include serine endopeptidases (e.g., chymases, cathepsin G, and tryptases), metallo-exopeptidases (e.g., carboxypeptidase A3), and thiol peptidases (e.g., dipeptidylpeptidase I/cathepsin C). There are potentially important differences between human and rodent mast cell and basophil peptidases in variety and functions. Some of these peptidases have anti-inflammatory as well as inflammatory potential, with roles in host defense. When originating from the secretory granule, most are active at the time of release, but their fates and potential for causing harm outside of the cell differ widely, with some enzymes remaining associated with the cell membrane, or being free but promptly inactivated, and others remaining active and capable of cleaving targets remote from the site of degranulation – indeed, acting systemically. Because of their abundance, several of the chymases and tryptases are biomarkers of anaphylaxis. Beyond their demonstrated utility in this regard, some of the peptidases may contribute to the pathology of anaphylaxis and are under investigation as targets for therapeutic inhibition.

**Keywords** Mast cell • Basophil • Protease • Peptidase • Chymase • Cathepsin G • Tryptase • Carboxypeptidase A3 • Dipeptidylpeptidase I • Cathepsin C • Proteoglycan • RMCPI • RMCPII • mMCP-1 • mMCP-4 • mMCP-6 • mMCP-7

## 6.1 Introduction

In retrospect, it is not surprising that mast cell peptidases came to be used experimentally and clinically as biomarkers of anaphylaxis. This is because they are by far the most abundant proteins of mast cell granules, are largely mast cell- and basophil-specific, are secreted in response to IgE-dependent degranulating stimuli, are detected conveniently in some instances by ELISA, and can have kinetics of appearance and disappearance in the bloodstream that offer a wider window of detection than

G.H. Caughey (✉)
University of California at San Francisco, Medicine and Cardiovascular Research Institute, San Francisco, CA, USA
e-mail: george.caughey@ucsf.edu

M.C. Castells (ed.), *Anaphylaxis and Hypersensitivity Reactions*,
DOI 10.1007/978-1-60327-951-2_6, © Springer Science+Business Media, LLC 2011

provided by more labile products, such as histamine and, especially, metabolites of arachidonic acid. However, significant caveats apply. Mast cell peptidases in a given mammal are unevenly distributed across mast cell and basophil populations in different tissues and tissue microenvironments, so that measuring the appearance of one peptidase in the bloodstream or a body cavity may disproportionately reflect activation of a particular type of mast cell or basophil. Moreover, there are fundamental differences between rats, mice, and humans in the types of peptidases that are useful as markers of systemic mast cell activation. The issue of species differences is just as significant, if not more so, in considering potential contributions of mast cell and basophil peptidases to the pathophysiology of anaphylaxis. The major peptidases of mast cell and basophil secretory granules are divided functionally into **endopeptidases** (the **chymases** and **tryptases** – a rubric first suggested by Lagunoff and Benditt [1,2] at a time when the nature, number, and varieties of these enzymes were only beginning to be appreciated) and **exopeptidases**, especially **mast cell carboxypeptidase A3** and **dipeptidylpeptidase I** (otherwise known as cathepsin C).

## 6.2 Chymase-like Peptidases

### *6.2.1 General Considerations*

Chymases are given top billing here because they were the first class of mast cell peptidase to be detected, characterized, and used as markers of anaphylaxis [3]. Because of the range of forms and functions, the chymases also exemplify some of the challenges in using peptidases to detect mast cell and basophil activation and in determining their contributions to the pathology of anaphylaxis. The major chymase-like peptidases of human mast cells are chymase (product of the CMA1 gene) and cathepsin G (product of CTSG). CMA1 and CTSG are related and are next to each other on chromosome 14q11.2 [4] and clearly arose by gene duplication early in mammalian evolution [5], probably more than 200 million years ago [6,7]. Immunohistochemical surveys [8–11] and studies of purified mast cell extracts suggest that chymase is expressed primarily or exclusively by mast cells [12,13]. Cathepsin G is expressed in the same mast cells that make chymase – and in similar amounts [14,15]. However, cathepsin G is also expressed in neutrophils, monocytes, and dendritic cells. Many more chymase-like genes are present in mice and rats, including several enzymes that have no clear functional or phylogenetic counterpart in humans [16] (see Table 6.1). Although the great majority of the scientific literature concerning systemic release of chymase derives from studies of rodents, human chymase recently was reported to circulate in an $\alpha$(alpha)$_2$-macroglobulin-bound form in which it can cleave peptides, like angiotensin I, from which it generates vasoactive angiotensin II [17].

### *6.2.2 Rat Chymases*

The first mast cell peptidases to be fully purified and characterized structurally and biochemically were chymases (RMCPI and II) from rats. It is perhaps a testament to the wide tissue distribution of mast cells and to their high storage capacity that RMCPI from skeletal muscle and RMCPII ("group-specific protease") from intestine were extensively purified and characterized, including crystallization, before recognition of their mast cell origins [18,19]. Fortunately, the investigations of biochemists pursuing proteases from a variety of tissue and purified mast cell sources converged in the late 1970s, resulting in recognition (1) that RMCPI and II are made and stored by serosal

**Table 6.1** Chymase-like peptidases in humans, mice, and rats

| | Peptidase | Gene | Features | References |
|---|---|---|---|---|
| Human | Chymase; aka α(alpha)-chymase | *CMA1* | Chymotryptic; expressed in $MC_{TC}$ | [4,8,41] |
| | Cathepsin G | *CTSG* | Tryptic, chymotryptic, and Met-ase activity; expressed in $MC_{TC}$, neutrophils, monocytes, and dendritic cells | [14,124] |
| Mouse | mMCP-5; aka α(alpha)-chymase | *Cma1* | Elastolytic, not chymotryptic; expressed in connective tissue MC; phylogenetically similar to human chymase but functionally dissimilar | [125,126] |
| | Cathepsin G | *Ctsg* | Chymotryptic; not tryptic; expressed in neutrophils and ?connective tissue MC | [45,127,128] |
| | mMCP-1 | *Mcpt1* | Chymotryptic β(beta)-chymase; no human ortholog; expressed in mucosal MC; appears in blood and in gut lumen after anaphylaxis | [129,130] |
| | mMCP-2 | *Mcpt2* | Expressed in mucosal MC but lacks chymotryptic activity; β(beta)-chymase with no human ortholog; appears in gut after antigen challenge | [40,129] |
| | mMCP-4 | *Mcpt4* | Chymotryptic, angiotensin II-generating, pro-MMP9-activating β(beta)-chymase; similar to human chymase in function and expression | [35,131,132] |
| | mMCP-8 | *Mcpt8* | Catalytically inactive; granzyme-like; no human ortholog; ? expressed mainly by basophils | [51] |
| | mMCP-9 | *Mcpt9* | Catalytic activity unknown; expressed by uterine MC; **not** an ortholog of rMCP-9 | [133] |
| Rat | rMCP-5; aka α(alpha)-chymase | *Cma1* | Elastolytic, not chymotryptic; expressed in connective tissue MC | [134,135] |
| | Cathepsin G | *Ctsg* | Likely similar to mouse but? not expressed in rat MC | [134] |
| | RMCPI aka rMCP-1 | *Mcpt1* | Chymotryptic β(beta)-chymase; heparin-bound; expressed in connective tissue MC; ortholog of mMCP-4; no human ortholog | [39,136] |
| | RMCPII aka rMCP-2 | *Mcpt2* | Chymotryptic; expressed in mucosal MC; β(beta)-chymase; no human ortholog; systemic release in anaphylaxis | [3,37,38,40] |
| | rMCP-4 | *Mcpt4* | Chymotryptic; ?MC expression; β(beta)-chymase; no human ortholog | [137] |
| | Vascular chymase | *VCH (Mcpt1)* | Chymotryptic; angiotensin II-generating β(beta)-chymase; ?MC expression; no human ortholog | [51] |
| | rMCP-8, 9, 10 | *Mcpt8, 9, 10* | Not characterized; likely catalytically inactive; no human ortholog; ?MC expression | [134] |

(termed "typical" at the time) and mucosal ("atypical") mast cells, respectively, and (2) that the enzymes are structurally and behaviorally distinct [20–26]. The destructive potential of these chymases was recognized early [20], including the possibility that they promote diffusion of plasma to sites of injury by breaking down "ground substance" [27], which is related to the pathophysiology of tissue edema and distributive shock in anaphylaxis. It was also correctly pointed out that as long as chymases remain within mast cells they can cause little harm and that granule heparin proteoglycan might play a role in controlling activity and limiting diffusion away from the mast cell following release [22], which may explain why chymase injected into skin increases the size of wheals caused by histamine [28]. The existence of activated forms of peptidases in mast cell granules was the means by which chymase and tryptase activity was first detected – as histochemical esterase activity [29,30]. This distinguished the mast cell enzymes from pancreatic enzymes like trypsin and chymotrypsinogen, which are released as inactive zymogens from acinar cell granules. It was not until after chymase and tryptase cDNAs were sequenced that it was determined that these enzymes also have zymogen forms, but that activation is essentially complete by the time peptidases are packaged in mature granules, given that there is no coupling of regulated secretion to peptidase activation [31] and that no zymogen forms have been detected in extracts of normal mast cells.

However, chymase pro-forms are observed in mast cells lacking their major activator, dipeptidyl-peptidase I [32]. Intriguingly, normal human mast cells constitutively secrete (but do not store) proenzyme forms of tryptases, and it is these secreted pro-forms that make up the majority of circulating immunoreactive tryptase under baseline conditions and in mastocytosis [33,34]. Whether chymases are secreted constitutively as proenzymes is not known.

More active chymase-like peptidases (and even more genes, some of which encode inactive peptidases) reside in mouse and rat mast cells than in human mast cells (Table 6.1). Furthermore, chymase-like peptidases are more widely distributed in rat and mouse mast cell populations. Chymases can be highly abundant, for example, 40% of soluble protein in cultured mast cells [35], so that chymases are prominent in extracts of tissues like skin and tongue [22,36], even though mast cells generally comprise only a few percentage of total cells in such tissues. In general, chymases have been more useful as biomarkers in rodents, and tryptases in humans – and not solely because of abundance. Differences in biophysical and enzymatic properties, including ability to form complexes with endogenous inhibitors, and differences in tissue distribution, which may affect access to stimulation by allergens, are also important. However, it is important to realize that in rats and mice, the chymase that has found use as a biomarker of anaphylaxis by virtue of systemic release, whether by classic allergen sensitization and challenge [37] or by Pavlovian conditioning [38], is largely confined to mucosal rather than serosal/connective tissue mast cells. Thus, it specifically reflects mucosal mast cell activation, which may or may not be associated with activation of connective tissue mast cells.

RMCPI, which may be regarded as candidate biomarker for systemic release of connective mast cell contents, faces several significant challenges in this regard. Highly cationic RMCPI is released from peritoneal mast cells as an insoluble complex with macromolecular heparin and chondroitin sulfate proteoglycan [39], from which histamine and perhaps tryptases diffuse away. While in this pellet, the chymase is protected from inactivation by circulating inhibitors, like serpins and $\alpha$(alpha)$_2$-macroglobulin. Thus, RMCPI diffuses only slowly away from the granule, does not tend to be spirited away from the extruded granule as a serpin complex, and has not been used as biomarker. On the other hand, RMCPII of mucosal mast cells is less cationic, binds weakly to sulfated glycosaminoglycans like heparin, and is much more soluble after release. It makes its way to the bloodstream and can also be detected by antibody-based techniques in gut secretions after intestinal antigen challenge. So it has been used extensively as a marker of systemic anaphylaxis. RMCPII appearing in rat blood after anaphylaxis is probably inactive and bound to inhibitors such as serpins, although this has not been fully established. It should be noted that RMCPII, which is made and stored nearly exclusively by mucosal mast cells, is not expected to reflect activation of mast cells in non-mucosal locations, such as the dermis and peritoneal cavity.

### *6.2.3 Mouse Chymases as Biomarkers*

The catalytic activity of chymases can affect clearance rates and therefore their utility as biomarkers. For example, the chymase-related peptides mMCP-1 and mMCP-2 are found in similar amounts in mucosal mast cells [20], and are thought to be released in similar quantities from activated mast cells.

However, mMCP-1 reaches far higher levels in blood after systemic release. This appears to be because mMCP-1 cleaves and forms soluble, circulating complexes with serpins [40], which are then detectable by ELISA. MMCP-1 thus is catalytically inactive in the circulating form in which it has found use as a biomarker. However, mMCP-2 is catalytically inactive, thanks to a mutation in a critical region of the substrate-binding site. Consequently, it is unable to complex with serpins (which are suicide inhibitors and must be cleaved before forming a stable complex), and is cleared more rapidly. Other mouse chymase-like peptidases (see Table 6.1), particularly those associated with connective tissue mast cells, have not been used as biomarkers. In the case of mMCP-4, which is the ortholog of RMCPI, there are likely to be similar issues relating to proteoglycan binding that affect diffusion into the systemic circulation.

### 6.2.4 *Human Chymase as a Biomarker*

Human chymase would seem to possess disadvantages relative to rodent chymases like RMCPII and mMCP-1 as biomarkers of anaphylaxis. First, it is a strongly cationic protein and is both attracted to and released with heparin proteoglycan. Second, it is mainly absent from the types of mast cells in mucosal locations that are the sources of the established blood and intestinal biomarkers (RMCPII and mMCP-1) of anaphylaxis in rodents, which is to say that human chymase principally is produced by connective tissue mast cells. On the other hand, exocytosed granules of human connective tissue mast cell are not as durable and insoluble as those of the often-studied rat peritoneal mast cell, apparently in part because the constituent proteoglycans are smaller. Consequently, human chymase may be more readily solubilized. In contrast to mMCP-1, human chymase is relatively resistant to serpins like $\alpha$(alpha)$_1$-antitrypsin and $\alpha$(alpha)$_1$-anti-chymotrypsin, but not because it is catalytically inactive (like mMCP-2); instead, when encountering plasma, chymase tends to be captured by $\alpha$(alpha)$_2$-macroglobulin into a cage-like structure in which it can still cleave small substrates like angiotensin I. Raymond and colleagues recently demonstrated that small concentrations of chymase circulate in human blood as an active enzyme bound to $\alpha$(alpha)$_2$-macroglobulin, in which form it can be detected by activity-based assay [17]. In this form, chymase may be increased in systemic mastocytosis but this is not yet studied in anaphylaxis. Other possibilities for detecting chymase release based on its activity include detection of selectively "nicked" albumin [41] and secretory leukocyte protease inhibitor [42]. Nonetheless, some progress has been made in establishing immunoassay-based techniques for detecting chymase in human serum [43–45]. The biochemical form of human chymase detected by immunoassay is unclear; potentially it is bound to inhibitors like serpins or $\alpha$(alpha)$_2$-macroglobulin, fragmented, or a pro-form.

### 6.2.5 *Chymases in Basophils*

Basophil expression of chymase-like peptidases has received scant attention relative to expression in mast cells. Little (if any) chymase is expressed in human basophils [46,47], at least in normal subjects. However, Li and colleagues found that a subset of subjects with asthma and/or allergy have circulating metachromatic cells that are chymase-positive, including chymase-like chloroacetyl esterase activity. However, some of these cells are c-kit-positive suggesting some may be mast cells or mast cell-like [48]. In basophils of mice, chymase-like activity has not been detected. However, mouse basophils express mMCP-8 [49], which was suggested to be the first basophil-specific differentiation marker in mice. mMCP-8 is more closely related to lymphocyte granzymes and cathepsin G than to chymase, has no human homologue [50], and may be proteolytically inactive [51].

### 6.2.6 Cathepsin G

This intriguing peptidase, which is often too narrowly described as "neutrophil cathepsin G," is stored in the same subset of human mast cells that make and store chymase, and in amounts similar to both chymase and tryptases [14,15]. In theory, cathepsin G is released from mast cells during systemic anaphylaxis, although this has not been reported. The human enzyme is unique in key ways. First, it is highly charged, and, indeed, is the most cationic immune peptidase known. Thus, it is likely to be strongly bound to polyanionic heparin and chrondroitin sulfate proteoglycans of the mast cell granule. Like human chymase, it probably diffuses only slowly from the site of exocytosis. Second, the human enzyme, although it has broad substrate preferences, including tryptic activity, is overall weak toward its best substrates compared with chymase [52]. Nonetheless, it is capable of cleaving a variety of peptide and protein targets potentially relevant to the pathology of anaphylaxis. These targets include complement, extracellular matrix, proteoglycans, proteinase-activated receptors, pro-urokinase, metalloproteinases, and angiotensin I (reviewed in [16]). Cathepsin G also stimulates secretion by airway gland cells [53], and, compared to chymase, is more prone to be inactivated by serpins (like $\alpha$(alpha)$_1$-antichymotrypsin) and less prone to react with $\alpha$(alpha)$_2$-macroglobulin, when released into serum [17,54,55]. Thus, its actions are likely to be brief and it is unlikely to contribute to $\alpha$(alpha)$_2$-macroglobulin-bound chymase-like activity in the bloodstream. On the other hand, cathepsin G, unlike chymase, is expressed in neutrophils, which are short-lived cells, a substantial fraction of which turn over every day. Thus, the body's total daily production of cathepsin G may exceed that of chymase. The functions of mast cell cathepsin G remain to be established. Studies in mice lacking cathepsin G expression suggest that it is important for host defense against bacteria and fungi, especially in combination with elastase [56,57]. The role of cathepsin G from mast cells relative to other cell sources, like neutrophils and dendritic cells, remains to be established.

## 6.3 Tryptase-like Peptidases

### 6.3.1 Mast Cell Tryptases in Rats and Mice

In rats, tryptases have received less attention than heavily scrutinized chymases like RMCPI and II and have not been studied in the context of anaphylaxis. This is mainly because tryptases in rat mast cells are less abundant than chymases – perhaps only 1/20 as abundant as chymases in peritoneal mast cells [21]. Also, rat tryptases appear to be more susceptible to endogenous inhibitors and less stabilized by heparin than the human soluble tryptases, which are relatively much more abundant. Nonetheless, rat tryptases exhibit a number of the properties that make such mast cell enzymes unique, including formation of oligomers [21,58–60]. It has not been reported whether rat tryptases are released systemically during anaphylaxis. On the other hand, as shown in Table 6.2, mouse mast cells harbor several more thoroughly characterized tryptase-like peptidases, include a membrane-anchored form (transmembrane/$\gamma$(gamma)-tryptase) of unknown function produced by the *Tpsg1* gene [61], and two to three soluble tryptases, depending on the strain of mouse. The two enzymes most closely resembling the classic soluble human $\beta$(beta)-tryptases are mMCP-6 and mMCP-7. mMCP-6 is heparin binding, oligomeric, and inhibitor resistant, and is most abundant in connective tissue mast cells. It provokes neutrophilic inflammation when injected into the peritoneum [62]. mMCP-7 is less inflammatory, less stabilized by heparin, and is not expressed in C57BL/6 mice because of a genetic mutation [63,64]. However, in mice in which it is expressed, it can be released systemically and appear in the blood in an active, fibrinolytic form [65] – but this has been demonstrated so far only in the V3 model of mastocytosis, in which the animal's body burden of mast cells and peptidases is very large [66]. Despite the fact that mMCP-6 and mMCP-7 are products of separate (though adjacent) genes and are biophysically distinct, in vitro they can mix and match to form heterotetramers [67], which is even more likely to occur among human β(beta)-tryptases, which are even more closely related to each other. Although the significance of mouse tryptase release to the pathophysiology of anaphylaxis is not yet clear, studies in mice lacking mMCP-6 or lacking both mMCP-6 and mMCP-7 suggest that they help to defend against certain bacteria and parasites [68], while contributing to inflammatory pathology in certain disease models, like immune arthritis [69–71]. Mouse mast cells also appear to express small amounts of the tryptase-like peptidase mMCP-11 [72,73], which is the ortholog of mastin, an enzyme abundantly expressed in dogs and pigs [74–76]. However, there is no expressed ortholog in humans, which contain only a pseudogene [77]. In mice, mMCP-11/mastin appears to be more abundant in basophils than in mast cells [73]. The rat genome also contains an intact mastin-like gene [76], although rat mast cells and basophil expression of MCP-11/mastin have not been examined. Potentially, mouse basophils contain more tryptase-like activity than some subsets of mast cells, although basophils and mast cell subsets remain to be compared in this regard. Overall, it can be concluded that mast cells and basophils of rats and mice express and release a variety of granule-associated tryptase-like peptidases, some of which are pro-inflammatory and may be pathogenic in anaphylaxis. However, compared to the corresponding cells in humans, the rodent mast cells and basophils express much lower amounts of classic soluble tryptases related to human β(beta) (see section below and Table 6.2), and much higher amounts (in basophils, particularly) of mastin-like MCP-11, which is not expressed at all in humans. Therefore, insights concerning the roles and relative importance of tryptase-like peptidases in anaphylaxis derived from rodent studies may not translate fluently to humans.

### *6.3.2 Mast Cell Tryptases in Humans: Roles in Anaphylaxis*

Human tryptases in mast cells are remarkable in abundance, variety, and genetic variation. As detailed elsewhere in this book, the measurement of immunoreactive mature tryptase in blood is clinically valuable and widely used to diagnose systemic mast cell degranulation in the cases of possible anaphylaxis. Tryptase immunoassays are also useful to detect local mast cell activation in a variety of biological samples, such as nasal secretions, tears, bronchoalveolar lavage, and skin blister fluid, and sputum, typically collected in the context of clinical research. Beyond their utility as markers of mast cell degranulation, tryptases may affect the clinical course of anaphylaxis, as suggested by multiple lines of indirect evidence. For example, (1) β(beta)-tryptases cleave and inactivate bronchodilating peptides, like vasoactive intestinal peptide, with the likely consequence of worsening bronchospasm [78]. (2) They also enhance airway smooth muscle contraction by bronchoconstrictor agonists, such as histamine [79,80]. (3) By fragmenting a procoagulant protein (fibrinogen) and activating pro-urokinase plasminogen activator – in association with the heparin with which they are released as a complex – β(beta)-tryptases oppose both the formation and persistence of fibrin clots at sites of mast cell activation [81,82]. In the context of anaphylaxis, this may have the effect of allowing fluid exiting vessels rendered leaky by histamine to travel farther and faster in various tissue sites before being obstructed by the formation of fibrin clots. (4) Tryptases may promote the spread of degranulation signals to other mast cells, by unclear mechanisms, as suggested by studies in experimental animals using tryptase inhibitors and exogenous tryptase [83,84]. Most of these effects are likely to be due to tryptase released at tissue sites at or near the site of mast cell degranulation, rather than effects of tryptases conveyed to remote systemic locations via the bloodstream. This is because tryptase in the bloodstream, although immunoreactive, has not been shown to be active, and because the timing of appearance of tryptase in the blood after an anaphylactic event does not conform well to kinetics of key signs and symptoms [85].

**Table 6.2** Tryptase-like peptidases in humans, mice, and rats

| | Peptidase | Gene locus | Features | Selected References |
|---|---|---|---|---|
| Human | α(alpha)-tryptase | *TPSAB1* | Activation-defective and catalytically impaired; constitutively secreted; not stored; often genetically absent; allelic partner is β(beta)I; forms haplotypes with β(beta)II | [34,38,95,99,100] |
| | β(beta)I-tryptase aka β(beta)1 | *TPSAB1* | Classic soluble tryptase; stored in MC granules and secreted; forms inhibitor-resistant tetramers; diglycosylated | [91] |
| | β(beta)II-tryptase aka β(beta)2 | *TPSB2* | Stored in MC granules and secreted; forms inhibitor-resistant tetramers; monoglycosylated | [91,139,140] |
| | β(beta)III-tryptase aka β(beta)III | *TPSB2* | Likely active, stored, and secreted; allelic partner is β(beta)II; forms haplotypes with β(beta)I; diglycosylated | [91,100] |
| | βIII(beta) $^{FS}$-tryptase | *TPSB2* | Inactive, frame-shifted variant of β(beta)III; common in some non-Asian populations | [100] |
| | γ(gamma)-tryptase aka transmembrane tryptase | *TPSG1* | Active with substrate preferences distinct from β(beta)-tryptases; attached to secretory granule membrane via peptide anchor; limited MC expression | [98,101,102] |
| | δ(delta)-tryptase aka mMCP-7-like | *TPSD1* | Chimeric, severely truncated, and nearly catalytically inactive; limited MC expression | [97,104,141] |
| Mouse | mMCP-6 aka Tryptase 1 | *Mcpt6* aka *Tpsb2* | Tryptic, soluble, tetrameric, heparin-binding; functionally most closely related to human β(beta)I ortholog of human α(alpha)- and β(beta)-tryptases | [66,96] |
| | mMCP-7 aka Tryptase 2 | *Mcpt7* aka *Tpsab1* | Tryptic, soluble, tetrameric; partly related to human δ(delta) not expressed in some mouse strains (e.g., C57BL/6J); can be released systemically during anaphylaxis | [64,66,97,104] |
| | mMCP-11 aka mastin, Prss34 | *Prss34* | Active; tryptic; expressed primarily in basophils; ortholog of mastin in dogs; no expressed human ortholog | [72,73,76] |
| | γ(gamma)-tryptase aka transmembrane tryptase | *Tpsg1* | Attached to secretory granule membrane via peptide anchor; limited MC expression | [61,103] |
| Rat | rMCP-6 aka Tryptase 1 | *Tpsb2* aka *Mcpt6* | Appears similar to mouse enzyme; expressed in connective tissue MC | [134,142] |
| | rMCP-7 aka Tryptase 2 | *Tpsab1* aka *Mcpt7* | Appears similar to mouse enzyme; expressed in some connective tissue MC | [60,134] |
| | rMCP-11 aka mastin, Prss34 | *Prss34* | Not characterized; appears similar to mouse enzyme | [76] |
| | γ(gamma) Tryptase aka transmembrane tryptase | *Tpsg1* | Not characterized; appears similar to mouse enzyme | [96] |

### 6.3.3 Human Mast Cell Tryptases: Variation of Form and Function

The presence of tryptases in human mast cells was suspected more than 50 years ago based on tryptic activity detected in histochemical surveys of mast cell-rich tissues [30]. In the early 1980s of the pre-genomic era, when human mast cell "tryptase" was extracted, purified, and characterized as a secretable mast cell enzyme distinct from then-known tryptic serine peptidases of digestion, coagulation, fibrinolysis, and complement activation [86–88], there was little inkling of the variety of forms and functions that would be revealed in the genomic era. In retrospect, most "tryptase" purified from mast cells or tissues is a mixture of β(beta)-type tryptases, which are products of two genes: *TPSB2* and *TSPAB1*, as summarized in Table 6.2. These are closely related to the classical soluble tryptases present in most mammalian genomes, of which human β(beta)I and β(beta)III are most representative. Additional variation of potential functional significance is generated by alternative mRNA splicing [89] and posttranslational processing, especially N-glycosylation, for which there can be differences between tissues and individuals [90]. However, even β(beta)-tryptase glycosylation variants can have a genetic basis: for example, β(beta)II has a single potential site of N-glycosylation, whereas β(beta) I and β(beta)III have two sites [91]. α(alpha)-tryptase, so named because it is translated from the first human tryptase mRNA to be sequenced [92], is anomalous and appears to be doubly defective in the sense that it possesses a proenzyme mutation that hinders proteolytic activation [92] and a catalytic domain mutation that greatly diminishes catalytic activity [93–95]. Furthermore, α(alpha) appears to be secreted constitutively by human mast cells, rather than being stored in secretory granules [34]. There are no α(alpha)-type tryptases in rodents or non-primates; indeed, phylogenetic analysis shows that the mutations arose separately – and very recently in the case of the processing mutation – in primate evolution. Thus, human α(alpha) genes are deficiency alleles. Although it was originally assumed that α(alpha)- and β(beta)-tryptases are products of separate gene loci, this is only partly correct, for α(alpha) is an allele at a site that also accepts functional β(beta)I alleles [97,98]. Because of this, many humans inheriting two β(beta)I alleles are completely α(alpha)-deficient [99,100]. In addition to *TPSB2* and *TSPAB1*, there are two more mast cell tryptase loci: *TPSG1* and *TPSD1*, which encode γ(gamma)- and δ(delta)-tryptases, respectively. Human γ(gamma)-tryptases are type I transmembrane peptidases that are similar to their rodent orthologs [98]. They are catalytically active tryptic enzymes with substrate preferences differing from those of β(beta)-tryptases [101,102]. Although human γ(gamma)-tryptases provoke airway hyperresponsiveness when introduced to mouse trachea [101], their function in their membrane-attached form is unknown. Unlike prostasin and some other related type I transmembrane peptidases, γ(gamma)-tryptases apparently do not exchange the peptide anchor for a lipid anchor [98,103], nor is there evidence of proteolytic shedding. Thus, γ(gamma) tryptase may remain associated with the cell surface after mast cell exocytosis. Phylogenetic analysis suggests that human β(beta) and other soluble mammalian tryptases evolved from membrane-anchored forms similar to γ(gamma) tryptase and to the epithelial transmembrane peptidase prostasin [96,98]. Potentially, γ(gamma) tryptases are an ancestral form of tryptases. In any case, they are absent in some mammalian genomes (e.g., in dogs) and thus lack a highly conserved function. δ(delta)-tryptases, on the other hand, are chimeric proteins generated recently in primate evolution by gene duplication, partial conversion, and point mutation [97,104]. In humans, mast cell expression of δ(delta) mRNA and protein is limited and the catalytic domain is severely truncated with minimal, if any, catalytic activity [105]. However, in some primates, like old-world monkeys, the δ(delta) tryptase catalytic domain is full length and active [104]. In summary, human mast cell tryptases are products of a cluster of four gene loci, and occur in membrane-anchored γ(gamma) and soluble α(alpha), β(beta), and δ(delta) forms. Of the soluble forms, only the β(beta) tryptases have the combined attributes of being catalytically active, stored in high concentrations in secretory granules, and released with mast cell degranulation. Thus, despite the confusing variety of human tryptase genes, alleles, and products, β(beta) tryptases should be regarded as the prime suspects in the pathogenesis of anaphylaxis [106].

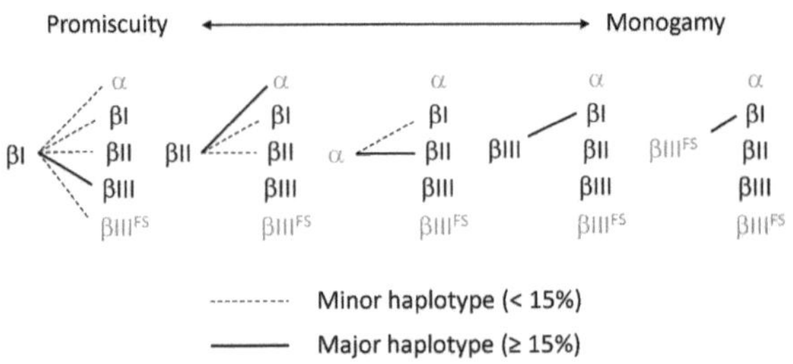


**Fig. 6.1** Haplotype associations among human soluble α(alpha)-/β(beta)-tryptase genes (at gene loci *TPSAB1* and *TPSB2*). Note that deficiency alleles (α(alpha) and β(beta)III$^{FS}$) are always paired with an active allele

### 6.3.4 Human Soluble Tryptases: Significance of Genetic Variation and Disequilibrium

Recent surveys reveal that individuals and indeed geographically separated human populations vary quite strikingly in the number of inherited active β(beta) tryptases, with individuals inheriting as few as two to as many as four active genes [100]. Because the two loci at which β(beta) alleles are found (*TPSAB1* and *TPSB2*) are only a few kilobases apart, not surprisingly they are in strong linkage disequilibrium, and the number and types of haplotypes are restricted (see Fig. 6.1). Consequently, deficiency alleles (which, like α(alpha) and recently described frame-shifted β(beta) III$^{FS}$ [100], are common), are always paired on the same chromosome with an allele encoding an active tryptase (β(beta) I, β(beta) II, or β(beta) III) [100]. In this manner, individuals are protected from complete deficiency of catalytically active tryptases – and this protection is observed in a variety of genetically distinct populations. This is indirect evidence that active tryptases play important and perhaps critical roles in humans, presumably related to host defense. However, if inheritance of two active tryptases is the minimum needed to preserved homeostatic functions, then perhaps inheritance of four active tryptases – as occurs in some individuals in all surveyed populations – is too many, that is, carries a cost such as overexuberant allergic and other inflammatory reactions, including anaphylaxis. This possibility is suggested by the observations that the majority of individuals in most surveyed populations inherit three active β(beta) tryptases, not two or four, which is evidence of so-called ambidirectional or "stabilizing" natural selection, in which inheritance of three active tryptases may be optimal in most environments and genetic backgrounds. This speculation aside, it remains to be established that there is a clinically or physiologically significant difference in mast cell tryptase content, host defense contributions, or phenotype in allergic or other diseases based on tryptase genotype. There are increases, albeit small, in baseline plasma levels of immunoreactive total tryptase (pro-α(alpha) plus pro-β(beta)) in healthy individuals inheriting β(beta) alleles [107], as well as possible decreases in mature tryptase levels in α(alpha)-positive subjects with mastocytosis [33]. These findings are consistent with available data from genetic studies and from studies of tryptase storage and release from isolated mast cells, which indicate that α(alpha) is unable to convert from proenzyme to mature form, that α(alpha)-tryptase is secreted constitutively rather than stored, and that humans lacking α(alpha) genes inherit β(beta) alleles instead.

### 6.3.5 Tryptase Expression in Human Basophils

Evidence from several investigators suggests that basophils express tryptases in variable (although usually small) amounts [46–48,108]. The basis of the heterogeneity, whether genetic, environmental, or an interaction between genes and environment, is presently unclear. On average, the level of stored, active tryptase in human basophils is <1% of levels in mast cells, and is best explained by comparatively low levels of tryptase mRNA content [46]. At one time, reverse transcriptase PCR studies suggested that basophils selectively express α(alpha)-tryptases [108]. However, further comparisons of tryptase mRNA and protein content in subjects of various α(alpha)-/β(beta)-tryptase genotypes, including α(alpha)-null [108], do not support the initial impressions. In light of these considerations, combined with the overwhelming numerical superiority of mast cell versus basophil numbers, it seems unlikely that basophils contribute significantly to increases in plasma tryptase content during systemic anaphylaxis.

## 6.4 Carboxypeptidase A3

Mast cell carboxypeptidase A (otherwise known as carboxypeptidase A3; gene symbol *CPA3*) appears to be expressed primarily if not exclusively in mast cells [109,110]. Like tryptases, chymases, and cathepsin G, it is stored with heparin and histamine as an activated enzyme in membrane-bound intracellular granules, from which it is released outside of the cell after stimulated exocytosis. Less is known of its fate outside of the cell after secretion. In humans, CPA3 expression appears to be confined primarily to chymase-containing ($MC_{TC}$) mast cells [111]. Indeed, analysis of macromolecular forms of exocytosed proteoglycan-peptidase complexes reveals that CPA3 tends to segregate with chymase-proteoglycan complexes rather than with β(beta)-tryptase-proteoglycan complexes [111]. Possibly, CPA3 associates with chymase because its substrate preferences are optimized for removing the neo-C-terminal aromatic and aliphatic amino acids generated by the action of chymotryptic enzymes like human chymase and mouse chymase MCP-4 [112]. Although it is capable of acting in tandem with chymases to break down peptide targets [113], CPA3 is unrelated to chymases, being a zinc-dependent metallo-exopeptidase similar to pancreatic carboxypeptidases [114]. Like other mast cell secretory granule peptidases, CPA3 is synthesized initially as an inactive zymogen, which is activated by proteolytic cleavage. Unlike chymases and tryptases, CPA3 does not appear to be activated by dipeptidylpeptidase I (DPPI), for protein levels and activity actually increase in cultured mouse mast cells lacking DPPI [115]. Rather, activation of CPA3 appears to be a function of an aspartyl peptidase cathepsin E [116]. Mast cell CPA3's roles and importance in anaphylaxis are not known. However, studies in mice engineered to selectively lack active CPA3 suggest that mast cell CPA3 can be a critical determinant in mice of survival from snake bite by inactivating venoms, notably sarafotoxins [117]. CPA3 also appears to pay a major role in limiting toxicity of endogenous sarafotoxin-related peptides such as endothelins, thereby limiting mortality from sepsis and acute bacterial peritonitis [117,118]. Whether detoxification is a more general function of CPA3 – and the extent to which CPA3 benefit from or require prior actions of mast cell-derived endopeptidases, like chymase and cathepsin G – remain to be determined (Fig. 6.2).

## 6.5 Dipeptidylpeptidase I (DPPI)/Cathepsin C

DPPI, which is also known as cathepsin C, is a thiol-class oligomeric peptidase [119]. Being expressed by most granulated leukocytes, DPPI is not a specific product of mast cells, but is particularly abundant in them. Although DPPI has some endoproteolytic activity, it is primarily an exopeptidase that removes amino acids in pairs from the amino terminus of peptides and proteins. This activity is particularly suited to removal of the pro-dipeptide from tryptases and chymases, which is indeed its major identified role in mast cells [138]. In mice, mast cells cultured from *Dppi* $^{-/-}$ bone marrow have little if any active chymase and have reduced levels of active tryptase [32].

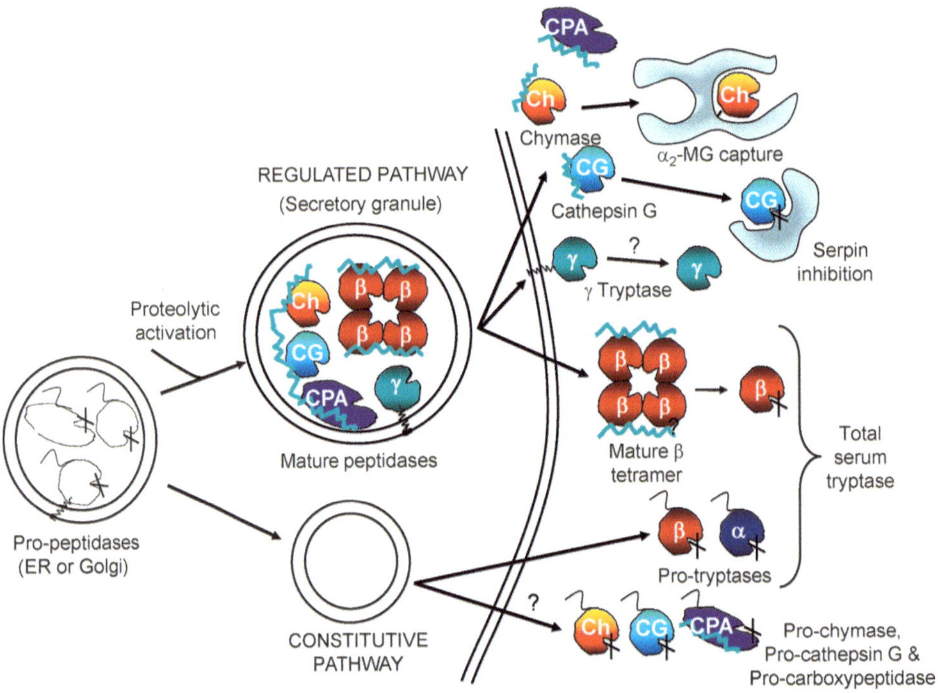


**Fig. 6.2** Activation, storage, secretion, and inactivation of mast cell peptidases. The peptidases are synthesized initially as inactive pro-peptidase zymogens. Activated forms are stored in classic secretory granules. Unprocessed, inactive forms may be diverted to constitutive pathways of secretion, and detected in blood by immunoassay. Secreted active peptidases are destined for a variety of fates, including $\alpha$(alpha)$_2$-macroglobulin capture (chymase, Ch), inactivation by serpins (cathepsin G, CG), dissociation into inactive monomers (β(beta)-tryptase), and (potentially) shedding from the cell surface (γ(gamma)-tryptase). The fate of mast cell carboxypeptidase A (CPA) after release is unclear. The extent to which proenzyme forms of chymase, cathepsin G, and carboxypeptidase A are secreted remains to be established

In contrast, they have increased levels of active carboxypeptidase A3 [115]. Thus, DPPI influences mast cell granule content in diverse ways, some of which remain to be explained on the basis of its enzymatic functions. Immunohistochemical surveys suggest that mast cells are the major source of DPPI in uninflamed tissues, like airway [120]. DPPI can be secreted from mast cells along with other constituents of the secretory granule [121], and unlike some thiol cathepsins, is active at the neutral to alkaline pH of most extracellular fluids. Although it is possible that extracellular release of DPPI in the context of local or systemic mast cell degranulation is pathophysiologically important, there is little present evidence of this possibility. Because DPPI is not mast cell-specific, it is not likely to be a useful biomarker of mast cell activation. Mice and humans lacking DPPI activity have a variety of immune deficits, which have been attributed to the absence of DPPI's contributions as an activator of mast cell, neutrophil, and lymphocyte serine peptidases [122,123].

## References

1. Lagunoff D, Benditt EP. Proteolytic enzymes of mast cells. *Ann NY Acad Sci.* 1963;103:185–198.
2. Lagunoff D. Mast cell proteases: a historical perspective. In: Caughey GH, ed. *Mast Cell Proteases in Immunology and Biology.* New York: Marcel Dekker; 1995:1–8.
3. Miller HRP, Woodbury RG, Huntley JF, Newlands G. Systemic release of mucosal mast-cell protease in primed rats challenged with *Nippostrongylus brasiliensis*. *Immunology.* 1983;49:471–479.

4. Caughey GH, Schaumberg TH, Zerweck EH, et al. The human mast cell chymase gene (CMA1): mapping to the cathepsin G/granzyme gene cluster and lineage-restricted expression. *Genomics.* 1993;15:614–620.
5. Caughey GH, Beauchamp J, Schlatter D, et al. Guinea pig chymase is leucine-specific: a novel example of functional plasticity in the chymase/granzyme family of serine peptidases. *J Biol Chem.* 2008;283:13943–13951.
6. Wouters MA, Liu K, Riek P, Husain A. A despecialization step underlying evolution of a family of serine proteases. *Mol Cell.* 2003;12:343–354.
7. Gallwitz M, Reimer JM, Hellman L. Expansion of the mast cell chymase locus over the past 200 million years of mammalian evolution. *Immunogenetics.* 2006;58:655–669.
8. Irani AA, Schechter NM, Craig SS, et al. Two types of human mast cells that have distinct neutral protease compositions. *Proc Natl Acad Sci USA.* 1986;83:4464–4468.
9. Irani AM, Bradford TR, Kepley CL, et al. Detection of MCT and MCTC types of human mast cells by immunohistochemistry using new monoclonal anti-tryptase and anti-chymase antibodies. *J Histochem Cytochem.* 1989;37:1509–1515.
10. Weidner N, Austen KF. Heterogeneity of mast cells at multiple body sites-fluorescent determination of avidin binding and immunofluorescent determination of chymase, tryptase, and carboxypeptidase content. *Path Res Pract.* 1993;189:156–162.
11. Buckley MG, McEuen AR, Walls AF. The detection of mast cell subpopulations in formalin-fixed human tissues using a new monoclonal antibody specific for chymase. *J Pathol.* 1999;189:138–143.
12. Schechter NM, Choi JK, Slavin DA, et al. Identification of a chymotrypsin-like proteinase in human mast cells. *J Immunol.* 1986;137:962–970.
13. Schwartz LB, Irani A-MA, Roller K, et al. Quantitation of histamine, tryptase, and chymase in dispersed human T and TC mast cells. *J Immunol.* 1987;138:2611–2615.
14. Schechter NM, Irani AM, Sprows JL, et al. Identification of a cathepsin G-like proteinase in the MCTC type of human mast cell. *J Immunol.* 1990;145:2652–2661.
15. Benyon RC, Enciso JA, Befus AD. Analysis of human skin mast cell proteins by two-dimensional gel electrophoresis: identification of tryptase as a sialylated glycoprotein. *J Immunol.* 1993;151:2699–2706.
16. Caughey GH. A pulmonary perspective on GASPIDs: granule-associated serine peptidases of immune defense. *Curr Resp Med Rev.* 2006;2:263–277.
17. Raymond WW, Su S, Makarova A, et al. $\alpha$ (alpha) $_2$-Macroglobulin capture allows detection of mast cell chymase in serum and creates a reservoir of angiotensin II-generating activity. *J Immunol.* 2009;182:5770–5777.
18. Woodbury RG, Katunuma N, Kobayashi K, et al. Covalent structure of a group-specific protease from rat small intestine. *Biochemistry.* 1978;17:811–819.
19. Sanada Y, Yasogawa N, Katunuma N. Crystallization and amino acid composition of a serine protease from rat skeletal muscle. *Biochem Biophys Res Commun.* 1978;82:108–113.
20. Pastan I, Almqvist S. Purification and properties of a mast cell protease. *J Biol Chem.* 1966;241:5090.
21. Lagunoff D, Pritzl P. Characterization of rat mast cell granule proteins. *Arch Biochem Biophys.* 1976;173:554–563.
22. Yurt R, Austen KF. Preparative purification of the rat mast cell chymase: characterization and interaction with granule components. *J Exp Med.* 1977;146:1405–1419.
23. Seppa HE. Rat skin main neutral protease: immunohistochemical localization. *J Invest Dermatol.* 1978;71:311–315.
24. Woodbury RG, Everitt M, Sanada Y, et al. A major serine protease in rat skeletal muscle: evidence for its mast cell origin. *Proc Natl Acad Sci USA.* 1978;75:5311–5313.
25. Woodbury RG, Gruzenski GM, Lagunoff D. Immunofluorescent localization of a serine protease in rat small intestine. *Proc Natl Acad Sci USA.* 1978;75:2785–2789.
26. Woodbury RG, Neurath H. Purification of an atypical mast cell protease and its levels in developing rats. *Biochemistry.* 1978;17:4298–4304.
27. Seppa H, Vaananen K, Korhonen K. Effect of mast cell chymase of rat skin on intercellular matrix: a histochemical study. *Acta Histochem (Jena).* 1979;64:64–70.
28. Rubinstein I, Nadel JA, Graf PD, Caughey GH. Mast cell chymase potentiates histamine-induced wheal formation in the skin of ragweed-allergic dogs. *J Clin Invest.* 1990;86:555–559.
29. Gomori G. Chloroacyl esters as histochemical substrates. *J Histochem Cytochem.* 1953;1:469–470.
30. Glenner GG, Cohen LA. Histochemical demonstration of a species-specific trypsin-like enzyme in mast cells. *Nature.* 1960;185:846–847.
31. Caughey GH, Lazarus SC, Viro NF, et al. Tryptase and chymase: comparison of extraction and release in two dog mastocytoma lines. *Immunology.* 1988;63:339–344.
32. Wolters PJ, Pham CT, Muilenburg DJ, et al. Dipeptidyl peptidase I is essential for activation of mast cell chymases, but not tryptases, in mice. *J Biol Chem.* 2001;276:18551–18556.
33. Akin C, Soto D, Brittain E, et al. Tryptase haplotype in mastocytosis: relationship to disease variant and diagnostic utility of total tryptase levels. *Clin Immunol.* 2007;123:268–271.

34. Schwartz LB, Min HK, Ren S, et al. Tryptase precursors are preferentially and spontaneously released, whereas mature tryptase is retained by HMC-1 cells, Mono-mac-6 cells, and human skin-derived mast cells. *J Immunol.* 2003;170:5667–5673.
35. Pemberton AD, Brown JK, Wright SH, et al. The proteome of mouse mucosal mast cell homologues: the role of transforming growth factor beta1. *Proteomics.* 2006;6:623–631.
36. Caughey GH, Raymond WW, Wolters PJ. Angiotensin II generation by mast cell α (alpha)- and β (beta)-chymases. *Biochim Biophys Acta.* 2000;1480:245–257.
37. Scudamore CL, Thornton EM, McMillan L, et al. Release of the mucosal mast cell granule chymase, rat mast cell protease-II, during anaphylaxis is associated with the rapid development of paracellular permeability to macromolecules in rat jejunum. *J Exp Med.* 1995;182:1871–1881.
38. MacQueen G, Marshall J, Perdue M, Siegel S, Bienenstock J. Pavlovian conditioning of rat mucosal mast cells to secrete rat mast cell protease ii. *Science.* 1989;243:83–85.
39. Le Trong H, Neurath H, Woodbury RG. Substrate specificity of the chymotrypsin-like protease in secretory granules isolated from rat mast cells. *Proc Natl Acad Sci USA.* 1987;84:364–367.
40. Pemberton AD, Wright SH, Knight PA, Miller HR. Anaphylactic release of mucosal mast cell granule proteases: role of serpins in the differential clearance of mouse mast cell proteases-1 and -2. *J Immunol.* 2006;176:899–904.
41. Raymond WW, Waugh Ruggles S, Craik CS, Caughey GH. Albumin is a substrate of human chymase: prediction by combinatorial peptide screening and development of a selective inhibitor based on the albumin cleavage site. *J Biol Chem.* 2003;278:34517–34524.
42. Belkowski SM, Boot JD, Mascelli MA, et al. Cleaved secretory leucocyte protease inhibitor as a biomarker of chymase activity in allergic airway disease. *Clin Exp Allergy.* 2009;39:1179–1186.
43. Satomura K, Shimizu S, Nagato T, et al. Establishment of an assay method for human mast cell chymase. *Hepatol Res.* 2002;24:361–367.
44. Nishio H, Takai S, Miyazaki M, et al. Usefulness of serum mast cell-specific chymase levels for postmortem diagnosis of anaphylaxis. *Int J Legal Med.* 2005;119:331–334.
45. Sun J, Zhang J, Lindholt JS, et al. Critical role of mast cell chymase in mouse abdominal aortic aneurysm formation. *Circulation.* 2009;120:973–982.
46. Xia H-Z, Kepley CL, Sakai K, et al. Quantitation of tryptase, chymase, $F_c$ε (epsilon) RIα (alpha), and $F_c$ε (epsilon) RIγ (gamma) mRNAs in human mast cells and basophils by competitive reverse transcription-polymerase chain reaction. *J Immunol.* 1995;154:5472–5480.
47. Foster B, Schwartz LB, Devouassoux G, et al. Characterization of mast-cell tryptase-expressing peripheral blood cells as basophils. *J Allergy Clin Immunol.* 2002;109:287–293.
48. Li L, Li Y, Reddel SW, et al. Identification of basophilic cells that express mast cell granule proteases in the peripheral blood of asthma, allergy, and drug-reactive patients. *J Immunol.* 1998;161:5079–5086.
49. Poorafshar M, Helmby H, Troye-Blomberg M, Hellman L. MMCP-8, the first lineage-specific differentiation marker for mouse basophils. Elevated numbers of potent Il-4-producing and MMCP-8- positive cells in spleens of malaria-infected mice. *Eur J Immunol.* 2000;30:2660–2668.
50. Lunderius C, Hellman L. Characterization of the gene encoding mouse mast cell protease 8 (mMCP-8), and a comparative analysis of hematopoietic serine protease genes. *Immunogenetics.* 2001;53:225–232.
51. Gallwitz M, Enoksson M, Hellman L. Expression profile of novel members of the rat mast cell protease (RMCP)-2 and (RMCP)-8 families, and functional analyses of mouse mast cell protease (MMCPO)-8. *Immunogenetics.* 2007;59:391–405.
52. Powers JC, Tanaka T, Harper JW, et al. Mammalian chymotrypsin-like enzymes. Comparative reactivities of rat mast cell proteases, human and dog skin chymases, and human cathepsin G with peptide 4-nitroanilide substrates and with peptide chloromethyl ketone and sulfonyl fluoride inhibitors. *Biochemistry.* 1985;24:2048–2058.
53. Sommerhoff CP, Nadel JA, Basbaum CB, Caughey GH. Neutrophil elastase and cathepsin G stimulate secretion from cultured bovine airway gland serous cells. *J Clin Invest.* 1990;85:682–689.
54. Travis J, Bowen J, Baugh R. Human alpha-1-antichymotrypsin: interaction with chymotrypsin-like proteinases. *Biochemistry.* 1978;17:5651–5656.
55. Schechter NM, Sprows JL, Schoenberger OL, et al. Reaction of human skin chymotrypsin-like proteinase chymase with plasma proteinase inhibitors. *J Biol Chem.* 1989;264:21308–21315.
56. Raptis SZ, Shapiro SD, Simmons PM, et al. Serine protease cathepsin G regulates adhesion-dependent neutrophil effector functions by modulating integrin clustering. *Immunity.* 2005;22:679–691.
57. Tkalcevic J, Novelli M, Phylactides M, et al. Impaired immunity and enhanced resistance to endotoxin in the absence of neutrophil elastase and cathepsin G. *Immunity.* 2000;12:201–210.
58. Lagunoff D, Rickard A, Marquardt C. Rat mast cell tryptase. *Arch Biochem Biophys.* 1991;291:52–58.
59. Kido H, Fukusen N, Katunuma N. Chymotrypsin- and trypsin-type serine proteases in rat mast cells: properties and functions. *Arch Biochem Biophys.* 1985;239:436–443.
60. Braganza VJ, Simmons WH. Tryptase from rat skin: purification and properties. *Biochemistry.* 1991;30:4997–5007.

61. Wong GW, Tang Y, Feyfant E, et al. Identification of a new member of the tryptase family of mouse and human mast cell proteases which possesses a novel COOH-terminal hydrophobic extension. *J Biol Chem.* 1999;274:30784–30793.
62. Huang C, Friend DS, Qiu WT, et al. Induction of a selective and persistent extravasation of neutrophils into the peritoneal cavity by tryptase mouse mast cell protease 6. *J Immunol.* 1998;160:1910–1919.
63. Hunt JE, Stevens RL, Austen KF, et al. Natural disruption of the mouse mast cell protease 7 gene in the C57BL/6 mouse. *J Biol Chem.* 1996;271:2851–2855.
64. Ghildyal N, Friend DS, Freelund R, et al. Lack of expression of the tryptase mouse mast cell protease 7 in mast cells of the C57BL/6J mouse. *J Immunol.* 1994;153:2624–2630.
65. Huang CF, Wong GW, Ghildyal N, et al. The tryptase, mouse mast cell protease 7, exhibits anticoagulant activity in vivo and in vitro due to its ability to degrade fibrinogen in the presence of the diverse array of protease inhibitors in plasma. *J Biol Chem.* 1997;272:31885–31893.
66. Ghildyal N, Friend DS, Stevens RL, et al. Fate of two mast cell tryptases in V3 mastocytosis and normal BALB/c mice undergoing passive systemic anaphylaxis: prolonged retention of exocytosed mMCP-6 in connective tissues, and rapid accumulation of enzymatically active mMCP-7 in the blood. *J Exp Med.* 1996;184:1061–1073.
67. Huang C, Morales G, Vagi A, et al. Formation of enzymatically active, homotypic, and heterotypic tetramers of mouse mast cell tryptases. Dependence on a conserved Trp-rich domain on the surface. *J Biol Chem.* 2000;275:351–358.
68. Thakurdas SM, Melicoff E, Sansores-Garcia L, et al. The mast cell-restricted tryptase mMCP-6 has a critical immunoprotective role in bacterial infections. *J Biol Chem.* 2007;282:20809–20815.
69. McNeil HP, Shin K, Campbell IK, et al. The mouse mast cell-restricted tetramer-forming tryptases mouse mast cell protease 6 and mouse mast cell protease 7 are critical mediators in inflammatory arthritis. *Arthritis Rheum.* 2008;58:2338–2346.
70. Shin K, Watts GF, Oettgen HC, et al. Mouse mast cell tryptase mMCP-6 is a critical link between adaptive and innate immunity in the chronic phase of *Trichinella spiralis* infection. *J Immunol.* 2008;180:4885–4891.
71. Shin K, Nigrovic PA, Crish J, et al. Mast cells contribute to autoimmune inflammatory arthritis via their tryptase/heparin complexes. *J Immunol.* 2009;182:647–656.
72. Wong GW, Yasuda S, Morokawa N, et al. Mouse chromosome 17a3.3 contains 13 genes that encode functional tryptic-like serine proteases with distinct tissue and cell expression patterns. *J Biol Chem.* 2004;279:2438–2452.
73. Ugajin T, Kojima T, Mukai K, et al. Basophils preferentially express mouse mast cell protease 11 among the mast cell tryptase family in contrast to mast cells. *J Leukoc Biol.* 2009;86:1417–1425.
74. Yezzi MJ, Hsieh IE, Caughey GH. Mast cell and neutrophil expression of dog mast cell proteinase-3, a novel tryptase-related serine proteinase. *J Immunol.* 1994;152:3064–3072.
75. Vanderslice P, Craik CS, Nadel JA, Caughey GH. Molecular cloning of dog mast cell tryptase and a related protease: structural evidence of a unique mode of serine protease activation. *Biochemistry.* 1989;28:4148–4155.
76. Raymond WW, Sommerhoff CP, Caughey GH. Mastin is a gelatinolytic mast cell peptidase resembling a mini-proteasome. *Arch Biochem Biophys.* 2005;435:311–322.
77. Caughey GH. Genetic insights into mast cell chymase and tryptase function. *Clin Exp All Rev.* 2004;4:96–101.
78. Tam EK, Caughey GH. Degradation of airway neuropeptides by human lung tryptase. *Am J Respir Cell Mol Biol.* 1990;3:27–32.
79. Sekizawa K, Caughey GH, Lazarus SC, et al. Mast cell tryptase causes airway smooth muscle hyperresponsiveness in dogs. *J Clin Invest.* 1989;83:175–179.
80. Johnson PRA, Ammit AJ, Carlin SM, et al. Mast cell tryptase potentiates histamine-induced contraction in human sensitized bronchus. *Eur Resp J.* 1997;10:38–43.
81. Stack MS, Johnson DA. Human mast cell tryptase activates single-chain urinary-type plasminogen activator (pro-urokinase). *J Biol Chem.* 1994;269:9416–9419.
82. Ren S, Lawson AE, Carr M, et al. Human tryptase fibrinogenolysis is optimal at acidic pH and generates anticoagulant fragments in the presence of the anti-tryptase monoclonal antibody B12. *J Immunol.* 1997;159:3540–3548.
83. Molinari JF, Moore WR, Clark J, et al. Role of tryptase in immediate cutaneous responses in allergic sheep. *J Appl Physiol.* 1995;79:1966–1970.
84. Molinari JF, Scuri M, Moore WR, et al. Inhaled tryptase causes bronchoconstriction in sheep via histamine release. *Am J Respir Crit Care Med.* 1996;154:649–653.
85. Schwartz LB, Yunginger JW, Miller J, et al. Time course of appearance and disappearance of human mast cell tryptase in the circulation after anaphylaxis. *J Clin Invest.* 1989;83:1551–1555.
86. Schwartz LB, Lewis RA, Austen KF. Tryptase from human pulmonary mast cells. Purification and characterization. *J Biol Chem.* 1981;256:11939–11943.
87. Schwartz LB, Lewis RA, Seldin D, Austen KF. Acid hydrolases and tryptase from secretory granules of dispersed human lung mast cells. *J Immunol.* 1981;126:1290–1294.
88. Smith TJ, Hougland MW, Johnson DA. Human lung tryptase. Purification and characterization. *J Biol Chem.* 1984;259:11046–11051.

89. Jackson NE, Wang HW, Bryant KJ, et al. Alternate mRNA splicing in multiple human tryptase genes is predicted to regulate tetramer formation. *J Biol Chem.* 2008;283:34178–34187.
90. Peng Q, McEuen AR, Benyon RC, Walls AF. The heterogeneity of mast cell tryptase from human lung and skin. *Eur J Biochem.* 2003;270:270v283.
91. Vanderslice P, Ballinger SM, Tam EK, et al. Human mast cell tryptase: multiple cDNAs and genes reveal a multigene serine protease family. *Proc Natl Acad Sci USA.* 1990;87:3811–3815.
92. Miller JS, Westin EH, Schwartz LB. Cloning and characterization of complementary DNA for human tryptase. *J Clin Invest.* 1989;84:1188–1195.
93. Huang C, Li L, Krilis SA, et al. Human tryptases α (alpha) and β (beta)/II are functionally distinct due, in part, to a single amino acid difference in one of the surface loops that forms the substrate-binding cleft. *J Biol Chem.* 1999;274:19670–19676.
94. Selwood T, Wang ZM, McCaslin DR, Schechter NM. Diverse stability and catalytic properties of human tryptase a (alpha) and b (beta) isoforms are mediated by residue differences at the S1 pocket. *Biochemistry.* 2002;41:3329–3340.
95. Marquardt U, Zettl F, Huber R, et al. The crystal structure of human α (alpha)1-tryptase reveals a blocked substrate-binding region. *J Mol Biol.* 2002;321:491–502.
96. Trivedi NN, Tong Q, Raman K, et al. Mast cell α (alpha) and β (beta) tryptases changed rapidly during primate speciation and evolved from γ (gamma)-like transmembrane peptidases in ancestral vertebrates. *J Immunol.* 2007;179:6072–6079.
97. Pallaoro M, Fejzo MS, Shayesteh L, et al. Characterization of genes encoding known and novel human mast cell tryptases on chromosome 16p13.3. *J Biol Chem.* 1999;274:3355–3362.
98. Caughey GH, Raymond WW, Blount JL, et al. Characterization of human γ (gamma)-tryptases, novel members of the chromosome 16p mast cell tryptase and prostasin gene families. *J Immunol.* 2000;164:6566–6575.
99. Soto D, Malmsten C, Blount JL, et al. Genetic deficiency of human mast cell α (alpha)-tryptase. *Clin Exp Allergy.* 2002;32:1000–1006.
100. Trivedi NN, Tamraz B, Chu C, et al. Human subjects are protected from mast cell tryptase deficiency despite frequent inheritance of loss-of-function mutations. *J Allergy Clin Immunol.* 2009;124:1099–1105.
101. Wong GW, Foster PS, Yasuda S, et al. Biochemical and functional characterization of human transmembrane tryptase (TMT)/tryptase g (gamma). TMT is an exocytosed mast cell protease that induces airway hyperresponsiveness in vivo via an interleukin-13/interleukin-4 receptor alpha/signal transducer and activator of transcription (STAT) 6-dependent pathway. *J Biol Chem.* 2002;277:41906–41915.
102. Yuan J, Beltman J, Gjerstad E, et al. Expression and characterization of recombinant γ (gamma)-tryptase. *Protein Expr Purif.* 2006;49:47–54.
103. Verghese GM, Gutknecht MF, Caughey GH. Prostasin regulates epithelial monolayer function: cell-specific Glpd1-mediated secretion and functional role for the GPI anchor. *Am J Physiol Cell Physiol.* 2006;291:1258–1270.
104. Trivedi NN, Raymond WW, Caughey GH. Chimerism, point mutation, and truncation dramatically transformed mast cell δ (delta)-tryptases during primate evolution. *J Allergy Clin Immunol.* 2008;121:1262–1268.
105. Wang HW, McNeil HP, Husain A, et al. δ (delta) Tryptase is expressed in multiple human tissues, and a recombinant form has proteolytic activity. *J Immunol.* 2002;169:5145–5152.
106. Caughey GH. Tryptase genetics and anaphylaxis. *J Allergy Clin Immunol.* 2006;117:1411–1414.
107. Min HK, Moxley G, Neale MC, Schwartz LB. Effect of sex and haplotype on plasma tryptase levels in healthy adults. *J Allergy Clin Immunol.* 2004;114:48–51.
108. Jogie-Brahim S, Min HK, Fukuoka Y, et al. Expression of α (alpha)-tryptase and β (beta)-tryptase by human basophils. *J Allergy Clin Immunol.* 2004;113:1086–1092.
109. Goldstein SM, Kaempfer CE, Proud D, et al. Detection and partial characterization of a human mast cell carboxypeptidase. *J Immunol.* 1987;139:2724–2729.
110. Reynolds DS, Gurley DS, Austen KF. Cloning and characterization of the novel gene for mast cell carboxypeptidase A. *J Clin Invest.* 1992;89:273–282.
111. Irani AM, Goldstein SM, Wintroub BU, et al. Human mast cell carboxypeptidase: selective localization to MCTC cells. *J Immunol.* 1991;147:247–253.
112. Lundequist A, Tchougounova E, Abrink M, Pejler G. Cooperation between mast cell carboxypeptidase A and the chymase mouse mast cell protease 4 in the formation and degradation of angiotensin II. *J Biol Chem.* 2004;279:32339–32344.
113. Kokkonen JO, Vartiainen M, Kovanen PT. Low density lipoprotein degradation by secretory granules of rat mast cells. Sequential degradation of apolipoprotein B by granule chymase and carboxypeptidase A. *J Biol Chem.* 1986;261:16067–16072.
114. Springman EB, Dikov MM, Serafin WE. Mast cell procarboxypeptidase A. Molecular modeling and biochemical characterization of its processing within secretory granules. *J Biol Chem.* 1995;270:1300–1307.
115. Henningsson F, Wolters P, Chapman HA, et al. Mast cell cathepsins C and S control levels of carboxypeptidase A and the chymase, mouse mast cell protease 5. *Biol Chem.* 2003;384:1527–1531.
116. Henningsson F, Yamamoto K, Saftig P, et al. A role for cathepsin E in the processing of mast-cell carboxypeptidase A. *J Cell Sci.* 2005;118:2035–2042.

117. Schneider LA, Schlenner SM, Feyerabend TB, et al. Molecular mechanism of mast cell mediated innate defense against endothelin and snake venom sarafotoxin. *J Exp Med.* 2007;204:2629–2639.
118. Maurer M, Wedemeyer J, Metz M, et al. Mast cells promote homeostasis by limiting endothelin-1-induced toxicity. *Nature.* 2004;432:512–516.
119. Turk D, Janjic V, Stern I, et al. Structure of human dipeptidyl peptidase I (cathepsin C): exclusion domain added to an endopeptidase framework creates the machine for activation of granular serine proteases. *EMBO J.* 2001;20:6570–6582.
120. Wolters PJ, Laig-Webster M, Caughey GH. Dipeptidyl peptidase I cleaves matrix-associated proteins and is expressed mainly by mast cells in normal dog airways. *Am J Respir Cell Mol Biol.* 2000;22:183–190.
121. Wolters PJ, Raymond WW, Blount JL, Caughey GH. Regulated expression, processing, and secretion of dog mast cell dipeptidyl peptidase I. *J Biol Chem.* 1998;273:15514–15520.
122. Mallen-St Clair J, Pham CT, Villalta SA, et al. Mast cell dipeptidyl peptidase I mediates survival from sepsis. *J Clin Invest.* 2004;113:628–634.
123. Pham CT, Ivanovich JL, Raptis SZ, et al. Papillon-Lefevre syndrome: correlating the molecular, cellular, and clinical consequences of cathepsin C/dipeptidyl peptidase I deficiency in humans. *J Immunol.* 2004;173:7277–7281.
124. Polanowska J, Krokoszynska I, Czapinska H, et al. Specificity of human cathepsin G. *Biochim Biophys Acta.* 1998;1386:189–198.
125. McNeil HP, Austen KF, Somerville LL, et al. Molecular cloning of the mouse mast cell protease-5 gene. A novel secretory granule protease expressed early in the differentiation of serosal mast cells. J Biol Chem. 1991;266:20316–20322.
126. Kunori Y, Koizumi M, Masegi T, et al. Rodent α (alpha)-chymases are elastase-like proteases. Eur J Biochem. 2002;269:5921–5930.
127. Nakamura N, Tsuru A, Hirayoshi K, Nagata K. Purification and characterization of a vimentin-specific protease in mouse myeloid leukemia cells. Regulation during differentiation and identity with cathepsin G. Eur J Biochem. 1992;205:947–954.
128. Raymond WW, Trivedi NN, Makarova A, Caughey GH. How peptidases evolve: acquisition of cathepsin G tryptic activity in primates by missense mutation. Am J Respir Crit Care Med. 2009;10:A.
129. Pemberton AD, Brown JK, Wright SH, et al. Purification and characterization of mouse mast cell proteinase-2 and the differential expression and release of mouse mast cell proteinase-1 and -2 in vivo. Clin Exp Allergy. 2003;33:1005–1012.
130. Andersson MK, Pemberton AD, Miller HR, Hellman L. Extended cleavage specificity of mMCP-1, the major mucosal mast cell protease in mouse-high specificity indicates high substrate selectivity. Mol Immunol. 2008;45:2548–2558.
131. Coussens LM, Raymond WW, Bergers G, et al. Inflammatory mast cells upregulate angiogenesis during squamous epithelial carcinogenesis. Genes Develop. 1999;13:1382–1397.
132. Tchougounova E, Pejler G, Abrink M. The chymase, mouse mast cell protease 4, constitutes the major chymotrypsin-like activity in peritoneum and ear tissue. A role for mouse mast cell protease 4 in thrombin regulation and fibronectin turnover. J Exp Med. 2003;198:423–431.
133. Hunt JE, Friend DS, Gurish MF, et al. Mouse mast cell protease 9, a novel member of the chromosome 14 family of serine proteases that is selectively expressed in uterine mast cells. J Biol Chem. 1997;272:29158–29166.
134. Lutzelschwab C, Pejler G, Aveskogh M, Hellman L. Secretory granule proteases in rat mast cells. Cloning of 10 different serine proteases and a carboxypeptidase A from various rat mast cell populations. J Exp Med. 1997;185:13–29.
135. Karlson U, Pejler G, Tomasini-Johansson B, Hellman L. Extended substrate specificity of rat mast cell protease 5, a rodent α (alpha)-chymase with elastase-like primary specificity. J Biol Chem. 2003;278:39625–39631.
136. Andersson MK, Karlson U, Hellman L. The extended cleavage specificity of the rodent β (beta)-chymases rMCP-1 and mMCP-4 reveal major functional similarities to the human mast cell chymase. Mol Immunol. 2007;45:766–775.
137. Karlson U, Pejler G, Froman G, Hellman L. Rat mast cell protease 4 is a β (beta)-chymase with unusually stringent substrate recognition profile. J Biol Chem. 2002;277:18579–18585.
138. Sakai K, Ren S, Schwartz LB. A novel heparin-dependent processing pathway for human tryptase: autocatalysis followed by activation with dipeptidyl peptidase I. J Clin Invest. 1996;97:988–995.
139. Miller JS, Moxley G, Schwartz LB. Cloning and characterization of a second complementary cDNA for human tryptase. J Clin Invest. 1990;86:864–870.
140. Pereira PJB, Bergner A, Macedo-Ribeiro S, et al. Human β (beta)-tryptase is a ring-like tetramer with active sites facing a central pore. Nature. 1998;392:306–311.
141. Min HK, Kambe N, Schwartz LB. Human mouse mast cell protease 7-like tryptase genes are pseudogenes. J Allergy Clin Immunol. 2001;107:315–321.
142. Ide H, Itoh H, Tomita M, et al. cDNA sequencing and expression of rat mast cell tryptase. *J Biochem.* 1995;118:210–215.

# Chapter 7
# Aspirin and NSAID Reactions: Diagnosis, Pathophysiology, and Management

**Andrew A. White, Tanya M. Laidlaw, and Katharine Woessner**

**Abstract** Nonsteroidal anti-inflammatory drugs (NSAIDS) and aspirin are commonly used medications that are not infrequently associated with severe adverse reactions. The approach to the patient with a reaction to a medication in this class can be challenging. Most reactions can be categorized into one of four different types: aspirin/NSAID-induced asthma and rhinitis in asthmatic patients, aspirin/NSAID-induced urticaria/angioedema in patients with chronic urticaria, aspirin/NSAID-induced cross-reacting urticaria in otherwise normal individuals, and single-NSAID-induced reactions in normal subjects. This classification system is useful in planning safe and accurate challenges as well as determining appropriate desensitization protocols. These reactions vary in their pathophysiology, with the role of cyclooxygenase 1, leukotrienes, and prostaglandins remaining dominant.

**Keywords** Aspirin • Cyclooxygenase 1 • Cyclooxygenase 2 • Nonsteroidal anti-inflammatory drugs (NSAIDS) • Aspirin-exacerbated respiratory disease (AERD) • Urticaria • Angioedema • Non-IgE-mediated anaphylaxis • Chronic sinusitis • Nasal polyps • Asthma • Leukotriene c4 • Leukotriene d4 • Leukotriene e4 • Prostaglandin e2 • Prostaglandin d2 • Thromboxane • Ketorolac • Desensitization • Lipoxin

## 7.1 Introduction

Reactions to aspirin (ASA) and nonsteroidal anti-inflammatory drugs (NSAIDs) continue to present a major problem for both patients and clinicians. For patients, the NSAIDs provide relief from pain, inflammation, and fever. In the case of aspirin, a potent antiplatelet effect makes it central in the primary and secondary prophylaxis of a variety of cardiovascular conditions. When adverse reactions occur, determining the mechanism of the reaction and, more importantly, counseling the patient on alternative medications that can be safely taken can be difficult for the clinician. In large part, this is because the diagnosis of nearly all NSAID-induced adverse reactions is made based on a precise history in combination with some form of drug challenge. For many, this can be seen as cumbersome, inconvenient, or too dangerous. This chapter focuses on critical aspects of the history

---

K. Woessner (✉)
Allergy, Asthma and Immunology Department, Scripps Clinic and Scripps Green Hospital, San Diego, CA, USA
e-mail: Woessner.katharine@scrippshealth.org

M.C. Castells (ed.), *Anaphylaxis and Hypersensitivity Reactions*,
DOI 10.1007/978-1-60327-951-2_7, © Springer Science+Business Media, LLC 2011

that can help to distinguish between the types of adverse reactions. Additionally, the chapter describes the options available for drug challenge and/or desensitization.

As a class, the NSAIDs are characterized by their blockade of the cyclooxygenase (COX) enzyme. It is through this inhibition that most of the anti-inflammatory and antiplatelet effects are produced. Inhibition of COX may be part of the mechanism involved in the "allergic" respiratory reactions to NSAIDs, and some reactions to NSAIDs can also occur through an IgE-mediated mechanism. COX inhibition and IgE-mediated mast cell activation explain the majority of reactions to NSAIDs. However, as they cause similar clinical manifestations, it can be quite difficult to distinguish between the types of reactions.

Various categories of NSAID reactions have been proposed in the literature. Identifying which of the four types of reactions is critical to determine which drug challenges should be performed in order to make a diagnosis. The categories are briefly described here and then will be discussed in detail.

**Type 1: ASA/NSAID-induced asthma and rhinitis in asthmatic patients.** Patients in this category invariably have a history of chronic rhinosinusitis with nasal polyposis and asthma. Reactions in this category are cross-reactive among all NSAIDs that inhibit the enzyme cyclooxygenase 1 (COX-1). This clinical condition is most accurately termed aspirin-exacerbated respiratory disease (AERD) and patients will generally have a combination of both upper and lower airway symptoms after NSAID exposure.

**Type 2: ASA/NSAID-induced urticaria/angioedema in patients with chronic urticaria.** Patients with underlying chronic urticaria are prone to flares of urticaria and angioedema after ingestion of ASA or NSAIDs. These reactions are somewhat dependent on the level of baseline urticaria at the time of NSAID ingestion. Reactions can be difficult to block, often requiring histamine receptor-1 and histamine receptor-2 antagonists as well as leukotriene receptor antagonists.

**Type 3: ASA/NSAID-induced cross-reacting urticaria in otherwise normal individuals**. This is seen in patients who experience urticaria/angioedema only after treatment with a COX-1 inhibitor. This is a cross-reactive phenomenon in that any COX-1 inhibitor can lead to the same clinical reaction. Patients with Type 3 reactions should be differentiated from Type 2, because desensitization options are described for Type 3 reactions, which may not be as effective in Type 2.

**Type 4. Single-NSAID-induced reactions in otherwise normal individuals**. These reactions are presumably mediated through an IgE-dependent mechanism. Cross-reactivity should not be widespread among all NSAIDs, because dissimilar structures would prevent immunologic cross-reactivity. In this category, reactions may present with a mild urticarial reaction or can be anaphylactic in nature. The unifying historical detail will be that these patients can tolerate other NSAIDs without difficulty. While single NSAID reactions are the rule, there exists the possibility that a minority of these patients experience non-IgE anaphylaxis mediated through the COX-1 pathway or that enough structural similarity exists among a particular family of NSAIDs that multiple NSAID anaphylaxis could occur. Fortunately, multiple-NSAID-induced anaphylaxis is very rare.

## 7.2 Aspirin-Exacerbated Respiratory Disease

Aspirin-exacerbated respiratory disease (AERD) has known several names since its first description by Widal. For decades, "aspirin triad," "aspirin-intolerant asthma," "aspirin-induced asthma," and "aspirin sensitivity" were used to describe the syndrome [1]. AERD has emerged as a more accurate description of the underlying disease mechanism. Individuals with AERD are characterized by ongoing airway inflammation even in the absence of ASA/NSAID ingestion. Many of them have both asthma and sinus disease, which generally includes nasal polyposis. The syndrome is characterized in all patients by exacerbation of airway complaints after the ingestion or exposure to any drug blocking the COX-1 enzyme.

AERD is thought to exist in 0.6–2.5% [2–5] of the general population. In asthmatics, as expected, the rates are much higher and range from 4.3% to 11% [2–4]. In a population of patients undergoing functional endoscopic sinus surgery, the rate of AERD was 4.8%. In those patients who have both asthma and nasal polyposis, the rate was 25.6% [6]. Unfortunately, many patients are unaware that they are vulnerable to the negative effects of ASA or NSAIDs and in patients with sinus disease and asthma as many as 15% may be unaware that ASA or NSAIDs pose a risk of reaction [7]. Because of this lack of recognition, self-reporting of AERD may underrepresent the true prevalence of the disorder. If instead ASA challenge studies are done, a higher prevalence of AERD is identified and in one meta-analysis an average of 21% of adult asthmatics had positive challenges to ASA [8].

## 7.3 Characteristics of AERD

AERD follows a typical course. Most patients experience the first onset of symptoms in the third to fourth decade of life, averaging 30–34 years of age [7,9]. Rhinitis is generally the presenting symptom that is followed by asthma in approximately 2 years. Reactions to ASA or NSAIDS develop another 4 years later and may coincide with the development of nasal polyposis [7].

A variety of symptoms have been reported as part of the reaction to ASA or NSAIDs in AERD. Most reactions include a significant respiratory component, often requiring the patient to seek care for asthma-related symptoms. The "classic" reaction includes both an asthmatic bronchoconstrictive reaction and accompanying nasal and ocular symptoms. This can consist of sneezing, nasal congestion, and rhinorrhea, as well as watering, tearing, erythema, and swelling of the eyes. In some patients the reaction may be exclusively upper respiratory in nature with only naso-ocular symptoms, or exclusively lower respiratory and cause only asthmatic symptoms [10]. Less-common manifestations include urticaria, angioedema, and/or non-IgE anaphylaxis with hypotension [7,11]. Other accompanying symptoms have included laryngospasm and cramping abdominal pain [11]. The average time to reaction upon ingestion of aspirin is 1.7 h [12].

Any compound that blocks COX-1 has the ability to cause a reaction in a patient with AERD. In the USA, the most common causes of reactions are aspirin (80%), ibuprofen (41%), naproxen (4%), and ketorolac (1%). Many patients have experienced reactions to more than one COX-1 inhibitor [9]. Similarly, in Europe, 82% have reacted to ASA with 9% reacting to one of the pyrazolone group of NSAIDs (phenylbutazone, oxyphenbutazone) [7]. The regional differences likely represent differences in availability and pattern of usage of these medications. Other COX-1 inhibitors that have been reported to cause reactions include a variety of oral compounds, parenterally administered ketorolac [13], and ocular ketorolac [14].

### *7.3.1 Acetaminophen and AERD*

There is a degree of cross-reactivity that exists between high doses of acetaminophen and the other NSAIDs in AERD. In one study, 34% of AERD patients reacted to acetaminophen at doses over 1,000 mg. It was noted in this study that these reactions were generally mild, and when bronchospasm occurred it was easily reversed [15]. In two previous studies challenging to a maximum dose of 600 and 650 mg of acetaminophen, reaction rates were 6% and 3%, respectively [16,17]. A meta-analysis of these and other studies found an overall positive challenge rate of 6.5% (CI – 0–16.4) [8]. Thus, most patients will be able to tolerate lower doses (<650 mg) of acetaminophen, while higher doses (>1,000 mg) should be used with greater caution.

### *7.3.2 COX-2 and AERD*

The package insert for celecoxib, a highly selective cyclooxygenase-2 (COX-2) inhibitor, continues to warn patients with AERD that the use of this drug could cause a serious adverse reaction. Yet several studies have conclusively shown that in the AERD population there is no risk of reacting to a pure COX-2-blocking drug [18–26]. Due to other safety concerns the only COX-2 inhibitor currently available in the USA is celecoxib. For AERD patients with a need for anti-inflammatory therapy, any specific COX-2 inhibitor can safely be used. Among traditional NSAIDs, there are drugs with much higher specificity for COX-2 than for COX-1. Meloxicam, nimesulide, and nabumetone all have demonstrated marked specificity of COX-2 enzyme blockade over the COX-1 isoform of the enzyme [27–29]. Studies of nimesulide, meloxicam, and nabumetone in the NSAID-intolerant population (also including cutaneous reactions) are generally favorable, but limited in number [30–32]. In one study of patients with AERD, all patients were able to tolerate routine doses of nimesulide. However, at higher doses, which likely cause some inhibition of COX-1 activity as well, there were mild reactions reported [33]. Nimesulide is not available in the USA. In specific circumstances it would be reasonable to administer the other two medications, but first dose observation in the office might be prudent.

## 7.4 AERD: An Aggressive Airway Disease

The presence of AERD generally predicts a more aggressive course of the sinus disease. Patients with AERD average ten times more previous sinus surgeries than those requiring functional endoscopic sinus surgery (FESS) without AERD [6]. In AERD, there is significantly greater hyperplasia on CT of sinuses than in aspirin-tolerant asthma, likely reflecting the increased inflammatory nature of the disease [34]. It is reasonable to conclude that patients with AERD have a higher baseline severity to their sinus disease, are much less likely to retain long-term benefit from FESS, and are more likely to undergo repeated sinus procedures [35–37].

The TENOR study showed that, among other variables, persistent airflow limitation was more likely in AERD patients than in those without aspirin sensitivity [38]. Additionally, when compared with aspirin-tolerant asthmatic individuals, patients with AERD tended to have more severe asthma and they were more likely to require high-dose inhaled corticosteroids, to receive bursts of systemic corticosteroids, and to have been intubated for asthma [39]. Of 92 asthmatics requiring mechanical ventilation, 8% had their attack precipitated by an NSAID [40]. In a Japanese population, AERD patients were much more likely to have multiple asthma exacerbations during the previous year (34.4% versus 5.4%) as well as near-fatal asthma [41]. As a group, AERD patients exhibit typical characteristics of severe asthma. In one US series, 22–51% required daily prednisone at an average dose of 7.5–8 mg per day [9,14].

## 7.5 AERD in Children

The classic triad of chronic sinusitis/nasal polyposis, asthma, and sensitivity to ASA or NSAIDs rarely exists in children. Despite this, ASA challenge studies in asthmatic children have demonstrated positive results in 0–28% of children [42–45]. In a recent study, 100 asthmatic children were challenged with ibuprofen and 2 had a positive challenge [46]. In a meta-analysis, the prevalence of a positive oral provocation test is 5% (0–14%). By history alone, the prevalence is estimated at 2%

(1–3%) [8]. The natural history of children with reactivity to ASA or NSAIDs is unclear. Because of these factors, it is not clear whether these pediatric patients would receive the same benefit from ASA desensitization as adults.

## 7.6 Mediators Involved in AERD

Several mediators are important in AERD or contribute to the reactions to ASA/NSAIDs in AERD, and most of these are eicosanoid lipid mediators. The eicosanoids, including prostaglandins and leukotrienes, are so named because they each have 20 carbon atoms and the Greek word for 20 is **eikosi.** These are generated and released from cell membranes through multiple enzymatic steps involving the hydrolysis of fatty acids from membrane phospholipids. Prostaglandin E2 ($PGE_2$), prostaglandin D2 ($PGD_2$), and thromboxane ($TXA_2$) have all been implicated in the pathogenesis of AERD and are all formed through actions of the COX enzyme pathway. This pathway involves two sequential catalytic reactions to convert arachidonic acid (AA) into prostaglandin H2 ($PGH_2$), the precursor for the prostanoids mentioned above. Both COX isoenzymes, COX-1 and COX-2, have two active enzymatic sites: a cyclooxygenase site that inserts two oxygen molecules into AA to transform it into prostaglandin $G_2$ ($PGG_2$), and a peroxidase site that reduces $PGG_2$ to $PGH_2$. Although both COX-1 and COX-2 act in very similar manners, they are expressed at varying levels in different cells.

One of the most investigated eicosanoids in regards to aspirin-precipitated reactions is $PGE_2$. Once $PGH_2$ is formed, there are then three discrete enzymes that can convert $PGH_2$ to $PGE_2$. These are the inducible microsomal PGE synthase-1 (mPGES-1), the constitutive microsomal PGE synthase-2 (mPGES-2), and the constitutive cytosolic PGE synthase (cPGES). The mechanisms by which $PGH_2$ is preferentially converted to one prostanoid product or another are poorly understood and there is some suggestion that the two COX isoforms may interact and couple differently with each particular PGE synthase. As is the case for all eicosanoids, the activity of $PGE_2$ is mediated through specific G-protein coupled receptors, and for $PGE_2$ they are termed E prostanoid receptors (EP1–EP4). Activation of the EP2 and EP4 receptors causes an increase in intracellular cAMP concentrations, whereas the EP1 receptor triggers an elevation of intracellular calcium levels [47]. The existence of these four subtypes of receptors and the potential for expression of multiple receptors in a single cell helps to explain the diversity of biological responses elicited by $PGE_2$ and how these responses might be distinct in different cells and tissues. Additionally, during episodes of inflammation, it is likely that the repertoire of receptors expressed in the inflamed tissue can change, leading to an even wider array of effects [48]. Within the lung, $PGE_2$ is a potent anti-inflammatory mediator and appears to be a key factor needed to control bronchoconstriction and the inflammation caused by asthma. Stimulation of the EP2 receptor by $PGE_2$ induces relaxation of airway smooth muscle and also inhibits the bronchoconstrictive response of the airway to methacholine [49]. Thereby, it is important to note that the peripheral blood cells of patients with AERD have a reduced capacity to release $PGE_2$ at baseline [50]. Additionally, it is known that if patients with AERD inhale $PGE_2$ prior to an aspirin challenge, their bronchoconstrictive response to the aspirin is almost entirely prevented [51]. In summary, AERD patients may have lower levels of the enzymes required to produce $PGE_2$ and therefore, despite the inflamed state of their asthmatic lung tissue, are more susceptible to the further inhibition of $PGE_2$ production that occurs when their COX-1 pathway is inhibited by an NSAID.

There is also mounting evidence that $PGD_2$ is an important mediator in AERD. Once released into the human circulation, $PGD_2$ is well known to induce bronchoconstriction, and it is the major eicosanoid produced by mast cells [52]. In 2003, a study investigated the baseline plasma levels of $9\alpha$(alpha),$11\beta$(beta)-$PGF_2$ (a $PGD_2$ metabolite) in patients with AERD and compared them to the same baseline levels in patients with aspirin-tolerant asthma. The patients with AERD had a significantly higher baseline plasma level of the $PGD_2$ metabolite, and upon precipitation of the respiratory reaction that accompanied a subsequent challenge with aspirin, most of these AERD patients developed a further rise in plasma levels of 9α(alpha),11β(beta)-$PGF_2$ [53]. Therefore, one hypothesis proposes that an increased circulating level of $PGD_2$ in patients with AERD contributes to their global symptoms of asthma. However, it is not clear how upon ingestion of a COX-1 inhibitor there would be an additional release of $PGD_2$ which then would cause the upper respiratory exacerbation and bronchoconstriction.

Among the eicosanoids formed from the metabolism of arachidonic acid, $TXA_2$ has also attracted attention as a potential mediator in the pathophysiology of asthma because of its potent bronchoconstrictive activity. A role for $TXA_2$ in asthma was first presented in 1980 [54], and it is believed to be involved in both late asthmatic responses and in the bronchial hyperresponsiveness that is a hallmark of asthma. There is data to suggest that $TXA_2$ may have specific applications for the subset of patients with AERD, as it has been found that monocytes isolated from patients with AERD released twice as much $TXA_2$ as monocytes from normal controls, when stimulated with calcium ionophore. And, as expected due to COX-1 inhibition, after desensitization and treatment with oral aspirin, the release of $TXA_2$ was almost completely abolished [55]. This decreased thromboxane production could contribute to the clinical improvement seen after aspirin desensitization and explain some of the mechanism underlying the therapeutic benefit of high-dose aspirin treatment.

Another group of principal mediators of AERD are the cysteinyl leukotrienes, which are also derivatives of AA, but are formed through the sequential actions of the enzymes 5-lipoxygenase and leukotriene $C_4$ synthase ($LTC_4S$), instead of the cyclooxygenase pathway. Eosinophils, basophils, mast cells, and macrophages each express the $LTC_4S$ enzyme and produce leukotriene $C_4$ ($LTC_4$), which is then converted to $LTD_4$ and $LTE_4$ extracellularly. $LTC_4$ and $LTD_4$ are known to be potent bronchoconstrictors, but $LTE_4$ is the more stable form, which is excreted into the urine and can be measured more easily. It has been known for more than 2 decades [56–62] that there are increased levels of $LTE_4$ at baseline in the nasal secretions, urine, and bronchoalveolar lavage fluid of patients with AERD and that these levels increase upon ingestion of aspirin. It has also been found that the patients who have the most severe respiratory reactions during oral aspirin challenge are also those patients with the most significantly elevated $LTE_4$ elevated at baseline [63]. Additionally, there are several studies suggesting that there is a genetic predisposition toward the overproduction of leukotrienes in this disorder. One group has found an overexpression of the $LTC_4S$ enzyme in the bronchial biopsies from patients with AERD [64], and another group found that 60% of their patients with AERD have a single-nucleotide polymorphism in the regulatory region of the $LTC_4S$ gene that leads to increased transcription of the enzyme [65]. This lipoxygenase pathway of leukotriene production and the COX-1 pathway of $PGE_2$ production do not act alone; in fact, both clinical and in vitro studies [51,66,67] have shown that $PGE_2$ functions as a "brake" on the 5-lipoxygenase enzyme and therefore inhibits the production of leukotrienes. An underproduction of $PGE_2$ in patients with AERD may explain part of the overproduction of leukotrienes in these patients.

Another group of lipoxygenase-derived eicosanoids are the lipoxins, but in contrast to leukotrienes, lipoxins inhibit bronchoconstriction [68] and are considered to be anti-inflammatory mediators. These mediators have been found in human bronchial tissue and nasal polyp tissue [69] and lipoxin A4 is known to inhibit both neutrophil and eosinophil migration. Interestingly, inhaled lipoxin $A_4$ inhibits $LTC_4$-induced bronchoconstriction in asthmatics [68], and, therefore, may play a protective role by balancing airway obstruction. Sanak et al. have shown that the stimulated whole blood of patients with AERD had a diminished capacity to generate lipoxins, and they suggest that this may contribute to their more severe clinical airway disease [70].

Taken together, it appears that during the aspirin-induced reaction, blockade of the COX-1 enzyme occurs and AERD patients lose the "braking" effect of $PGE_2$, thus leading to a marked increase in leukotriene production. Leukotrienes, along with other inflammatory mediators such as

$PGD_2$ and $TXA_2$, lead to the symptoms of an acute ASA-induced attack in a group of patients who at baseline may have lower levels of the protective pulmonary mediators such as $PGE_2$ and lipoxin $A_4$. That this same pathway of unregulated leukotriene production does not occur in normal individuals with COX-1 enzyme blockade remains a mystery.

## 7.7 AERD and Diagnostics

The gold standard for the diagnosis of AERD remains oral ASA challenge. The importance of the oral challenge is underscored by the fact that the negative challenge rate consistently remains 15%. In other words, 15% of patients with a presumptive diagnosis of AERD and at least one historical reaction thought to be from ASA or an NSAID did not in fact have the disease [9,10]. Several variables, including multiple and severe prior asthma reactions to ASA or NSAIDs, anosmia and age less than 40, were significantly associated with a positive oral aspirin challenge [71]. The timing and dosing of a recommended aspirin challenge protocol is outlined in Table 7.2. Various starting doses have been recommended. We favor starting at 30 mg of ASA as reactions to less than this dose are extremely unlikely. Some low-risk patients can be started at a dose of 40–60 mg of ASA [12]. Stopping a challenge at 325 mg of ASA is also reasonable, as in a series of 420 challenges, no patient who tolerated 325 mg ASA went on to react to 650 mg of ASA [12]. A variety of schedules have been used to determine how quickly the challenges can be given. Since mean reactions occur at 1.7 h after the offending dose of ASA, a 3-h schedule between doses seems safe and reasonable. Pulmonary function testing should be done hourly to monitor for early evidence of a reaction. A drop in FEV1 from baseline of >15% is the definition of a lower respiratory tract reaction [72].

For the purpose of an ASA challenge, the goal is to find the provoking dose and not necessarily to desensitize the patient. Thus, after the provoking dose is determined, the reaction is reversed and the challenge is over. Treatment options are outlined in Table 7.1. The symptoms should be recorded as well as any change in pulmonary function.

## 7.8 Routes of Challenge: Inhaled, Intranasal, and Intravenous

The current gold standard in the diagnosis of AERD in the USA remains a supervised oral ASA challenge. In Europe and Japan, the availability of ASA-lysine, a form of ASA which can be easily diluted in liquid, has allowed intranasal, bronchial, and intravenous challenges to be explored [73–75]. These challenges do not quite equal the sensitivity and specificity of an oral ASA challenge yet can be very useful. Intranasal challenges with ASA-lysine, when compared with oral ASA challenge have a sensitivity and specificity of 73–86.7% and 92.5–95.7%, respectively [76–78]. One of the main advantages of using nasal challenges is localizing the reaction to the nasal membranes.

**Table 7.1** Treatment options for aspirin-induced reactions

| |
|---|
| Ocular – Topical antihistamine |
| Nasal – Oral antihistamine or diphenhydramine, 50 mg administered intravenously, topical decongestant |
| Bronchial – Five inhalation of beta-agonist every 5 min until comfortable |
| Laryngeal – Racemic epinephrine nebulization 2.5 mg/2 mL |
| Gastrointestinal cramping – Intravenous ranitidine, 50 mg |
| Urticaria/angioedema – Intravenous diphenhydramine, 50 mg |
| Hypotension – Epinephrine 1:1,000 0.3 mL administered intramuscularly |

**Table 7.2** Aspirin desensitization protocol [93]

| |
|---|
| Prior to desensitization: |
| 1. Document airway stability with FEV1 >60–70% predicted (>1.5 L absolute) |
| 2. FEV1 every hour × 3 h with <10% variability |
| 3. Start montelukast 10 mg daily for 7 days prior |
| 4. Adequately control underlying airway disease with ICS/LABA |
| 5. If evidence of low FEV1 or instability start systemic corticosteroids |
| 6. No antihistamines 48 h prior to challenge |
| Protocol: |
| 1. Start intravenous line with heparin lock |
| 2. First dose 20.25–40.5 mg (prepared by using a pill cutter on an 81 mg aspirin tablet) |
| 3. Subsequent doses: 60, 81, 101, 162.5 (1/2 of 325 mg), and 325 mg |
| 4. Doses are administered every 90 min to 3 h with clinical assessment and FEV1 each hour |
| 5. Provoking dose: between 20–00 mg (see Table 7.1 for treatment) |
| 6. After the patient has stabilized, re-administer the "provoking dose" |
| 7. If time limits the readministration of the provoking dose, it can be given at the beginning of day 2 |
| 8. The desensitization is complete when the patient tolerates 325 mg with no reaction |
| 9. Increase to 650 mg twice daily if tolerated |

This would be a safer way of doing a diagnostic challenge in a less-stable asthmatic. However, lower respiratory reactions from nasal ASA-lysine challenge can occur [79]. In the USA, the availability of ketorolac in an intravenous formulation has led to preliminary work exploring the use of this as a local method to challenge the nasal membranes, theoretically leading to fewer pulmonary reactions. This appears to compare favorably with intranasal challenges done with ASA-lysine [80].

Bronchial challenges are routinely used in European studies of AERD patients. These are done primarily with ASA-lysine, although other NSAIDs have been described [81,82]. The bronchial challenge may have a slightly lower sensitivity, but it provides a relatively safe and efficient method of diagnosing AERD [74,83–86]. Distinguishing characteristics of the bronchial response in inhalational challenge include an early but prolonged decrease in pulmonary function, with the notable absence of a late reaction [87]. Due to the unavailability of ASA-lysine in the USA, bronchial challenges are not currently able to be performed for the diagnosis of AERD.

As with any drug challenge, the appropriate setting and patient selection should be made before embarking. According to a recent practice paper, patients should have stable baseline pulmonary function, generally with FEV1 greater than 70% (>1.5 L) [72]. It is reasonable to have an intravenous line in place before the challenge is started, and the patient should have given informed consent. All available treatments to reverse a severe pulmonary reaction should be available, including nebulized short-acting beta-agonists, intravenous corticosteroids, intramuscular epinephrine, and nebulized racemic epinephrine. Considerations should be made for transfer to a higher level of care in the rare case that it is necessary. In most situations, in the hands of an experienced clinician, an outpatient setting is appropriate for this challenge.

## 7.9 AERD and Desensitization

Desensitization to ASA in AERD is an integral part of treatment for many of these patients. In this setting, desensitization refers to the regular administration of ASA in order to maintain a desensitized state. The benefits from ASA desensitization occur only in the setting of regular daily administration of ASA and are lost 48 h after the last dose is taken. For most patients, desensitization is undertaken in an effort to better control underlying airway inflammation or nasal polyposis.

Patients with a compelling need for ASA therapy, such as for cardiovascular disease [88] or those with rheumatologic conditions requiring regular NSAIDs, gain both the respiratory disease benefits as well as the benefits from ASA or NSAIDs on the other coexistent diseases.

Numerous studies quantify the benefit from ASA therapy in AERD [89–92]. Improvement in sinus disease, decreased requirements for sinus surgery, decrease in sinus infections, and improvement in sense of smell have all been shown in the upper airways. Lower airway benefits include decreased need for systemic corticosteroids, fewer emergency room visits and hospitalizations for asthma, and overall improvement in asthma symptom scores. Another obvious benefit of ASA desensitization is the ability to use this medication daily for cardiovascular indications [88]. Thus, ASA desensitization is well suited for the individual with need for unacceptably high doses of systemic corticosteroids, recalcitrant sinus disease requiring repeated surgical interventions, or those with persistent ongoing symptoms that have not responded to other conventional therapies [93]. In one study, ASA desensitization was also shown to be cost effective in the treatment of AERD [94].

The dose of ASA necessary to treat the airway disease is in the range of 650–1,300 mg of ASA per day (325 mg tablets, one tablet twice daily to two tablets twice daily). In one smaller study, 100 mg of daily ASA was ineffective, while 300 mg was effective at controlling sinus disease [95]. It would appear from the existing literature that 300–325 mg of daily ASA therapy represents the lower limits of effectiveness of chronic ASA therapy in AERD. Doses of 325 mg per day are less likely to give clinical benefit when compared with higher doses [96]. A recent report identified the difficulty in predicting the dose of ASA that patients will have an optimum response to. In this study, patients were randomly assigned to 650 or 1,300 mg cumulative daily ASA dose. While both doses were effective, about half of the patients in the high-dose arm were able to decrease to a 650 mg daily dose, while half of the group initially randomized to the 650 mg daily dose found it necessary to increase to the high dose (1,300 mg daily dose) due to inadequate symptom control [92]. This suggests the presence of a dose-effect of ASA therapy in AERD. While some patients may have benefit from ASA doses in the 300 mg daily range, many of these would likely enjoy greater benefit to their respiratory tree by increasing the ASA dose.

## 7.10 Side Effects

Chronic ASA therapy is not without risk. Dyspepsia ranks as the most common reason that patients discontinue or reduce the dose of ASA [92]. Bleeding or ecchymosis and urticaria/angioedema were also some of the more common reasons for ASA cessation. Another less common but more severe adverse effect is gastric bleeding (2/172) [89]. At the end of 1 year, between 14% and 16% of patients will discontinue ASA due to adverse effects [89,92]. Another adverse effect of ASA or NSAID therapy is acute kidney injury. Many patients are on angiotensin converting enzyme inhibitors or angiotensin receptor blockers at the time of ASA desensitization. Co-therapy with either of these antihypertensives and ASA can increase the risk of acute kidney injury and should be taken into consideration if long-term treatment with ASA is planned [97].

## 7.11 ASA Desensitization Specifics

ASA desensitization is carried out in much the way that the ASA challenge is done. Patients are selected with stable airway disease and an FEV1 > 70%. Doses are administered starting at 30–60 mg ASA. The dose that causes the reaction is called the “provoking dose.” The reaction is treated, and then the same dose is then repeated. In most cases, the reaction to the second dose is attenuated if not absent altogether. Subsequent dosing is outlined in Table 7.2. The desensitization is completed when the patient has received 325 mg of ASA without reaction. The desensitized state lasts approximately 48 h. After this time, if no more ASA is administered desensitization will be lost completely by 96 h. It is incumbent on the patient to understand that ASA desensitization is an ongoing treatment.

## 7.12 Leukotriene-Modifying Drugs (LTMDs) in AERD and During Desensitization

Given the dramatic outpouring of leukotriene mediators in the AERD reaction, the use of pharmacologic therapy targeting this particular pathway would seem to offer promise in treatment of the underlying disease and attenuation of the acute reaction to ASA in AERD. In the USA, the leukotriene receptor antagonists montelukast and zafirlukast are available, as is the 5-lipoxygenase inhibitor zileuton. In treatment of the underlying inflammatory airway disease in AERD, both zileuton and montelukast have been evaluated. Zileuton was associated with improvement in pulmonary function, need for less rescue inhaler use, and improvement in sense of smell [98]. In a similar double-blinded, placebo-controlled trial of 80 patients, montelukast was shown to improve several measures of asthma including FEV1 [99]. Similarly, an improvement in nasal symptoms and function was observed after a 4-week trial of montelukast when compared with placebo [100]. What is unexpected is that AERD patients do not have an enhanced response to leukotriene modifier drugs. The response to treatment appears to be roughly similar to the non-AERD asthmatic population [101,102].

However, during the reaction from ingested ASA, LTMDs, particularly montelukast, have an important modulatory role. Montelukast has been studied the most, likely due to its ready availability in the USA. It is clear that the use of montelukast during ASA challenges changes the nature of the reaction. Reactions shift from involving both the upper and lower airways to primarily upper airway reactions [103,104]. This has been shown to decrease the magnitude drop in FEV1, thereby enhancing the safety of these reactions [11]. In these studies, the negative challenge rate remained unchanged from historical rates prior to the introduction of LTMDs to the market, or to the negative challenge rate in those patients not taking an LTMD. Thus, there does not appear to be a significant risk that the entire ASA reaction could be completely masked by the use of montelukast. One study challenged ten patients with ASA before and then while using montelukast. In one of these ten patients, the reaction appeared to be blocked completely by montelukast [105]. So, while likely very rare, there may be patients who undergo a "silent" challenge or desensitization to ASA while taking an LTMD.

In other studies, pranlukast use during ASA challenge led to diminished respiratory reactions, but did not decrease aspirin-induced leukotriene production [106]. In studies evaluating the nasal response, montelukast pretreatment protected against local effects from nasal ASA-lysine challenge with no difference observed between a 10 or 40 mg montelukast dose [107]. In a 4-week placebo-controlled trial, montelukast significantly improved nasal flow and symptoms during nasal ASA-lysine challenge [100]. Discordant results evaluating zileuton in protection of the ASA-induced reaction exist. Israel and colleagues found zileuton to completely protect the upper and lower airways from ASA challenge at a predetermined provoking dose [108]. Increasing doses of ASA were not investigated. Pauls et al. found that zileuton did not offer complete protection to any of six patients undergoing ASA challenge and desensitization [109]. The authors conclude that zileuton may offer a degree of benefit by shifting the response to a higher dose of ASA, but that complete blockade of the ASA-induced reaction by zileuton is uncommon.

These studies demonstrate that LTMD therapy can be considered as part of the maintenance therapy for the AERD patient, recognizing that benefit to the airways would not be any different than in aspirin-tolerant asthma. But, during the acute desensitization process, concomitant LTMD therapy, specifically with montelukast, should be strongly considered as a means of increasing the safety of the oral challenge.

## 7.13 Local Nasal Desensitization

Several studies have evaluated a role of ASA-lysine in desensitization, primarily to treat nasal polyposis [110–113]. Of these, two have demonstrated an improvement in outcomes with intranasal chronic ASA-lysine administration, yet the only double-blinded controlled trial failed to show significant clinical benefit [113]. Further studies in this regard are recommended to address this important issue.

## 7.14 Desensitization Events

The mechanism behind ASA desensitization remains unclear. It certainly represents a uniquely different desensitization process when compared with traditional allergen immunotherapy, which effects a long-term immunological change or standard antibiotic desensitization that allows continued use of the drug on a regular basis, but leads to no long-term immunological effect. In ASA desensitization, the continued use of ASA exerts a disease modifying effect, yet permanent effects are not seen in that the ability to safely take ASA is lost after 48–96 h have elapsed from the last dose [114]. The beneficial effects of ASA desensitization are thought to rapidly wane after that time.

Several concepts have shaped the degree to which the mechanism of ASA desensitization is understood. Leukotriene B4, one of the products of AA metabolism, is reduced after ASA desensitization to levels seen in normal controls [115]. In AERD patients after acute and chronic desensitization, a rise in urinary $LTE_4$ still occurred with administration of ASA, but this rise was less intense than during the ASA-provoked reaction. Despite the increase in urinary $LTE_4$, there was no concomitant decrease in FEV1 [116]. Airway responsiveness to inhaled $LTE_4$ decreases markedly on the day following ASA desensitization [117,118]. Cys-LT1 receptors are elevated at baseline in AERD patients, and may decrease to levels seen in ASA-tolerant asthmatics after chronic desensitization [119]. These findings support a conclusion that in the desensitized individual, although leukotrienes are still produced, they no longer cause such pronounced inflammatory changes.

## 7.15 Cutaneous Reactions

In chronic idiopathic urticaria (CIU), it is well known that ingestion of ASA or NSAIDs can lead to precipitous worsening of cutaneous symptoms. The incidence of aspirin sensitivity in the chronic urticaria population is likely between 5% and 40% [120–122]. In a population of patients without chronic urticaria, urticaria and angioedema from ASA occurs in 0.07–0.2% [8]. There is not a clear distinction between those patients with respiratory reactions (AERD) and those with cutaneous reaction. Some patients with AERD will experience hives and or urticaria during aspirin challenge. Typically, these AERD patients can be successfully desensitized to ASA/NSAIDs, which distinguishes them from CIU patients in whom desensitization is not as successful. Similarly, in a population of patients with CIU and reactions to NSAIDS, about 10% may also have respiratory symptoms [123].

The underlying mechanism of cutaneous reactions to cross-reacting NSAIDs or ASA and AERD reactions is similar. COX-1 blockade is central to the mechanism as demonstrated by the following findings: COX-2 selective medications are well tolerated in these individuals, and urinary leukotriene levels are elevated at the time of reaction and correlate with severity of symptoms [123]. There is one report of possible cross-reactivity between COX-1 and COX-2 inhibitors in COX-1-induced urticaria or angioedema. In this report, 1/26 patients reacted to valdecoxib and 2/26 to rofecoxib [124]. This is difficult to explain, given the bulk of evidence that exists demonstrating safety of COX-2 inhibitors in COX-1-mediated urticaria [125–127].

NSAID reactions have been observed to precede chronic urticaria [128]. This suggests that cross-reacting cutaneous reactions to ASA and NSAIDs may represent a spectrum. At one end, there are individuals without chronic urticaria who experience urticaria only after ASA or NSAID ingestion. At the other end are individuals with chronic daily urticaria who develop significant worsening of their symptoms after NSAID or ASA ingestion.

## 7.16 Desensitization

Several protocols exist for desensitization to COX-1-mediated reactions to NSAIDs or ASA. These, in part, reflect the clinical scenario prompting desensitization whether urgent [129–132] or routine [133]. An example desensitization protocol can be found in Table 7.3. In the authors' experience, desensitization in the setting of chronic urticaria is generally unsuccessful, but a report of a successful desensitization has been published [134].

## 7.17 Isolated NSAID Reactions

In some patients, a reaction only occurs to one NSAID while a variety of other COX-1 inhibitors are tolerated with adverse reaction. Generally, clinical history provides the diagnosis in patients with proven tolerance to multiple NSAIDs and an isolated reaction to only one. Four general patterns of isolated NSAID reactions have been described: (1) single-NSAID-induced urticaria/

**Table 7.3** Rapid desensitization for aspirin-related urticaria-angioedema [132]

Prior to desensitization:

Antihistamine pretreatment
Prepare aspirin dilutions as follows: disperse 81 mg ASA tablet in 81 mL of water
Desensitization:
Start intravenous line
Administer every 15–20 min orally

| Dose (mg) | mL | Total dose (mg) |
|---|---|---|
| 0.1 mg ASA | 0.1 | 0.1 |
| 0.3 mg ASA | 0.3 | 0.4 |
| 1 | 1 | 1.4 |
| 3 | 3 | 4.4 |
| 10 | 10 | 14.4 |
| 20 | 20 | 34.4 |
| 40 | 40 | 74.4 |
| 81 | 81 | 155.4 |
| Can increase to 325 mg | | |

angioedema, (2) single-NSAID-induced anaphylaxis or non-IgE anaphylaxis, (3) aseptic meningitis from a specific NSAID, and (4) hypersensitivity pneumonitis caused by a specific NSAID [135]. The absence of cross-reactivity among the COX-1 inhibitors rules out this pathway in the etiology of the reaction. In general, these reactions are less well characterized, but likely immune mediated. Type 1 and 2 reactions are likely to be IgE mediated in many cases.

Given the wide usage of NSAIDs, it is not surprising that the prevalence of single NSAID urticarial or anaphylaxis reactions is between 0.1% and 3.6% [5,136,137]. These reactions have occurred most commonly with diclofenac, naproxen, and ibuprofen [138]. These authors concluded that there may be an increased risk for anaphylactic reactions among the heteroaryl acetic acid group of NSAIDs, comprised of diclofenac, tolmetin, and ketorolac. Strom and colleagues suggested that the risk of allergic sensitization was not associated with the specific drug, but rather with the reason for the use of the NSAID [139].

Unfortunately, clinical history alone may not be able to help confirm the diagnosis in patients who react to one NSAID and immediately discontinue the use of any further NSAIDs. If an isolated NSAID reaction is suspected, confirmation can be made by oral challenge with a structurally dissimilar NSAID or ASA [140,141]. Unfortunately, neither skin prick testing nor specific IgE assays are helpful in identifying a specific diagnosis in these individuals. While rare, there are individuals who likely have IgE-mediated reactions to a single class of NSAIDs and thus may react to several NSAIDs in the same group, but tolerate unrelated COX-1 blockers [137]. Table 7.4 lists the classes of NSAIDs.

**Table 7.4** Classification of nonsteroidal anti-inflammatory drugs by structural class (Adapted from [146])

| | | |
|---|---|---|
| ***Enolic acids*** | | |
| *Oxicams* | | *Pyrazolones* |
| Piroxicam | | Phenylbutazone |
| Meloxicam | | Oxyphenbutazone |
| ***Carboxylic acids*** | | |
| ***Acetic acids*** | | |
| *Phenylactic acids* | | *Carbo- and heterocyclic acids* |
| Diclofenac | | Indomethacin |
| | | Etodolac |
| | | Sulindac |
| | | Tolmetic |
| | | Ketorolac |
| ***Propionic acids*** | ***Fenamic acids*** | ***Salicyclic acids*** |
| Motrin, Rufen (ibuprofen) | Meclofenamate | Aspirin |
| Naprosyn (naproxen) | Mefanimic acid | Salsalate |
| Anaprox (naproxen sodium) | | Diflunisal |
| Oraflex (benoxaprofen) | | Sodium salicylate |
| Nalfon (fenoprofen) | | Trisalicylate |
| Orudis (ketoprofen) | | |
| **Nonacidic compounds** | | |
| Nabumetone | | |

This article was published in Ballou et al. [146].

## 7.18 Desensitization

Given the hypothesis that these single-drug reactions are likely IgE mediated, desensitization should be effective. Since most patients are able to tolerate alternative NSAIDs, it is uncommon for these patients to required desensitization to the specific drug they have reacted to. If desensitization is performed, it should start at very low doses of the drug and be performed in an intensive care unit with an intravenous line in place. A protocol similar to that given in Table 7.3 would likely be appropriate.

## 7.19 COX-2 Isolated Reactions

As outlined above, COX-2 inhibitors should not cross-react with NSAID and ASA-induced airway and urticarial reactions, as these are mediated through COX-1. There are however cases of COX-2 inhibitor-induced anaphylaxis [142–144]. These are best treated as single-drug allergic reactions. There is a single report of reaction to both rofecoxib and diclofenac-misoprostol [145]. While there may be some rare cross-reacting immunogen similar between these medications, another explanation is that given the high rate of use of these medications, rare patients may develop allergic reactions to two separate molecules.

## References


1. Stevenson DD, Simon RA, Zuraw BL. Sensitivity to aspirin and nonsteroidal anti-inflammatory drugs. In: Adkinson NF, Yunginger JW, et al., eds. *Middleton's Allergy Principles and Practice,* 6th edition. Philadelphia, PA: Mosby; 2003:1695–1710.
2. Hedman J, Kaprio J, Poussa T, et al. Prevalence of asthma, aspirin intolerance, nasal polyps and chronic obstructive pulmonary disease in a population-based study. *Int J Epidemiol.* 1999;28:717–722.
3. Vally H, Taylor M, Thompson PJ. The prevalence of aspirin intolerant asthma in Australian asthmatic patients. *Thorax.* 2002;57:569–574.
4. Kasper L, Sladek K, Duplaga M, et al. Prevalence of asthma with aspirin hypersensitivity in the adult population of Poland. *Allergy.* 2003;58:1064–1066.
5. Gomes E, Cardoso MF, Praca F, et al. Self-reported drug allergy in a general adult Portuguese population. *Clin Exp Allergy.* 2004;34:1597–1601.
6. Kim J, Kountakis SE. The prevalence of Samter's triad in patients undergoing functional endoscopic sinus surgery. *Ear, Nose, Throat J.* 2007;86(7):396–399.
7. Szczeklik A, Nizankowska E, Duplaga M. Natural history of aspirin-induced asthma. AIANE Investigators. European Network on Aspirin-Induced Asthma. *Eur Respir J.* 2000;16:432–436.
8. Jenkins C, Costello J, Hodge L. Systematic review of prevalence of aspirin-induced asthma and its implications for clinical practice. *Br Med J.* 2004;328:434–437
9. Berges-Gimeno MP, Simon RA, Stevenson DD. The natural history and clinical characteristics of aspirin-exacerbated respiratory disease. *Ann Allergy Asthma Immunol.* 2002;89:474–478.
10. Pleskow WW, Stevenson DD, Mathison DA, Simon RA, Schatz M, Zeiger RS. Aspirin-sensitive rhinosinusitis/asthma: spectrum of adverse reactions to aspirin. *J Allergy Clin Immunol.* 1983:71;574–579.
11. White A, Ludington E, Mehra P, Stevenson DD, Simon RA. Effect of leukotriene modifier drugs on the safety of oral aspirin challenges. *Ann Allergy Asthma Immunol.* 2006;97:688–693.
12. Hope AP, Woessner KA, Rimon RA, Stevenson DD. Rational approach to aspirin dosing during oral challenges and desensitization or patients with aspirin-exacerbated respiratory disease. *J Allergy Clin Immunol.* 2009;123:406–410.
13. Chen A, Bennett C. Ketorolac-induced bronchospasm in an aspirin-intolerant patient. *Anesth Prog.* 1994;41:102–107.

14. Sitenga GL, Ing EB, Van Dellen RG, Younge BR, Leavitt JA. Asthma caused by topical application of ketorolac. *Ophthalmology.* 1996;103:890–892.
15. Settipane RA, Schrank PJ, Simon RA, Mathison DA, Christiansen SC, Stevenson DD. Prevalence of cross-sensitivity with acetaminophen in aspirin-sensitive asthmatic subjects. *J Allergy Clin Immunol.* 1995;96:480–485.
16. Szczeklik A, Gryglewski RJ, Czerniawska-Mysik G. Clinical patterns of hypersensitivity to nonsteroidal anti-inflammatory drugs and their pathogenesis. *J Allergy Clin Immunol.* 1977;60:276–284.
17. Delaney JC. The diagnosis of aspirin idiosyncrasy by analgesic challenge. *Clin Allergy.* 1976;6:177–181.
18. Stevenson DD, Simon RA. Lack of cross-reactivity between rofecoxib and aspirin in aspirin-sensitive patients with asthma. *J Allergy Clin Immunol.* 2001;108:47–51.
19. Woessner KM, Simon RA, Stevenson DD. Safety of high-dose rofecoxib in patients with aspirin-exacerbated respiratory disease. *Ann Allergy Asthma Immunol.* 2004;93:339–344.
20. Woessner KM, Simon RA, Stevenson DD. The safety of celecoxib in aspirin exacerbated respiratory disease. *Arthritis Rheum.* 2002;46:2201–2206.
21. Gyllfors BG, Overholt J, Drupka D, et al. Biochemical and clinical evidence that aspirin-intolerant asthmatic subjects tolerate the cyclooxygenase 2-selective analgetic drug celecoxib. *J Allergy Clin Immunol.* 2003;111:1116–1121.
22. Yoshida S, Ishizaki Y, Onuca K, et al. Selective cyclo-oxygenase 2 inhibitor in patients with aspirin-induced asthma. *J Allergy Clin Immunol.* 2000;106:1201–1202.
23. Micheletto C, Tognella S, Guerriero M, Dal Negro R. Nasal and bronchial tolerability of rofecoxib in patients with aspirin induced asthma. *Eur Ann Allergy Clinical Immunol.* 2006;38:10–14.
24. Celik G, Pasaoglu G, Bavbek S, et al. Tolerability of selective cyclooxygenase inhibitor, celecoxib, in patients with analgesic intolerance. *J Asthma.* 2005;42:127–131.
25. Martin-Garcia C, Hinojosa M, Berges P, et al. Celecoxib, a highly selective COX-2 inhibitor, is safe in aspirin-induced asthma patients. *J Invest Allergol Clin Immunol.* 2003;13:20–25.
26. Szczeklik A, Nizankowska E, Bochenek G, et al. Safety of a specific COX-2 inhibitor in aspirin-induced asthma. *Clin Exp Allergy.* 2001;31:219–225.
27. Patrono C, Patrignani P, Garcia Rodriguez LA. Cyclooxygenase-selective inhibition of prostanoid formation: transducing biochemical selectivity into clinical read-outs. *J Clin Invest.* 2001;108:7–13.
28. Patrignani P, Panara MR, Sciulli MG, et al. Differential inhibition of human prostaglandin endoperoxide synthase-1 and -2 by nonsteroidal anti-inflammatory drugs. *J Physiol Pharmacol.* 1997; 48:623–632.
29. Kirchner T, Argentieri DC, Barbone AG, et al. Evaluation of the Anti-inflammatory activity of a dual cyclooxygenase-2 selective/5-lipoxygenase inhibitor, RWJ 63556, in a canine model of inflammation. *J Pharmacol Exper Therapeutics.* 1997;282:1094–1101.
30. Prieto A, De Barrio M, Martin E, et al. Tolerability to nabumetone and meloxicam in patients with nonsteroidal anti-inflammatory drug intolerance. *J Allergy Clin Immunol.* 2007;119:960–964.
31. Senna G, Bilo MB, AntonicelliL, et al. Tolerability of three selective cyclo-oxygenase-2 inhibitors, meloxicam, celecoxib and rofecoxib in NSAID-sensitive patients. *Eur Ann Allergy Clinl Immunol.* 2004;36:215–218.
32. Bavbek S, Celik G, Ozer F, Mungan D, Misirligil Z. Safety of selective COX-2 inhibitors in aspirin/nonsteroidal anti-inflammatory drug intolerant patients: comparison of nimesulide, meloxicam, and rofecoxib. *J Asthma.* 2004;41:67–75.
33. Bianco S, Robuschi M, Petrigni G, et al. Efficacy and tolerability of nimesulide in asthmatic patients intolerant to aspirin. *Drugs.* 1993;46:115–120.
34. Mascia K, Borish L, Patrie J, et al. Chronic hyperplastic eosinophilic sinusitis as a predictor of aspirin-exacerbated respiratory disease. *Ann Allergy Asthma Immunol.* 2005;94:652–657.
35. Young J, Frenkiel S, Tewfik MA, Mouadeb DA. Long-term outcome analysis of endoscopic sinus surgery for chronic sinusitis. *Am J Rhinol.* 2007;21:743–747.
36. Garrel R, Gardiner Q, Khudjadze M, et al. Endoscopic surgical treatment of sinonasal polyposis-medium term outcomes (mean follow-up of 5 years). *Rhinology.* 2003;41:91–96.
37. Vento SI, Ertama LO, Hytonen ML, Wolff CH, Malmberg CH. Nasal polyposis: clinical course during 20 years. *Ann Allergy Asthma Immunol.* 2000;85:209–214.
38. Lee JH, Haselkorn T, Borish L, et al. Risk factors associated with perstent airflow limitation in severe or difficult-to-treat asthma: insights from the TENOR study. *Chest.* 2007;132(6):1882–1889.
39. Mascia K, Haselkorn T, Deniz YM, et al. Aspirin sensitivity and severity of asthma: evidence for irreversible airway obstruction in patients with severe or difficult-to-treat asthma. *J Allergy Clin Immunol.* 2005;116:970–975.
40. Picado C, Castillo JA, Montserrat JM, Agusti-Vidal A. Aspirin-intolerance as a precipitating factor of life-threatening attacks of asthma requiring mechanical ventilation. *Eur Respir J.* 1989;2:137–139.
41. Koga T, Oshita Y, Kamimura T et al. Characterization of patients with frequent exacerbation of asthma. *Respir Med.* 2006;100:273–278.

42. Rachelefsky GS, Coulson A, Siegel SC, Stiehm ER. Aspirin intolerance in childhood asthma: detected by oral challenge. *Pediatrics.* 1975;56:443–448.
43. Vedanthan PK, Menon MM, Bell TD, Bergin D. Aspirin and tartrazine oral challenge: incidence of adverse response in chronic childhood asthma. *J Allergy Clin Immunol.* 1977;60:8–13.
44. Fischer TJ, Guilfoile TD, Kesarwala HH, et al. Adverse pulmonary responses to aspirin and acetaminophen in chronic childhood asthma. *Pediatrics.* 1983;71:313–318.
45. Towns SJ, Mellis CM. Role of acetyl salicylic acid and sodium metabisulfite in chronic childhood asthma. *Pediatrics.* 1984;73:631–637.
46. Debley JS, Carter ER, Gibson RL, Rosenfeld M, Redding GJ. The prevalence of ibuprofen-sensitive asthma in children: a randomized controlled bronchoprovocation challenge study. *J Pediatr.* 2005;147:233–238.
47. Tilley SL, Coffman TM, Koller BH. Mixed messages: modulation of inflammation and immune responses by prostaglandins and thromboxanes. *J Clin Invest.* 2001;108:15–23.
48. Vancheri C, Mastruzzo C, Sortino MA, Crimi N. The lung as a privileged site for the beneficial actions of PGE2. *Trends Immunol.* 2004;25(1):40–46.
49. Sheller JR, Mitchell D, Meyrick B, Oates J, Breyer R. EP2 receptor mediates bronchodilation by PGE2 in mice. *J Appl Physiol.* 2000; 88: 2214–2218.
50. Schafer D, Schmid M, Gode UC, Baenkler V. Dynamics of eicosanoids in peripheral blood cells during bronchial provocation in aspirin-intolerant asthmatics. *Eur Respir J.* 1999;13:638–646.
51. Sestinini P, Armetti L, Gambaro G, et al. Inhaled PGE2 prevents aspirin-induced bronchoconstriction and urinary LTE4 excretion in aspirin-sensitive asthma. *Am J Respir Crit Care Med.* 196;572–577.
52. Roberts LJ, Sweetman BJ, Lewis RA, et al. Increased production of prostaglandin D2 in patients with systemic mastocytosis. *N Engl J Med.* 1980;303:1400–1404.
53. Bochenek G, Nagraba K, Nizankowska E, Szczeklik A. A controlled study of 9alpha,11beta-PGF2 (a prostaglandin D2 metabolite) in plasma and urine of patients with bronchial asthma and healthy controls after aspirin challenge. *J Allergy Clin Immunol.* 2003;111(4):743–749.
54. Morris HG, Sherman NA, Shepperdson FT, Selner JC. Radioimmunoassay of thromboxane B2 in plasma of normal and asthmatic subjects. *Adv Prostaglandin & Thromboxane Res.* 1980;8:1759–1764.
55. Juergens UR, Christiansen SC, Stevenson DD, Zuraw BL. Inhibition of monocyte leukotriene B4 production after aspirin desensitization. *J Allergy Clin Immunol.* 1995;96(2):148–56.
56. Antczak A, Montuschi P, Kharitonow S, Gorski P, Barnes PJ. Increased exhaled cysteinyl-leukotrienes and 8-isoprostane in aspirin-induced asthma. *Am J Respir Crit Care Med.* 2002;166:301–306.
57. Ferreri NR, Howland WC, Stevenson DD, et al. Release of leukotrienes, prostaglandins and histamine into nasal secretions of aspirin-sensitive asthmatics during reaction to aspirin. *Am Rev Respir Dis.* 1988;137:847–854.
58. Fischer AR, Rosenberg MA, Lilly CM, et al. Direct evidence for a role of the mast cell in the nasal response to aspirin in aspirin-sensitive asthma. *J Allergy Clin Immunol.* 1994;94:1046–1056.
59. Kowalski ML, Sliwinska-Kowalska M, Igarashi Y, et al. Nasal secretions in response to acetylsalicylic acid. *J Allergy Clin Immunol.* 1993;91:580–598.
60. Picado C, Ramis I, Rosello J, et al. Release of peptide leukotriene into nasal secretions after local instillation of aspirin in aspirin-sensitive asthmatic patients. *Am Rev Respir Dis.* 1992;145:65–69.
61. Christie PE, Tagari P, Ford-Hutchinson AW, Charlesson S, Chee P, Arm JP. Lee TH, et al. Urinary leukotriene E4 concentrations increase after aspirin challenge in aspirin-sensitive asthmatic subjects. *Am Rev Respir Dis.* 1991;143(5 Pt 1):1025–1029.
62. Sladek K, Dworski R, Soja J, et al. Eicosanoids in bronchoalveolar lavage fluid of aspirin-intolerant patients with asthma after aspirin challenge. *Am J Respir Crit Care Med.* 1994;149:940–946.
63. Daffern PJ, Muilenburg D, Hugli T. Stevenson DD. Association of urinary leukotriene E4 excretion during aspirin challenges with severity of respiratory responses. *J Allergy Clin Immunol.* 1999;104:559–564.
64. Cowburn AS, Sladek K, Soja J, et al: Overexpression of leukotriene C4 synthase in bronchial biopsies from patients with aspirin-intolerant asthma. *J Clin Invest.* 1998;101:834–846.
65. Szczeklik A, Sanak M, Nizankowska E, et al. Leukotriene C4 synthase genetic polymorphism directs urinary cyteinyl-leukotriene response to aspirin challenge in asthma, *Allergy.* 1998;53:61–67.
66. Celik G, Bavbek S, Misirligi Z, et al. Release of cysteinyl leukotrienes with aspirin stimulation and the effect of prostaglandin E2 on this release from peripheral blood leucocytes in aspirin-induced asthmatic patients. *Clin Exp Allergy.* 2001;31:1615–1622.
67. Szczeklik A, Mastalerz L, Nizankowska E, et al. Protective and bronchodilator effects of prostaglandin E and salbutamol in aspirin-induced asthma. *Am J Resp Crit Care Med.* 1996;152:571–576.
68. Christie PE, Spur BW, Lee TH. The effects of lipoxin A4 on airway responses in asthmatic subjects. *Am Rev Respir Dis.* 1992;145:1281–1284.
69. Edenius C, Kumlin M, Bjork T, Anggard A, Lindgren JA. Lipoxin formation in human nasal polyps and bronchial tissue. *FEBS Lett.* 1990; 272: 25–28.
70. M Sanak, BD Levy, CB Clish, et al. Aspirin-tolerant asthmatics generate more lipoxins than aspirin-intolerant asthmatics. *Eur Respir J.* 2000;16:44–49.

71. Dursun AB, Woessner KA, Simon RA, Karasoy D, Stevenson DD. Predicting outcomes of oral aspirin challenges in patients with asthma, nasal polyps, and chronic sinusitis. *Ann Allergy Clin Immunol.* 2008;100:420–425.
72. Macy E, Bernstein J, Castells MC, et al. Aspirin challenge and desensitization for aspirin exacerbated respiratory disease: a practice paper. *Ann Allergy Asthma Immunol.* 2007;98:172–174.
73. Melillo G, Balzano G, Blanco S, et al. Report of the INTERASMA Working Group on standardization of inhalation provocation tests in Aspirin-Induced Asthma: oral and inhalation provocation tests for the diagnosis of aspirin-induced asthma. *Allergy.* 2001;56:899–911.
74. Nizankowska-Mogilnicka E, Bochenek G, Mastalerz L, et al. EAACI/GA2LEN guideline: aspirin provocation tests for the diagnosis of aspirin hypersensitivity. *Allergy.* 2007;62:1111–1118.
75. Mita H, Higashi N, Taniguchi M, Higashi A, Akiyama K. Increase in urinary leukotriene B4 glucuronide concentration in patients with aspirin-intolerant asthma after intravenous aspirin challenge. *Clin Exp Allergy.* 2004;34:1262–1269.
76. Milewski M, Mastalez L, Nizankowska E, Szczeklik A. Nasal provocation test with lysine-aspirin for diagnosis of aspirin-sensitive asthma. *J Allergy Clin Immunol.* 1998;101:581–586.
77. Alonso-Llamazares A, Martinez-Cocera C, Dominguez-Ortega J, et al. Nasal provocation test (NPT) with aspirin: a sensitive and safe method to diagnose aspirin-induced asthma (AIA). *Allergy.* 2002;57:632–635.
78. Casadevall J, Ventura P-J, Mullol J, Picado C. Intranasal challenge with aspirin in the diagnosis of aspirin intolerant asthma: evaluation of nasal response by acoustic rhinometry. *Thorax.* 2000;55:921–924.
79. Pawlowicz A, Williams WR, Davies BH. Inhalation and nasal challenge in the diagnosis of aspirin-induced asthma. *Allergy.* 1991;46:405–409.
80. White A, Bigby T, Stevenson D. Intranasal ketorolac challenge for the diagnosis of aspirin-exacerbated respiratory disease. *Ann Allergy Asthma Immunol.* 2006;97:190–195.
81. Martelli NA. Bronchial and intravenous provocation tests with indomethacin in aspirin-sensitive asthmatics. *Am Rev Respir Dis.* 1979;120:1073–1079.
82. Melillo E, LoSchiavo M, DeFelice A. Cross sensitivity to aspirin, noramidopyrine and naproxen in a patient with asthma detected by inhalation test with the three drugs. *Allergy.* 1993;48 Suppl 16:A2325.
83. Melillo G, Balzano G, Bianco S, et al. Oral and inhalation provocation tests for the diagnosis of aspirin-induced asthma. *Allergy.* 2001:56:899–911.
84. Nizankowska E, Bestynska-Krypel A, Cmiel A, et al. Oral and bronchial provocation tests with aspirin for diagnosis of aspirin-induced asthma. *Eur Respir J.* 2000;15:863–869.
85. Phillips GD, Foord R, Holgate ST. Inhaled lysine-aspirin as a bronchoprovocation procedure in aspirin-sensitive asthma, its repeatability, absence of a late-phase reaction, and the role of histamine. *J Allergy Clin Immunol.* 1989;84:232–241.
86. Dahlen B, Zetterstrom O. Comparison of bronchial and per oral provocation with aspirin in aspirin-sensitive asthmatics. *Eur Respir J.* 1990;3:527–534.
87. Melillo G, Padovano A, Masi C, et al. Aspirin-intolerance in asthma: detection by a new dosimeter inhalation test. *Aerosol Med.* 1991;4:865.
88. Gollapudi RR, Teirstein PS, Stevenson DD, Simon RA. Aspirin sensitivity: implications for patients with coronary artery disease. *JAMA.* 2004;292:3017–3023.
89. Berges-Gimeno MP, Simon RA, Stevenson DD. Long-term treatment with aspirin desensitization in asthmatic patients with aspirin-exacerbated respiratory disease. *J Allergy Clin Immunol.* 2003;111:180–186.
90. Stevenson DD, Hankammer MA, Mathison DA, Christiansen SC, Simon RA. Aspirin desensitization treatment of aspirin-sensitive patients with rhinosinusitis-asthma: long term outcomes. *J Allergy Clin Immunol.* 1996;98:751–758.
91. Berges Gimeno MP, Simon RA, Stevenson DD. Early effects of aspirin desensitization treatment in asthmatic patients with aspirin-exacerbated respiratory disease. *Ann Allergy Asthma Immunol.* 2003;90:338–341.
92. Lee JY, Simon RA, Stevenson DD. Selection of aspirin dosages for aspirin desensitization treatment in patients with aspirin-exacerbated respiratory disease. *J Allergy Clin Immunol.* 2007;119:157–164.
93. Stevenson DD, Simon RA. Selection of patients for aspirin desensitization treatment. *J Allergy Clin Immunol.* 2006;118:801–804.
94. Shaker M, Lobb A, Jenkins P, et al. An economic analysis of aspirin desensitization in aspirin-exacerbated respiratory disease. *J Allergy Clin Immunol.* 2008;121:81–87.
95. Rozsasi A, Polzehl D, Deutschle T, et al. Long-term treatment with aspirin desensitization: a prospective clinical trial comparing 100 and 300mg aspirin daily. *Allergy.* 2008;63:1228–1234.
96. Stevenson DD, Pleskow WW, Simon RA, et al. Aspirin-sensitive rhinosinusitis asthma: a double-blind crossover study of treatment with aspirin. *J Allergy Clin Immunol.* 1984;73:500–507.
97. Whelton A. Nephrotoxicity of nonsteroidal anti-inflammatory drugs: physiologic foundations and clinical implications. *Am J Med.* 1999;106:13S–24S.
98. Dahlen B, Nizankowska E, Szczeklik A, et al. Benefits from adding the 5-lipoxygenase inhibitor zileuton to conventional therapy in aspirin-sensitive asthmatics. *Am J Resp Crit Care Med.* 1998;157:1187–1194.

99. Dahlen S, Malstrom K, Nizankowska E, et al. Improvement of aspirin-intolerant asthma by montelukast, a leukotriene antagonist: a randomized, double blind, placebo controlled trial. *Am J Respir Crit Care Med.* 2002;165:9–14.
100. Micheletto C, Tognella S, Visconti M,. Montelukast 10 mg improves nasal function and nasal response in ASA-sensitive asthmatics: a controlled study vs placebo. *Allergy.* 2004;59:284–294.
101. Israel E, Cohn J, Dube L, Drazen J. Effect of treatment with zileuton, a 5-lipoxygenase inhibitor, in patients with asthma: a randomized controlled trial. *JAMA.* 1996;275:931–936.
102. Joos S, Miksch A, Szecsenyi J, et al. Montelukast as add-on therapy to inhaled corticosteroids in the treatment of mild to moderate asthma: a systematic review. *Thorax.* 2008;63:453–462.
103. Berges-Gimeno MP, Simon RA, Stevenson DD. The effect of leukotriene-modifier drugs on aspirin-induced asthma and rhinitis reactions. *Clin Exp Allergy.* 2002;32:1491–1496.
104. White AA, Stevenson DD, Simon RA. The blocking effect of essential controller medications during aspirin challenges in patients with aspirin-exacerbated respiratory disease. *Ann Allergy Asthma Immunol.* 2005;95:330–335.
105. Stevenson DD, Simon RA, Mathison DA, Christiansen SC. Montelukast is only partially effective in inhibiting aspirin responses in aspirin-sensitive asthmatics. *Ann Allergy Asthma Immunol.* 2000;85:477–482.
106. Obase Y, Shimoda T, Tomari S, et al. Effects of pranlukast on aspirin-induced bronchoconstriction: differences in chemical mediators between aspirin-intolerant and tolerant asthmatic patients. *Ann Allergy Asthma Immunol.* 2001;87:74–79.
107. Lee DKC, Haggart K, Robb FM, Lipworth BJ. Montelukast protects against nasal lysine-aspirin challenge in patients with aspirin-induced asthma. *Eur Respir J.* 2004;24:226–230.
108. Israel E, Fischer AR, Rosenberg MA, et al. The pivotal role of 5-lipoxygenase products in the reaction of aspirin-sensitive asthmatics to aspirin. *Am Rev Respir Dis.* 1993;148:1447–1451.
109. Pauls JD, Simon RA, Daffern PJ, Stevenson DD. Lack of effect of the 5-lipoxygenase inhibitor zileuton in blocking oral aspirin challenges in aspirin-sensitive asthmatics. *Ann Allergy Asthma Immunol.* 2000;85:40–45.
110. Ogata N, Darby Y, Scadding G. Intranasal lysine-aspirin administration decreases polyp volume in patients with aspirin-intolerant asthma. *J Laryngol Otol.* 2007;121:1156–1160.
111. Patriarca G, Bellioni P, Nucera E, et al. Intranasal treatment with lysine acetylsalicylate in patients with nasal polyposis. *Ann Allergy.* 1991;67:588–592.
112. Nucera E, Shiavino D, Milani A, et al. Effects of lysine-acetylslicylate (LAS) treatment in nasal polyposis: two controlled long term prospective follow up studies. *Thorax.* 2000;55:S75–S78.
113. Parikh AA, Scadding GK. Intranasal lysine-aspirin in aspirin-sensitive nasal polyposis: a controlled trial. *Laryngoscope.* 2005;115:1385–1390.
114. Pleskow WW, Stevenson DD, Mathison DA, Simon RA, Schatz M, Zeiger RS. Aspirin desensitization in aspirin-sensitive asthmatic patients: clinical manifestations and characterization of the refractory period. *J Allergy Clin Immunol.* 1982;69:11–19.
115. Juergens UR, Christiansen SC, Stevenson DD, Zuraw BL. Inhibition of monocyte leukotriene B4 production following aspirin desensitization. *J Allergy Clin Immunol.* 1995;96:148–156.
116. Nasser SM, Patel M, Bell GS, Lee TH. The effect of aspirin desensitization on urinary leukotriene E4 concentrations in aspirin-sensitive asthma. *Am J Respir Crit Care Med.* 1995;15:1326–1330.
117. Arm JP, Austen KF. Leukotriene receptors and aspirin sensitivity. *N Engl J Med.* 2002;347:1524–1526.
118. Arm JP, ÓHickey Sp, Spur BW, Lee TH. Airway responsiveness to histamine and leukotriene E(4) in subjects with aspirin-induced asthma. *Am Rev Respir Dis.* 1989;140:148–153.
119. Sousa AR, Parikh A, Scadding G, Corrigan CJ, Lee TH. Leukotriene-receptor expression on nasal mucosal inflammatory cells in aspirin-sensitive rhinosinusitis. *N Eng J Med.* 2002;347:1493–1499.
120. Szczeklik A, Nizankowska-Mogilnicka E, Sanak M. Hypersensitivity to Aspirin and Non-Steroidal Antiinflammatory Drugs. In: Adkinson NF, Bochner BS, Busse WW, et al., eds. *Middleton's Allergy: Principles and Practice,* 7th ed. Philadelphia, PA: Mosby; 2008:1227–1239.
121. Champion RH, Roberts SO, Carpenter RG, Roger JH. Urticaria and angioedema: a review of 554 patients. *Br J Dermatol.* 1969;81:588–597.
122. Juhlin L. Recurrent urticaria: clinical investigation of 330 patients. *Br J Dermatol.* 1981;104:369–381.
123. Mastalerz L Setkowicz M, Sanak M, Szczeklik A. Hypersensitivity to aspirin: common eicosanoid alterations in urticaria and asthma. *J Allergy Clin Immunol.* 2004;113:771–775.
124. Sanchez-Borges M, Caballero-Fonseca F, Capriles-Hulett A. Tolerance of nonsteroidal anti-inflammatory drug-sensitive patients to the highly specific cyclo-oxygenase 2 inhibitors rofecoxib and valdecoxib. *Ann Allergy Asthma Immunol.* 2005;94:34–38.
125. Sanchez-Borges M, Capriles-Hulett A, Caballero-Fonseca F, Perez CR. Tolerability to new COX-2 inhibitors in NSAID-sensitive patients with cutaneous reactions. *Ann Allergy Asthma Immunol.* 2001;87:201–204.
126. Pacor M, Di Lorenzo G, Biasi D, Barbagallo M, Corrocher R. Safety of rofecoxib in subjects with a history of adverse cutaneous reactions to aspirin and/or non-steroidal anti-inflammatory drugs. *Clin Exp Allergy.* 2002;32:397–400.

127. Zembowicz A, Mastalerz L, Setkowicz M, Radziszewski W, Szczeklik A. Safety of cyclo-oxygenase 2 inhibitors and increased leukotriene synthesis in chronic idiopathic urticaria with sensitivity to nonsteroidal anti-inflammatory drugs. *Arch Dermatol.* 2003;139:1577–1582.
128. Asero R. Intolerance to nonsteroidal anti-inflammatory drugs might precede by years the onset of chronic urticaria. *J Allergy Clin Immunol.* 2003;111:1095–1098.
129. Rossini R, Angiolillo DJ, Musumeci G, et al. Aspirin desensitization in patients undergoing percutaneous coronary interventions with stent implantation. *Am J Cardiology.* 2008;101:786–789.
130. Dalmau G, Gaig P, Gazquez V, Merce J. Rapid desensitization to acetylsalicylic acid in acute coronary syndrome patients with NSAID intolerance. *Rev Esp Cardiol.* 2009;62:224–225.
131. Silberman S, Neukirch-Stoop C, Steg PG. Rapid desensitization procedure for patients with aspirin hypersensitivity undergoing coronary stenting. *Am J Cardiol.* 2005;95;509–510.
132. Wong JT, Nagy CS, Krinzman SJ et al. Rapid oral challenge-desensitization for patients with aspirin-related urticaria-angioedema. *J Allergy Clin Immunol.* 2000;105:997–1001.
133. Grzelewska-Rzymowska I, Rozniecki J, Szmidt M. Aspirin "desensitization" in patients with aspirin-related urticaria-angioedema. *Allergol Immunopathol.* 1988;16:305–308.
134. Slowik SM, Slavin RG. Aspirin desensitization in a patient with aspirin sensitivity and chronic idiopathic urticaria. *Ann Allergy Asthma Immunol.* 2009;102:171–172.
135. Stevenson DD, Sanchez-Borges M, Szczeklik A. Classification of allergic and pseudoallergic reactions to drugs that inhibit cyclo-oxygenase enzymes. *Ann Allergy Asthma Immunol.* 2001;87:1–4.
136. van der Klauw MM, Stricker BH, Herings RM, et al. A population based case-cohort study of drug-induced anaphylaxis. *Br J Clin Pharmacol.* 1993;35:400–408.
137. Berkes EA. Anaphylactic and anaphylactoid reactions to aspirin and other NSAIDs. *Clin Rev Allergy Immunol.* 2003;24:137–148.
138. Van Puijenbroek EPEA, Meyboom RH, Leufkens HG. Different risks for NSAID-induced anaphylaxis. *Ann Pharmacother.* 2002;36:24–29.
139. Strom BL, Carson JL, Schinnar R. The effect of indication on the risk of hypersensitivity reactions associated with tolmetin sodium versus other nonsteroidal anti-inflammatory drugs. *J Rheumatol.* 1988;15:695–699.
140. Asero R. Oral aspirin challenges in patients with a history of intolerance to single non-steroidal anti-inflammatory drugs. *Clin Exp Allergy.* 2005;35:713–716.
141. Asero R. Use of ketoprofen oral challenges to detect cross-reactors among patients with a history of aspirin-induced urticaria. *Ann Allergy Asthma Immunol.* 2006;97:187–189.
142. Gagnon R, Julien M, Gold P. Selective celecoxib-associated anaphylactoid reaction. *J Allergy Clin Immunol.* 2003;111:1404–1405.
143. Levy MB, Fink JN. Anaphylaxis to celecoxib. *Ann Allergy Asthma Immunol.* 2001;87:72–73.
144. Grob M, Pichler WJ, Wuthrich B. Anaphylaxis to celecoxib. *Allergy.* 2002;57:264–265.
145. Schellenberg R, Isserow SH. Anaphylactoid reaction to a cyclo-oxygenase-2 inhibitor in a patient who had a reaction to a cyclo-oxygenase-1 inhibitor. *N Engl J Med.* 2001;345:1856.
146. Ballou LR, Wang BWE. Nonsteroidal Anti-inflammatory Drugs. In: Firestein GF, Budd RC, et al., eds. *Kelley's Textbook of Rheumatology,* 8th edition. Philadelphia, PA: W.B Saunders; 2008:843.

# Chapter 8
# IgE-Dependent and Independent Effector Mechanisms in Human and Murine Anaphylaxis

**Fred D. Finkelman**

**Abstract** Anaphylaxis is shock mediated by cells of the innate immune system. Studies in murine models demonstrate at least three pathways: (1) antigen cross-linking of IgE bound to Fcε(epsilon)RI leads to mast cell degranulation with release of histamine and PAF; (2) antigen-IgG complexes cross-link Fcγ(gamma)RIII on mast cells and basophils with secretion of PAF; and (3) complement activation leads to production of C3a and C5a, which activate mast cells, basophils, and macrophages. C3a and C5a appear unable to induce shock by themselves in the murine models, but can exacerbate anaphylaxis induced by the other mechanisms. Anaphylaxis can also be exacerbated by IL-4 and IL-13, which increase effector cell responsiveness to vasoactive mediators, and by β(beta)-adrenergic receptor antagonists, which decrease ability to compensate for vascular leak and decreased intravascular volume. IgG-dependent anaphylaxis requires much higher concentrations of antibody and antigen than IgE-mediated anaphylaxis; consequently, IgG antibodies can block the development of anaphylaxis when antigen quantity is low by binding to antigen before it can cross-link mast cell-associated IgE, but can mediate anaphylaxis when antigen quantity is high. Inhibitory receptors, such as Fcγ(gamma)RIIb, can suppress mast cell activation and anaphylaxis, but this effect is less important in our models than IgG neutralization of antigen. Although human IgE anaphylaxis is well established, the existence of IgG-mediated human anaphylaxis is unproven. However, we believe that studies of human anaphylaxis associated with infusion of large quantities of foreign proteins, such as chimeric monoclonal antibodies, make it likely that this type of human anaphylaxis can occur. Elucidation of these mechanisms suggests prophylactic and therapeutic approaches and goals for future anaphylaxis research.

**Keywords** IgE • IgG • Complement • Anaphylatoxin • Rodent • Histamine • PAF • Mast cell • Macrophage • Basophil • Fcε(epsilon)RI • Fcγ(gamma)RIII

## Abbreviations

| | |
|---|---|
| Ab | Antibody |
| Ag | Antigen |
| Fcε(epsilon)RI | High-affinity receptor for IgE |
| Fcγ(gamma)RIII | Low-affinity receptor 3 for IgG |
| IgE | Immunoglobulin E |
| IgG | Immunoglobulin G |

F.D. Finkelman (✉)
University of Cincinnati College of Medicine, Cincinnati, OH, USA
e-mail: ffinkelman@pol.net

M.C. Castells (ed.), *Anaphylaxis and Hypersensitivity Reactions*,
DOI 10.1007/978-1-60327-951-2_8, 

| | |
|---|---|
| mAb | Monoclonal antibody |
| PAF | Platelet-activating factor |
| PCA | Passive cutaneous anaphylaxis |
| R | Receptor |
| TNP | Trinitrophenyl |

## 8.1 Introduction

This chapter discusses IgE-, IgG-, and complement-dependent mechanisms involved in the pathogenesis of anaphylaxis in mouse and man and highlights similarities and differences in these mechanisms in the two species.

## 8.2 Definition of Anaphylaxis

No definition of anaphylaxis has been universally accepted. Some clinicians and investigators reserve "anaphylaxis" for shock that is mediated by IgE and refer to other immune-mediated forms of shock as anaphylactoid reactions. Others define "anaphylaxis" as antibody (Ab)-mediated shock, and use "anaphylactoid" to refer to Ab-independent shock that clinically resembles anaphylaxis. This chapter will use an even more inclusive definition of anaphylaxis: shock mediated by the innate and/or adaptive immune system. This is consistent with the nomenclature recommended by the World Health Organization, which divides anaphylaxis into immunologic (antibody)-mediated and non-immunologic (non-antibody)-mediated disease and then subdivided immunologic anaphylaxis into IgE- and non-IgE-mediated disease. I justify this broad definition of anaphylaxis with evidence that different immune mechanisms can simultaneously contribute to the development of shock; use of a narrower definition of anaphylaxis can lead to semantic problems when considering these "mixed" responses.

## 8.3 Murine Models of Anaphylaxis

### *8.3.1 Advantages and Disadvantages*

Most early animal model studies of anaphylaxis were performed with species, such as the guinea pig, that develop anaphylaxis more easily than the mouse [1]. More recently, however, murine studies have dominated the field. This reflects the availability of reagents for murine studies, including mice themselves, which are available on multiple inbred genetic backgrounds with deletion or overexpression of many genes pertinent to the sensitization and/or effector phases of anaphylaxis. These include mice that specifically lack IgE [2], Fcε(epsilon)RIα(alpha) [3] (the IgE binding chain of Fcε(epsilon)RI, the high-affinity IgE receptor), FcRγ(gamma) [4] (a component of all stimulatory Ig receptors in the mouse, as well as some additional receptors); the IgG binding chains of the stimulatory high-affinity (Fcγ(gamma)RI [5]) and low-affinity (Fcγ(gamma)RIII [6]) IgG receptors (Rs), the inhibitory IgGR (Fcγ(gamma)RIIb [7]), or any of several components of the complement system and their receptors. In addition, mice are available in which greatly decreased expression of c-kit, the receptor for stem cell factor, prevents nearly all mast cell development [8, 9] and antibodies and other reagents have been developed that deplete mast cells by neutralizing c-kit [10], or selectively deplete basophils [11, 12] or macrophages [13, 14]. Together, use of these reagents has made the mouse an excellent tool for defining pathogenic mechanisms that contribute to anaphylaxis.

In addition to these advantages, the general similarity of the murine and human immune systems suggests that murine studies are likely to have human relevance (Table 8.1). Mouse and man both make IgE Abs that bind with high affinity to homologous high-affinity receptors on mast cells and basophils and intermediate affinity receptors on B cells (Fcε(epsilon)RII) [15–19]. Cross-linking of the high-affinity receptor activates mast cells and basophils in both species [18] and IgE binding to the intermediate affinity receptor contributes in both species to antigen (Ag) presentation [15, 20]. Ag/IgE-induced mast cell and basophil activation causes the release of vasoactive mediators, including histamine and PAF, and the production of several cytokines in both species [11, 21–29], leading to bronchospasm and increased vascular permeability that can cause shock (generally detected in mice as decreased motility and hypothermia) through intravascular fluid depletion. Both mouse and man also produce IgG antibodies that induce macrophage production of PAF by binding to Fcγ(gamma) RIII [27, 30, 31] and that activate complement, with the production of the anaphylatoxins C3a and C5a [32, 36]. Anaphylatoxin binding to specific receptors on mast cells and macrophages can also induce vasoactive mediator production [37–40]. Thus, three mechanisms known to stimulate vasoactive mediator production are generally similar in mouse and man.

There are, however, some significant differences between the murine and human immune systems that could affect anaphylaxis (Table 8.1). The most abundant IgG isotype, which is labeled IgG1 in both species (although mouse and human IgG1 are neither homologous nor analogous), activates complement in man, but not in mice and may also be a better Fcγ(gamma)R activator in humans [41]. In contrast, humans, but not mice, produce two other IgG isotypes, IgG2 and IgG4, which have little ability to activate complement [41], and a subset of mouse IgG1, but not human IgG molecules, has some ability to activate mast cells [42, 43]. Fcε(epsilon)RI is more broadly distributed in humans than in mice, with expression on macrophages and dendritic cells as well as mast cells and basophils [18, 44–46], while only mast cells and basophils are known to express

**Table 8.1** Similarities and differences of the murine and human immune systems that are relevant to anaphylaxis

| | Murine | Human |
|---|---|---|
| Reagenic IgE antibodies | + | + |
| High-affinity IgER on mast cells and basophils | + | + |
| High-affinity IgER on macrophages and dendritic cells | – | + |
| Low-affinity IgER on B cells and dendritic cells | + | + |
| Low-affinity IgER on additional cell types | – | + |
| Low-affinity stimulatory IgGR on mast cells, basophils, macrophages | + | + |
| High-affinity IgGR on myeloid cells | + | + |
| Low-affinity inhibitory IgGR on mast cells, basophils, macrophages | – | + |
| Histamine production by mast cells | + | + |
| Histamine production by basophils | – | + |
| IL-4/IL-13 production by basophils | + | + |
| PAF production by macrophages | + | + |
| PAF production by basophils | + | ? |
| Complement-activating IgG antibodies | + | + |
| IL-4-induced non-complement-activating antibodies | + | + |
| Anaphylatoxin receptors on mast cells, basophils, macrophages | + | + |
| Predominant IgG isotype activates complement | – | + |
| Predominant IgG isotype can activate mast cells | + | – |

Fcε(epsilon)RI in the mouse. Fcε(epsilon)RII, which is only expressed on B cells and dendritic cells in mice, is also more broadly expressed in humans [19]. Human basophils have large numbers of granules that release considerable quantities of histamine following IgE/Fcε(epsilon)RI-dependent activation, while mouse basophils have relatively few granules and release little histamine following IgE/Fcε(epsilon)RI-dependent activation [47]. In contrast, murine basophils secrete considerable quantities of PAF following IgG/Fcγ(gamma)R-dependent activation [11], while IgG/Fcγ(gamma)R-induced PAF secretion by human basophils is less well characterized. Additionally, although some mouse and human FcRs (Fcε(epsilon)RI, Fcε(epsilon)RII, Fcγ(gamma)RI, Fcγ(gamma)RIIb, and mouse Fcγ(gamma)RIV/human Fcγ(gamma)RIIIA are homologous and, except as previously noted, expressed by similar cell types in mouse and man, humans express some Fcγ(gamma)Rs that are not expressed by mice [48]; it is not known whether these nonhomologous Fcγ(gamma)Rs play a role in anaphylaxis. Taken together, these considerations suggest that mechanisms that induce anaphylaxis will be generally similar in mouse and man, although there is a potential for murine anaphylaxis to be more IgG/Fcγ(gamma)R-dependent and less IgE/Fcε(epsilon)RI-dependent than human anaphylaxis.

### *8.3.2 Murine IgE-Mediated Anaphylaxis*

Both passive and active models of murine IgE-dependent anaphylaxis have been demonstrated. Passive anaphylaxis can be induced by sensitizing mice with an IgE monoclonal Ab (mAb), such as IgE anti-trinitrophenyl (TNP), followed by challenge with a TNP-protein conjugate that has at least two molecules of hapten per molecule of protein (to allow cross-linking of Fcε(epsilon)RI-bound IgE). This mechanism is both Fcε(epsilon)RI- and mast cell-dependent, as demonstrated by studies with Fcε(epsilon)RI-deficient and c-kit hypomorphic W/W$^v$ mice [3, 49]. IgE/Fcε(epsilon)RI/mast cell-dependent systemic anaphylaxis is mediated primarily by histamine, although PAF also contributes [27]. IgE-mediated passive anaphylaxis is an exquisitely sensitive process; shock in mice sensitized with IgE anti-TNP mAb can be triggered by as little as 10 ng of TNP-ovalbumin [50]. Passive IgE-mediated anaphylaxis, which has characteristics similar to anaphylaxis induced by Ag-specific IgE followed by Ag, can also be induced in mice by injecting an anti-IgE mAb, such as EM-95 [51], which is functionally bivalent and thus, capable of cross-linking IgE. As little as 10 μ(mu)g of EM-95, injected IV, can induce hypothermia [24]. Although EM-95, a rat IgG2a mAb, might also be expected to have some capacity to induce IgG-mediated anaphylaxis by forming a complex with IgE that can interact with Fcγ(gamma)Rs, this does not seem to occur in practice, inasmuch as unpublished research in our laboratory shows that EM-95 fails to cause shock when injected into Fcε(epsilon)RIα(alpha)-deficient mice. Anti-IgE mAb-induced anaphylaxis requires only very small quantities of IgE; it can be demonstrated even in mice deficient in both IL-4 and IL-13, in which serum IgE is difficult to detect [52].

IgE, Fcε(epsilon)RI and mast cells can also mediate active anaphylaxis in models in which mice are immunized with peptide Ags or haptens such as penicillin or TNP conjugated to an immunogenic carrier, then challenged with the immunogen [53]. However, because these models can also induce Ag-specific IgG responses and IgG can mediate anaphylaxis in the mouse as well as inhibit IgE-dependent anaphylaxis (see below), demonstration that active anaphylaxis is IgE mediated requires studies that show that anaphylaxis fails to develop in mast cell-deficient c-kit hypomorphic mice, anti-c-kit mAb-treated mice, IgE-deficient mice, anti-IgE mAb-treated mice, or Fcε(epsilon)RIα(alpha)-deficient mice (Table 8.2). Studies with IL-4- IL-4Rα(alpha)-, or Stat6-deficient mice are inadequate for this purpose, because these strains are not totally IgE deficient [52, 54] and very small quantities of IgE can mediate anaphylaxis, as noted above.

**Table 8.2** Discriminators of IgE- and IgG-dependent anaphylaxis

| | *IgE-dependent* | *IgG-dependent* |
|---|---|---|
| IgE-deficient mice | Absent | Normal |
| Fcε(epsilon)RI-deficient mice | Absent | Normal or increased |
| Anti-IgE mAb-treated mice | Absent | Normal |
| Mast cell-deficient mice | Absent | Normal |
| Anti-c-kit mAb-treated mice | Absent | Normal |
| FcRγ(gamma)-deficient mice | Absent | Absent |
| Fcγ(gamma)RIII-deficient mice | Normal | Absent |
| Anti-Fcγ(gamma)RII/RII-mAb-treated mice | Normal or increased | Absent |
| Fcγ(gamma)RIIb-deficient mice | Increased | Increased |
| Anti-histamine-treated mice | Decreased | Normal |
| PAF antagonist-treated mice | Slightly decreased | Greatly decreased |
| Gadolinium-treated mice | Normal | Decreased |
| Clodronate liposome-treated mice | Normal | Decreased |

### *8.3.3 Murine IgG-Mediated Anaphylaxis*

Anaphylaxis can also be induced in mice by a process that depends on IgG rather than IgE. Anaphylaxis induced by the IgG-dependent pathway is mast cell-independent (it occurs normally in c-kit hypomorphic mice) [27] and Fcε(epsilon)RI-independent [55], but is Fcγ(gamma)RIII-dependent [56]. Consistent with the ability of mouse IgG1, IgG2a, and IgG2b to bind to Fcγ(gamma)RIII, any of these isotypes can mediate IgG-dependent anaphylaxis [57], although, in practice, IgG1 usually has a dominant role, presumably because immunization with protein Ags generally stimulates a predominantly IgG1 response [41]. IgG-dependent anaphylaxis can be induced passively, by sensitizing mice with a hapten-specific IgG mAb, then challenging them with a polyvalent conjugate of the relevant hapten [11, 57], or by injecting unprimed mice with 2.4G2 [27], a rat IgG2b mAb that binds to both Fcγ(gamma)RIIb and, FcγRIII and can cross-link these receptors in vivo [58]. As would be expected, anaphylaxis in the latter system depends on the ability of 2.4G2 to bind to the stimulatory Fcγ(gamma)R, Fcγ(gamma)RIII, rather than the inhibitory Fcγ(gamma)R, Fcγ(gamma)RIIb, and is exacerbated in Fcγ(gamma)RIIb-deficient mice [7, 48]. Although murine IgE- and IgG-dependent shock (revealed as hypothermia and hypomotility [27]) develop with similar kinetics, they differ in that IgG-mediated anaphylaxis is histamine-independent and considerably more PAF-dependent than IgE-mediated anaphylaxis [27]. In addition, the induction of pure IgG-mediated anaphylaxis requires ~100-fold more Ag than the induction of pure IgE-mediated anaphylaxis [50]. This is consistent with the much higher affinity of Fcε(epsilon)RI for IgE than Fcγ(gamma)RIII for IgG [48, 59, 60]; indeed, while Ag activates mast cells and basophils by binding to Ag-specific, Fcε(epsilon) RI-associated IgE on the surface of these cells, Ag and Ag-specific IgG most likely form complexes in blood or lymph that then achieve sufficient avidity for Fcγ(gamma)RIII to activate PAF production by cross-linking this receptor. The main differences between IgE- and IgG-dependent anaphylaxis are summarized in Table 8.3.

Stoichiometric considerations become complex when Ag-specific IgE and IgG are present in the same animal; these conditions can actually make IgG-dependent anaphylaxis occur at a lower concentration than IgE-mediated anaphylaxis [50] (see Fig. 8.1 and discussion below). IgG- and IgE-mediated murine anaphylaxis have also been reported to differ in the speed of development of tachycardia and decreased airway dynamic compliance [56], although this may depend on the genetic background of the mice used for these studies as well as concentrations of Ag and Ab and Ab affinity.

**Table 8.3** Differences between IgE- and IgG-dependent murine anaphylaxis

| | *IgE-dependent* | *IgG-dependent* |
|---|---|---|
| Cells | Mast cells | Macrophages, basophils |
| Receptor | Fcε(epsilon)RI | Fcγ(gamma)RIII |
| Mediators | Histamine > PAF | PAF |
| Required Ag quantity | Small | ~100× larger |
| Required Ab quantity | Very small | Considerably larger |

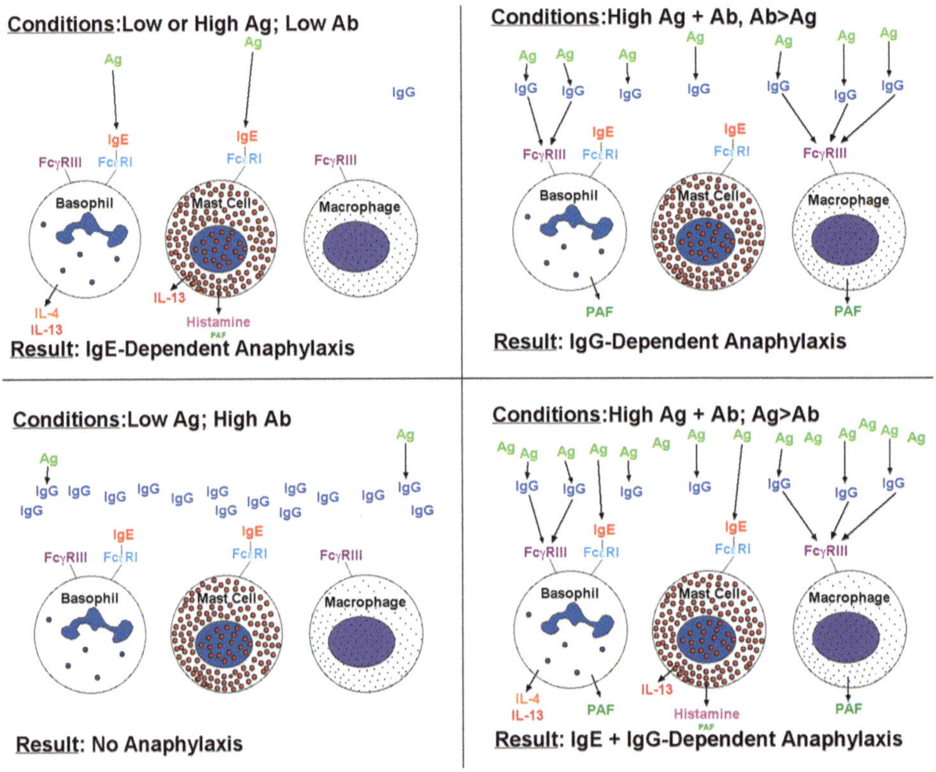


**Fig. 8.1** Effects of interactions between IgE and IgG on the development of murine anaphylaxis. Diagrams show how low-specific Ab levels favor IgE-dependent anaphylaxis (*upper left panel*), low antigen and high Ab levels prevent anaphylaxis (*lower left panel*), high antigen and Ab levels with an excess of Ab favor IgG-dependent anaphylaxis (*upper right panel*), and high antigen and Ab levels with an excess of antigen favor combined IgE- and IgG-dependent anaphylaxis (*lower right panel*) when specific IgE and IgG antibodies are both present

Active IgG-mediated anaphylaxis, like active IgE-mediated anaphylaxis, can be induced by immunization with a protein Ag followed by challenge with the same Ag [27]. Demonstration that active anaphylaxis in the mouse is IgG-mediated requires evidence that it fails to occur in Fcγ(gamma)RIII-deficient mice or mice pretreated with 2.4G2, but still occurs in mice with deficiencies in c-kit, IgE, or Fcε(epsilon)RI, or mice pretreated with antibodies to these molecules [6, 7, 27, 61] (Table 8.2).

Although IgG-mediated anaphylaxis is mast cell-independent, there is controversy about the cell type(s) that secretes the PAF that is the key mediator for this type of anaphylaxis. Initial studies, including some performed in the author's laboratory [27], identified macrophages as the cell type responsible for IgG-dependent anaphylaxis, on the basis of inhibition by treatment with the macrophage inhibitor gadolinium [62]. In contrast, a convincing, more recent study failed to reproduce this observation, found that IgG-mediated anaphylaxis could be profoundly suppressed by pretreating mice with a basophil-depleting mAb and demonstrated that basophils are an especially potent source of PAF [11]. This apparent conflict appears to result from differences in the mouse strain and IgG-dependent anaphylaxis protocol used. It is our unpublished observation that macrophages contribute considerably more to IgG-mediated anaphylaxis in BALB/c than in C57BL/6 mice, that an active IgG-mediated anaphylaxis protocol is considerably more macrophage-dependent than passive anaphylaxis protocols in both strains and that C57BL/6 mice are considerably more sensitive than BALB/c mice to injected PAF. Specifically, basophil depletion almost totally suppresses passive IgG-mediated anaphylaxis in C57BL/6 mice and partially suppresses active IgG-mediated anaphylaxis in C57BL/6 mice and passive IgG-mediated anaphylaxis in BALB/c mice, but has almost no effect on active IgG-mediated anaphylaxis in BALB/c mice (at least in the model used, in which mice are sensitized by injection of a goat IgG Ab to mouse IgD and challenged IV 2 weeks later with goat IgG). The mechanisms responsible for these BALB/c–C57BL/6 and passive–active anaphylaxis differences have not yet been determined.

### 8.3.4 The Multiple Roles of Basophils in Anaphylaxis

In addition to its ability to contribute directly to IgG-dependent anaphylaxis by secreting PAF in response to Fcγ(gamma)RIII-mediated activation, the mouse basophil can contribute less directly to IgE-mediated anaphylaxis. Although the mouse basophil is a poor source of histamine and Fcγ(gamma)RI cross-linking does not induce basophil PAF secretion [11, 27, 47], Fcε(epsilon)RI cross-linking stimulates basophils to rapidly synthesize and secrete large quantities of IL-4 and IL-13 [24, 63], which sensitize mice to the effects of PAF and histamine [64]. Furthermore, basophils are activated to secrete IL-4 by ~ one-tenth the quantity of anti-IgE mAb (or Ag) that is required to activate mast cell degranulation [24]. Although the mechanisms responsible for the considerably greater sensitivity of IgE-mediated basophil than mast cell activation are not known, IgE-dependent basophil IL-4 and IL-13 secretion have the potential ability to contribute to anaphylaxis by increasing target cell sensitivity to mast cell-secreted PAF and histamine [64]. IgE-mediated stimulation of basophil IL-4 production also promotes the sensitization phase of anaphylaxis by increasing: (1) B cell isotype switching to IgE [65, 66], and (2) naïve T cell differentiation into Th2 cells [67–71]. The latter effect of basophils may be particularly potent and important, inasmuch as basophils express MHC class II and can process and present Ag to T cells at the same time as they promote Th2 differentiation by secreting IL-4 [69–71]. Basophil contributions to anaphylaxis are listed in Table 8.4.

**Table 8.4** Roles of basophils in murine anaphylaxis

1. Secrete PAF in response to Fcγ(gamma)RIII stimulation
2. Secrete IL-4 and IL-13, in response to Fcε(epsilon)RI stimulation, that:
   a. Increases responsiveness to vasoactive mediators
   b. Stimulates B cell isotype switching to IgE
   c. Promotes Th2 differentiation
3. Present Ag in fashion that activates naïve T cells

### 8.3.5 Complement-Dependent Anaphylaxis

The role of complement in murine anaphylaxis is less well defined than the roles of IgE and IgG. Although complement activation generates the anaphylatoxins C3a and C5a, which can activate mast cells, basophils, and macrophages [37, 39], studies with complement-deficient mice demonstrate that complement is not required for IgG- or IgE-dependent anaphylaxis [27]. Injection of mice with *Klebsiella pneumoniae* LPS, which activates complement through the lectin pathway, rapidly induces shock that is C3-, C5a-, platelet-, and macrophage-dependent and toll-like receptor 4-, B, T, and mast cell-independent, but only if mice are pretreated with muramyl dipeptide, which activates NOD2 [72–74]. Injection of mice with a soluble peanut extract also activates complement and rapidly induces LPS-independent, C3-, C3aR-, macrophage-, PAF-dependent shock, but only if mice are pretreated with IL-4, which increases sensitivity to PAF, and a β(beta)-adrenergic antagonist, which decreases ability to compensate for decreased intravascular volume [75]. More importantly, complement activation by peanut extract synergizes with IgE-mediated mast cell activation to induce severe anaphylaxis in mice that have not been pretreated with IL-4 or a β(beta)-adrenergic antagonist. Thus, it seems unlikely that complement activation is generally, by itself, sufficient to induce murine anaphylaxis, but likely that complement activation can contribute to the severity of anaphylaxis induced by Ab-dependent mechanisms. This synergy is most likely to be observed in mice inoculated with Ags that can activate complement through innate immune mechanisms or in the unusual circumstances that anaphylaxis is mediated by the complement-activating IgG2a and IgG2b isotypes, but unlikely to be important when anaphylaxis is induced by an Ag that does not directly activate complement and is mediated by IgE or IgG1, which activate complement poorly if at all [41].

### 8.3.6 IgE–IgG Interactions in Murine Anaphylaxis

Taken together, the much lower Ag and Ab requirements for induction of IgE- than IgG-mediated anaphylaxis and the possibility for IgG to intercept Ag before it can be bound by mast cell-associated IgE create a complex set of different possible ways in which Ag interactions with the two isotypes can influence the development and severity of anaphylaxis (Fig. 8.1). When Ag concentrations are sufficient to trigger "pure" IgE-mediated anaphylaxis but insufficient to trigger IgG-mediated anaphylaxis, IgG antibodies block anaphylaxis development [50]. In contrast, the simultaneous presence of higher concentrations of Ag and IgG antibodies can trigger IgG-mediated anaphylaxis while simultaneously preventing IgE-mediated anaphylaxis [50]. Once Ag concentrations are sufficient to saturate IgG, however, IgE- and IgG-mediated anaphylaxis can occur simultaneously [50]. Thus, "pure" IgE-mediated anaphylaxis is most likely to occur when IgE and IgG Ab responses are small (sufficient for some Ag-specific IgE to bind to mast cell Fcε(epsilon)RI, but insufficient for IgG Ab to intercept Ag effectively), "pure" IgG-mediated anaphylaxis is most likely to occur even in the presence of IgE antibodies when Ab and Ag levels are both high but Ag is insufficient to saturate IgG, and mixed IgE/IgG-dependent responses, which can be additive [76], are most likely to occur when Ag and IgG levels are both relatively high but Ag concentration exceeds the neutralizing capacity of IgG.

The relative importance of IgE- versus IgG-mediated anaphylaxis is also affected, for stoichiometric reasons, by the site of Ag administration. Although Ag most potently and rapidly induces anaphylaxis when injected intravenously, intracutaneous administration (e.g.,, an insect sting) may allow immediate access to skin mast cell IgE with less rapid neutralization by IgG, facilitating IgE-mediated anaphylaxis. Oral Ag administration is even more likely to favor IgE-mediated systemic as well as intestinal anaphylaxis [77] because: (1) enteral concentrations of IgG and even IgA are unlikely to be sufficient to neutralize most ingested Ag, (2) the amount of Ag absorbed through the gut is unlikely to be sufficient to trigger IgG-mediated anaphylaxis, and (3) absorbed Ag has immediate access to intraepithelial mast cells in intestinal villi. It is not known, however, whether the induction of systemic shock by ingested Ag requires activation of vascular mast cells or whether activation of gut mucosal mast cells is sufficient.

### 8.3.7 *Fcγ(gamma)RIIb-Dependent Inhibition of IgE-Mediated Anaphylaxis by IgG*

In addition to its ability to intercept Ag before it can bind to mast cell Fcε(epsilon)RI-associated IgE, IgG has the potential to inhibit IgE-mediated anaphylaxis by interacting with the inhibitory receptor Fcγ(gamma)RIIb, which activates phosphatases that interrupt the stimulatory signaling pathways initiated when Fcε(epsilon)RI activates kinases [78]. Studies with Fcγ(gamma)RIIb-deficient mice have demonstrated increased sensitivity to IgE-mediated anaphylaxis [7] and mAb inhibition of Fcγ(gamma)RIIb can have similar effects. Our own studies, however, suggest that Fcγ(gamma)RIIb-mediated inhibition of IgE-dependent anaphylaxis is a rather subtle process, that becomes significant in the relatively narrow range of Ag and IgG Ab concentrations at which IgG Ab incompletely intercepts Ag before it can bind to mast cell-associated IgE [50]. This relatively subtle inhibition, however, may have considerable clinical importance when IgG is present at relatively low concentration and the dose of Ag is low. In addition, linkage of Ag with Fcγ(gamma) or Fcγ(gamma) with Fcε(epsilon) provides an interesting possibility for inhibiting IgE-mediated anaphylaxis by cross-linking Fcγ(gamma)RIIb to Fcε(epsilon)RI on mast cells and basophils [79–81].

The ability of IgG to inhibit IgE-mediated anaphylaxis by cross-linking Fcε(epsilon)RI to Fcγ(gamma)RIIb raises the question of how IgG can trigger anaphylaxis through Fcγ(gamma)RIII when it also activates Fcγ(gamma)RIIb. Most likely, this reflects considerably greater presence of Fcγ(gamma)RIII than Fcγ(gamma)RIIb on murine macrophages, and possibly, basophils. Consistent with this, the mAb 2.4G2, which binds to both Fcγ(gamma)RIIb and Fcγ(gamma)RIII [58], induces PAF/macrophage/basophil/Fcγ(gamma)RIII-dependent anaphylaxis when injected in vivo [27], but induces more severe disease in Fcγ(gamma)RIIb-deficient mice than in wild-type mice [7].

### 8.3.8 *Controversial and Confusing Issues in Murine Anaphylaxis*

Issues that confuse a comprehensive understanding of murine anaphylaxis result from studies of: (1) IgG1-mediated passive cutaneous anaphylaxis (PCA); (2) anaphylaxis in Fcε(epsilon)RI-deficient mice; (3) anaphylaxis in IL-4, IL-4Rα(alpha)- and Stat6-deficient mice; and (4) anaphylaxis mediated by IgE and Fcγ(gamma)RIV. Intracutaneous injection of mice with some, but not all IgG1 mAbs or IgG1 polyclonal antisera sensitizes mast cells to degranulate in response to specific Ag challenge [42]. The ability of IgG1 Abs to have this effect is, to a great extent, IL-4-dependent and has been found to reflect the presence of terminal sialic acid residues on polysaccharide moieties covalently linked to the Fc part of the γ(gamma)1 polypeptide [43]. IgG1 sensitization of mast cells for PCA is considerably less efficient than IgE sensitization and, unlike long-lasting IgE sensitization, is gone within 24 h [57, 82]. It is not settled whether IgG1 mast cell sensitization involves Fcγ(gamma)RIII or Fcε(epsilon)RI; I favor the latter possibility because IgG1 is the only IgG isotype that has been described to sensitize mast cells in normal mice while IgG2b and IgG2a bind at least as well as IgG1 to Fcγ(gamma)RIII [59]. In contrast to its ability to sensitize mice for mast cell-mediated PCA, it seems unlikely that IgG1 is important in mast cell-mediated systemic anaphylaxis, because IgG-mediated anaphylaxis is c-kit- (and therefore, mast cell-) independent [27] but is macrophage- and basophil-dependent, as described above.

These conclusions may seem to conflict with studies in Fcε(epsilon)RIα(alpha)-deficient mice, which show increased severity of IgG-mediated anaphylaxis as well as IgG-mediated mast cell degranulation [55]. This most likely represents an unphysiological situation, however. Because the FcR common γ(gamma) chain is a necessary constituent of both Fcγ(gamma)RIII and Fcε(epsilon) RIα(alpha) and appears to be present in quantities low enough to limit the function of both receptors, the absence of Fcε(epsilon)RI allows increased Fcγ(gamma)RIII functionality in cells that normally express large quantities of Fcε(epsilon)RIα(alpha) (mast cells and basophils). Consequently, Fcγ(gamma)RIII gains the ability to trigger mast cell degranulation in Fcε(epsilon)RIα(alpha)-deficient mice, even though it has little ability to do that (or to trigger basophil cytokine secretion) in Fcε(epsilon)RIα(alpha)-sufficient mice [55].

Studies that demonstrate Ag-specific cutaneous anaphylaxis in IL-4/IL-13- and IL-4Rα(alpha)-deficient mice might also appear to promote the conclusion that IgG can induce mast cell-dependent anaphylaxis by demonstrating that Ag-specific mast cell degranulation can occur in these mice in the absence of IgE. However, although IgE production is greatly decreased in these mice, it is not totally absent, and the small quantity that is produced is sufficient to mediate mast cell degranulation [52]. Consequently, it is preferable to use IgE-deficient mice rather than Fcε(epsilon)RIα(alpha)-, IL-4-, Stat6- or IL-4Rα(alpha)-deficient mice to determine whether mast cell-mediated anaphylaxis can be induced by an IgE-independent, IgG-dependent mechanism.

Finally, recent studies show that murine IgE can bind to and signal through Fcγ(gamma)RIV, a receptor that is homologous to human Fcγ(gamma)RIIIa and is present on murine macrophages and neutrophils (there is disagreement, however, about whether all allotypes of murine IgE, or only IgE of the *b*, but not the *a* allotype bind [83, 84]). Studies also demonstrate that murine IgE can signal through Fcγ(gamma)RIV and induce macrophage cytokine and mediator release [83, 84]. As a result, it has been argued that macrophage Fcγ(gamma)RIV in the mouse is analogous to macrophage Fcγ(gamma)RI in man [83]. This view, however, seems incompatible with affinity considerations; while Fcγ(gamma)RI on human macrophages binds IgE with high affinity and does not bind IgG, mouse Fcγ(gamma)RIV binds IgE less avidly than it binds IgG2a and IgG2b [59, 84, 85], which are generally present in considerably higher concentration than IgE. Consequently, with the possible exception of a pure Th2 response that induces IgE but neither IgG2a nor IgG2b Ab against a specific Ag, it is difficult to think of a situation in which IgE would replace or significantly supplement IgG in activating murine macrophages.

Taken together, the four issues discussed in this section appear to illustrate potential immune mechanisms that can occur and possibly do occur in vivo under very restricted circumstances. On balance, however, it seems likely that murine mast cell-mediated systemic anaphylaxis is normally IgE-dependent and murine macrophage-mediated anaphylaxis is normally IgG-dependent.

## 8.4 Human Anaphylaxis

### *8.4.1 Human IgE-Mediated Anaphylaxis*

Most human anaphylaxis that has been well characterized is mediated by IgE, Fcε(epsilon)RI, and Fcε(epsilon)RI-expressing cells, particularly mast cells and basophils (which can secrete large amounts of histamine in humans [28]). IgE-, Fcε(epsilon)RI-, and mast cell/basophil-dependence of most human anaphylaxis has been demonstrated by in vitro studies with purified polyclonal and monoclonal antibodies and normal cell populations and cell lines, in vivo PCA studies and the frequent association of human anaphylaxis with increased serum levels of tryptase, which is released by degranulating mast cells [86, 87]. More recently, the existence of IgE-mediated human anaphylaxis has been confirmed by studies in which an anti-IgE mAb that blocks IgE binding to Fcε(epsilon)RI and cannot cross-link Fcε(epsilon)RI-bound IgE reduced the frequency and severity of anaphylactic responses during rapid Ag desensitization to ragweed Ag [88] and increased tolerance for peanuts in peanut-allergic patients [89]. IgE binding to Fcε(epsilon)RI on macrophages and dendritic cells may also contribute to anaphylaxis by inducing mediator and cytokine release and through IgE-mediated focusing of Ag onto these cells, which promotes Ag presentation and T cell activation [49, 90].

### 8.4.2 IgE-Independent Human Anaphylaxis

Ag-induced anaphylaxis also occurs with considerable frequency in individuals who lack detectable Ag-specific serum IgE and show no elevations in serum tryptase [91]. This does not prove that these responses are not mediated by IgE and mast cells; the high affinity of Fcε(epsilon)RI for IgE and the small number of Fcε(epsilon)RI molecules that need to be cross-linked to induce mast cell or basophil degranulation make it possible for sufficient Ag-specific IgE to be on these cells to mediate degranulation even in the absence of clinically detectable Ag-specific IgE in serum [52]. Furthermore, the approximately 2 h in vivo half-life of serum tryptase can cause it to be reduced to baseline concentrations in serum samples obtained several hours after an anaphylactic response [87]. Nevertheless, repeated observations of anaphylaxis developing after administration of specific drugs or procedures in the absence of detectable IgE, mast cell degranulation, and tryptase makes it likely that human anaphylaxis can be triggered by IgE-independent mechanisms. As in the mouse, evidence favors anaphylaxis induction by IgG- and complement-dependent mechanisms. In addition, some agents appear to induce human anaphylactic responses that are both Ig- and complement-independent.

### 8.4.3 IgG-Dependent Human Anaphylaxis

Although not definitively proven, humans most likely can develop IgG-mediated anaphylaxis. At least four situations have been described in which anaphylaxis develops in the absence of detectable Ag-specific IgE or tryptase and in the presence of relatively large serum concentrations of Ag-specific IgG antibodies: infusion of dextran [92], aprotinin [93], and von Willebrand factor (to patients deficient in this factor) [94] and infusion of the chimeric anti-TNF mAb, infliximab, to individuals with Crohn's disease or rheumatoid arthritis [95]. It is striking that each of these conditions involves the IV administration of large quantities of the putative Ag; the same situation that is required to trigger IgG-mediated anaphylaxis in the mouse. It is also noteworthy that human anaphylaxis has been associated with increased blood levels of PAF, the predominant mediator responsible for murine IgG-dependent anaphylaxis, and occurs with increased severity in individuals who have decreased ability to catabolize PAF [96].

Humans also share with mice the possibility for IgG antibodies to protect against IgE-dependent anaphylaxis. In humans, IgG4 is the "blocking Ab" isotype most associated with protection against IgE-mediated anaphylaxis [20, 97]. Like the mouse blocking Ab isotype, IgG1, human IgG4 is induced by the cytokine IL-4 [98] and fails to activate complement [99]. Interestingly, class switching to human IgG4 is induced by simultaneous stimulation of B cells with IL-4 or IL-13 and the anti-inflammatory cytokine, IL-10 [100], which is produced by regulatory T cells in addition to other cell types [101], and thus, is likely to be part of a regulatory, rather than an inflammatory response. In the absence of IL-10 production by Tregs or other cells, IL-4 and IL-13 induce isotype switching to IgE, while the addition of IL-10 inhibits IgE isotype switching and promotes IgG4 production [100].

Murine and human IgG-mediated anaphylaxis may differ, however, in the importance of the role played by complement. Complement activation and anaphylatoxin production is well described in human IgG-associated anaphylaxis [32, 92, 94] but not in murine IgG-dependent anaphylaxis. This most likely reflects the ability of human IgG1, but not murine IgG1, to activate complement [41]. Until pharmaceuticals that block complement or Fcγ(gamma)R activation and have little toxicity are clinically available, it will be difficult, if not impossible, to ethically determine the relative importance of complement- and Fcγ(gamma)R-dependent mechanisms in human IgG-mediated anaphylaxis.

### *8.4.4 Complement-Dependent Human Anaphylaxis*

In addition to complement activation by the classical pathway in human IgG-mediated anaphylaxis, complement activation by the alternative and lectin pathways has been associated with human anaphylactic responses (usually referred to as anaphylactoid responses) in which there is no evidence for Ab participation. Relatively common examples include anaphylaxis in association with complement activation by hemodialysis membranes (particularly with initial use of new membranes) [102, 103], by protamine neutralization of heparin [104], by liposomal drugs [105], and by polyethylene glycols [106]. It is not known whether complement activation and anaphylatoxin production is sufficient, by itself, to induce clinical shock or, as in the mouse, must be associated with other, still undefined stimuli, to induce shock. One human example of the latter possibility appears to be anaphylaxis induced by wasp stings. Although a critical component of wasp sting-induced anaphylaxis is IgE-dependent [107, 108], some of the toxins in wasp venom activate complement and severe wasp sting-induced anaphylaxis in humans is usually associated with evidence of complement activation [109]. Additionally, evidence that peanut extract activates complement in human plasma in vitro [75] supports the possibility that complement activation by peanut molecules may synergize with peanut-stimulated, IgE-mediated mast cell activation to promote human peanut-induced anaphylaxis, as appears to be the case for the mouse. Some of the more common stimuli for human anaphylaxis that appears to be primarily dependent on IgG or complement are listed in Table 8.5.

### *8.4.5 Other Mechanisms of Human Anaphylaxis*

Not all human anaphylactic responses are associated with the presence of detectable IgE or IgG Ag-specific Abs or with evidence of complement activation. For example, although initial reports of the relatively common anaphylactic responses induced by intravenous administration of iodinated radiological contrast media suggested dependence on complement activation, more recent studies

**Table 8.5** Drugs and procedures that induce human IgG- and complement-mediated anaphylaxis

| |
|---|
| **IgG-mediated anaphylaxis** |
| Infusion of dextran |
| Infusion of aprotinin |
| Infusion of von Willebrand factor |
| Infusion of monoclonal chimeric, humanized, or human therapeutic mAbs |
| **Complement-mediated anaphylaxis** |
| Hemodialysis |
| Protamine neutralization of heparin |
| Liposomal drugs |
| Polyethylene glycols |

provide evidence that this is not the case. These studies suggest instead that the pathogenesis of iodinated radiological contrast medium-induced shock involves either direct basophil and/or mast cell activation or bradykinin production via the contact-dependent clotting system [110–112]. These conclusions, however, are still tentative.

## 8.5 Conclusions and Clinical Implications

The studies described in this chapter demonstrate several similarities between murine and human anaphylaxis: (1) IgE-mediated anaphylaxis involves mast cells, Fcε(epsilon)RI, and histamine in both species; (2) IgG-mediated anaphylaxis, which involves Fcγ(gamma)RIII, macrophages, and basophils and PAF in mice, appears to also occur in humans and to require inoculation with relatively large quantities of Ag in both species; (3) complement activation with anaphylatoxin production can exacerbate anaphylaxis in mice and appears to contribute to anaphylaxis in humans; and (4) Fcγ(gamma)RIIb can downregulate inflammatory cell activation that leads to anaphylaxis in both species. There are also differences between murine and human anaphylaxis, however, including: (1) greater ability of human basophils to secrete histamine and probably, less ability of human basophils to secrete PAF; and (2) expression of Fcε(epsilon)RI on human, but not murine macrophages and dendritic cells, suggesting the possibility for mechanisms of IgE-mediated anaphylaxis in humans that do not occur in mice. In addition, IgE-independent mechanisms that have been definitively demonstrated in mice are probable, but not proven in humans, where they are based predominantly on correlative studies.

Assuming that humans can develop anaphylaxis caused by these IgE-independent mechanisms and that these mechanisms operate similarly in humans and mice, the observations discussed here suggest that one goal of immunotherapy directed against IgE-mediated anaphylaxis should be induction of Ab responses, such as IgG4, that do not activate complement. Additionally, because human IgG4, like mouse IgG1, has some ability to induce Fcγ(gamma)R-mediated immunopathology [113], immunotherapy that promotes the production of IgG "blocking antibodies" should be a goal only for patients who have anaphylaxis induced by small quantities of Ag; increasing Ag-specific IgG Ab responses might well exacerbate IgG-mediated anaphylactic responses that are induced by inoculation of large quantities of Ag.

The observations made in this chapter also suggest key goals for further anaphylaxis research that could lead to advances in the diagnosis, prevention and, possibly, treatment of anaphylaxis (Table 8.6). These include: (1) the development of markers for IgE-mediated anaphylaxis that are more sensitive and persistent than mast cell-released proteases; (2) development of markers for IgG-mediated anaphylaxis that can be used to identify putative human IgG-mediated anaphylaxis; (3) testing of PAF antagonists in humans (particularly as prophylaxis during IV infusion of large quantities of Ags that have been associated with IgG-mediated anaphylaxis); (4) development of improved inhibitors of mast cell, basophil, and macrophage activation, including inhibitors of stimulatory FcRs and stimulators of inhibitory receptors, such as Fcγ(gamma)RIIb; and (5) possibly

**Table 8.6** Goals for future anaphylaxis research

| |
|---|
| 1. Development of markers for IgE-mediated anaphylaxis that are more sensitive and persistent than mast cell-released proteases. |
| 2. Development of markers for IgG-mediated anaphylaxis that can be used to identify putative human IgG-mediated anaphylaxis. |
| 3. Testing PAF antagonists as prophylaxis and possibly therapy for human anaphylaxis. |
| 4. Development of improved inhibitors of mast cell, basophil, and macrophage activation. |
| 5. Optimizing combined use of Ag nonspecific inhibitors with Ag-specific desensitization. |

combined use of Ag nonspecific inhibitors with Ag-specific desensitization, as has been shown already with a non-stimulatory anti-IgE mAb [88].

**Acknowledgments** This work was supported by a merit award from the US Department of Veterans Affairs and NIH grant R21AI079947. I thank my colleagues Marat Khodoun, Suzanne Morris, and Richard Strait, who performed much of the work described in this review.

## References

1. Verdier F, Chazal I, Descotes J. Anaphylaxis models in the guinea-pig. *Toxicology* 1994;93:55–61.
2. Oettgen HC, Martin TR, Wynshaw-Boris A, Deng C, Drazen JM, Leder P. Active anaphylaxis in IgE-deficient mice. *Nature* 1994;370:367–370.
3. Dombrowicz D, Flamand V, Brigman KK, Koller BH, Kinet JP. Abolition of anaphylaxis by targeted disruption of the high affinity immunoglobulin E receptor α(alpha) chain gene. *Cell* 1993;75: 969–976.
4. Takai T, Li M, Sylvestre D, Clynes R, Ravetch JV. FcRγ(gamma) chain deletion results in pleiotrophic effector cell defects. *Cell* 1994;76:519–529.
5. Fossati-Jimack L, Ioan-Facsinay A, Reininger L, et al. Markedly different pathogenicity of four immunoglobulin G isotype-switch variants of an antierythrocyte autoantibody is based on their capacity to interact in vivo with the low-affinity Fcγ(gamma) receptor III. *J Exp Med* 2000;191:1293–1302.
6. Hazenbos WL, Gessner JE, Hofhuis FM, et al. Impaired IgG-dependent anaphylaxis and Arthus reaction in Fcγ(gamma)RIII (CD16) deficient mice. *Immunity* 196;5:181–188.
7. Takai T, Ono M, Hikida M, Ohmori H, Ravetch JV. Augmented humoral and anaphylactic responses in Fcγ(gamma)RII-deficient mice. *Nature* 1996;379:346–349.
8. Ha TY, Reed ND, Crowle PK. Delayed expulsion of adult *Trichinella spiralis* by mast cell-deficient W/W$^v$ mice. *Infect Immun* 1983;41:445–447.
9. Grimbaldeston MA, Chen CC, Piliponsky AM, Tsai M, Tam SY, Galli SJ. Mast cell-deficient W-sash c-kit mutant Kit W-sh/W-sh mice as a model for investigating mast cell biology in vivo. *Am J Pathol* 2005;167:835–848.
10. Nishikawa S, Kusakabe M, Yoshinaga K, et al. In utero manipulation of coat color formation by a monoclonal anti-c-kit antibody: two distinct waves of c-kit-dependency during melanocyte development. *Embo J* 1991;10:2111–2118.
11. Tsujimura Y, Obata K, Mukai K, et al. Basophils play a pivotal role in immunoglobulin-G-mediated but not immunoglobulin-E-mediated systemic anaphylaxis. *Immunity* 2008;28:581–589.
12. Sokol CL, Barton GM, Farr AG, Medzhitov R. A mechanism for the initiation of allergen-induced T helper type 2 responses. *Nat Immunol* 2008;9:310–318.
13. Husztik E, Lazar G, Szilagyi S. Study on the mechanism of Kupffer cell phagocytosis blockade induced by gadolinium chloride. In: Wisse E, Knook D, eds. *International Kupffer Cell Symposium.* Noordwijkerhout, Netherlands: Elsevier/North-Holland Biomedical Press; 1977:387–395.
14. Van Rooijen N, Kors N, vd Ende M, Dijkstra CD. Depletion and repopulation of macrophages in spleen and liver of rat after intravenous treatment with liposome-encapsulated dichloromethylene diphosphonate. *Cell Tissue Res* 1990;260:215–222.
15. Kehry MR, Yamashita LC. Low-affinity IgE receptor (CD23) function on mouse B cells: role in IgE- dependent antigen focusing. *Proc Natl Acad Sci USA* 1989;86:7556–7560.
16. Ra C, Jouvin MH, Kinet JP. Complete structure of the mouse mast cell receptor for IgE (Fcε(epsilon)RI) and surface expression of chimeric receptors (rat–mouse–human) on transfected cells. *J Biol Chem* 1989;264:15323–15327.
17. Squire CM, Studer EJ, Lees A, Finkelman FD, Conrad DH. Antigen presentation is enhanced by targeting antigen to the Fcε(epsilon)RII by antigen-anti-Fcε(epsilon)RII conjugates. *J Immunol* 1994;152:4388–4396.
18. Kinet JP. The high-affinity IgE receptor (Fcε(epsilon)RI): from physiology to pathology. *Annu Rev Immunol* 1999;17:931–972.
19. Yokota A, Kikutani H, Tanaka T, et al. Two species of human Fc ε(epsilon) receptor II (Fcε(epsilon)RII/CD23): tissue-specific and IL-4-specific regulation of gene expression. *Cell* 1988;55:611–618.
20. van Neerven RJ, Wikborg T, Lund G, et al. Blocking antibodies induced by specific allergy vaccination prevent the activation of CD4$^+$ T cells by inhibiting serum-IgE-facilitated allergen presentation. *J Immunol* 1999;163:2944–2952.
21. Seder RA, et al. Production of interleukin-4 and other cytokines following stimulation of mast cell lines and in vivo mast cells/basophils. *Int Arch Allergy Appl Immunol* 1991;94:137–140.

22. Seder RA, Paul WE, Ben-Sasson SZ, et al. Mouse splenic and bone marrow cell populations that express high-affinity Fcε(epsilon) receptors and produce interleukin 4 are highly enriched in basophils. *Proc Natl Acad Sci USA* 1991;88:2835–2839.
23. MacGlashan D Jr, White JM, Huang SK, Ono SJ, Schroeder JT, Lichtenstein LM. Secretion of IL-4 from human basophils. The relationship between IL-4 mRNA and protein in resting and stimulated basophils. *J Immunol* 1994;152:3006–3016.
24. Khodoun MV, Orekhova T, Potter C, Morris S, Finkelman FD. Basophils initiate IL-4 production during a memory T-dependent response. *J Exp Med* 2004;200:857–870.
25. Gessner A, Mohrs K, Mohrs M. Mast cells, basophils, and eosinophils acquire constitutive IL-4 and IL-13 transcripts during lineage differentiation that are sufficient for rapid cytokine production. *J Immunol* 2005;174:1063–1072.
26. Fox PC, Basciano LK, Siraganian RP. Mouse mast cell activation and desensitization for immune aggregate-induced histamine release. *J Immunol* 1982;129:314–319.
27. Strait RT, Morris SC, Yang M, Qu XW, Finkelman FD. Pathways of anaphylaxis in the mouse. *J Allergy Clin Immunol* 2002;109:658–668.
28. Camussi G, Aglietta M, Coda R, Bussolino F, Piacibello W, Tetta C. Release of platelet-activating factor (PAF) and histamine. II. The cellular origin of human PAF: monocytes, polymorphonuclear neutrophils and basophils. *Immunology* 1981;42:191–199.
29. Ishizaka T, Conrad DH. Binding characteristics of human IgE receptors and initial triggering events in human mast cells for histamine release. *Monogr Allergy* 1983;18:14–24.
30. Mencia-Huerta JM, Benveniste J. Platelet-activating factor and macrophages. I. Evidence for the release from rat and mouse peritoneal macrophages and not from mastocytes. *Eur J Immunol* 1975;9:409–415.
31. Benveniste J. Paf-acether, an ether phospho-lipid with biological activity. *Prog Clin Biol Res* 1988;282:73–85.
32. Bergamaschini L, Santangelo T, Faricciotti A, Ciavarella N, Mannucci PM, Agostoni A. Study of complement-mediated anaphylaxis in humans. The role of IgG subclasses (IgG1 and/or IgG4) in the complement-activating capacity of immune complexes. *J Immunol* 1996;156:1256–1261.
33. Hugli TE. The structural basis for anaphylatoxin and chemotactic functions of C3a, C4a, and C5a. *Crit Rev Immunol* 1981;1:321–366.
34. Carroll MC. The role of complement and complement receptors in induction and regulation of immunity. *Annu Rev Immunol* 1998;16:545–568.
35. Walport MJ. Complement. Second of two parts. *N Engl J Med* 2001;344:1140–1144.
36. Walport MJ. Complement. First of two parts. *N Engl J Med* 2001;344:1058–1066.
37. Klos A, Tenner AJ, Johswich KO, Ager RR, Reis ES, Köhl J. The role of the anaphylatoxins in health and disease. *Mol Immunol* 2009;46:2753–2766.
38. Damerau B. Biological activities of complement-derived peptides. *Rev Physiol Biochem Pharmacol* 1987;108:151–206.
39. Kownatzki E. Triggering of mast cells. *Mol Immunol* 1982;19:1297–1300.
40. Dias Da Silva W, Lepow IH. Complement as a mediator of inflammation. II. Biological properties of anaphylatoxin prepared with purified components of human complement. *J Exp Med* 1967;125:921–946.
41. Snapper C, Finkelman F. Immunoglobulin Class Switching. In: Paul WE, ed. *Fundamental Immunology*. Philadelphia: Lippincott-Raven; 1999.
42. Faquim-Mauro EL, Coffman RL, Abrahamsohn IA, Macedo MS. Cutting edge: mouse IgG1 antibodies comprise two functionally distinct types that are differentially regulated by IL-4 and IL-12. *J Immunol* 1999;163:3572–3576.
43. Silva SR, Casabuono A, Jacysyn JF, et al. Sialic acid residues are essential for the anaphylactic activity of murine IgG1 antibodies. *J Immunol* 2008;181:8308–8314.
44. Bieber T, de la Salle H, Wollenberg A, et al. Human epidermal Langerhans cells express the high affinity receptor for immunoglobulin E (Fcε(epsilon)RI). *J Exp Med* 1992;175:1285–1290.
45. Maurer D, Fiebiger E, Reininger B, et al. Expression of functional high affinity immunoglobulin E receptors (Fcε(epsilon)RI) on monocytes of atopic individuals. *J Exp Med* 1994;179:745–750.
46. Maurer D, Fiebiger S, Ebner C, et al. Peripheral blood dendritic cells express Fcε(epsilon)RI as a complex composed of Fcε(epsilon)RI alpha- and Fcε(epsilon)RIγ(gamma)-chains and can use this receptor for IgE-mediated allergen presentation. *J Immunol* 1996;157:607–616.
47. Lee JJ, McGarry MP. When is a mouse basophil not a basophil? *Blood* 2007;109:859–861.
48. Ravetch JV, Bolland S. IgG Fc receptors. *Annu Rev Immunol* 2001;19:275–290.
49. Ando A, Martin TR, Galli SJ. Effects of chronic treatment with the c-kit ligand, stem cell factor, on immunoglobulin E-dependent anaphylaxis in mice. Genetically mast cell-deficient Sl/Sld mice acquire anaphylactic responsiveness, but the congenic normal mice do not exhibit augmented responses. *J Clin Invest* 1993;92:1639–1649.
50. Strait RT, Morris SC, Finkelman FD. IgG-blocking antibodies inhibit IgE-mediated anaphylaxis in vivo through both antigen interception and Fcγ(gamma)RIIb cross-linking. *J Clin Invest* 2006;116:833–841.

51. Eshhar Z, Ofarim M, Waks T. Generation of hybridomas secreting murine reaginic antibodies of anti-DNP specificity. *J Immunol* 1980;124:775–780.
52. Fish SC, Donaldson DD, Goldman SJ, Williams CM, Kasaian MT. IgE generation and mast cell effector function in mice deficient in IL-4 and IL-13. *J Immunol* 2005;174:7716–7724.
53. Park JS, Choi IH, Lee DG, et al. Anti-IL-4 monoclonal antibody prevents antibiotics-induced active fatal anaphylaxis. *J Immunol* 1997;158:5002–5006.
54. Morawetz RA, Gabriele L, Rizzo LV, Noben-Trauth N, Kühn R, Rajewsky K, Morawetz RA, et al. Interleukin (IL)-4-independent immunoglobulin class switch to immunoglobulin (Ig)E in the mouse. *J Exp Med* 1996;184:1651–1661.
55. Dombrowicz D, Flamand V, Miyajima I, Ravetch JV, Galli SJ, Kinet JP. Absence of Fcε(epsilon)RIα(alpha) chain results in upregulation of Fcγ(gamma)RIII-dependent mast cell degranulation and anaphylaxis. Evidence of competition between Fcε(epsilon)RI and Fcγ(gamma)RIII for limiting amounts of FcR β(beta) and γ(gamma) chains. *J Clin Invest* 1997;99:915–925.
56. Miyajima I, Dombrowicz D, Martin TR, Ravetch JV, Kinet JP, Galli SJ. Systemic anaphylaxis in the mouse can be mediated largely through IgG1 and Fcγ(gamma)RIII. Assessment of the cardiopulmonary changes, mast cell degranulation, and death associated with active or IgE- or IgG1-dependent passive anaphylaxis. *J Clin Invest* 1997;99:901–914.
57. Hirayama N, Hirano T, Köhler G, Kurata A, Okumura K, Ovary Z. Biological activities of antitrinitrophenyl and antidinitrophenyl mouse monoclonal antibodies. *Proc Natl Acad Sci USA* 1982;79:613–615.
58. Unkeless J. Characterization of a monoclonal antibody directed against mouse macrophage and lymphocyte Fc receptors. *J Exp Med* 1979;150:580–596.
59. Nimmerjahn F, Ravetch JV. Divergent immunoglobulin γ(gamma) subclass activity through selective Fc receptor binding. *Science* 2005;310:1510–1512.
60. Kinet JP, Blank U, Brini A, et al. The high-affinity receptor for immunoglobulin E: a target for therapy of allergic diseases. *Int Arch Allergy Appl Immunol* 1991;94:51–55.
61. Hazenbos WL, Heijnen IA, Meyer D, et al. Murine IgG1 complexes trigger immune effector functions predominantly via Fcγ(gamma)RIII (CD16). *J Immunol* 1998;161:3026–3032.
62. Lázár G Jr, Lázár G, Kaszaki J, Oláh J, Kiss I, Husztik E. Inhibition of anaphylactic shock by gadolinium chloride-induced Kupffer cell blockade. *Agents Actions* 1994;41:C97–98.
63. Gibbs BF, et al. Purified human peripheral blood basophils release interleukin-13 and preformed interleukin-4 following immunological activation. *Eur J Immunol* 1996;26:2493–2498.
64. Strait RT, Morris SC, Smiley K, Urban JF Jr, Finkelman FD. IL-4 exacerbates anaphylaxis. *J Immunol* 2003;170:3835–3842.
65. Coffman RL, Ohara J, Bond MW, Carty J, Zlotnik A, Paul WE. B cell stimulatory factor-1 enhances the IgE response of lipopolysaccharide-activated B cells. *J Immunol* 1986;136:4538–4541.
66. Finkelman FD, Katona IM, Urban JF Jr, et al. IL-4 is required to generate and sustain in vivo IgE responses. *J Immunol* 1988;141:2335–2341.
67. Swain SL, Weinberg AD, English M, Huston G. IL-4 directs the development of Th2-like helper effectors. *J Immunol* 1990;145:3796–3806.
68. Shimoda K, van Deursen J, Sangster MY, et al. Lack of IL-4-induced Th2 response and IgE class switching in mice with disrupted Stat6 gene. *Nature* 1996;380:630–633.
69. Yoshimoto T, Yasuda K, Tanaka H, et al. Basophils contribute to T(H)2-IgE responses in vivo via IL-4 production and presentation of peptide-MHC class II complexes to $CD4^+$ T cells. *Nat Immunol* 2009;10:706–712.
70. Sokol CL, Chu NQ, Yu S, Nish SA, Laufer TM, Medzhitov R. Basophils function as antigen-presenting cells for an allergen-induced T helper type 2 response. *Nat Immunol* 10, 713–720 (2009).
71. Perrigoue JG, Saenz SA, Siracusa MC, et al. MHC class II-dependent basophil-$CD4^+$ T cell interactions promote $T_H2$ cytokine-dependent immunity. *Nat Immunol* 2009;10:697–705.
72. Kawabata Y, Yang TS, Yokochi TT, et al. Complement system is involved in anaphylactoid reaction induced by lipopolysaccharides in muramyldipeptide-treated mice. *Shock* 2000;14:572–577.
73. Murch O, Abdelrahman M, Kapoor A, Thiemermann C. Muramyl dipeptide enhances the response to endotoxin to cause multiple organ injury in the anesthetized rat. *Shock* 2008;29:388–394.
74. Yamaguchi K, Yu Z, Kumamoto H, et al. Involvement of Kupffer cells in lipopolysaccharide-induced rapid accumulation of platelets in the liver and the ensuing anaphylaxis-like shock in mice. *Biochim Biophys Acta* 2006;1762:269–275.
75. Khodoun M, Strait R, Orekov T, et al. Peanuts can contribute to anaphylactic shock by activating complement. *J Allergy Clin Immunol* 2009;123:342–351.
76. Liu E, Moriyama H, Abiru N, et al. Anti-peptide autoantibodies and fatal anaphylaxis in NOD mice in response to insulin self-peptides B:9-23 and B:13-23. *J Clin Invest* 2002;110:1021–1027.
77. Brandt EB, Strait RT, Hershko D, et al. Mast cells are required for experimental oral allergen-induced diarrhea. *J Clin Invest* 2003;112:1666–1677.

78. Ravetch JV. Fc receptors. *Curr Opin Immunol* 1997;9:121–125.
79. Zhang K, Kepley CL, Terada T, Zhu D, Perez H, Saxon A. Inhibition of allergen-specific IgE reactivity by a human Ig Fcγ(gamma)-Fcε(epsilon) bifunctional fusion protein. *J Allergy Clin Immunol* 2004;114:321–327.
80. Van Scott MR, Mertsching E, Negrou E, et al. Systemic administration of an Fcg(gamma)-Fce(epsilon)-fusion protein in house dust mite sensitive nonhuman primates. Clin Immunol 2008;128:340–348.
81. Mertsching E, Bafetti L, Hess H, et al. A mouse Fcg(gamma)-Fce(epsilon) protein that inhibits mast cells through activation of Fcg(gamma)RIIB, SH2 domain-containing inositol phosphatase 1, and SH2 domain-containing protein tyrosine phosphatases. J Allergy Clin Immunol 2008;121:441–447, e445.
82. Arimura A, Nagata M, Takeuchi M, Watanabe A, Nakamura K, Harada M. Active and passive cutaneous anaphylaxis in WBB6F1 mouse, a mast cell-deficient strain. Immunol Invest 1990;19:227–233.
83. Mancardi DA, Iannascoli B, Hoos S, England P, Daëron M, Bruhns P. Fcg(gamma)RIV is a mouse IgE receptor that resembles macrophage Fce(epsilon)RI in humans and promotes IgE-induced lung inflammation. J Clin Invest 2008;118:3738–3750.
84. Hirano M, et al. IgEb immune complexes activate macrophages through Fcg(gamma)RIV binding. Nat Immunol 2007;8:762–771.
85. Nimmerjahn F, Bruhns P, Horiuchi K, Ravetch JV. Fcg(gamma)RIV: a novel FcR with distinct IgG subclass specificity. Immunity 2005;23:41–51.
86. Worobec A. Metcalfe DD. Anaphylactic Syndrome. In: Austen KF, Frank MM, Atkinson JP, Cantor H, eds. Samter's Immunologic Diseases. Philadelphia: Lippincott Williams & Wilkins; 2001:825–836.
87. Schwartz LB, Yunginger JW, Miller J, Bokhari R, Dull D. Time course of appearance and disappearance of human mast cell tryptase in the circulation after anaphylaxis. J Clin Invest 1989;83:1551–1555.
88. Casale TB, Busse WW, Kline JN, et al. Omalizumab pretreatment decreases acute reactions after rush immunotherapy for ragweed-induced seasonal allergic rhinitis. J Allergy Clin Immunol 2006;117:134–140.
89. Leung DY, Sampson HA, Yunginger JW, et al. Effect of anti-IgE therapy in patients with peanut allergy. N Engl J Med 2003;348:986–993.
90. Ochiai K, Kagami M, Umemiya K, Matsumura R, Kawashima T, Tomioka H. Expression of high-affinity IgE receptor (Fce(epsilon)RI) on human alveolar macrophages from atopic and non-atopic patients. Int Arch Allergy Immunol 1996;111Suppl 1:55–58.
91. Simons FE, Frew AJ, Ansotegui IJ, et al. Risk assessment in anaphylaxis: current and future approaches. J Allergy Clin Immunol 2007;120:S2–S24.
92. Hedin H, Richter W, Messmer K, Renck H, Ljungström KG, Laubenthal H. Incidence, pathomechanism and prevention of dextran-induced anaphylactoid/anaphylactic reactions in man. Dev Biol Stand 1980;48:179–189.
93. Umeda Y, Fukumoto Y, Miyauchi T, Imaizumi M, Shimabukuro K, Mori Y, et al. Anaphylactic shock related to aprotinin induced by anti-aprotinin immunoglobulin G antibody alone; report of a case. Kyobu Geka 2007;60:69–71.
94. Bergamaschini L, Mannucci PM, Federici AB, Coppola R, Guzzoni S, Agostoni A. Posttransfusion anaphylactic reactions in a patient with severe von Willebrand disease: role of complement and alloantibodies to von Willebrand factor. J Lab Clin Med 125, 348–355 (1995).
95. Cheifetz A, Smedley M, Martin S, Reiter M, Leone G, Mayer L, et al. The incidence and management of infusion reactions to infliximab: a large center experience. Am J Gastroenterol 2003;98:1315–1324.
96. Vadas P, Gold M, Perelman B, Liss GM, Lack G, Blyth T, et al. Platelet-activating factor, PAF acetylhydrolase, and severe anaphylaxis. N Engl J Med 2008;358:28–35.
97. Till J, Francis JN, Nouri-Aria K, Durham SR. Mechanisms of immunotherapy. J Allergy Clin Immunol 2004;113:1025–1034, quiz 1035.
98. Punnonen J, Aversa G, Cocks BG, et al. Interleukin 13 induces interleukin 4-independent IgG4 and IgE synthesis and CD23 expression by human B cells. Proc Natl Acad Sci USA 1993;90:3730–3734.
99. van der Zee JS, van Swieten P, Aalberse RC. Inhibition of complement activation by IgG4 antibodies. Clin Exp Immunol 1986;64:415–422.
100. Jeannin P, Lecoanet S, Delneste Y, Gauchat JF, Bonnefoy JY. IgE versus IgG4 production can be differentially regulated by IL-10. *J Immunol* 1998;160:3555–3561.
101. Lochner M, Peduto L, Cherrier M, et al. In vivo equilibrium of proinflammatory IL-17+ and regulatory IL-10+ Foxp3+ RORg(gamma)t+ T cells. J Exp Med 2008;205:1381–1393.
102. Hakim RM, Breillatt J, Lazarus JM, Port FK. Complement activation and hypersensitivity reactions to dialysis membranes. N Engl J Med 1984;311:878–882.
103. Suzuki Y, Uchida J, Tsuji H, et al. Acute changes in C3a and C5a in an anaphylactoid reaction in hemodialysis patients. Tohoku J Exp Med 1987;152:35–45.
104. Westaby S, Turner MW, Stark J. Complement activation and anaphylactoid response to protamine in a child after cardiopulmonary bypass. Br Heart J 1985;53:574–576.
105. Szebeni J. Complement activation-related pseudoallergy: a new class of drug-induced acute immune toxicity. Toxicology 2005;216:106–121.

106. Hamad I, Hunter AC, Szebeni J, Moghimi SM. Poly(ethylene glycol)s generate complement activation products in human serum through increased alternative pathway turnover and a MASP-2-dependent process. Mol Immunol 2008;46:225–232.
107. Kemeny DM, Lessof MH, Patel S, Youlten LJ, Williams A, Lambourn E. IgG and IgE antibodies after immunotherapy with bee and wasp venom. Int Arch Allergy Appl Immunol 1989;88:247–249.
108. Hoffman DR, Wood CL, Hudson P. Demonstration of IgE and IgG antibodies against venoms in the blood of victims of fatal sting anaphylaxis. J Allergy Clin Immunol 1983;71:193–196.
109. van der Linden PW, Hack CE, Kerckhaert JA, Struyvenberg A, van der Zwan JC. Preliminary report: complement activation in wasp-sting anaphylaxis. Lancet 1990;336:904–906.
110. Vik H, Froysa A, Sonstevold A, Toft K, Stov PS, Ege T. Complement activation and histamine release following administration of roentgen contrast media. Acta Radiol Suppl 1995;399:83–89.
111. Morcos SK. Review article: acute serious and fatal reactions to contrast media: our current understanding. Br J Radiol 2005;78:686–693.
112. Idee JM, Pines E, Prigent P, Corot C. Allergy-like reactions to iodinated contrast agents. A critical analysis. Fundam Clin Pharmacol 2005;19:263–281.
113. Bruhns P, Iannascoli B, England P, et al. Specificity and affinity of human Fcg(gamma) receptors and their polymorphic variants for human IgG subclasses. Blood 2009;113:3716–3725.

# Chapter 9
# Food-Induced Anaphylaxis

**Kirsi M. Järvinen-Seppo and Anna Nowak-Węgrzyn**

**Abstract** Food allergy is the most common single cause of anaphylaxis. About 4–6% of children and 3% of adults suffer from confirmed food allergy, which places a huge population at risk for anaphylaxis. This chapter provides an overview of the epidemiology, pathophysiology, clinical presentation, pediatric considerations, risk factors, treatment, diagnosis, prevention, and natural history of food-induced anaphylaxis. With a growing population of food-allergic children and adults, who appear to have more severe and more persistent food allergies, new therapies are vigorously sought and are also reviewed here.

**Keywords** Abdominal pain • Adolescents • Allergenicity • Allergic reaction • Anaphylactic reaction • Anaphylaxis • Angioedema • Antigen • Asthma • Atopic eczema • Autoinjectible • Autoinjector • Basophils • Biphasic • Bronchodilators • CD23 • Children • Clinical presentation • Conformational Epitopes • Corticosteroids • Cow's Milk Allergy • Cpg motifs • Cutaneous • Degranulation • Desensitization • Diagnosis • Diarrhea • Diphenhydramine • Effector cells • Egg allergy • Epidemiology • Epinephrine • Exercise • Fatal • FcεRi • Fish allergy • Food allergens • Food allergy • Food-dependent exercise-induced anaphylaxis • Food-induced • Food-specific ige • Future therapy • Gastrointestinal • Heated • Heat-Killed *E. Coli* • Histamine • Hives • Humanized monoclonal anti-ige • Hypersensitivity • Immunostimulatory sequences • Immunotherapy • Incidence • Infants • Intestinal Uptake • Lethargy • Mast cells • Medical identification bracelet • Murine models • Natural history • Near-fatal • Oral • Oral food challenge • Outgrow • Paf acetylhydrolase • Paracellular • Pathophysiology • Peanut allergy • Peptide • Plasmid dna • Platelet activating factor • Precautionary labeling • Prevalence • Prevention • Prick skin test • Protracted • Recombinant proteins • Rhinitis • Risk factors • Route of exposure • Sequential epitopes • Shellfish allergy • Soy allergy • Sublingual • Tolerance • Traditional Chinese medicine • Transcellular • Transport • Treatment • Tree nut allergy • Tryptase • Unheated • Uniphasic • Urticaria • Vomiting • Wheat allergy • Wheezing

## 9.1 Introduction

Anaphylaxis, the most severe manifestation of an allergic reaction, has been recently defined by an expert panel as "a serious allergic reaction that is rapid in onset and may cause death" [1]. Food allergy is the most common single cause of anaphylaxis. About 4–6% of children and 3% of adults

A. Nowak-Węgrzyn (✉)
Mount Sinai School of Medicine, New York, NY, USA
e-mail: anna.nowak-wegrzyn@mssm.edu

M.C. Castells (ed.), *Anaphylaxis and Hypersensitivity Reactions*,
DOI 10.1007/978-1-60327-951-2_9, © Springer Science+Business Media, LLC 2011

suffer from confirmed food allergy, which places a huge population at risk for anaphylaxis. With a growing population of food-allergic children and adults, who appear to have more severe and more persistent food allergies, new therapies are being vigorously sought.

## 9.2 Epidemiology

Food allergy is an increasing problem in Westernized countries around the world [2]. Food allergy has been reported in 4–6% of children and 3.7% of adults [2–4]. In general, the prevalence of reported food allergy in the USA increased 18% from 1997 to 2007 [4]. The incidence of food allergy to peanuts about doubled within the last decade, with over 1% of school children in the USA, the UK, Canada, and Australia being affected [5–8]. Asthma and other atopic diseases have likewise increased within the same time period [9]. Food-induced anaphylaxis is the leading single cause of anaphylaxis treated in emergency departments in the USA, especially in childhood. Food-induced anaphylaxis represents 15–57% of cases of anaphylaxis presenting to the emergency department [3] and up to 50–80% of anaphylactic reactions in children [10, 11].

The incidence of anaphylaxis has been reported to be between 8.4 and 21 per 100,000 person-years [3] and occurrence rate to be 30 per 100,000 person-years [12]. Two population studies based in the Olmsted County in Minnesota, Rochester, USA, reported the doubling of the average annual incidence rate from 21 cases per 100,000 person-years from 1983 to 1987 to 49.8 cases per 100,000 from 1990 to 2000 [12, 13]. There was also an increase in the annual incidence rate during the study period from 46.9 per 100,000 persons in 1990 to 58.9 per 100,000 persons in 2000 ($P=.03$) [13]. Hospitalization for anaphylaxis has increased in the UK by 700% [14, 15]. In New York State, hospital admissions for anaphylaxis in children showed a fourfold increase between 1990 and 2006 [16]. This increase parallels the increases in peanut allergy and atopic diseases in children.

In the study by Yocum et al. [12], the annual incidence of food-induced anaphylaxis was 7.6 cases per 100,000 person-years and food-induced anaphylaxis occurrence rate was 10.8 per 100,000 person-years. Based on these figures it has been estimated that there are 25,000–30,000 food-induced anaphylactic reactions treated in ED, 2,000 hospitalizations, and 150–200 deaths in the USA each year [17]. These numbers assumed no increase in the prevalence of food allergy since the late 1980s. However, despite an increase in the prevalence of food allergy, food-induced-anaphylaxis mortality rates, based on death certificates, were recently shown to remain stable between 2000 and 2009 in a report from Australia [18]. Extrapolations from a recent emergency department (ED) data from The National Electronic Injury Surveillance System (NEISS) predicts 2,333 ED visits and 418 hospitalizations for food-related anaphylaxis for a 2-month study period, but deaths cannot be estimated as none were identified [19]. The rate of hospital admissions for severe food-induced reactions has been reported 0.89 per 100,000 children per year in the UK and Ireland [11]. A report from the UK estimated, based on data from death certificates and clinical reports, an incidence of fatal reactions in children less than 16 years to be 0.006 deaths per 100,000 children per year [20].

In a registry of a fatal food-induced anaphylaxis, the majority of cases were adolescents and young adults [21, 22]. Food anaphylaxis has been reported as often in females and males in reports from the USA, [21] although more females reported in some studies [23, 24] and male preponderance in others [25]. The rates are probably affected by the proportion of children in the cohort, as food allergies are common in boys, whereas more women reported anaphylactic reactions than men [23].

Most cases of anaphylaxis are reported to occur in the home [23, 26, 27]. In a study of self-reported anaphylactic reactions due to foods in the United Kingdom, nearly one-fifth of the reactions in children occurred at school [23].

## 9.3 Food Allergens and Route of Exposure

In the developed countries, the major food allergens include milk, egg, wheat, soy, peanut, tree nuts, fish, shellfish, and seeds, such as sesame. Food allergens differ between countries probably due to local eating habits. Peanut allergy is one of the most common food allergies in the USA, seafood is a common food allergy in Hong Kong and Southern Europe [25, 27–29], and sesame is a major food allergen in Israeli children [30].

The most common food allergens causing allergic reactions in children include milk, egg, wheat, soy, peanuts, tree nuts, fish and shellfish, whereas allergies to peanut, tree nuts, fish, and shellfish are more commonly found in adults. Though any food can cause anaphylaxis, peanut, tree nuts, and shellfish are the most commonly implicated foods in anaphylaxis, recently milk and egg have also emerged among the most common foods inducing anaphylactic reactions especially in children [11, 31] (Table 9.1). In addition, lipid transfer protein (LTP) has been reported as the most common food allergen to induce anaphylaxis in Southern Europe [32].

Although prior exposure is necessary for the development of sensitization, 72% of peanut and/or tree nut allergic patients reported symptoms during their first known exposure [33]. These patients may have had previous unknown exposures through breast feeding, as hidden allergens, or use of topical products containing food oils, e.g., peanut [34]. However, the majority of patients (40–90%) with food-induced anaphylaxis had prior history of reaction to the food allergen in question [21, 23, 35].

Although most of the anaphylactic reactions occur to ingested food allergens, reports on anaphylaxis to inhaled food allergens also exist. Published reports have described anaphylaxis from inhalation of allergens from fish, shellfish, seeds, soybeans, cereal grains, egg, milk, and other foods when the subject has been exposed to airborne allergens such in the form of allergen flour in the air and vapors during cooking or roasting [36]. However, inhalation of or skin exposure to peanut butter in highly peanut-sensitized children did not result in systemic or respiratory reactions [37].

**Table 9.1** Foods implicated in anaphylaxis

| Authors | Population | No of subjects | Country | Most common foods (% of reactions) |
|---|---|---|---|---|
| Asero et al. [32] | Adults | 58 | Italy | LTP 33%, shrimp 17%, tree nut 16%, legumes 7%, seed 3% |
| Jarvinen et al. [31] | Children | 95 | USA | Peanut 25%, milk 19%, tree nut 13%, nut 4%, wheat 9%, fish/shellfish 3%, soy 2%, seed 2% |
| Colver et al. [11] | Children | 229 | UK, Ireland | Peanut 21%, tree nut 16%, milk 10%, egg 7% |
| Oren et al. [82] | Mixed age | 19 | USA | Peanut, tree nut |
| Uguz [23] | Mixed age | 126 | UK | Peanut ~25%, tree nut ~25%, milk 10%, egg ~5% |
| Moneret-Vautrin et al. [68] | Mixed age | 107 | France | Tree nut 15%, peanut 13%, shellfish 10%, lupine flour 9%, wheat 7% |

## 9.4 Pathophysiology of Food-Induced Anaphylaxis

Human food-induced anaphylaxis is triggered by food allergen binding to allergen-specific IgE [38]. Food allergic reactions require transfer of allergen across the epithelial and/or endothelial barrier and contact with specific IgE antibodies that are bound by sensitized effector cells such as mast cells (in tissues) and basophils (in peripheral blood), as well as several other cell types, through the high-affinity Fcε RI receptors on the cell surface. Aggregation and cross-linking of the Fcε RI leads to a signaling cascade triggering the release of pre-formed and newly synthesized mediators from mast cell and basophil granules. These mediators exert effects on a host of different target organs leading to the clinical manifestations of food-induced anaphylaxis. Children possessing IgE antibodies directed at more numerous epitopes on major peanut allergens had history of more severe peanut-induced reactions than the children with IgE antibodies directed at fewer epitopes [39]. In their study, greater diversity of recognized allergenic epitopes was associated with more efficient cross-linking of the IgE receptors and effector cells' degranulation.

Pathophysiology of food-induced anaphylaxis may differ from other causes of anaphylaxis [3]. Whereas fatal venom and drug-induced anaphylaxis typically is caused by cardiovascular shock, food-induced anaphylaxis is most often caused by respiratory compromise. It has been suggested that basophils as opposed to mast cells are the predominant cells involved in food-induced anaphylaxis [17].

### 9.4.1 *Murine Models*

Murine models of oral sensitization with peanut and cow's milk protein been established and induction of anaphylaxis by the same route of antigen exposure has been correlated with the presence of antigen-specific IgE [40, 41]. Elevations in plasma histamine levels as well as degranulation of tissue mast cells suggests that the anaphylactic reactions were due to IgE-mediated activation of mast cells. The importance of IgE and mast cells in food-induced anaphylaxis was recently confirmed by Sun et al. [42] in a peanut-induced anaphylaxis model in mast cell deficient mice (knock-out mice). These mice had detectable peanut-specific IgE, IgG1, and IgG2a after sensitization but were protected from anaphylaxis upon intraperitoneal peanut challenge. B-cell knock-out and CD40L knock-out mice were unable to produce peanut-specific immunoglobulin during sensitization and were protected from peanut-induced anaphylaxis, whereas Fcε RI -deficient mice (Fcε RI α-chain knock-out mice) were only partially protected from anaphylaxis, which could be due to the presence of an IgG-mediated "alternative pathway" of food-induced anaphylaxis, as recently published [43] and presented elsewhere in this book. It is not proven that an alternative pathway of anaphylaxis (i.e., IgG-mediated reactions) exists in human, although food-induced anaphylaxis in the absence of detectable food-specific IgE has occasionally been reported [38]. Concurrent blockade of the mast cell mediators, histamine and platelet activating factor prevented severe anaphylaxis in a mouse model of peanut anaphylaxis [44]. Taken together, these results suggest that mast cells and antigen-specific immunoglobulin are essential for peanut-induced anaphylaxis [45].

### 9.4.2 *Intestinal Antigen Uptake*

In patients sensitized to foods, alterations in gut permeability may play a role in the effector phase of the food-induced reactions. In animal models, normal uptake of food proteins includes two routes, transcellular transport (a small amount of food protein is taken up by the gut epithelium through endocytosis and is degraded in cellular lysosomes) and paracellular transport (regulated by tight junctions) [46, 47]. In the food-allergic host, food allergen uptake via the transcellular route is enhanced by the presence of food-specific IgE [48]. CD23, the low affinity IgE receptor, facilitates the bidirectional transcytosis of IgE [45]. Luminal IgE-antigen complexes are bound by CD23, endocytosed, shunted away from cellular lysosomes and transported intact across the cell to activate gut mast cells, followed by local mast cell activation, which leads to disruption of epithelial cell tight junctions with resultant increased gut permeability. This increase in gut permeability allows greater paracellular transport of a large number of molecules, including food allergens. Increased levels of food-specific IgE and soluble CD23 were found in the stool of food-allergic patients after oral food challenges suggesting that this mechanism is also important in humans [48].

Food-dependent exercise-induced anaphylaxis (FDEIA) is also thought to be due to increased gut permeability with resultant increased food allergen uptake [49, 50]. Increased intestinal uptake of food allergens has been shown after exercise and intake of nonsteroidal anti-inflammatory medications or alcohol [50]. Patients with FDEIA typically have low-level food-specific IgE titers and are tolerant to the implicated food unless stressed by exercise [50, 51].

### *9.4.3 Allergenicity of Food Antigens*

Most known food allergens are proteins that are resistant to thermal processing and enzymatic digestion. Allergenicity of food proteins can be modified by the degree of enzymatic digestion and thermal processing [45]. Underdigestion of food proteins places food-allergic patients at higher risk for more severe allergic reactions, such as anaphylaxis [52, 53]. In a cohort of adult patients taking an antacid medication for 3 months, a quarter of patients showed an increase in food-specific IgE formation and 15% showed de novo food-specific IgE formation [52]. Codfish-allergic patients were at greater risk for more severe allergic reactions when underdigested (with digestive enzymes at higher pH) codfish was ingested during a double-blinded placebo controlled food challenge (DBPCFC) [53]. In wheat-dependent, exercise-induced anaphylaxis, exercise induces the activation of tissue transglutaminase, which results in generation of high molecular weight complexes of omega-5 gliadin, a wheat allergen that bind IgE with increased intensity leading to mast cell activation and anaphylaxis [51]. Furthermore, as compared with frying or boiling peanuts, dry roasting peanut is associated with increased quantities of Ara h1 as well as increased IgE binding to the Ara h2 and Ara h3, major peanut proteins [54]. These results may explain the high prevalence of peanut allergy in the USA, Canada, UK, and Australia where dry roasting is the predominant form of thermal processing of peanut. In contrast, extensive heating of egg and milk proteins (e.g., baked goods such as muffins and waffles) causes modification of the protein structure which results in tolerance by 70–75% of subjects who otherwise react to lightly heated egg (e.g., French toast, scrambled eggs) or non-cooked milk [55, 56]. In Nowak-Wegrzyn et al. study, tolerance to extensively heated milk appeared to be a marker of a less severe milk allergy [55]. Children reactive to extensively heated (baked) milk were at higher risk for systemic reactions treated with epinephrine than those children tolerant to heated milk but reactive to unheated milk, 30% versus 0%. In contrast, the rate of systemic reactions treated with epinephrine was similar in children reactive to extensively heated egg and in children tolerant of extensively heated egg but reactive to unheated egg. This suggested that unlike in milk allergy, tolerance to extensively heated egg would not be a marker for decreased risk of severe reaction to lightly cooked egg [56].

Carbohydrate moieties frequently encountered in food are able to elicit IgE responses, but their clinical significance is unclear. Commins et al. [57] identified 24 patients with history of anaphylaxis or urticaria 3-6 hr after the ingestion of meat with IgE antibodies to galactose-α-1,3-galactose a carbohydrate commonly expressed on non-primate mammalian proteins. Mammalian meat extracts produced small wheals on skin prick tests (SPT) whereas intradermal or fresh-food SPT gave larger responses. Serum specific IgE antibodies to beef, pork, lamb, cow's milk, cat, and dog but not turkey, chicken, or fish were detected. Absorption experiments indicated that this pattern of sensitivity was explained by an IgE antibody specific for galactose-α-1,3-galactose, although it is currently not clear why the reactions had a delayed onset [57].

## 9.5 Clinical Presentation

The symptoms of food-induced anaphylaxis are most commonly seen in the skin (urticaria, angioedema, pruritus, flushing) in about 80% of cases and respiratory tract (cough, difficulty, wheezing) [27] (Table 9.2). Symptoms from the gastrointestinal tracts (vomiting, diarrhea, abdominal cramps) are more common in adults, 41% versus 5% in children [27]. In food-induced-anaphylaxis cardiovascular system (hypotension, loss of consciousness, shock) is less often affected than in anaphylaxis of other causes [28], especially in children (17% in adults versus 34% in children) [27].

The clinical presentation including the onset of symptoms, clinical severity, and sequence of symptom progression varies between individuals and between reactions in the same individual. This variability is likely dependent on numerous variables such as: the amount of food ingested, consumption of food on an empty versus full stomach, concurrent illness, exercise, consumption of alcohol or medications, etc. In childhood, more severe symptoms become more common as children get older and develop asthma.

### 9.5.1 *Onset of Symptoms*

The majority of reactions manifest within 1 hr of exposure, but the onset of symptoms from food-induced anaphylaxis may occur a few hours after exposure to the food allergen. A slower symptoms onset may be related to a less severe reaction or delayed absorption of the food [17]. Reactions to ingested allergens, such as foods, have a slower onset than injected allergens. In nonfatal reactions presenting to the emergency room or allergist's office, the average onset of reaction was 15 min–2 hr [27, 35].

**Table 9.2** Clinical presentation of food-induced anaphylaxis

| | |
|---|---|
| Cutaneous | Skin pruritus, urticaria, flushing, morbilliform rash, angioedema |
| Ocular | Pruritus, eye lid edema and erythema, conjunctival injection and tearing |
| Respiratory Tract Nasal | Nasal and ear pruritus, rhinorrhea, sneezing, congestion |
| Laryngeal | Throat pruritus and/or tightness, stridor, hoarseness, dysphonia, barky cough |
| Pulmonary | Cough, wheezing, dyspnea, chest tightness, cyanosis |
| Gastrointestinal Oral | Pruritus and or edema of the lips/mouth/tongue, metallic taste, dysphagia |
| Lower GI | Nausea, vomiting, crampy abdominal pain, diarrhea |
| Cardiovascular | Tachycardia, arrhythmia, dizziness, syncope, chest pain, hypotension, shock |
| Neurologic | Anxiety, headache, seizure, altered consciousness |
| Other | Urinary/fecal incontinence, diaphoresis, lower back pain and uterine contractions in women, sense of "pending doom" |

Modified from [84]

### *9.5.2 Patterns of Anaphylaxis*

In addition to uniphasic reaction, delayed onset, protracted (symptoms not responding to treatment and lasting up to 72 hr), and biphasic reactions (initial symptomatic period followed by an asymptomatic period of 30 min–72 hr) have been described [58, 59]. The pathophysiologic mechanisms involved in different patterns of anaphylaxis have not been identified. Biphasic and protracted course has been reported in fatal and near-fatal anaphylaxis [59].

### *9.5.3 Differential Diagnosis*

Symptoms of anaphylaxis may be confused with many illnesses. Skin manifestations including hives and angioedema may be due to other causes such as acute urticaria due to viral infections commonly seen in children and urticarial syndromes (covered elsewhere in this book), hereditary, and acquired angioedema and can also mimic those seen with insect bites. Flushing can be seen with mastocytosis, pheochromocytoma, and carcinoid syndrome (covered elsewhere). Respiratory symptoms similar to those seen in anaphylaxis may be also seen in asthma exacerbations, bronchiolitis, foreign body aspiration (especially in children), laryngospasms, and vocal cord dysfunction. Food poisoning, in particular from scombroid fish, and ingestion of monosodium glutamate or sulfites may be misdiagnosed as food-induced anaphylaxis. Features of vasovagal reaction, panic attack, somatiform disorder, mastocytosis and mast cell activation syndromes (covered elsewhere in this book) also mimic those of anaphylaxis.

## 9.6 Risk Factors for Food-Induced Anaphylaxis

Asthma has been shown to be a universal risk factor for severe food anaphylaxis [17, 31, 60]. In one study, the severity of coexisting other atopic diseases has also been associated with likelihood of developing life-threatening allergic reactions to peanut and tree nuts [61]. A history of severe rhinitis was associated with an increased risk for severe pharyngeal edema, severe asthma with increased risk of bronchospasm and severe eczema with increased risk of unconsciousness during an acute allergic reaction.

Age is another important factor with adolescents and young adults being more likely to develop a severe food-induced reaction [17, 61]. It has been appreciated that reactions generally worsen as children get older and with development of asthma [62].

Some other factors considered associated with severity of reactions include physical exertion, alcohol, acute illness, and menstruation [63, 64]. Food-dependent, exercise-induced anaphylaxis (FDEIA) occurs when ingestion of food 2–4 hr of exercise. Symptoms do not occur in the absence of exercise or if the food was not ingested before exercise.

In anaphylaxis generally, alcohol, aspirin, concurrent infection, use of β-blockers, and angiotensin converting enzyme inhibitors are additional factors that may increase the severity of anaphylactic reactions or diminish the efficacy of epinephrine [62]. Recently, it was shown that angiotensin-converting enzyme concentrations were significantly lower in peanut and tree nut-induced anaphylactic reactions, which progressed into severe pharyngeal edema [61] but not to other conditions such as severe bronchospasm. ACE is involved in the breakdown of bradykinin, the mediator that has been associated with life-threatening angioedema in patients with hereditary angioedema. An observation that patients taking enalapril, an inhibitor of ACE are more prone to develop angioedema further supports the importance of bradykin pathway in angioedema and potentially anaphylaxis.

Although allergy tests correlate with the likelihood of reactivity to foods, they do not correlate with the severity of reactions. Correlation has been made between the number of IgE-binding epitopes recognized by patients' specific IgE antibodies and the likelihood of a severity of reactions [39]. There is controversy over whether the amount of food triggering an allergic reaction correlates with the severity of a reaction [65, 66]. Perry et al. reported that more severe reactions were caused by smaller doses of food during oral food challenges [66]. In contrast, our own data do not support this observation [65, 66]. However, oral food challenges are conducted in a highly controlled environment and according to a strict dosing schedule and may not accurately reflect the potential for severe anaphylaxis in the real life scenario [9].

## 9.7 Pediatric Considerations

Features of anaphylaxis differ between children and adults [67]. Although generalized allergic reactions occur more commonly in children, adults more often experience anaphylaxis [24], including food-induced anaphylaxis [68]. Pediatric cases are more often triggered by foods, which may be explained by the presentation of food allergies at an earlier age, while drugs and insect venom are relatively more common triggers for adults.

### *9.7.1 Clinical Presentation*

Clinical presentation of anaphylaxis of any etiology differs slightly in children from adults. More than 90% of adults have cutaneous symptoms with anaphylaxis; this rate is lower in children (80%) [67]. The prevalence of asthma is higher in children with anaphylaxis as compared to adults (36.8% versus 23.2%) and children, indeed, more often experience respiratory symptoms, whereas adults are more frequently affected by cardiovascular compromise [67], which may be due to their increased age and a higher frequency of comorbid conditions. Whereas adults reported severe symptoms, including cardiovascular collapse more often, severe abdominal pain, hives, rhinitis, conjunctivitis and flushing were reported more often in children [23].

### *9.7.2 Risk Factors*

Within the pediatric population, previously identified risk factors for food-induced anaphylaxis include the following: older age, asthma, prior reactions involving the respiratory tract, peanut-tree nut allergy, and reactions to trace exposures [21, 60]. Peanut, tree nuts and milk have been found responsible for the majority of reactions. Asthma, similarly to adults, is a risk factor for food-induced anaphylaxis [23, 31], although severity of asthma did not correlate with severity of food-induced anaphylaxis [23]. Children also used a second dose of epinephrine less often than adults [31, 32].

### *9.7.3 Anaphylaxis in Infants*

The rate of anaphylaxis in infants is unknown, but it is likely underdiagnosed [69]. Food-induced anaphylactic reactions have been reported in infants starting from the age of 1 month [69]. Common allergens are cow's milk and egg, but any food can be a trigger [69]. Respiratory symptoms [70, 71] and anaphylaxis [72, 73] have been reported even in exclusively breastfed infants due to occult ingestion of food allergens in the mother's diet, such as cow's milk and fish. It is not known which factors increase the risk of anaphylaxis in infants [69]. Anaphylaxis in infants may have atypical presentation with lethargy, cyanosis, and hypotension with the lack of cutaneous symptoms [72] fussing, irritability, and seizures, and otherwise common in infants (drowsiness, regurgitation). The diagnosis of food-induced anaphylaxis may be missed [69] unless there is a suspicion or an already established diagnosis of food allergy. Food-induced anaphylaxis could be the first and last sign of food allergy in case of a fatal outcome. Furthermore, an elevated serum tryptase level may not indicate anaphylaxis as it has been found elevated in some infants with sudden infant syndrome without evidence of food sensitization [74]. In terms of treatment, the initial dose of 0.01 mg/kg epinephrine is empirical, and autoinjectable devices are not available for infants less that 15 kg. Signs of overdose including pulmonary edema may furthermore be difficult to detect in infants [69]. Furthermore, orally administered H1-antihistamines can lead to respiratory arrest in infants [69].

## 9.8 Biphasic Reactions

Biphasic reactions are those with recurrence of symptoms after resolution of the initial event in 1–78 hr [75]. Limited published data suggest that most late phase reactions develop within 8 hr of resolution of the initial reaction but may occur up to 72 hr later [58]. These late phase reactions are not uncommon, especially in food-induced anaphylaxis and in particular nut- and seafood-induced anaphylaxis. They have been reported in 3–20% of anaphylactic reactions in adult and mixed age populations to both oral and parenteral agents [75]. In one pediatric population, the incidence of biphasic reactions has been lower (6%) [26]. Foods responsible were fish and nuts. In our series of food-induced anaphylaxis provoked during in-patient oral food challenges, the incidence of biphasic reactions was even lower, 2% of anaphylactic reactions, and occurred to milk [31, 65]. The severity of the late-phase symptoms is highly variable and could be either less or more severe than the initial reaction [58].

There are no distinguishing signs or symptoms that would allow one to predict whether or not a biphasic response might occur. Tole and Lieberman [75] have extrapolated information from previous studies to identify risk factors for a biphasic response, which included: food- (or other orally administered antigen) allergen induced allergic reaction, delayed onset of initial symptoms after antigen exposure (>30 min), prior β-blockade, a delay in the administration of epinephrine, an inadequate amount of epinephrine given for the first response, or the requirement of larger doses of epinephrine. Failure to administer corticosteroids seemed to predispose to a biphasic response, although data are controversial. A report from Hong Kong noted that respiratory features were less common in those reactions that had a biphasic pattern [25].

The mechanisms of biphasic reactions are largely unknown [45]. It has been suggested that biphasic reactions may be due to insufficient treatment of the initial symptoms leading to only temporary amelioration of the reaction, cytokine-mediated influx of inflammatory cells and mediators into tissues, waves of absorption of orally administered antigens and delayed basophil degranulation [58]. Whereas undertreatment of the initial symptoms may explain late phase reactions occurring within hours of the initial reaction, it seem unlikely to be related to those occurring many hours or even days after the initial anaphylactic response [45]. Histologic findings in patients with fatal anaphylactic reactions have not identified inflammatory cells, except for eosinophils, in post-mortem specimens from patients suffering fatal biphasic anaphylactic reactions [58] and therefore do not support the cytokine-mediated influx of inflammatory cells. Delayed absorption of orally administered antigens could theoretically cause waves of mast cell degranulation leading to late phase responses, although human late phase respiratory responses are basophil-generated [45]. Delayed absorption would naturally not explain biphasic reactions induced by parenterally administered antigens, suggesting alternate pathogenic mechanisms [58].

## 9.9 Fatal Food-Induced Anaphylaxis

The rate of fatal anaphylaxis due to foods, although rare but probably underreported, is unknown [76]. The risk of a fatal outcome from food-induced anaphylaxis has been estimated to be less than 1 per million population per year [76] or less than 1 per 20 million population per year in children [77]. In other series using data from fatality registries, the rate of a fatal outcome despite prompt treatment with epinephrine has been estimated at 7–10% [21, 78]. In the United Kingdom, food allergens were responsible for up to 30% of fatal cases of anaphylaxis [79], but a more recent study from Australia identified foods responsible for only 6% of anaphylactic fatalities, with all food-induced anaphylactic fatalities occurring between 8 and 35 yr of age [18].

Fatal and near-fatal reactions due to foods occur within 30 min of ingesting the triggering food allergen [59, 62]. In contrast, median time intervals for fatal anaphylaxis to medications and insect venom are shorter, ranging from 5 to 15 min.

Unfortunately, most life-threatening/fatal anaphylaxis is unpredictable. The most common risk factors are asthma (any severity, but possibly more so when asthma is poorly controlled), failure to identify a known food allergen in the meal and previous allergic reactions to the food in question [11, 21, 59, 79, 80]. The majority of fatal food-induced anaphylactic reactions are associated with peanut and tree nuts, with seafood, milk, and egg accounting for the rest [21, 79] (Table 9.3). Adolescents and young adults are the peak age group identified in fatality registries [21, 22, 79]. Lack of timely treatment with epinephrine is a universal risk factor for a fatal food-induced anaphylaxis [21, 59, 79, 80], although fatalities have occurred also after timely administration of epinephrine [79]. Between 70% and 90% did not have epinephrine available at the time of the reaction [21, 22]. Although previous life-threatening or severe reaction after an ingestion of a small amount of the allergen is also associated with an increased risk of fatal anaphylaxis in the future, severe reactions are usually associated with exposure to larger doses of the allergen [76].

Rapid onset and reaction progression are associated with more severe reactions [76]. First reactions to foods commonly occur at home, but the following ones often happen outside home. In one series, one-third of cases occurred at home, 25% in restaurants and 15% at school or work. Commercial catering accounted for 68% of nut reactions [79].

**Table 9.3** Foods implicated in fatal or near-fatal food-induced anaphylaxis

| Authors | Population | No of subjects | Country | Most common foods |
|---|---|---|---|---|
| Bock et al. [22] | Mixed age | 31 | USA | Peanut 55%, tree nut 26%, milk 13%, shrimp 6% |
| Pumphrey et al. [78] | Mixed age | 48 | UK | Peanut 19%, nuts 9%, milk 13% |
| Moneret-Vautrin et al. [68] | Mixed age | 2 | France | Peanut 50%, soy 50% |
| Pumphrey et al. [79] | Mixed age | 6 | UK | Peanut 16%, tree nut 35%, milk 8%, fish 3%, shellfish 3% |
| Bock et al. [21] | Mixed age | 53 | USA | Peanut 36%, tree nut 15%, nut[a] 4%, milk 2%, fish 2% |
| Pumphrey et al. [145] | Mixed age | 37 | UK | Peanut 27%, tree nut 14%, nut 27%, seafood 8%, milk 5% |
| Colver et al. [11] | Children | 3 | UK, Ireland | Milk 67%, peanut 33% |
| Sampson et al. [59] | Children | 13 | USA | Peanut 30%, nuts 46%, eggs 8%, milk 15% |

[a]Unclear whether it was peanut or tree nut

The time interval from the ingestion of the food allergen to demise has been reported to be approximately 25–35 min (range: 10 min–6 hr) [79]. Fatal food reactions are more commonly associated with bronchospasm, respiratory symptoms, and asphyxia, which is in contrast to insect sting or medication reactions that present with shock. Interestingly, lack of cutaneous symptoms may be risk factor for fatal anaphylaxis [59]. A movement to an upright position with reduced venous return is associated with fatalities in cases of food-induced anaphylactic shock, and therefore keeping a supine position during treatment of an anaphylactic reaction is encouraged [62] unless prevented by profuse vomiting.

## 9.10 Treatment of a Food-Induced Anaphylactic Reaction

Pharmacologic treatment of anaphylaxis is reviewed elsewhere in this book (Chapter 18). The principles of treatment for food-induced anaphylaxis are same as for other types of anaphylaxis. While H1-antihistamine may relieve skin symptoms and rhinorrhea, the mainstay of treatment of any anaphylactic reaction is the timely administration of epinephrine. A rapidly absorbed H1 antihistamine is preferable. The time to peak plasma level after single oral dose is 1.0 +/− 0.5 hr for cetirizine and 1.7 +/−1 hr for diphenhydramine [81]. In most series of fatal anaphylaxis, epinephrine administration was delayed for the majority of patients and may have contributed to the fatal outcome [58]. Therapies directed toward slowing or preventing further absorption of food protein from the gastrointestinal tract after accidental ingestion have not been a routine part of management. It has been shown that activated charcoal forms complexes with peanut protein, effectively competing for binding with peanut-specific IgG in an in vitro assay [81]. While removal of the ingested food or binding with an activated charcoal to prevent intestinal absorption is logical, the practical application of such approaches is limited by the potential serious side effect of induced emesis or gastric lavage-aspiration. Administration of activated charcoal by oral route is extremely difficult due to poor palatability and frequent induction of emesis (authors' own unpublished experience).

Food-induced anaphylaxis may require more than one dose of epinephrine in 10–19% of anaphylactic reactions in mixed and pediatric populations [23, 31, 82]. In a retrospective survey of self-reported anaphylaxis in children with food allergies, the second dose of epinephrine was administered by health care professional in 94% of reactions, with favorable outcomes. The children requiring epinephrine were significantly older than those not treated with epinephrine [31]. Milk, egg and peanut were responsible for the majority of reactions and asthma found more often in those reactions treated with multiple doses of epinephrine [31]. The need for multiple doses of epinephrine did not appear to be associated with a delay in administration of epinephrine. Increased symptom severity has also been associated with the need for multiple doses [83]. Corticosteroids are often given to patients with anaphylaxis although their role in anaphylaxis has not been determined. Certainly corticosteroids are not effective in treating the acute reaction given their onset of action of several hours, but they are given with the goal of preventing or ameliorating a late phase reaction. Bronchodilators can also be given to help reverse bronchoconstriction (see Chapter 18).

## 9.11 Diagnosis of Food-Induced Anaphylaxis

Making a diagnosis of anaphylaxis, and in particular food-induced anaphylaxis, can be difficult at times for a variety of reasons; this is especially true if there is no known history of food allergy. Of note, a large percentage of patients experiencing food-induced anaphylaxis report a positive history of food allergy [84]. However, most patients are unaware that the foods they are eating and that trigger the anaphylactic reaction contain the known allergen due to the hidden, undeclared food ingredient or due to unintentional cross-contact with food allergen during food processing or serving.

The diagnosis of food-induced anaphylaxis is often over-looked because of the absence of cutaneous manifestations. Up to 20% of patients, and in particular children, with food-induced anaphylaxis do not have cutaneous involvement, making the diagnosis considerably less obvious [84]. The diagnosis can also be difficult to make because of transience of symptoms due to endogenous production of cathecholamines or pre-hospital administration of medications such as anti-histamines or epinephrine.

There have been immense research efforts to identify reliable laboratory markers to aid in the diagnosis of anaphylaxis. Currently, total tryptase level is most commonly measured to establish a diagnosis of anaphylaxis. Tryptase levels increase immediately, peak at 1–2 hr after the onset of anaphylaxis and return to baseline 24 hr after complete resolution of symptoms. Levels are ideally obtained within 3 hours of onset of symptoms and serial measurements may help establish a diagnosis of anaphylaxis [38]. In 19 cases of fatal anaphylaxis, elevated serum tryptase levels (12 ng/ml–150 μg/ml) were detected in 17 subjects, including 6 of 8 who died of food-induced anaphylaxis. Lack of tryptase elevation does not, however, rule-out the diagnosis of anaphylaxis, especially food-induced anaphylaxis. In a study by Sampson et al. [59] 4 out of 5 of patients with fatal and near-fatal food-induced anaphylaxis, in whom measurements were available, did not have detectable increases in serum tryptase. Sampson and colleagues also failed to demonstrate elevated tryptase levels in patients with symptoms of anaphylaxis undergoing food challenges even though samples were obtained in the ideal time frame [85].

There are several theories as to why tryptase levels are often not elevated in food-induced anaphylaxis [45]. First, food-induced anaphylactic reactions tend to be slower in onset, more protracted and more likely to be biphasic as compared to anaphylaxis secondary to a systemic exposure, such as insect venom or intravenous medication. This may result in a slower release of tryptase and a decreased peak. Secondly, mucosal mast cells, the major effector cells in food-induced anaphylaxis, often contain less tryptase compared to skin mast cells. Finally, basophils, which do not contain tryptase, may play a significant role in food-induced anaphylaxis.

Another laboratory marker of anaphylaxis is serum histamine. Histamine levels typically peak within 10 min of onset of symptoms and decrease to baseline by 60 min [45]. Unfortunately, this is not a clinically useful marker as the majority of patients with anaphylaxis, and in particular food-induced anaphylaxis, do not present to the emergency room in time to capture the histamine peak. However, urinary histamine metabolites remain elevated for up to 24 h after anaphylaxis and may be helpful in establishing the diagnosis.

Research efforts are under way to find alternative clinically useful markers of anaphylaxis. PAF levels have been shown increased and PAF acetylhydrolase (PAF-AH), the enzyme that inactivates PAF, levels decreased in fatal cases of peanut-induced anaphylaxis as compared with healthy controls, patients with nonfatal peanut allergic reactions and non-anaphylactic fatalities [86]. Recent studies suggest that other granule mast cell mediators such as chymase and carboxipeptidase and acid arachidonic products such as prostaglandins and leukotrienes may be potential markers of anaphylaxis [87]. Further studies are required to determine if these mast cell enzymes or urinary lipid metabolites could be useful markers for food-induced anaphylaxis.

Oral food challenges (OFCs) are the gold standard for the diagnosis of food allergy. Naturally, anaphylactic reactions can be elicited in OFCs. Reactive (i.e., failed or positive) challenges can elicit skin, respiratory, or gastrointestinal symptoms that may be severe and require medications [65, 66]. In one study, the rate of epinephrine administration in failed OFCs is 11%, with 6% of anaphylactic reactions requiring multiple doses of epinephrine [65]. Presumptive diagnoses are more often made based on a convincing clinical history of anaphylaxis within 2 h of ingestion of a particular food allergen and detection of food allergen-specific IgE by means of prick skin tests (PST) or serum allergen-specific IgE. Unfortunately, these tests are not always sensitive or highly specific. Several studies have demonstrated that less than 40% of patients with histories of food allergy have positive PSTs or detectable food-specific IgE and that less than 40% of patients with positive PSTs or food-specific IgE have OFC-proven food allergy [45]. However, in our series of anaphylactic reactions elicited during oral food challenges, food-specific IgE was detected by either PST or measurement of serum allergen-specific IgE in all but one subject [65]. Furthermore, the fact that many foods are usually consumed at the same time, may obscure identification of the triggering allergen.

## 9.12 Prevention, Education and Emergency Treatment Plan

All patients with food allergy, and especially food-induced anaphylaxis, should be educated about the signs and symptoms of anaphylaxis and the correct use of an epinephrine autoinjector together with written instructions on its proper administration and an anaphylaxis treatment plan.

Epinephrine is available in autoinjectable devices containing pre-set doses of either 0.15 mg (junior) or 0.3 mg (adult) of epinephrine per injection. The devices are designed for self-treatment or for administration by a companion, and their use is not meant to be a substitute for prompt professional treatment, but rather as a "first-aid" measure. Intramuscular injection of epinephrine into the lateral thigh (vastus lateralis) is the preferred route for therapy in first-aid treatment. On the basis of current data, it is recommended that autoinjectors with 0.15 mg of epinephrine are prescribed for otherwise healthy young children who weigh 10–25 kg (22–55 lb) and autoinjectors with 0.30 mg of epinephrine for those who weigh approximately 25 kg (55 lb) or more [88]. For children who weigh less than 10 kg (22 lb), the physician and family should weigh the risks of delay in dosing and dosing errors when an ampule/syringe/needle is used against accepting non-ideal autoinjector doses. Multiple doses of epinephrine may be needed in anaphylactic reactions resulting from foods [23, 31, 82]. It has been suggested that patients at risk for severe anaphylaxis should always carry two doses of epinephrine [89], but currently there are no consensus guidelines on when to prescribe more than one autoinjectable epinephrine device. The second dose of epinephrine should be administered if anaphylactic symptoms persist or worsen following the first dose administration. However, they are not substitute for emergency medical attention and every patient should be seen by a medical professional and observed under medical supervision for a minimum of 4 h after resolution of symptoms.

Also of the utmost importance is educating the patient regarding dietary avoidance of the food allergen(s) known to cause allergic reaction/anaphylaxis. This includes careful reading of package labels and advisory labeling and asking questions regarding the food to be consumed. The Food Allergen and Consumer Protection Plan (FALCPA) since 2006 requires that package labels identify any of the eight major allergens (peanut, tree nuts, milk, egg, soy, wheat, fish, and crustaceans) in plain English. Precautionary labeling ("may contain," "manufactured on shared equipment/facility with") is not regulated, but indicates the potential for cross-contamination and in general identifies foods that should be avoided by patients with history of anaphylaxis. Patients should be educated about the potential for severe reactions even in the absence of previous severe reactions, although it is not shown that each subsequent reaction would necessarily be more severe than the preceding one. Effective care also requires a comprehensive management approach involving schools, camps, and other youth organizations and education of supervising adults with regard to recognition and treatment of anaphylaxis. A medical identification bracelet or necklace is also recommended. The anticipation of unforeseen accidental exposures together with the knowledge of potential fatal outcome of an anaphylactic reaction have significant bearing on the quality of life in individuals with food allergies and their families [90].

## 9.13 Natural History

The resolution of food allergy is variable and depends on the specific food allergen. Of children with cow's milk allergy, 19% will become tolerant by age 4 year, 42% by age 8 year, 64% by age 12 year, and 79% by 16 year [91]. Resolution of egg allergy occurs in 4% by age 4 year, 12% by age 6 year, 37% by age 10 year, and 68% by age 16 year [92]. For wheat, the rates of resolution were 29% by 4 year, 56% by 8 year, and 65% by 12 year [93]. In contrast, only 20% of children with peanut allergy and 9% with tree nut allergy will develop tolerance [94, 95]. Recurrence of food allergy is very uncommon; to the best of our knowledge it has been reported in about 8% of peanut allergic individuals [96].

Currently, there are no reliable predictors to determine when and in whom resolution of allergy will occur, hence, periodic follow-up with measurement of serum specific IgE levels and prick skin testing can help determine when oral food challenges would be appropriate utilizing the 95% predictive food-specific IgE levels. For milk, egg, and wheat allergy, the highest specific-IgE level for each patient was found to be highly predictive of outcome. Children with cow's milk-, egg white-, or wheat-specifc IgE antibody level greater than 50 $kU_A/L$ generally had persistent allergy. It should be noted that many children outgrew wheat allergy with even the highest levels of wheat IgE [91–93]. Coexisting asthma and allergic rhinitis were also significant associated with persistence of milk allergy into teenage years. Predictors of outcome for milk allergy [91] and presence of other atopic disease, and presence of other food allergy were significantly related to egg allergy persistence [92]. History of anaphylaxis was not identified as a risk factor for persistence of food allergy.

It has been demonstrated that patients with persistent egg and milk allergy recognize a greater number of sequential (linear) egg-protein epitopes as compared with patients who had developed clinical tolerance to egg ("outgrown" their egg allergy) [97, 98]. Microarray technology utilizing the presence of such epitope-specific IgE could be applied could be used to identify those patients who will likely develop clinical tolerance versus those patients with persistent allergy.

## 9.14 Future Therapies

Currently the only treatment for food-induced anaphylaxis is strict dietary avoidance. Development of therapies to prevent food-induced anaphylaxis is a vigorous research area. Promising therapies under investigation are both allergen-specific and nonspecific. Nonspecific therapies for food-induced anaphylaxis under investigation include anti-IgE, which increased the threshold dose for peanut in peanut-allergic individuals [99] and Chinese herbal medications, which have been shown to prevent peanut anaphylaxis in an animal model, for which human studies are under way [100]. Allergen-specific therapies include oral, sublingual, and cutaneous immunotherapy (desensitization), mutated recombinant proteins, which are deficient their IgE-binding activity, coadministered with heat-killed *E. coli* to generate maximum immune response, which is under way, and peptide immunotherapy [101].

### *9.14.1 Non-Allergen-Specific Therapy*

#### 9.14.1.1 Humanized Monoclonal Anti-IgE

Humanized monoclonal anti-IgE antibodies bind to the constant region (third domain of the Fc region) of IgE molecules and prevent the IgE from binding to receptors ($Fc_\varepsilon$ RI and $Fc_\varepsilon$ RII).

Anti-IgE cannot interact with IgE molecules when they are bound to the IgE receptor and is less likely to induce mast cell or basophil degranulation by cross-linking IgE. Anti-IgE also downregulates the expression of $Fc_{\varepsilon}$ RI receptor on mast cells and decreases basophil histamine release [102]. A multi-center randomized trial evaluated humanized monoclonal anti-IgE mouse $IgG_1$ antibody (TNX-901) in 84 patients with a history of immediate hypersensitivity to peanut [99]. Peanut hypersensitivity was confirmed and the threshold dose of peanut protein established by a double-blind placebo-controlled food challenge at screening. Subjects were randomly assigned to receive either humanized monoclonal antibody TNX-901 (150, 300, or 450 mg) or placebo subcutaneously every 4 week for 4 doses. They underwent a second oral peanut challenge within two to four weeks after the fourth dose.

The mean baseline sensitivity threshold increased in all groups, with an apparent dose response, but was statistically significant only in the 450 mg group. In this group, the sensitivity threshold increased from a level equal to approximately half a peanut (178 mg) to one equal to almost nine peanuts (2,805 mg). However, approximately 25% of subjects treated even with the highest dose of TNX-901, were not protected. A controlled trial of different anti-IgE humanized $IgG_1$ antibody (omalizumab) in children older than 6 year with peanut anaphylaxis was discontinued prematurely because of safety issues related to anaphylactic reactions. Further studies are currently on hold as alternative study designs are considered.

Combined treatment with anti-IgE and specific food allergen immunotherapy is also a consideration because of the potential of anti-IgE to decrease life-threatening side effects of allergen immunotherapy. Evaluation of combination therapy has begun with environmental allergens, but has not yet been assessed for food allergens [103].

#### 9.14.1.2 Traditional Chinese Medicine (TCM)

Traditional Chinese medicine (TCM) has been used in Asia for centuries and is reported to be effective, safe, and affordable. The mechanism of action of TCM is largely unknown and it has not been evaluated in randomized clinical trials. Xiu-Min Li and colleagues have conducted most of the work that provided insight into the mechanism of TCM in food allergy. Food allergy herbal formula-1 (FAHF-1, a mixture of 11 herbs), was tested in a mouse model of peanut allergy [104]. FAHF-1 abolished peanut-induced anaphylaxis, reduced mast cell degranulation and histamine release. Peanut-specific serum IgE levels significantly decreased by 2 week of treatment, and remained lower four weeks following discontinuation of treatment. FAHF-1 reduced peanut-induced lymphocyte proliferation as well as IL-4, IL-5, and IL-13 production, but not IFN-γ synthesis. FAHF-1 had no toxic effects on liver or kidneys.

A modified formula, FAHF-2, containing nine herbs completely blocked anaphylaxis to peanut challenge up to five weeks following therapy [100]. This therapeutic effect was in large part mediated by interferon-γ producing CD8+ T cells [105, 106]. Examination of the individual herbs revealed that each had some effect, but none offered equivalent protection from anaphylaxis compared with FAHF-2 [107]. Safety studies in humans are currently under way.

### *9.14.2 Allergen-Specific Immunotherapy*

#### 9.14.2.1 Subcutaneous Peanut Immunotherapy

The evidence that immunotherapy may induce tolerance to a food allergen was provided by two controlled studies that evaluated subcutaneous immunotherapy with peanut extract. In the initial study, three treated subjects displayed a 67–100% decrease in symptoms during double-blind, placebo-controlled food challenge, and had a 2- to 5-log reduction in end-point skin prick skin test reactivity to peanut [108]. One placebo-treated subject completed the study and had no change in DBPCFC symptoms or skin prick test sensitivity to peanut. In a follow up study of 12 subjects, 6 were treated with a maintenance dose of 0.5 ml of 1:100 wt/vol peanut extract [109]. All treated subjects experienced increased tolerance to peanut oral food challenge and decreased sensitivity on titrated peanut skin prick test, whereas controls experienced no changes. However, anaphylaxis with respiratory involvement occurred a mean of 7.7 times during 12 months, with an average of 9.8 epinephrine injections per study subject. Only three subjects achieved the intended maintenance dose due to adverse events. This important study demonstrated that injected food allergen could be successfully used to induce tolerance but clinical application was limited by safety concerns.

#### 9.14.2.2 Oral Immunotherapy

A successful oral immunotherapy was first reported in the early twentieth century in a boy with anaphylactic allergy to egg [110]. Currently, oral immunotherapy (OIT) to food is a focus of many ongoing studies. As food allergy most likely results from the failure of development or the breakdown of normal oral tolerance, the oral route of administration is a logical choice for food allergens because it involves cells and immune pathways involved in induction of oral tolerance. Animal studies suggest that high-dose feeding of an antigen results in anergy or deletion of antigen-specific T lymphocytes, whereas continuous low dose ingestion may induce protective suppressive responses from regulatory T cells [111, 112]. In contrast, intermittent feedings or non-oral exposures (e.g., cutaneous) may induce sensitization and allergy [113]. A distinction should be made between approaches that induce "desensitization," where the allergen is ingested without symptoms during treatment but maintenance requires daily, uninterrupted ingestion. Possible mechanisms of oral desensitization include increased food-specific IgG and decreased food-specific IgE antibodies, and decreased activation of mast cells and basophils. When oral tolerance is accomplished, the food may be ingested without allergy symptoms despite periods of abstinence. The mechanism of persistent tolerance likely involves development of regulatory T cells and immunologic deviation away from Th2 response.

During OIT, food is mixed in a vehicle and ingested in gradually increasing doses. The dose escalation occurs in a controlled setting; regular ingestion of a maximal tolerated dose occurs at home. Early reports were limited to case series and uncontrolled trials; nevertheless they provided evidence that at least a subset of food allergic subjects could be "desensitized" to a variety of foods, including milk, egg, fish, fruit, peanut, and celery [114–120]. These studies did not distinguish the effects of oral desensitization versus the natural resolution of food allergy and did not evaluate the permanency of the desensitized state. In some subjects who ultimately tolerated a maintenance dose, even for a significant period of time, allergic symptoms re-developed if the food was not ingested on a regular basis, highlighting a concern that permanent tolerance was not achieved [121]. In the first randomized trial of OIT, children with challenge proven IgE-mediated cow's milk (CM) allergy or hen's egg (HE) allergy were randomly assigned to OIT or elimination diet as a control group. OIT treatment was performed at home on a daily basis according to a study protocol with fresh CM or lyophilized HE protein. Children were re-evaluated by food challenge after a median of 21 months. Children in the OIT group received a secondary elimination diet for 2 months prior to follow-up challenge to evaluate persistence of induced oral tolerance. At follow-up challenge, nine of 25 children (36%) showed permanent tolerance in the OIT group, three of 25 (12%) were tolerant with regular intake and four of 25 (16%) were partial responders. In the control group, seven of 20 children (35%) were tolerant. Allergen-specific immunoglobulin E decreased significantly both in children who developed natural tolerance during the elimination diet ($P<0.05$) and in those with OIT ($P < 0.001$). Although the rate of permanent tolerance was not different between the groups, some children were tolerant with regular intake and some were tolerant to smaller maintenance dose and were protected from inadvertent exposures as they continued to ingest the daily dose of the food in question.

In the first randomized and placebo-controlled trial of OIT, 20 children with IgE-mediated milk allergy were randomized to milk or placebo OIT (2:1 ratio) [122]. Dosing included three phases: the build-up day (initial dose, 0.4 mg of milk protein; final dose, 50 mg), daily doses with 8 weekly in-office dose increases to a maximum of 500 mg, and continued daily maintenance doses for 3–4 months. Double-blind, placebo-controlled food challenges; end-point titration skin prick tests; and milk protein serologic studies were performed before and after OIT. Nineteen patients, 6–17 year of age, completed treatment: 12 in the active group and 7 in the placebo group. The median milk threshold dose in both groups was 40 mg at the baseline challenge. After OIT, the median cumulative dose inducing a reaction in the active treatment group was 5,140 mg (range 2,540–8,140 mg), whereas all patients in the placebo group reacted at 40 mg ($P = .0003$). Among 2,437 active OIT doses versus 1,193 placebo doses, there were 1,107 (45.4%) versus 134 (11.2%) total reactions, with local symptoms being most common. Milk-specific IgE levels did not change significantly in either group. Milk-Specific IgG levels increased significantly in the active treatment group, with a predominant milk-specific $IgG_4$ level increase.

Longo and colleagues recently assessed the safety and efficacy of OIT for children with severe cow's milk protein-induced anaphylaxis [123]. Sixty children with history of a severe milk-induced anaphylaxis reacted to very small amounts of milk during an oral milk challenge and were randomly divided in two groups. Thirty children began OIT with 10-day rush phase including 3–10 daily doses up to 20 ml of undiluted milk in the hospital and a slow dose escalation phase at home (increasing by 1 ml every second day). The remaining 30 continued on a milk-free diet and were followed for 1 year. Adverse reactions were common in both groups but no child had severe anaphylaxis. During the rush phase, intramuscular epinephrine was administered 4 times in 4 children. During the home phase, 2 children required treatment including epinephrine in the emergency department. Another study explored rush OIT in 9 children with persistent milk allergy [124]. Six children reached the maximum dose of 120 ml cow's milk within 3–7 days; all of them experienced mild side effects that were not treated with epinephrine or steroids. A smaller study confirmed that OIT can be successfully used to induce tolerance to increased doses of peanut in subjects with severe peanut allergy [125].

### Mechanism of OIT

A recent study provided more insight into the mechanism of OIT [126]. Of the 29 children with peanut allergy who completed the protocol, 27 ingested 3.9 g peanut protein during the final food challenge. Most symptoms noted during OIT resolved spontaneously or with antihistamines. By 6 months, titrated skin prick tests and activation of basophils decreased significantly. Peanut-specific IgE decreased by 12–18 months whereas $IgG_4$ increased significantly. Serum factors inhibited IgE-peanut complex formation in an IgE-facilitated allergen binding assay. Secretion of IL-10, IL-5, IFN-γ, and TNF-α from peripheral blood mononuclear cells increased over a period of 6–12 months. Peanut-specific forkhead box protein-3 (Fox P3)-positive T cells increased until 12 months and decreased thereafter. In addition, T-cell microarrays showed down-regulation of genes in apoptotic pathways.

### Safety of OIT Home Dosing

Among the children who participated in a trial of peanut OIT, 20 completed all phases of the study [127]. During the initial escalation, the risk of mild wheezing was 18%. The probability of having any symptoms after a build-up phase dose was 46%, with a risk of 29% for upper respiratory tract and 24% for skin symptoms. The risk of reaction with any home dose was 3.5%; upper respiratory tract (1.2%) and skin (1.1%) symptoms being most common. Treatment was given for 0.7% of home doses. Two subjects received epinephrine after 1 home dose each. Allergic reactions during home dosing were more common in the open-label maintenance after milk OIT, from 2.55% to 96.4% of doses per subject in the first 3 months compared with 0–79.8% in the subsequent 3 months [128]. Local and multisystem reactions whereas all other reactions remained unchanged. Several systemic reactions occurred at previously tolerated doses in the setting of exercise or viral illness. As highlighted by a recent paper from Wesley Burks' group, the risk of an allergic reaction to a previously tolerated dose of food is associated with physical exertion after dosing, dosing on empty stomach, dosing during menses, concurrent febrile illness, and sub-optimally controlled asthma [124, 128–130].

#### 9.14.2.3 Sublingual Immunotherapy

Another approach to reduce hypersensitivity or induce tolerance is sublingual immunotherapy (SLIT) with food. An initial case report described modified SLIT with fresh kiwi pulp extract in a 29-yr-old woman with history of kiwi anaphylaxis [131]. The extract or kiwi cube was kept under the tongue for 1 min before swallowing (e.g., combined SLIT and oral therapy). There was a diminished IgE-reactivity to the major kiwi allergen, Act c 1 (30 kD), in western blots with kiwi extract. Five years into kiwi modified SLIT, treatment was interrupted for 4 months and then resumed without any problems [132].

Subsequently, a randomized, double-blind, placebo-controlled trial of SLIT for treatment of hazelnut allergy was conducted [133]. Adults with hazelnut allergy (54.5% with history of oral allergy symptoms), confirmed by double-blind placebo-controlled food challenge (DBPCFC), were randomly assigned to two groups, hazelnut immunotherapy ($n=12$) or placebo ($n=11$). Subjects kept the hazelnut extract solution in the mouth for at least 3 min and then discharged. All subjects receiving hazelnut immunotherapy reached the planned maximum dose with a 4 day rush protocol, followed by a daily maintenance dose (containing 188.2 μg of Cor a 1 and 121.9 μg of Cor a 8, major hazelnut allergens). Systemic reactions were observed in 0.2% of the total doses administered, were limited to the rush build up phase and were treated successfully with oral antihistamines. Local reactions, mainly in the form of immediate oral itching, were observed in 7.4% (109 reactions/1,466 doses). Four patients in the active group reported abdominal pain several hours after dosing on one occasion each and only during the build-up phase. All local reactions during the maintenance phase were limited to oral itching and only occurred in one patient. After 5 months of SLIT, the mean threshold dose of ingested hazelnut provoking allergic symptoms increased from 2.3 to 11.6 g in active group ($P=0.02$) versus 3.5–4.1 g in placebo (NS). Almost 50% of treated subjects tolerated the highest dose (20 g) of hazelnut during follow-up DBPCFC, compared to 9% in the placebo group. Levels of serum hazelnut-specific $IgG_4$ antibody and total serum IL-10 increased only in the active group, but there were no differences in hazelnut-specific IgE antibody levels pre- and post-immunotherapy.

Another study evaluated SLIT in eight children with cow's milk allergy [134]. A day after an initial positive milk food challenge, children started SLIT with 0.1 ml of milk for the first 2 week, increasing by 0.1 ml every 15 days until 1 ml/day was given. Milk was kept in the mouth for 2 min and then discharged. Seven subjects completed the protocol, one subject withdrew due to oral symptoms. After 6 months of treatment, the provocative dose of milk increased from a mean of 39 ml at baseline to 143 ml ($P<0.01$). Recently, a randomized double-blind placebo-controlled trial of sublingual OIT with a Pru p 3 (major peach allergen) quantified peach extract was reported. After 6 months of SLIT, the active group tolerated a significantly higher amount of peach, had significantly decreased skin prick test and significantly increased Pru p 3-specific IgE and $IgG_4$. In contrast, no significant changes were observed in the placebo group [135].

These preliminary data on OIT and SLIT are encouraging, especially with regard to safety. However, additional studies must address multiple factors including optimal dose, ideal duration of immunotherapy, degree of protection, efficacy for different ages, severity and type of food allergy responsive to treatment and need for patient protection during home administration. In view of the recent reports of the reactions to the tolerated doses of OIT at home, it may be necessary to hold doses during acute febrile illness, avoid exercise within two hours following dosing, and take daily OIT dose with meal or snack [128]. Rhinitis and asthma should be maintained under optimal control.

#### 9.14.2.4 Immunotherapy with Recombinant Engineered Food Proteins

Point mutations introduced by site-directed mutagenesis in the known IgE-binding epitopes of major food allergens and polymerization result in decreased IgE activation during immunotherapy. In vivo efficacy of the engineered recombinant peanut proteins was tested in the mouse model of peanut anaphylaxis [136, 137]. Mice were sensitized to whole peanut and then desensitized by intranasal administration of engineered recombinant Ara h 2 (three doses a wk for 4 week). Desensitization with the engineered recombinant Ara h 2 protein suppressed synthesis of Ara h 2-specific IgE and resulted in significantly decreased severity of anaphylactic reactions following oral peanut challenge compared to a control group. Modified food allergens may be combined with bacterial adjuvants to further reduce specific IgE production. Initially, heat-killed *Listeria moncytogenes* (HKLM) combined with engineered peanut allergens (mAra a 1–3) has been tested [138]. Peanut-allergic C3H/HeJ mice were treated subcutaneously 10 week following sensitization with a mixture of the recombinant, modified major peanut allergens and HKLM [modified (m)Ara h 1–3 plus HKLM]. All mice in the sham-treated group developed anaphylactic symptoms, whereas only 31% of mice in the mAra h 1–3 plus HKLM group developed mild anaphylaxis on a post-treatment oral peanut challenge. This protective effect was more potent than in the mAra h 1–3 protein alone-treated group. Though the approach of injecting heat-killed bacteria with modified proteins was effective, safety concerns about using potentially pathogenic bacteria in humans were raised. Therefore, in subsequent studies, a nonpathogenic strain of *Escherichia coli* was used as an adjuvant. In addition, considering potential complications from the subcutaneous route of administration in humans, rectal route of delivery was tested. It was assumed that rectal delivery would provide superior safety regarding possible infectious complications as well as limit severe adverse reactions because nonpathogenic *E. coli* bacteria reside in the colon. Peanut-allergic C3H/HeJ mice received 0.9 (low dose), 9 (medium dose), or 90 (high dose) μg of heat killed *E. coli* expressing modified proteins Ara h 1–3 (HKE-MP123) per rectum, HKE-containing vector (HKE-V) alone, or vehicle alone (sham) weekly for 3 week [139]. Mice were challenged with peanut 2 week later. Second and third peanut challenges were performed at 4-week intervals. After the first peanut challenge, all 3 HKE-MP123 and HKE-V-treated groups had reduced severity of anaphylaxis ($P<0.01$, 0.01, 0.05, 0.05, respectively) compared with the sham-treated group. However, only the medium- and high-dose HKE-MP123-treated mice remained protected for up to 10 week after treatment. Peanut specific-IgE levels were significantly lower in all HKE-MP123-treated groups ($P<0.001$); they were most reduced in the high-dose HKE-MP123-treated group at the time of each challenge. Peanut-stimulated splenocytes from the high-dose HKE-MP123-treated mice produced in vitro significantly less IL-4, IL-13, IL-5 and IL-10 ($P<0.01$, 0.001, 0.001, and 0.001, respectively). IFN-γ and TGF-β production was significantly increased ($P<0.001$ and 0.01, respectively) compared with sham-treated mice at the time of the last challenge. Phase I clinical safety and efficacy studies are currently enrolling adult subjects with peanut allergy.

#### 9.14.2.5 Other Approaches

Three additional immunomodulatory approaches to peanut allergy were evaluated in the animal studies but subsequently were abandoned in favor of other treatments. In peptide immunotherapy, the vaccine consists of overlapping peptides (10–20-amino acid long) that represent the entire sequence of a specific protein. The antigen presenting cells are provided with all possible T-cell epitopes, but mast cells are not activated because the short peptides are unable to cross-link two IgE molecules. Pre-treatment with two doses of the major peanut protein Ara h2 peptide mixture prior to peanut challenge has been shown to prevent anaphylactic reactions in peanut sensitized mice [139, 140]. Although peptide immunotherapy allows for formulation of vaccines against any food in which major allergenic proteins are known because IgE binding sites for each food protein do not have to be mapped, allergen-specific DNA does not need to be mutated, and engineered recombinant proteins are not required, the cost of generating the peptides is significant. Perhaps peptide immunotherapy will be revisited when the most relevant peptides are identified.

Immunization with bacterial plasmid DNA (pDNA) that encodes specific antigens can induce prolonged humoral and cellular immune TH 1 responses, attributable to immunostimulatory sequences (ISSs) consisting of un-methylated cytosine and guanine motifs (CpG motifs) in the pDNA backbone. An early study found that the intramuscular immunization of naïve AKR/J (H-$2^K$) and C3H/HeJ (H-$2^K$) mice with pDNA ecoding Ara h 2 prior to intraperitoneal peanut sensitization had some protective effect in AKR/J mice, but induced anaphylactic reactions in C3H/HeN mice upon peanut challenge [141]. In another study, oral chitosan embedded Ara h 2 had a protective effect in AKR mice [142]. Xiu-Min Li at Mount Sinai School of Medicine, New York (Li et al., unpublished data), tested therapeutic effect of pDNA-expressing Ara H 2 in peanut-allergic mice and found no reduction in peanut-specific IgE antibody levels. Taken together, these data indicate that pDNA-based immunotherapy may not be effective in reversing IgE-mediated hypersensitivity.

A different approach to DNA-based immunotherapy is based on the synthetic immunostimulatory oligodeoxynucleotides containing unmethylated CpG motifs (ISS). ISS-conjugated allergen administration was more effective than a mixture of antigen and ISS in the suppression of allergic airway responses probably due to the enhanced dendritic cell uptake of ISS-allergen. Li et al. investigated the use of ISS-conjugated-Ara h 2 (ISS-Ara h 2) in the peanut-allergic mice. C3H/HeJ mice were immunized intradermally with ISS-linked Ara h 2, or ISS-linked Amb a 1 (ISS-Amb a 1) as a control [143]. Four weeks after immunization, mice were intragastrically sensitized with peanut and then challenged with Ara h 25 week later. ISS-Ara h 2 treated mice did not develop symptoms and had significantly lower plasma histamine levels following oral challenge compared to ISS-Amb a 1-treated mice that became symptomatic. Nguyen et al. [144] found that intradermal immunization with a mixture of ISS and β-galactosidase (β-gal), but not with ISS alone or β-gal alone, provided protection against fatal anaphylaxis induced by intraperitoneal β–gal sensitization and challenge that was associated with an increase in IgG2a/IFN-γ and a reduction in IgE/IL-4, IL-5 patterns. This effect was comparable to immunization with the pDNA-encoding β-gal. Therefore, antigen-ISS immunization may have a prophylactic effect against food allergy, however, the ability to reverse established food allergy remains to be determined.

## 9.15 Conclusion

Food-induced anaphylaxis is an increasingly prevalent problem in westernized countries. As our understanding of the pathophysiology of food anaphylaxis increases, so does our ability to identify therapies which may aid not only in the diagnosis of, but also the treatment and prevention of, food-induced anaphylaxis.

# References

1. Sampson HA, Munoz-Furlong A, Campbell RL, et al. Second symposium on the definition and management of anaphylaxis: summary report – second national institute of allergy and infectious disease/food allergy and anaphylaxis network symposium. *J Allergy Clin Immunol.* 2006;117:391–397.
2. Sicherer SH, Sampson HA. Food allergy. *J Allergy Clin Immunol.* 2006;117:S470–S475.
3. Keet CA, Wood RA. Food allergy and anaphylaxis. *Immunol Allergy Clin North Am.* 2007;27:193–212, vi.
4. Branum AM, Lukacs SL. Food allergy among children in the United States. *Pediatrics.* 2009;124:1549–1555.
5. Grundy J, Matthews S, Bateman B, Dean T, Arshad SH. Rising prevalence of allergy to peanut in children: data from 2 sequential cohorts. *J Allergy Clin Immunol.* 2002;110:784–789.
6. Sicherer SH, Munoz-Furlong A, Sampson HA. Prevalence of peanut and tree nut allergy in the United States determined by means of a random digit dial telephone survey: a 5-year follow-up study. *J Allergy Clin Immunol.* 2003;112:1203–1207.
7. Kagan RS, Joseph L, Dufresne C, et al. Prevalence of peanut allergy in primary-school children in Montreal, Canada. *J Allergy Clin Immunol.* 2003;112:1223–1228.
8. Mullins RJ, Dear KB, Tang ML. Characteristics of childhood peanut allergy in the Australian capital territory, 1995 to 2007. *J Allergy Clin Immunol.* 2009;123:689–693.
9. Downs SH, Marks GB, Sporik R, Belosouva EG, Car NG, Peat JK. Continued increase in the prevalence of asthma and atopy. *Arch Dis Child.* 2001;84:20–23.
10. Simons FER, Chad ZH, Gold M. Anaphylaxis in children: real-time reporting from a national network. *Allergy Clin Immunol Int-J World Allergy Org.* 2004:242–244.
11. Colver AF, Nevantaus H, Macdougall CF, Cant AJ. Severe food-allergic reactions in children across the UK and Ireland, 1998–2000. *Acta Paediatr.* 2005;94:689–695.
12. Yocum MW, Butterfield JH, Klein JS, Volcheck GW, Schroeder DR, Silverstein MD. Epidemiology of anaphylaxis in Olmested County: a population-based study. *J Allergy Clin Immunol.* 1999;104:452–456.
13. Decker WW, Campbell RL, Manivannan V, et al. The etiology and incidence of anaphylaxis in Rochester, Minnesota: a report from the Rochester Epidemiology Project. *J Allergy Clin Immunol.* 2008;122:1161–1165.
14. Gupta R, Sheikh A, Strachan DP, Anderson HR. Time trends in allergic disorders in the UK. *Thorax.* 2007;62:91–96.
15. Sheikh A, Alves B. Hospital admissions for acute anaphylaxis: time trend study. *Br Med J.* 2000;320:1441.
16. Lin RY, Anderson AS, Shah SN, Nurruzzaman F. Increasing anaphylaxis hospitalizations in the first 2 decades of life: New York state, 1990–2006. *Ann Allergy Asthma Immunol.* 2008;101:387–393.
17. Sampson HA. Anaphylaxis and emergency treatment. *Pediatrics.* 2003;111:1601–1608.
18. Liew WK, Williamson E, Tang ML. Anaphylaxis fatalities and admissions in Australia. *J Allergy Clin Immunol.* 2009;123:434–442.
19. Ross MP, Ferguson M, Street D, Klontz K, Schroeder T, Luccioli S. Analysis of food-allergic and anaphylactic events in the national electronic injury surveillance system. *J Allergy Clin Immunol.* 2008;121:166–171.
20. Macdougall CF, Cant AJ, Colver AF. How dangerous is food allergy in childhood? The incidence of severe and fatal allergic reactions across the UK and Ireland. *Arch Dis Child.* 2002;86:236–239.
21. Bock SA, Munoz-Furlong A, Sampson HA. Fatalities due to anaphylactic reactions to foods. *J Allergy Clin Immunol.* 2001;107:191–193.
22. Bock SA, Munoz-Furlong A, Sampson HA. Further fatalities caused by anaphylactic reactions to food, 2001–2006. *J Allergy Clin Immunol.* 2007;119:1016–1018.
23. Uguz A, Lack G, Pumphrey R, et al. Allergic reactions in the community: a questionnaire survey of members of the anaphylaxis campaign. *Clin Exp Allergy.* 2005;35:746–750.
24. Brown AF, McKinnon D, Chu K. Emergency department anaphylaxis: a review of 142 patients in a single year. *J Allergy Clin Immunol.* 2001;108:861–866.
25. Smit DV, Cameron PA, Rainer TH. Anaphylaxis presentations to an emergency department in Hong Kong: incidence and predictors of biphasic reactions. *J Emerg Med.* 2005;28:381–388.
26. Lee JM, Greenes DS. Biphasic anaphylactic reactions in pediatrics. *Pediatrics.* 2000;106:762–766.
27. Novembre E, Cianferoni A, Bernardini R, et al. Anaphylaxis in children: clinical and allergologic features. *Pediatrics.* 1998;101:E8.
28. Cianferoni A, Novembre E, Mugnaini L, et al. Clinical features of acute anaphylaxis in patients admitted to a university hospital: an 11-year retrospective review (1985–1996). *Ann Allergy Asthma Immunol.* 2001;87:27–32.
29. Crespo JF, Pascual C, Burks AW, Helm RM, Esteban MM. Frequency of food allergy in a pediatric population from Spain. *Pediatr Allergy Immunol.* 1995;6:39–43.
30. Dalal I, Binson I, Reifen R, et al. Food allergy is a matter of geography after all: sesame as a major cause of severe IgE-mediated food allergic reactions among infants and young children in Israel. *Allergy.* 2002;57:362–365.

31. Jarvinen KM, Sicherer SH, Sampson HA, Nowak-Wegrzyn A. Use of multiple doses of epinephrine in food-induced anaphylaxis in children. *J Allergy Clin Immunol.* 2008;122:133–138.
32. Asero R, Antonicelli L, Arena A, et al. Causes of food-induced anaphylaxis in Italian adults: a multi-centre study. *Int Arch Allergy Immunol.* 2009;150:271–277.
33. Sicherer SH, Burks AW, Sampson HA. Clinical features of acute allergic reactions to peanut and tree nuts in children. *Pediatrics.* 1998;102:e6.
34. Lack G, Fox D, Northstone K, Golding J. Avon Longitudinal Study of Parents and Children Study Team. Factors associated with the development of peanut allergy in childhood. *N Engl J Med.* 2003;348:977–985.
35. Clark S, Bock SA, Gaeta TJ, et al. Multicenter study of emergency department visits for food allergies. *J Allergy Clin Immunol.* 2004;113:347–352.
36. James JM, Crespo JF. Allergic reactions to foods by inhalation. *Curr Allergy Asthma Rep.* 2007;7:167–174.
37. Simonte SJ, Ma S, Mofidi S, Sicherer SH. Relevance of casual contact with peanut butter in children with peanut allergy. *J Allergy Clin Immunol.* 2003;112:180–182.
38. Simons FE, Frew AJ, Ansotegui IJ, et al. Risk assessment in anaphylaxis: current and future approaches. *J Allergy Clin Immunol.* 2007;120:S2–24.
39. Shreffler WG, Beyer K, Chu TH, Burks AW, Sampson HA. Microarray immunoassay: association of clinical history, in vitro IgE function, and heterogeneity of allergenic peanut epitopes. *J Allergy Clin Immunol.* 2004;113:776–782.
40. Li XM, Schofield BH, Huang CK, Kleiner GI, Sampson HA. A murine model of IgE-mediated cow's milk hypersensitivity. *J Allergy Clin Immunol.* 1999;103:206–214.
41. Li XM, Serebrisky D, Lee SY, et al. A murine model of peanut anaphylaxis: T- and B-cell responses to a major peanut allergen mimic human responses. *J Allergy Clin Immunol.* 2000;106:150–158.
42. Sun J, Arias K, Alvarez D, et al. Impact of CD40 ligand, B cells, and mast cells in peanut-induced anaphylactic responses. *J Immunol.* 2007;179:6696–6703.
43. Khodoun M, Strait R, Orekov T, et al. Peanuts can contribute to anaphylactic shock by activating complement. *J Allergy Clin Immunol.* 2009;123:342–351.
44. Arias K, Baig M, Colangelo M, et al. Concurrent blockade of platelet-activating factor and histamine prevents life-threatening peanut-induced anaphylactic reactions. *J Allergy Clin Immunol.* 2009;124:307–314.
45. Lemon-Mule H, Nowak-Wegrzyn A, Berin C, Knight AK. Pathophysiology of food-induced anaphylaxis. *Curr Allergy Asthma Rep.* 2008;8:201–208.
46. Berin MC, Kiliaan AJ, Yang PC, Groot JA, Kitamura Y, Perdue MH. The influence of mast cells on pathways of transepithelial antigen transport in rat intestine. *J Immunol.* 1998;161:2561–2566.
47. Yang PC, Berin MC, Yu LC, Conrad DH, Perdue MH. Enhanced intestinal transepithelial antigen transport in allergic rats is mediated by IgE and CD23 (Fcε RII). *J Clin Invest.* 2000;106:879–886.
48. Li H, Nowak-Wegrzyn A, Charlop-Powers Z, et al. Transcytosis of IgE-antigen complexes by CD23a in human intestinal epithelial cells and its role in food allergy. *Gastroenterology.* 2006;131:47–58.
49. Yano H, Kato Y, Matsuda T. Acute exercise induces gastrointestinal leakage of allergen in lysozyme-sensitized mice. *Eur J Appl Physiol.* 2002;87:358–364.
50. Matsuo H, Morimoto K, Akaki T, et al. Exercise and aspirin increase levels of circulating gliadin peptides in patients with wheat-dependent exercise-induced anaphylaxis. *Clin Exp Allergy.* 2005;35:461–466.
51. Palosuo K, Varjonen E, Nurkkala J, et al. Transglutaminase-mediated cross-linking of a peptic fraction of omega-5 gliadin enhances IgE reactivity in wheat-dependent, exercise-induced anaphylaxis. *J Allergy Clin Immunol.* 2003;111:1386–1392.
52. Untersmayr E, Bakos N, Scholl I, et al. Anti-ulcer drugs promote IgE formation toward dietary antigens in adult patients. *FASEB J.* 2005;19:656–658.
53. Untersmayr E, Vestergaard H, Malling HJ, et al. Incomplete digestion of codfish represents a risk factor for anaphylaxis in patients with allergy. *J Allergy Clin Immunol.* 2007;119:711–717.
54. Beyer K, Morrow E, Li XM, et al. Effects of cooking methods on peanut allergenicity. *J Allergy Clin Immunol.* 2001;107:1077–1081.
55. Nowak-Wegrzyn A, KA B, SH S, et al. Tolerance to extensively heated milk in children with cow's milk allergy. *J Allergy Clin Immunol.* 2008;122:342–347.
56. Lemon-Mule H, Sampson HA, Sicherer SH, Shreffler WG, Noone S, Nowak-Wegrzyn A. Immunologic changes in children with egg allergy ingesting extensively heated egg. *J Allergy Clin Immunol.* 2008;122:977–983.e1.
57. Commins SP, Satinover SM, Hosen J, et al. Delayed anaphylaxis, angioedema, or urticaria after consumption of red meat in patients with IgE antibodies specific for galactose-α-1,3-galactose. *J Allergy Clin Immunol.* 2009;123:426–433.
58. Lieberman P. Biphasic anaphylactic reactions. *Ann Allergy Asthma Immunol.* 2005;95:217–226; quiz 226, 258.
59. Sampson HA, Mendelson L, Rosen JP. Fatal and near-fatal anaphylactic reactions to food in children and adolescents. *N Engl J Med.* 1992;327:380–384.

60. Kemp AS. EpiPen epidemic: suggestions for rational prescribing in childhood food allergy. *J Paediatr Child Health*. 2003;39:372–375.
61. Summers CW, Pumphrey RS, Woods CN, McDowell G, Pemberton PW, Arkwright PD. Factors predicting anaphylaxis to peanuts and tree nuts in patients referred to a specialist center. *J Allergy Clin Immunol*. 2008;121:632–638.e2.
62. Pumphrey R. Anaphylaxis: can we tell who is at risk of a fatal reaction? *Curr Opin Allergy Clin Immunol*. 2004;4:285–290.
63. Calvani M, Alessandri C, Frediani T, et al. Correlation between skin prick test using commercial extract of cow's milk protein and fresh milk and food challenges. *Pediatr Allergy Immunol*. 2007;18:583–588.
64. Caminiti L, Passalacqua G, Vita D, Ruggeri P, Barberio G, Pajno GB. Food-exercise-induced anaphylaxis in a boy successfully desensitized to cow milk. *Allergy*. 2007;62:335–336.
65. Jarvinen KM, Amalanayagam S, Shreffler WG, et al. Epinephrine treatment is infrequent and biphasic reactions are rare in food-induced reactions during oral food challenges in children. *J Allergy Clin Immunol*. 2009;124:1267–1272.
66. Perry TT, Matsui EC, Conover-Walker MK, Wood RA. Risk of oral food challenges. *J Allergy Clin Immunol*. 2004;114:1164–1168.
67. Braganza SC, Acworth JP, Mckinnon DR, Peake JE, Brown AF. Paediatric emergency department anaphylaxis: different patterns from adults. *Arch Dis Child*. 2006;91:159–163.
68. Moneret-Vautrin DA, Kanny G, Morisset M, Rance F, Fardeau MF, Beaudouin E. Severe food anaphylaxis: 107 cases registered in 2002 by the allergy vigilance network. *Eur Ann Allergy Clin Immunol*. 2004;36:46–51.
69. Simons FE. Anaphylaxis in infants: can recognition and management be improved? *J Allergy Clin Immunol*. 2007;120:537–540.
70. Isolauri E, Tahvanainen A, Peltola T, Arvola T. Breast-feeding of allergic infants. *J Pediatr*. 1999;134:27–32.
71. Jarvinen KM, Makinen-Kiljunen S, Suomalainen H. Cow's milk challenge through human milk evokes immune responses in infants with cow's milk allergy. *J Pediatr*. 1999;135:506–512.
72. Lifschitz CH, Hawkins HK, Guerra C, Byrd N. Anaphylactic shock due to cow's milk protein hypersensitivity in a breast-fed infant. *J Pediatr Gastroenterol Nutr*. 1988;7:141–144.
73. Monti G, Marinaro L, Libanore V, Peltran A, Muratore MC, Silvestro L. Anaphylaxis due to fish hypersensitivity in an exclusively breastfed infant. *Acta Paediatr*. 2006;95:1514–1515.
74. Buckley MG, Variend S, Walls AF. Elevated serum concentrations of beta-tryptase, but not alpha-tryptase, in sudden infant death syndrome (SIDS). an investigation of anaphylactic mechanisms. *Clin Exp Allergy*. 2001;31:1696–1704.
75. Tole JW, Lieberman P. Biphasic anaphylaxis: review of incidence, clinical predictors, and observation recommendations. *Immunol Allergy Clin North Am*. 2007;27:309–326, viii.
76. Atkins D, Bock SA. Fatal anaphylaxis to foods: epidemiology, recognition, and prevention. *Curr Allergy Asthma Rep*. 2009;9:179–185.
77. Pumphrey RS, Stanworth SJ. The clinical spectrum of anaphylaxis in north-west England. *Clin Exp Allergy*. 1996;26:1364–1370.
78. Pumphrey RS, Gowland MH. Further fatal allergic reactions to food in the United Kingdom, 1999–2006. *J Allergy Clin Immunol*. 2007;119:1018–1019.
79. Pumphrey RS. Fatal anaphylaxis in the UK, 1992–2001. *Novartis Found Symp*. 2004;257:116–128; discussion 128–132, 157–160, 276–285.
80. Yunginger JW, Sweeney KG, Sturner WQ, et al. Fatal food-induced anaphylaxis. *J Am Med Assoc*. 1988;260:1450–1452.
81. Vadas P, Perelman B. Activated charcoal forms non-IgE binding complexes with peanut proteins. *J Allergy Clin Immunol*. 2003;112(1):175–179.
82. Oren E, Banerji A, Clark S, Camargo CA, Jr. Food-induced anaphylaxis and repeated epinephrine treatments. *Ann Allergy Asthma Immunol*. 2007;99:429–432.
83. Korenblat P, Lundie MJ, Dankner RE, Day JH. A retrospective study of epinephrine administration for anaphylaxis: how many doses are needed? *Allergy Asthma Proc*. 1999;20:383–386.
84. Wang J, Sampson HA. Food anaphylaxis. *Clin Exp Allergy*. 2007;37:651–660.
85. Sampson HA, Jolie PL. Increased plasma histamine concentrations after food challenges in children with atopic dermatitis. *N Engl J Med*. 1984;311:372–376.
86. Vadas P, Gold M, Perelman B, et al. Platelet-activating factor, PAF acetylhydrolase, and severe anaphylaxis. *N Engl J Med*. 2008;358:28–35.
87. Nishio H, Takai S, Miyazaki M, et al. Usefulness of serum mast cell-specific chymase levels for postmortem diagnosis of anaphylaxis. *Int J Leg Med*. 2005;119:331–334.
88. Sicherer SH, Simons FE, Section on Allergy and Immunology, American Academy of Pediatrics. Self-injectable epinephrine for first-aid management of anaphylaxis. *Pediatrics*. 2007;119:638–646.
89. Kelso JM. A second dose of epinephrine for anaphylaxis: how often needed and how to carry. *J Allergy Clin Immunol*. 2006;117:464–465.

90. Sicherer SH, Noone SA, Munoz-Furlong A. The impact of childhood food allergy on quality of life. *Ann Allergy Asthma Immunol.* 2001;87:461–464.
91. Skripak JM, Matsui EC, Mudd K, Wood RA. The natural history of IgE-mediated cow's milk allergy. *J Allergy Clin Immunol.* 2007;120:1172–1177.
92. Savage JH, Matsui EC, Skripak JM, Wood RA. The natural history of egg allergy. *J Allergy Clin Immunol.* 2007;120:1413–1417.
93. Keet CA, Matsui EC, Dhillon G, Lenehan P, Paterakis M, Wood RA. The natural history of wheat allergy. *Ann Allergy Asthma Immunol.* 2009;102:410–415.
94. Fleischer DM, Conover-Walker MK, Matsui EC, Wood RA. The natural history of tree nut allergy. *J Allergy Clin Immunol.* 2005;116:1087–1093.
95. Skolnick HS, Conover-Walker MK, Koerner CB, Sampson HA, Burks W, Wood RA. The natural history of peanut allergy. *J Allergy Clin Immunol.* 2001;107:367–374.
96. Fleischer DM, Conover-Walker MK, Christie L, Burks AW, Wood RA. Peanut allergy: recurrence and its management. *J Allergy Clin Immunol.* 2004;114:1195–1201.
97. Cooke SK, Sampson HA. Allergenic properties of ovomucoid in man. *J Immunol.* 1997;159:2026–2032.
98. Jarvinen KM, Beyer K, Vila L, Bardina L, Mishoe M, Sampson HA. Specificity of IgE antibodies to sequential epitopes of hen's egg ovomucoid as a marker for persistence of egg allergy. *Allergy.* 2007;62:758–765.
99. Leung DY, Sampson HA, Yunginger JW, et al. Effect of anti-IgE therapy in patients with peanut allergy. *N Engl J Med.* 2003;348:986–993.
100. Srivastava KD, Kattan JD, Zou ZM, et al. The Chinese herbal medicine formula FAHF-2 completely blocks anaphylactic reactions in a murine model of peanut allergy. *J Allergy Clin Immunol.* 2005;115:171–178.
101. Sicherer SH, Sampson HA. Peanut allergy: emerging concepts and approaches for an apparent epidemic. *J Allergy Clin Immunol.* 2007;120:491–503; quiz 504–505.
102. MacGlashan DW Jr, Bochner BS, Adelman DC, et al. Down-regulation of Fcε RI expression on human basophils during in vivo treatment of atopic patients with anti-IgE antibody. *J Immunol.* 1997;158:1438–1445.
103. Kuehr J, Brauburger J, Zielen S, et al. Efficacy of combination treatment with anti-IgE plus specific immunotherapy in polysensitized children and adolescents with seasonal allergic rhinitis. *J Allergy Clin Immunol.* 2002;109:274–280.
104. Li XM, Zhang TF, Huang CK, et al. Food allergy herbal formula -1 (FAHF-1) blocks peanut-induced anaphylaxis in a murine model. *J Allergy Clin Immunol.* 2001;108:639–646.
105. Qu C, Srivastava K, Ko J, Zhang TF, Sampson HA, Li XM. Induction of tolerance after establishment of peanut allergy by the food allergy herbal formula-2 is associated with up-regulation of interferon-γ. *Clin Exp Allergy.* 2007;37:846–855.
106. Srivastava KD, Qu C, Zhang T, Goldfarb J, Sampson HA, Li XM. Food allergy herbal formula-2 silences peanut-induced anaphylaxis for a prolonged posttreatment period via IFN-γ-producing CD8+ T cells. *J Allergy Clin Immunol.* 2009;123:443–451.
107. Kattan JD, Srivastava KD, Zou ZM, Goldfarb J, Sampson HA, Li XM. Pharmacological and immunological effects of individual herbs in the food allergy herbal formula-2 (FAHF-2) on peanut allergy. *Phytother Res.* 2008;22:651–659.
108. Oppenheimer JJ, Nelson HS, Bock SA, Christensen F, Leung DY. Treatment of peanut allergy with rush immunotherapy. *J Allergy Clin Immunol.* 1992;90:256–262.
109. Nelson HS, Lahr J, Rule R, Bock A, Leung D. Treatment of anaphylactic sensitivity to peanuts by immunotherapy with injections of aqueous peanut extract. *J Allergy Clin Immunol.* 1997;99:744–751.
110. AT S. A case of egg poisoning. *Lancet.* 1908;1:716.
111. Schofield AT, Scurlock AM, Burks AW, Jones SM. Oral immunotherapy for food allergy. *Curr Allergy Asthma Rep.* 2009;9:186–193.
112. Chehade M, Mayer L. Oral tolerance and its relation to food hypersensitivities. *J Allergy Clin Immunol.* 2005;115:3–12; quiz 13.
113. Strid J, Hourihane J, Kimber I, Callard R, Strobel S. Epicutaneous exposure to peanut protein prevents oral tolerance and enhances allergic sensitization 1. *Clin Exp Allergy.* 2005;35:757–766.
114. Patriarca C, Romano A, Venuti A, et al. Oral specific hyposensitization in the management of patients allergic to food. *Allergol Immunopathol.* 1984;12:275–281.
115. Patriarca G, Schiavino D, Nucera E, Schinco G, Milani A, Gasbarrini GB. Food allergy in children: results of a standardized protocol for oral desensitization. *Hepatogastroenterology.* 1998;45:52–58.
116. Patriarca G, Nucera E, Roncallo C, et al. Oral desensitizing treatment in food allergy: clinical and immunological results. *Aliment Pharmacol Ther.* 2003;17:459–465.
117. Patriarca G, Nucera E, Pollastrini E, et al. Oral rush desensitization in peanut allergy: a case report. *Dig Dis Sci.* 2006;51:471–473.
118. Rueff F, Eberlein-Konig B, Przybilla B. Oral hyposensitization with celery juice. *Allergy.* 2001;56:82–83.

119. Buchanan AD, Scurlock AM, Jones SM, et al. Oral desensitization and induction of tolerance in peanut-allergic children. *J Allergy Clin Immunol.* 2006;117:S327–S327.
120. Buchanan AD, Green TD, Jones SM, et al. Egg oral immunotherapy in nonanaphylactic children with egg allergy. *J Allergy Clin Immunol.* 2007;119:199–205.
121. Rolinck-Werninghaus C, Staden U, Mehl A, Hamelmann E, Beyer K, Niggemann B. Specific oral tolerance induction with food in children: transient or persistent effect on food allergy? *Allergy.* 2005;60:1320–1322.
122. Skripak JM, Nash SD, Rowley H, et al. A randomized, double-blind, placebo-controlled study of milk oral immunotherapy for cow's milk allergy. *J Allergy Clin Immunol.* 2008;122:1154–1160.
123. Longo G, Barbi E, Berti I, et al. Specific oral tolerance induction in children with very severe cow's milk-induced reactions. *J Allergy Clin Immunol.* 2008;121:343–347.
124. Staden U, Rolinck-Werninghaus C, Brewe F, Wahn U, Niggemann B, Beyer K. Specific oral tolerance induction in food allergy in children: efficacy and clinical patterns of reaction. *Allergy.* 2007;62:1261–1269.
125. Clark AT, Islam S, King Y, Deighton J, Anagnostou K, Ewan PW. Successful oral tolerance induction in severe peanut allergy. *Allergy.* 2009;64:1218–1220.
126. Jones SM, Pons L, Roberts JL, et al. Clinical efficacy and immune regulation with peanut oral immunotherapy. *J Allergy Clin Immunol.* 2009;124:292–300.
127. Hofmann AM, Scurlock AM, Jones SM, et al. Safety of a peanut oral immunotherapy protocol in children with peanut allergy. *J Allergy Clin Immunol.* 2009;124:286–291.
128. Narisety SD, Skripak JM, Steele P, et al. Open-label maintenance after milk oral immunotherapy for IgE-mediated cow's milk allergy. *J Allergy Clin Immunol.* 2009;124:610–612.
129. Varshney P, Steele PH, Vickery BP, et al. Adverse reactions during peanut oral immunotherapy home dosing. *J Allergy Clin Immunol.* 2009;124:1351–1352.
130. Meglio P, Bartone E, Plantamura M, Arabito E, Giampietro PG. A protocol for oral desensitization in children with IgE-mediated cow's milk allergy. *Allergy.* 2004;59:980–987.
131. Mempel M, Rakoski J, Ring J, Ollert M. Severe anaphylaxis to kiwi fruit: immunologic changes related to successful sublingual allergen immunotherapy. *J Allergy Clin Immunol.* 2003;111:1406–1409.
132. Kerzl R, Simonowa A, Ring J, Ollert M, Mempel M. Life-threatening anaphylaxis to kiwi fruit: protective sublingual allergen immunotherapy effect persists even after discontinuation. *J Allergy Clin Immunol.* 2007;119:507–508.
133. Enrique E, Pineda F, Malek T, et al. Sublingual immunotherapy for hazelnut food allergy: a randomized, double-blind, placebo-controlled study with a standardized hazelnut extract. *J Allergy Clin Immunol.* 2005;116:1073–1079.
134. de Boissieu D, Dupont C. Sublingual immunotherapy for cow's milk protein allergy: a preliminary report. *Allergy.* 2006;61:1238–1239.
135. Fernandez-Rivas M, Garrido FS, Nadal JA, et al. Randomized double-blind, placebo-controlled trial of sublingual immunotherapy with a Pru p 3 quantified peach extract. *Allergy.* 2009;64:876–883.
136. Bannon GA, Cockrell G, Connaughton C, et al. Engineering, characterization and in vitro efficacy of the major peanut allergens for use in immunotherapy. *Int Arch Allergy Immunol.* 2001;124:70–72.
137. Li XM, Srivastava K, Huleatt JW, Bottomly K, Burks AW, Sampson HA. Engineered recombinant peanut protein and heat-killed *Listeria monocytogenes* coadministration protects against peanut-induced anaphylaxis in a murine model. *J Immunol.* 2003;170:3289–3295.
138. Li XM, Srivastava K, Grishin A, et al. Persistent protective effect of heat-killed *Escherichia coli* producing "engineered," recombinant peanut proteins in a murine model of peanut allergy. *J Allergy Clin Immunol.* 2003;112:159–167.
139. Li S, Li XM, Burks AW, Sampson HA. Modulation of peanut allergy by peptide-based immunotherapy. *J Allergy Clin Immunol.* 2001;107:S233.
140. Horner AA, Nguyen MD, Ronaghy A, Cinman N, Verbeek S, Raz E. DNA-based vaccination reduces the risk of lethal anaphylactic hypersensitivity in mice. *J Allergy Clin Immunol.* 2000;106:349–356.
141. Roy K, Mao HQ, Huang SK, Leong KW. Oral gene delivery with chitosan – DNA nanoparticles generates immunologic protection in a murine model of peanut allergy. *Nat Med.* 1999;5:387–391.
142. Srivastava K, Li XM, Bannon GA, et al. Investigation of the use of ISS-linked ara h2 for the treatment of peanut-induced allergy [abstract]. *J Allergy Clin Immunol.* 2001;107:S233–S233.
143. Nguyen MD, Cinman N, Yen J, Horner AA. DNA-based vaccination for the treatment of food allergy. *Allergy.* 2001;56 Suppl 67:127–130.
144. Simons FE. Advances in H1-antihistamines. *N Engl J Med.* 2004;351:2203–2217.

# Chapter 10
# Antibiotic-Induced Anaphylaxis

**Pascal Demoly, Philippe Jean Bousquet, and Antonino Romano**

**Abstract** An antibiotic allergic reaction represents one of the side effects of drugs and is a daily worry for the clinician. If urticaria and maculo–papular eruptions are the most frequent manifestations, then anaphylaxis can occur. The tools allowing a definite diagnosis are validated for some antibiotics and include the following procedures: a thorough clinical history, standardized skin tests, reliable biological tests, and drug provocation tests. When properly performed in specialized centers, a firm diagnosis is often possible and safe alternative medication can be proposed. This is particularly the case for β-lactam antibiotics, considering their wide prescription and utility.

**Keywords** Drug allergy/hypersensitivity • Anaphylaxis • Antibiotic allergy • β(beta)-lactams • Skin tests • Provocation tests • Specific IgE

## 10.1 Introduction

Drug hypersensitivity, which includes allergic reaction, represents the adverse effects of certain drugs, when taken at a dose tolerated by normal subjects. Drug hypersensitivity clinically resembles allergy [1] and is one of the side effects of drugs and a daily worry for the clinician. This is particularly the case for antibiotics considering their utility and large population exposure. Drug hypersensitivities may affect up to 20% of hospitalized patients [2] and up to 7% of outpatients [3]; they can be life threatening [2]. In the UK, for example, where hospital admissions for acute anaphylaxis are increasing (from 56 per million in 1991 to 102 per million in 1995) [4], drugs are the leading cause of fatal anaphylaxis (88 deaths out of 202) followed by food and insect stings [5]. In this survey, antibiotic reactions had been caused by cephalosporins [8], penicillins [5], ciprofloxacin [1], amphoteracin [1], and vancomycin [1].

By definition, drug allergies are adverse reactions whereby antibodies and/or activated T-cells are directed against the drug or one of its metabolites [1]. Drug intake can indeed induce drug sensitization, and further exposures possibly drug allergies. The exact mechanisms are not fully understood. Moreover, numerous reactions with symptoms suggestive of allergy are often erroneously considered to be real drug allergies, especially in the case of antibiotics.

The revised nomenclature for allergy classifies allergic reactions to drugs as IgE-mediated or non-IgE-mediated [1]. They can further be classified as immediate or non-immediate according to

P. Demoly (✉)
Hôpital Arnaud de Villeneuve, University Hospital of Montpellier, Montpellier, France
e-mail: pascal.demoly@inserm.fr

M.C. Castells (ed.), *Anaphylaxis and Hypersensitivity Reactions*,
DOI 10.1007/978-1-60327-951-2_10, 

the time interval between the last drug administration and the onset [6]. Immediate reactions occur within 1 h and are manifested by urticaria, angioedema, bronchospasm and anaphylactic shock. Anaphylactic shock is one of the severe reactions. It is usually an IgE-mediated reaction and is the most frightening and potentially lethal allergic event. Symptoms are produced by a rapid release of histamine and other vasoactive inflammatory mediators immediately after hapten-antibody interaction. It requires prompt treatment and a firm diagnosis to avoid relapses.

When properly performed in specialized centers, a firm diagnosis is often possible and safe alternative medication can be proposed. The clinical tools allowing a definite diagnosis are few in number and include the following procedures: a thorough clinical history, standardized skin tests, reliable biological tests and drug provocation tests. New diagnostic tools, such as the basophil activation test and the lymphocyte activation test, have been developed and are under validation. All of these tools, although not always validated or predictive at the individual level and sometimes dangerous, have been carefully evaluated [6–11].

## 10.2 Drug Allergy Workup

### *10.2.1 Clinical History*

The diagnosis of drug allergy and anaphylaxis always starts with complete details of the episode. Clinical history should be very thoroughly examined, addressing the symptomatology (compatible with an allergy), the chronology of the symptoms (previous exposure, delay between the last dose and the onset of symptoms, effect of stopping treatment), other medication taken (both at the time of the reaction as well as other drugs of the same class taken since) and the medical background of the patient (any suggestion of a previous allergy whether associated with medication or not). Data should be recorded in a uniform format and, a questionnaire [7] is available in many different languages (on http://www.eaaci.net/site/content.php?l1=91&sel=480). Diagnosis is more difficult when patients are not seen during the acute phase, in which case photographs and medical reports are helpful. Even in the case of anaphylaxis where the responsibility of the drug might appear obvious, the complete drug allergy workup is mandatory.

The history is often not reliable since different drugs are frequently taken simultaneously and can account for the symptoms. The more severe the reaction, the more likely it will be drug related. History can also be imprecise in many cases. Thus, for drug allergy diagnosis, many doctors rely on history and various reference manuals. They do not attempt to prove the relationship between the drug intake and the symptoms or to clarify the underlying pathomechanism of the reaction. Such attitude could lead to a misunderstanding of the epidemiology and the pathophysiology of this highly relevant field. In cases where a hypersensitivity reaction is suspected, if the drug is essential and/or frequently prescribed (e.g., β(beta)-lactams, quinolones), a certified diagnosis should be performed and tests should be carried out in a specialist centre. Only a formal diagnosis of drug allergy allows the measures required for prevention and treatment to be brought into play. For these drugs, the prudent principle of eviction may be insufficient. This procedure could lead to the elimination of drugs which do not necessarily give rise to reactions and which are widely used. In the case of antibiotics, this may really lead to a loss of chance for future infection treatments. This may lead to extra costs and other unnecessary side effects. However, this is a valid option until a specialist consultation can be scheduled.

The specific allergy diagnosis should be carried out 4 weeks after the complete clearing of all clinical symptoms and signs. On the other hand, after a time interval of more than 6–12 months, some drug tests may already have turned negative resulting in false negative results.

### 10.2.2 Skin Tests

The diagnostic value of skin tests has not been fully evaluated for all drugs, and the exchange of experience within different centers has only recently started. Skin tests have to be applied depending on the suspected pathomechanism of the hypersensitive drug reactions. Skin prick tests and intradermal tests are particularly important for reactive haptens in order to demonstrate an IgE-dependent mechanism, which is the case for most anaphylaxis [8]. They should be performed 4–6 weeks after the reaction. The prick test is recommended for initial screening due to its simplicity, rapidity, low cost and high specificity. Intracutaneous tests consist of injecting a sterile, diluted allergen extract superficially into the dermis, and then reading the results after 20 min [8].

Their sensitivity, specificity and negative predictive value vary, depending on the culprit drug, from excellent (penicillins, cephalosporins) to satisfactory, poor or unknown (sulfonamides, quinolones, macrolides and other anti-infectious agents). The positive predictive value has rarely been tested, mostly for ethical reasons. The tests should follow standard operation procedures and should be performed by trained staff. Unfortunately, apart from allergic reactions to several antibiotics, for most drug allergens, standardized and validated test concentrations and vehicles have not been elucidated. Sometimes the drug is not available in an adequate reactive form—generally because it is a metabolic derivative which is immunogenic and for which provocation tests are required to confirm the diagnosis.

### 10.2.3 Provocation Tests

A drug provocation test has become the gold standard for the identification of an eliciting drug. It is independent of the pathogenesis and takes individual factors into account such as the metabolism and genetic disposition of an individual. Provocation tests have the finest sensitivity, but can only be performed under the most rigorous surveillance conditions and are therefore restricted to certain specialist centers with on-site intensive care facilities [9]. These tests are particularly required for antibiotics other than β(beta)-lactams, or for β(beta)-lactams when skin tests are negative. They should be performed after a certain time interval following the hypersensitivity reaction (at least 1 month) using the same drug as in the initial case. The route of administration depends on the suspected drug. The precise challenge procedure varies a great deal from one team to the next and guidelines for the performance of provocation tests in drug allergies have been proposed [9]. Provocation tests should not be performed if the offending drug is infrequently used or if several safe alternatives exist. Anaphylaxis is not a contra-indication for drug provocation [9] since it can be manage by opposition to severe cutaneous reactions such as toxic epidermal necrolysis and Steven Johnson syndrome. An extensive study of more than 1,000 drug provocations has validated this means of diagnosis, not only allowing drug hypersensitivity to be diagnosed, but also excluding it in more than 80% of the reactions suffered by patients displaying negative results in skin tests [11]. In this study, some patients had severe reactions, according to the referring doctor, including 43 episodes of anaphylactic shock and 42 episodes of anaphylaxis without shock. In these test-negative cases, we attributed the symptoms to vaso–vagal faint (61%), nonspecific histamine release (37%), or food allergy (2%).

### 10.2.4 Biological Tests

It would be highly advantageous to have discriminating biological tests available to establish the nature of the culprit agent, especially for the patient receiving several drugs simultaneously.

However, these tests are few in number and, for the most part, not fully validated. It should also be remembered that the interpretation of the results needs to be determined with caution. A negative test does not exclude the responsibility of the drug while a positive result shows sensitivity to the drug but does not confirm its responsibility.

The demonstration of isolated drug-specific IgE (e.g., to penicillins [12] and quinolones [13]) does not enable the diagnosis of a drug allergy. However, in conjunction with clinical findings (e.g., typical symptoms of rapid onset), the IgE-dependent mechanism can be pinpointed (particularly if the skin tests to the drug are also positive) [12]. Cross-reactivity among several drugs using quantitative inhibition may also be explored, but mostly in research laboratories. The absence of specific circulating IgE does not rule out a diagnosis of anaphylaxis and this assay is not available for all drugs. The usefulness of measuring sulphidopeptide leukotrienes still requires further validation but does not appear to be very sensitive [14]. Tests involving basophil degranulation are not trustworthy given the low numbers of circulating basophils. These tests have been replaced by basophil activation tests, which hold great promise and which are currently undergoing strong evaluation [15]. At present, the most commonly used antibody is anti-CD63 and, to a lesser extent, anti-CD203c. Although it does not enable the differentiation between IgE-dependent and IgE-independent basophil activation, it is anticipated that it might constitute a unique tool for the diagnosis of IgE-mediated anaphylaxis when a specific IgE assay is unavailable [16]. Studies involving T-lymphocytes (lymphocyte transformation/activation tests) are performed by only a few laboratories and, for diagnosis purposes, usually deal only with non-immediate type IV reactions [17].

During anaphylaxis, basophils and mast cells are activated and then degranulate and release mediators into intracellular fluids. These mediators can be measured in the patient's serum and have proved to be useful for the diagnosis of perioperative anaphylaxis, in which antibiotics have become the third leading cause [18]. Again, the absence of increased serum histamine or tryptase does not rule out an allergic reaction.

### *10.2.5 Standard Operating Procedures and Preventive Measures*

The diagnosis of hypersensitivity reactions to drugs is often difficult and requires a stereotypic attitude no matter which drug is involved. It remains largely clinical with the help of certain allergy tests that are available for some of the drug classes (Table 10.1). Provocation tests are the gold standard but, being cumbersome and possibly harmful, are limited to highly specialized centers. New and validated biological tools for diagnosis, available to all clinicians, are necessary in order to improve care for these patients. Although difficult, the allergy diagnosis of reactions to drugs has been standardized, and standard operating procedures have been published [19].

A definite diagnosis of hypersensitivity reactions to antibiotics is required in order to institute proper preventive measures. Whatever the intensity of the clinical reaction, a state of hypersensitivity is shown towards the particular drug, with the possibility of an even more serious reaction in the future.

**Table 10.1** Recommendations for the diagnosis of antibiotic anaphylaxis

| |
|---|
| **A. Confirm the responsibility of the antibiotic by:** |
| 1. Clinical history and tryptase level if available during the initial reaction |
| 2. Skin testing when validated |
| 3. Drug provocation test if skin tests are negative |
| **B. Evaluate risk for cross reactivity** by skin tests |
| **C. Find safe alternative(s)** |
| 1. In the same chemical class by skin tests and drug provocation if skin tests are negative |
| 2. In another chemical class |

General preventive measures include a declaration to the Committee on Safety of Medicine Reports. Individual measures include the issue of an "Allergy Card" specifying the culprit agent(s), the delivery of a list of drugs to avoid and the delivery of a list of possible alternatives. The patient is also asked to make his allergies known prior to all prescriptions and surgical operations and to read the package insert on any drugs to be taken. The lists can never be completely exhaustive, are only indicative and should be frequently updated. Similarly, the questioning (to elicit any history of allergy) of every patient by every clinician prior to issuing a prescription is essential from both a medical and a medicolegal point of view. Preventive measures by pre-medication (e.g., slow injection and preparations with glucocorticoids and antihistamines) mainly concern non-allergic hypersensitivity reactions (for example to vancomycin). The possibility of desensitization should always be considered when the offending drug is essential and when no alternatives exist or are unsatisfactory, as in the following cases: sulfonamides in HIV-infected patients [21], quinolone allergies in some cystic fibrosis patients [22, 23], serious infections especially in cystic fibrosis patients with allergy to penicillins [22, 24] and antituberculosis drugs [25].

## 10.3 Antibiotic Anaphylaxis Diagnosis

### *10.3.1 β(beta)-Lactams*

β(beta)-lactams are by far the most widely used antibiotics. During the last 15 years there has been a definite change in the pattern of their use: the consumption of benzylpenicillin and first-generation cephalosporins has decreased and that of amoxicillin and second- and third-generation cephalosporins has increased [24, 27]. Over time, these changes have entailed modifications of the immune response, mainly because of the differences among the side-chain antigenic determinants of the various β(beta)-lactams. Allergic reactions to β(beta)-lactams are the most common cause of adverse drug reactions mediated by specific immunological mechanisms. Reactions may be induced by all β(beta)-lactams currently available, ranging from benzylpenicillin to other more recently introduced β(beta)-lactams (Fig. 10.1). They all share the β(beta)-lactam ring (azetidine-2-ione). They may cause all kinds of allergic reactions [28], anaphylaxis probably not being the most frequent [2, 3]. Many people (up to 4.5% of the general population in one study [3]) having experienced a drug hypersensitivity reaction while taking a β(beta)-lactam antibiotic are classified as allergic to the drug without any further investigation and are then denied β(beta)-lactam antibiotics. These reactions can indeed be life-threatening [2] and drug reintroduction in these cases may cause reactions that may be more severe than the initial ones. This is the case in the perioperative setting, where antibiotic-induced anaphylaxis has increased over the last 20 years. At present antibiotic-induced anaphylaxis represent 12–15% of the perioperative reactions observed in France [18], penicillins and cephalosporins being the most frequently involved. On the other hand, overdiagnosis due to common fear of anaphylaxis is frequent [29, 30], which entails depriving non-hypersensitive patients of potentially useful drugs. It is therefore important to diagnose β(beta)-lactam hypersensitivity reactions. Confirmation of the diagnosis should be rigorous and follow the standard operating procedures described above, always starting with a thorough clinical history.

Since the reagents used for diagnostic tests have changed [31] and many new data have been published over the past 5 years, guidelines [6] have recently been updated in Europe [10]. For presumed IgE-mediated allergic reactions, skin tests are performed by prick, and if responses are negative, intradermal tests are carried out. The β(beta)-lactams to be tested have to be freshly reconstituted. In both the European position guidelines [6, 32] and the American practice parameters [32], skin testing with benzylpenicilloyl-poly-L-lysine (PPL) and minor determinant mixture (MDM)

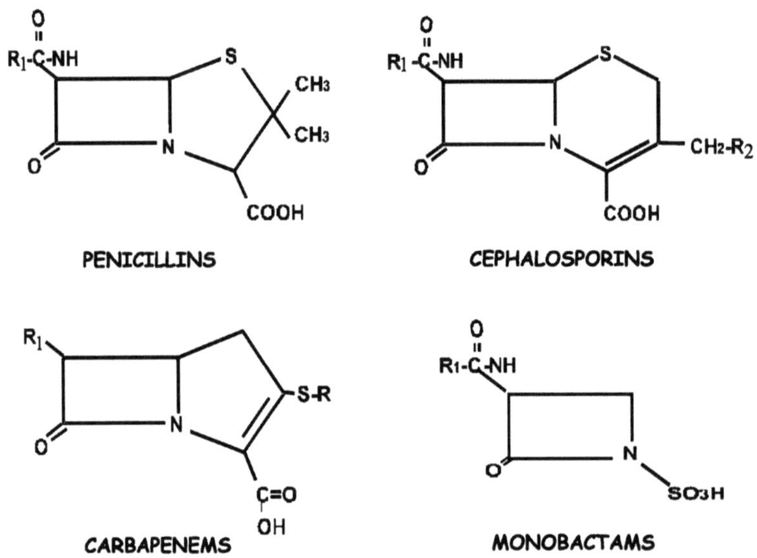


**Fig. 10.1** β(beta)-lactam chemical structure

represents the first-line method for diagnosing immediate hypersensitivity reactions to β(beta)-lactams. After the production of PPL and MDM in 2004 ceased, there was the danger that physicians would be set back by more than 25 years in managing patients with hypersensitivity reactions to β(beta)-lactams. However, PPL and MDM have been sold in Europe since 2003 and a study of has shown a good concordance between two different commercially available reagents [33]. PPL has also become available in the USA recently since 2009. In evaluating subjects with immediate reactions to β(beta)-lactams, the aforesaid guidelines [6, 10, 32] recommend the use of benzyl-penicillin, amoxicillin, ampicillin, and any other suspect β(beta)-lactam, in addition to PPL and MDM. Techniques and concentrations (Table 10.2) are validated in terms of sensitivity and specificity [6]. Higher concentrations may cause false positives. In patients reporting severe reactions, tests should begin with concentrations as low as 1,000th of those shown in the table, which can be gradually increased. Patients should be kept under close surveillance [34]. Readings should be taken after 15–20 min. In skin prick tests, a wheal larger than 3 mm accompanied by erythema is considered positive, as long as the negative control saline presents no wheal and flare reaction. In intradermal tests, an increase in the initial wheal diameter greater than 3 mm with a negative response to the control saline is considered positive. Some drugs have to be discontinued prior to undertaking immediate-reading skin tests, such as antihistamines (1 week) and β(beta)-blockers (48 h) in cooperation with the prescribing physician and under monitoring of the blood pressure. The patient should be free of any infectious disease, fever or inflammatory reactions at the time of testing. It is difficult to calculate the sensitivity of skin testing because drug provocation cannot always be used as a gold standard for ethical reasons. In one study involving 290 patients [35], the sensitivity of skin testing in patients with a clinical history of urticaria and/or anaphylaxis was 22% for PPL, 21% for MDM, 43% for amoxicillin, 33% for ampicillin and 70% for the combination of all four of the allergens; the specificity was 97%. However, in the case of type-I allergy to β(beta)-lactams, skin-test sensitivity decreases with time. Moreover, skin-test negativization has been observed in subjects with penicillin allergy, retested after at least 1 year [36, 37], with some subjects tolerating penicillin again [36]. With regard to cephalosporins, further studies in larger numbers of subjects are still required even if skin test sensitivity in two recent studies were rather similar: 76.4% (39 out of 51 persons) [38] and 69.7% (53 of 76) [39]. Cephalosporin skin tests are also useful in finding safe alternatives in penicillin-allergic subjects. In a study involving 128

**Table 10.2** Maximum concentrations accepted for both prick and intradermal testing of patients with a suspicion of allergic reactions to β(beta)-lactams Adapted from [6]

| Hapten | Dose | Unit |
|---|---|---|
| **BPO-PPL**[a] | $5 \times 10^{-5}$ | mMol/L |
| **MDM** | $2 \times 10^{-2}$ | mMol/L |
| **Amoxicillin** | 20–25 | mg/mL |
| **Benzylpenicillin** | 10–25,000 | IU/mL |
| **Culprit Drug** | | |
| Amoxicillin-clavulanic | 20–25 | mg/mL |
| Ampicillin | 20–25 | mg/mL |
| Piperacillin | 20–25 | mg/mL |
| Ticarcillin | 20–25 | mg/mL |
| Cephalosporin | 1–2 | mg/mL |
| Imipenem-cilastin | 1–2 | mg/mL |
| Aztreonam | 1–2 | mg/mL |

[a]BPO-PPL, benzylpenicilloyl poly-L-lysine; MDM, minor determinant mixture

patients with a well-established IgE-mediated allergy to penicillins, mainly to aminopenicillins [40], all 101 patients who displayed negative skin tests for cephalosporins (cefuroxime, ceftazidime, ceftriaxone, and cefotaxime) and underwent graded challenges with cefuroxime axetil and ceftriaxone tolerated them. Two recent studies [41, 42] proved that skin tests with native carbapenems are also useful in finding safe alternatives in subjects with a well-demonstrated IgE-mediated hypersensitivity to penicillins. In these studies [41, 42], all penicillin-allergic subjects who displayed negative results in skin tests with imipenem/cilastatin and meropenem and agreed to undergo imipenem/cilastatin and/or meropenem challenges tolerated them (specifically, 44 subjects tolerated imipenem/cilastatin, 35 meropenem, and 68 both imipenem/cilastatin and meropenem). In the aforesaid studies [40–42], more than 60% of penicillin-allergic subjects had experienced anaphylactic shocks. Previous consensus recommendation [32, 43] for the administration of a cephalosporin to subjects with IgE-mediated hypersensitivity to penicillins included choosing a cephalosporin with a different side chain and performing a graded challenge in an intensive care unit without previous skin tests with the relevant cephalosporin. More recent guidelines do not exclude the use of skin testing prior to drug challenge and favor rapid desensitization if the skin test is positive and there is no substitute [11]. European studies [40–42] recommend skin testing before graded challenges with alternative β(beta)-lactams, including carbapenems.

Serum-specific IgE assays (radioallergosorbent tests, or RAST, and immunoenzymatic assays, or ELISA) have been evaluated for the diagnosis of β(beta)-lactam allergic reactions. Although they appear to be less sensitive than skin testing [12], they are recommended [6, 10] in cases with the most severe reactions in order to avoid provocation tests, which is the next step in the diagnosis procedure. The sensitivity and specificity of the flow cytometric evaluation of CD63 on blood basophils was 50% and 93.3% respectively in 70 patients with immediate reactions to β(beta)-lactams [15].

Recent publications have reinforced the need to perform drug provocations in the diagnostic work-up of patients with allergic reactions to β(beta)-lactams [10]. They are carried out under the most rigorous surveillance conditions and only when skin tests are negative. They are important, since even if all possible reagents are used in skin testing, sensitivity is not 100%. Indeed, 8–17% of patients with negative skin tests have a positive provocation test [11, 35]. Therefore, in subjects with positive histories, the formal assumption according to which negativity of skin tests to major and minor determinants of benzylpenicillin is accompanied by a high probability of tolerance is no longer valid [10, 44]. In the case of positive allergologic tests, drug provocations to other β(beta)-lactams also allow an alternative to be found. This is of great importance in situations where exclusion of the whole class may result in more harm than benefit because of the potential adverse consequences of untreated infections or the choice of another possibly more toxic and expensive antibiotic. However, as mentioned above, it is advisable to perform prophylactic skin tests with alternative β(beta)-lactam antibiotics in allergic subjects before challenges.

Changes in the prescribed β(beta)-lactam antibiotics over time have modified the allergic determinants to which our patients are sensitized. This has justified a revision of past diagnostic guidelines [10]. The diagnosis is based on positive skin tests and/or specific IgE assays or, when negative, on a positive provocation. In the case of positive reactions, β(beta)-lactam therapy should be avoided until a safe alternative, which may often be in the same class, has been found or desensitization is recommended.

### *10.3.2 Quinolones*

Quinolones are broad spectrum synthetic antibiotics derived from nalidixic acid. Their basic structure is composed of a pyridine cycle and an aromatic. Even if quinolones generally have a good safety profile, there are reports of anaphylaxis. Even though allergy to quinolones is considered rare (0.1–2%), it is probably underestimated [45]. From 1984 to 1992, 76 cases of serious anaphylactic reactions (47 shocks) were registered at the French Regional Centres of Pharmacovigilance [46]. This figure consisted of 59 women (the principal indication being urinary infections) and 17 men. Flumequine was blamed in 30 cases, pefloxacin in 16, ofloxacin in 11, pipedimic acid in 9, nalidixic acid, norfloxacine and ciprofloxacin in 3 each and rosoxacin in 1 case. The notion of a previous absorption of quinolones was only found in 32 cases (42%) of which 22 concerned the same quinolone and 10 cases another quinolone (not necessarily of the same generation). This posed the problem of the origin of the sensitization (other quinoleins, contaminated food) and confirmed the possibility of cross-reactions between the different generations of quinolones. In their systematic review [45] identified 384 reports of unpredictable adverse reactions to quinolones, suggesting an immune mechanism. Ciprofloxacin, now the most widely used quinolone, was the most frequently involved. Immediate reactions, including urticaria, angioedema and anaphylactic shock, were the most frequent. This suggests a type 1 (IgE-mediated) allergic mechanism for most of these reactions, as has since been demonstrated in a series of cases where 30 out of 55 Italian patients (44 female, 11 men) had specific IgE [13]. A high degree of cross-reactivity among quinolones also was shown.

No in vivo or in vitro method of diagnostics can be advised as this has not been validated in a sufficient number of proven cases. The above-described stepwise strategy should be applied. As always in drug allergy, the diagnosis relies on the clinical history, which must be of evocative semiology and chronology. The reliability of skin tests (prick tests and intradermal) is unknown. These have, in fact, only been carried out in small numbers of patients and there are both false negatives [47] and false positives [48]. The latter are probably triggered by a direct histamine release by quinolones [49]. However, these tests should be performed since Manfredi et al. [13] demonstrated an IgE-mediated pathogenic mechanism, using a radioimmunoassay (RIA) with epoxy-activated sepharose 6B as the solid phase. A further development of this specific IgE assay (ELISA instead of RIA) might make it more widely available and a helpful tool in the diagnosis of quinolone hypersensitivity. Meanwhile, the drug provocation test remains the only type of testing that can prove the responsibility of the drug in a suspicion of quinolone immediate allergy [11].

### *10.3.3 Macrolides*

Macrolides are characterized by their basic structure which is made up of a lactonic cycle with two osidic chains. They are classified according to the number of carbon atoms in the cycle: 14 membered macrolides (erythromicin, roxithromycin, dirithromycin, clarithromycin, etc.), 15 membered (azithromycin) and 16 membered (spiramycin, josamycin, midecamycin, etc.) macrolides. Epidemiological studies show that macrolides are amongst the safest antibiotics. In a recent systematic review [50], 199 hypersensitivity reactions to macrolides were reported, with erythromycin [77] followed by spiramycin [47] and azythromycin being the most implicated drugs. Urticaria (35 cases) was the most common reported clinical reaction, anaphylaxis being rare [44]. In these series, no drug allergy workup was performed. An immediate IgE-dependent hypersensitivity has been shown with erythromycin in some cases [51]. The mechanism is frequently unknown and the skin tests are negative in most other cases. It would appear that the macrolide allergies are unlikely to be class allergies.

There is little information, which does not allow a conclusion with regard to the diagnostic tests [50]. Skin tests are more often negative, so drug provocation tests [52] performed in specialized centers should be regarded as the gold standard for macrolide allergy diagnosis.

### *10.3.4 Other Antibiotics*

Sulfonamide antibiotics have a sulfanilamide basic core and are responsible for frequent allergic reactions (10% of treatments). However, most of these reactions are delayed cutaneous reactions (after 1–3 weeks of treatment) and not anaphylaxis. There are a few cases of co-trimoxazole induced anaphylaxis, with positive skin tests and/or specific IgE to either trimethoprim [53] or sulfamethoxazole [54]. Specifically, in the latter study [54] skin tests with multivalent sulfamethoxazole-poly-L-tyrosine revealed an IgE-mediated pathogenic mechanism in 10 (29.4%) of 34 patients with immediate reactions to sulfamethoxazole.

Vancomycin has also been incriminated in some cases of anaphylaxis with positive skin tests [55]. However, in most cases, the adverse reactions observed are related to the histamine-release mediated red-man syndrome associated with rapid vancomycin administration [56]. The other glycopeptide teicoplanin has also been involved in anaphylaxis [57], but cross-reactivity is not mandatory.

There are several reports of single cases of anaphylactic reactions related to aminoglycosides—such as gentamicin [58], streptomycin [57–61], bacitracin [62–65], tobramycin [66], ribostamycin [67], and polymixin B [64], rifamycin SV [68], antituberculosis drugs [61, 69, 70], telithromycin [71], metronidazole [72], clindamycin [73], amphotericin B [74], fosfomycin [75], chloramphenicol [76], and pristinamycin [77, 78]. They were not all fully evaluated as described above and, if there is no alternative, a complete drug allergy workup should still be applied.

**Acknowledgement** The authors would like to thank Ms. Anna Bedbrook for the correction of the English.

## References

1. Johansson S, Bieber T, Dahl R, et al. Revised nomenclature for allergy for global use: Report of the Nomenclature Review Committee of the World Allergy Organization, October 2003. *J Allergy Clin Immunol* 2004;113:832–836.
2. Gomes ER, Demoly P. Epidemiology of hypersensitivity drug reactions. *Curr Opin Allergy Clin Immunol* 2005;5:309–316.
3. Gomes E, Cardoso MF, Praça F, et al. Self reported drug allergy in a general adult Portuguese population. *Clin Exp Allergy* 2004;34:1597–1601.
4. Sheikh A, Alves B. Hospital admissions for acute anaphylaxis: time trend study. *Br Med J* 2000;320:1441.
5. Pumphrey RS. Lessons for management of anaphylaxis from a study of fatal reactions. *Clin Exp Allergy* 2000;30:1144–1150.

6. Torres MJ, Blanca M, Fernandez J, et al. Diagnosis of immediate allergic reactions to β(beta)-lactam antibiotics. *Allergy* 2003;58:961–972.
7. Demoly P, Kropf R, Bircher A, Pichler WJ. Drug hypersensitivity questionnaire. *Allergy* 1999;54:999–1003.
8. Brochow K, Romano A, Blanca M, Ring J, Pichler WJ, Demoly P. General considerations for skin test procedures in the diagnosis of drug hypersensitivity. *Allergy* 2002;57:45–51.
9. Aberer W, Bircher A, Romano A, et al. Drug provocation testing in the diagnosis of drug hypersensitivity reactions: general considerations. *Allergy* 2003;58:854–863.
10. Blanca M, Romano A, Torres MJ, et al. Update on the evaluation of hypersensitivity reactions to β(beta)lactams. *Allergy* 2009;64:183–193.
11. Cephalosporin administration to patients with a history of penicillin allergy. The American Academy of Allergy, Asthma and Immunology. http://www.aaaai.org/members/academy_statements/. Accessed April 20, 2010.
12. Messaad D, Sahla H, Benahmed S, et al. Drug provocation tests in patients with a history suggesting an immediate drug hypersensitivity reaction. *Ann Intern Med* 2004;42:1001–1006.
13. Fontaine C, Mayorga L, Bousquet PJ, et al. Relevance of the determination of serm-specific IgE antibodies in the diagnosis of immediate β(beta)-lactam allergy. *Allergy* 2007;62:47–52.
14. Manfredi M, Severino M, Testi S, et al. Detection of specific IgE to quinolones. *J Allergy Clin Immunol* 2004;113:155–160.
15. Lebel B, Messaad D, Kvedariene V, Rongier M, Bousquet J, Demoly P. Cysteinyl-leukotriene release test (CAST) in the diagnosis of immediate drug reactions. *Allergy* 2001;56:688–692.
16. Torres MJ, Padial A, Mayorga C, et al. The diagnostic interpretation of basophil activation test in immediate allergic reactions to β(beta)lactams. *Clin Exp Allergy* 2004;34:1768–1775.
17. De Week AL, Sanz ML, Gamboa PM, et al. Diagnostic tests based on human basophils: more potentials and perspectives than pitfalls. II. Technical issues. *J Investig Allergol Clin Immunol* 2008;18:143–155.
18. Nyfeler B, Pichler WJ. The lymphocyte transformation test for the diagnosis of drug allergy: sensitivity and specificity. *Clin Exp Allergy* 1997;27:175–181.
19. Mertes PM, Alla F, Laxenaire MC. Anaphylactic and anaphylactoid reactions occurring during anesthesia in France in 1999–2000. *Anesthesiology* 2003;99:536–545.
20. Bousquet PJ, Demoly P, Romano A, et al. Pharmacovigilance of drug allergy and hypersensitivity using the ENDA-DAHD database and the GA²LEN platform. The Galenda Project. *Allergy* 2009;64:194–203.
21. Demoly P, Messaad D, Sahla H, et al. Six-hour trimethoprim-sulfamethoxazole graded challenge in HIV-infected patients. *J Allergy Clin Immunol.* 1998;102:1033–1036.
22. Legere III HJ, Palis RI, Rodriguez Bouza T, Uluer AZ, Castells M. A safe protocol for rapid desensitization in patients with cystic fibrosis and antibiotic hypersensitivity. *J Cyst Fibros* 2009;8:418–424.
23. Lantner RR. Ciprofloxacin desensitization in a patient with cystic fibrosis. *J Allergy Clin Immunol* 1995;96:1001–1002.
24. Moss RB, Babin S, Hsu Y, Blessing-Moore J, Levinston NJ. Allergy to semisynthetic penicillins in cystic fibrosis. *J Pediatr* 1984;104:460–466.
25. Matz J, Borish LC, Routes JM, Rosenwasser L. Oral desensitization to rifampicin and ethmabutol in Mycobacterial disease. *Am J Respir Crit Care Med* 1994;149:815–817.
26. Cars O, Molstad S, Melander A. Variation in antibiotic use in the European Union. *Lancet* 2001;357:1851–1853.
27. Guillemot D, Maison P, Carbon C, et al. Trends in antimicrobial drug use in the community-France, 1981–1992. *J Infect Dis* 1998;177:492–497.
28. Demoly P, Romano A. Update on β(beta)-lactam allergy diagnosis. *Curr Allergy Asthma Rep* 2005;5:9–14.
29. Rebelo Gomes E, Fonseca J, Araujo L, Demoly P. Drug allergy claims in children: from self-reporting to confirmed diagnosis. *Clin Exp Allergy* 2008;38:191–198.
30. Apter AJ, Kinman JL, Bilker WB, et al. Represcription of penicillin after allergic-like events. *J Allergy Clin Immunol* 2004;113:764–770.
31. Blanca M, Mayorga C, Torres MJ, et al. Side chain specific reactions to β(beta)lactams: Fourteen years later. *Clin Exp Allergy* 2002;32:192–197.
32. Executive summary of disease management of drug hypersensitivity: a practice parameter. Joint Task Force on Practice Parameters, the American Academy of Allergy, Asthma and Immunology, the American College of Allergy, Asthma and Immunology, and the Joint Council of Allergy, Asthma and Immunology. *Ann Allergy Asthma Immunol* 1999;83:665–700.
33. Romano A, Viola M, Bousquet PJ, et al. A comparison of the performance of two penicillin reagent kits in the diagnosis of β(beta)-lactam hypersensitivity. *Allergy* 2007;62:53–58.
34. Co Minh HB, Bousquet PJ, Fontaine C, et al. Systemic reactions during skin tests with β(beta)-lactams: a risk factor analysis. *J Allergy Clin Immunol* 2006;117:466–468.
35. Torres MJ, Romano A, Mayorga C, et al. Diagnostic evaluation of a large group of patients with immediate allergy to penicillins: the role of skin testing. *Allergy* 2001;56:850–856.

36. Chandra RK, Joglekar SA, Tomas E. Penicillin allergy: anti-penicillin IgE antibodies and immediate hypersensitivity skin reactions employing major and minor determinants of penicillin. *Arch Dis Child* 1980;55:857–860.
37. Blanca M, Torres MJ, García JJ, et al. Natural evolution of skin test sensitivity in patients allergic to β(beta)-lactam antibiotics. *J Allergy Clin Immunol* 1999;103:918–924.
38. Antunez C, Blanca-Lopez N, Torres MJ, et al. Immediate allergic reactions to cephalosporins: Evaluation of cross-reactivity with a panel of penicillins and cephalosporins. *J Allergy Clin Immunol* 2006;117:424–410.
39. Romano A, Guéant-Rodriguez RM, Viola M, et al. Diagnosing immediate reactions to cephalosporins. *Clin Exp Allergy* 2005;35:1234–1242.
40. Romano A, Guéant-Rodriguez RM, Viola M, et al. Cross-reactivity and tolerability of cephalosporins in patients with immediate hypersensitivity to penicillins. *Ann Intern Med* 2004;141:16–22.
41. Romano A, Viola M, Guéant-Rodriguez RM, et al. Imipenem in patients with immediate hypersensitivity to penicillins. *N Engl J Med* 2006;354:2835–2837.
42. Romano A, Viola M, Guéant-Rodriguez RM, et al. Brief communication: tolerability of meropenem in patients with IgE-mediated hypersensitivity to penicillins. *Ann Intern Med* 2007;146:266–269.
43. Gruchalla RS, Pirmohamed M. Antibiotic allergy. *N Engl J Med* 2006;354:601–609.
44. Bousquet PJ, Pipet A, Bousquet-Rouanet L, Demoly P. Oral challenges are needed in the diagnosis of β(beta)-lactam hypersensitivity. *Clin Exp Allergy* 2008;38:185–190.
45. Campi P, Pichler WJ. Quinolone hypersensitivity. *Curr Opin Allergy Clin Immunol* 2003;3:275–281.
46. Blayac JP, Hillaire-Buys D, Pinzani V. Fluoroquinolone and anaphylaxis. *Thérapie* 1996;51:417–418.
47. Valdivieso R, Pola J, Losada E, Subiza J, Armentia A, Zapata C. Severe anaphylactoid reaction to nalidixic acid. *Allergy* 1988;43:71–73.
48. Davila I, Diez ML, Quirce S, Fraj J, De La Hoz B, Lazaro M. Cross-reactivity between quinolones. Report of three cases. *Allergy* 1993;48:388–390.
49. Kurata M, Kasuga Y, Nanba E, Nakamura H, Asano T, Haruta K. Flush induced by fluoroquinolones in canine skin. *Inflamm Res* 1995;44:461–465.
50. Araújo L, Demoly P. Macrolides allergy. *Curr Pharm Des* 2008;14:2842–2862.
51. Pascual C, Crespo JF, Quiralte J, Lopez C, Wheeler G, Martin-Esteban M. In vitro detection of specific IgE antibodies to erythromycin. *J Allergy Clin Immunol* 1995;95:668–671.
52. Benahmed S, Scaramuzza C, Messaad D, Sahla H, Demoly P. The accuracy of the diagnosis of suspected macrolide antibiotic hypersensitivity: results of a single-blinded trial. *Allergy* 2004;59:1130–1133.
53. Cabañas R, Caballero MT, Vega A, Martín-Esteban M, Pascual C. Anaphylaxis to trimethoprim. *J Allergy Clin Immunol* 1996;97:137–138.
54. Gruchalla RS, Sullivan TJ. Detection of human IgE to sulfamethoxazole by skin testing with sulfamethoxazoyl-poly-L-tyrosine. *J Allergy Clin Immunol* 1991;8:784–792.
55. Anne' S, Middleton E Jr, Reisman RE. Vancomycin anaphylaxis and successful desensitization. *Ann Allergy* 1994;73:422–424.
56. Renz CL, Laroche D, Thurn JD, Finn HA, Lynch JP, Thisted R, Moss J. Tryptase levels are not increased during vancomycin-induced anaphylactoid reactions. *Anesthesiology* 1998;89:620–625.
57. Asero R. Teicoplanin-induced anaphylaxis. *Allergy* 2006;61:1370.
58. Schulze S, Wollina U. Gentamicin-induced anaphylaxis. *Allergy* 2003;58:88–89.
59. Abeck D, Kuwert C, Segnini-Torres M, Przybilla B, Ring J. Streptomycin-induced anaphylactic reaction during in vitro fertilization (IVF). *Allergy* 1994;49:388–389.
60. Iikura M, Yamaguchi M, Hirai K, et al. Case report: streptomycin-induced anaphylactic shock during oocyte retrieval procedures for in vitro fertilization. *J Allergy Clin Immunol* 2002;109:571–572.
61. Romano A, Viola M, Di Fonso M, Rosaria Perrone M, Gaeta F, Andriolo M. Anaphylaxis to streptomycin. *Allergy* 2002;57:1087–1088.
62. Dyck ED, Vadas P. Anaphylaxis to topical bacitracin. *Allergy* 1997;52:870–871.
63. Saryan JA, Dammin TC, Bouras AE. Anaphylaxis to topical bacitracin zinc ointment. *Am J Emerg Med* 1998;16:512–513.
64. Fox KA. Anaphylaxis caused by polymixin B sulfate and zinc bacitracin ointment. *J Emerg Nurs* 1994;20:262–264.
65. Sharif S, Goldberg B. Detection of IgE antibodies to bacitracin using a commercially available streptavidin-linked solid phase in a patient with anaphylaxis to triple antibiotic ointment. *Ann Allergy Asthma Immunol* 2007;98:563–566.
66. Earl HS, Sullivan TJ. Acute desensitization of a patient with cystic fibrosis allergic to both β(beta)-lactam and aminoglycoside antibiotics. *J Allergy Clin Immunol* 1987;79:477–483.
67. Lee YD, Cho Y, Han MS. Anaphylaxis to ribostamycin. *Allergy* 2004;59:1134–1135.
68. Magnan A, Venemalm L, Porri F, et al. Anaphylactic reaction to rifamycin SV: presence of specific IgE antibodies. *J Allergy Clin Immunol* 1999;103:954–956.
69. Crook MJ. Isoniazid-induced anaphylaxis. *J Clin Pharmacol* 2003;43:545–546.

70. Harland RW, Lindblom SS, Munnell MO. Anaphylaxis from rifampin. *Am J Med* 1992;92:581–582.
71. Bottenberg MM, Wall GC, Hicklin GA. Apparent anaphylactoid reaction after treatment with a single dose of telithromycin. *Ann Allergy Asthma Immunol* 2007;98:89–91.
72. Asensio Sánchez T, Dávila I, Moreno E, et al. Anaphylaxis due to metronidazole with positive skin prick test. *J Investig Allergol Clin Immunol* 2008;18:138–139.
73. Chiou CS, Lin SM, Lin SP, Chang WG, Chan KH, Ting CK. Clindamycin-induced anaphylactic shock during general anesthesia. *J Chin Med Assoc* 2006;69:549–551.
74. Vaidya SJ, Seydel C, Patel SR, Ortin M. Anaphylactic reaction to liposomal amphotericin B. *Ann Pharmacother* 2002;36:1480–1481.
75. Rosales MJ, Vega F. Anaphylactic shock due to fosfomycin. *Allergy* 1998;53:905–907.
76. Palchick BA, Funk EA, McEntire JE, Hamory BH. Anaphylaxis due to chloramphenicol. *Am J Med Sci* 1984;288:43–45.
77. Bensaid B, Rozieres A, Berard F, Bienvenu J, Nicolas JF. IgE-mediated allergy to pristinamycin: the value of skin tests and basophil activation tests. *Allergy* 2009;64:1694.
78. Rubio M, Bousquet PJ, Demoly P. IgE-mediated anaphylaxis to pristinamycin—report of a case. *Allergy* 2010; in press. *Allergy* 2010;65:1198–9.

# Chapter 11
# Anaphylaxis During Radiological Procedures and in the Peri-operative Setting

**Pascale Dewachter and David L. Hepner**

**Abstract** IgE-mediated anaphylaxis remains one of the rare but significant events specifically related to contrast agents or drugs used during the perioperative period that can lead to morbidity and mortality. Its clinical diagnosis, initially presumptive, is not always obvious. However, anesthesiologists and radiologists must know the different clinical symptoms heralding anaphylaxis in order to provide the appropriate care management according to the severity of the clinical reaction. Clinical signs are described by the *Ring and Messmer* four-step grading scale, which also helps to guide care according to the severity of the reaction. Grade I and II reactions are usually not life-threatening. Conversely, Grade III and IV reactions are likely to be life threatening and require immediate resuscitative measures including epinephrine and fluid therapy. Early administration of epinephrine remains the cornerstone of anaphylaxis treatment; the appropriate dose should be administered according to the clinical picture. Biochemical tests, either in vivo or in vitro, including at least tryptase level are measured following the clinical reaction, and may help to prove its pathomechanism. Skin tests remain the *gold standard* for the detection of IgE-mediated reactions and should be performed according to strict rules. Skin tests remain the cornerstone of the allergological assessment in order to identify the culprit agent, prove the pathomechanism of the reaction and provide advice for further procedures. Accordingly, this review also focuses on the clinical pathway used to reintroduce a contrast agent or a neuromuscular blocking agent in patients having presented a documented anaphylactic response to one of these drugs.

Finally, as no preemptive therapeutic strategies have been proven to prevent anaphylaxis during the perioperative or radiological settings, an allergological follow-up in patients having presented an immediate reaction, either in the radiological or in the perioperative settings, is highly recommended in order to prevent further recurrences.

**Keywords** Anaphylaxis • Anesthesia • Contrast media • Epinephrine • Histamine • Hypersensitivity • Immediate • Premedication • Skin tests • Tryptases

## 11.1 Introduction

Anaphylaxis remains one of the rare but significant events specifically related to contrast agents or anesthetic drugs that can lead to morbidity and mortality, even in previously healthy patients. In the perioperative and radiological settings, clinical presentations of anaphylaxis may be very rapid,

D.L. Hepner (✉)
Harvard Medical School, Brigham and Women's Hospital, Boston, MA, USA
e-mail: dhepner@partners.org

M.C. Castells (ed.), *Anaphylaxis and Hypersensitivity Reactions*,
DOI 10.1007/978-1-60327-951-2_11, © Springer Science+Business Media, LLC 2011

variable in clinical features and diagnosis might be missed altogether. The aims of this chapter are to describe the different clinical expressions suggestive of anaphylaxis occurring during the perioperative period and radiological procedures and to detail the allergological assessment. This evaluation should include at least skin tests performed in order to prove the pathophysiological mechanism of the reaction and to identify the suspected agent in order to prevent further recurrences. As no preemptive therapeutic strategies have been proven to prevent anaphylaxis, this review also focuses on the clinical pathway used to reintroduce a contrast agent or a neuromuscular blocking agent in patients having presented a documented anaphylactic response to one of these drugs. Finally, the management of the different clinical expressions of anaphylaxis will also be detailed.

## 11.2 Definition

Anaphylaxis occurring during the perioperative or in the radiological settings is a potential life-threatening condition that may be difficult to identify because multiple drugs and substances are used for anesthesia and surgical/radiological procedures. It is a clinical syndrome involving multiple organ systems. The clinical expressions are the consequences of the immediate release of preformed inflammatory mediators from mast cells and basophils.

In the early 2000s, the European Academy of Allergology and Clinical Immunology Task Force published a revised nomenclature for allergic and related reactions [1]. The aim of this report was to propose a revised nomenclature for these reactions that can be used independent of target organ or patient age group. According to this, hypersensitivity reactions correspond to the "reproducible signs or symptoms, initiated by exposure to a defined stimulus at a dose tolerated by normal subjects." Immediate reactions with clinical signs suggesting allergy were called immediate hypersensitivity reactions and were subdivided into "non-allergic hypersensitivity" reactions (where an immune mechanism is excluded) and "allergic hypersensitivity" reactions (where a specific immune mechanism is proven or is highly suspected). In vivo and in vitro procedures can be used to differentiate between allergic and non-allergic immediate hypersensitivity reactions.

However, the concept of immediate reaction remains undefined by the European Academy of Allergology and Clinical Immunology in terms of onset delay between the introduction of the suspected agent and the initiation of the reaction [1]. Nevertheless, it is generally admitted that immediate reactions occur within 60 min following the injection/introduction of the culprit drug/agent [2]. Because the term anaphylaxis had been applied to different entities, a clinical definition regardless of the target organ failure was used. Thus, anaphylaxis has been defined as "a severe life-threatening generalized or systemic hypersensitivity reaction" [1] (Table 11.1). While "allergic anaphylaxis" refers to an immunologic mechanism including IgE-mediated mechanism, "non-allergic anaphylaxis" refers to "all other situations." Nevertheless, it was underlined that hypotension and severe bronchospasm do not have to be present for a reaction to be classified as anaphylaxis [1], thus indicating that not only severe reactions may be IgE-mediated. This nomenclature published as the official European Academy of Allergology and Clinical Immunology Position Statement was updated in 2003 by the Nomenclature Review Committee of the World Allergy Organization [3]. More recently, the Joint Task Force representing the American Academy of Allergy, Asthma and Immunology, the American College of Allergy, Asthma and Immunology and the Joint Council of Allergy, Asthma and Immunology proposed an updated practice parameter on anaphylaxis [4]. As previously suggested by the European Academy of Allergology and Clinical Immunology [1], anaphylaxis was also defined as a clinical event, i.e., "an acute, life-threatening systemic reaction with varied mechanisms, clinical presentations, and severity that results from the sudden systemic release of mediators from mast cells and basophil mediators." This definition is also being described independent of target organ or patient age group [4]. In 2006, the second National Institute of

**Table 11.1** Nomenclature based on the present knowledge of the mechanisms that initiate and mediate allergic reactions according to the European Academy of Allergology and Clinical Immunology (*EAACI*) [1] updated by the World Allergy Organization (*WAO*) [3] and compared to the updated practice parameter proposed by the American Academy of Allergy, Asthma and Immunology (*AAAAI*) [4] and the second National Institute of Allergy and Infectious Disease/Food Allergy and Anaphylaxis Network (*NIAID* and *FAAN*) [5]

| | EAACI 2001 [5] | WAO 2003 [4] | AAAAI 2005 [3] | NIAID and FAAN 2006 [5] |
|---|---|---|---|---|
| Statement | *Hypersensitivity* causes reproducible symptoms or signs initiated by exposure to a defined stimulus at a dose tolerated by normal subjects<br>Distinction between *allergic* (immunologic defined or strongly suspected) and *non-allergic hypersensitivity* (when immunologic mechanism cannot be proven) | Same as EAACI [3] | The term *hypersensitivity* [4] has not been defined | The term *hypersensitivity* has not been defined |
| Definition of Anaphylaxis | Severe, life-threatening, generalized or systemic hypersensitivity reaction | Same as EAACI | An acute, life-threatening systemic reaction with varied mechanisms, clinical presentations, and Severity | Serious allergic reaction that is rapid in onset and may cause death |
| Mechanism | *Allergic anaphylaxis* when an immunologic mechanism can be shown *or non-allergic anaphylaxis* where an immunologic mechanism can be ruled out | Same as EAACI | Condition caused by an IgE-mediated reaction | Condition caused by an IgE-mediated reaction |
| Anaphylactoïd | This term should not be used | Not precise | Reactions that produce the same clinical picture as anaphylaxis but are not IgE-mediated | Non-IgE-mediated anaphylactic reactions |
| Precision | Hypotension and severe bronchospasm do not have to be present for a reaction to be classified as anaphylaxis | Not precise | Not precise | Not precise |

Allergy and Infectious Disease/Food Allergy and Anaphylaxis Network symposium recommended the following definition "Anaphylaxis is a serious allergic reaction that is rapid in onset and may cause death" [5].

Finally, while anaphylaxis is mostly defined as an IgE-mediated condition, anaphylactoid reactions correspond to those that produce the same clinical features without being IgE-mediated [4, 5]. Nevertheless, although the European Academy of Allergology and Clinical Immunology committee recommended to no longer utilize the term *anaphylactoid* [1], other organizations did not follow suit [4, 5].

Allergic hypersensitivity is initiated by an immune mechanism due, in most cases, to specific IgE-antibodies bound to high affinity $F_C$RI receptors located in the membrane of tissue mast cells and blood basophils. If reintroduced, the allergen binds specifically to the corresponding IgEs, creating a bridge, which then aggregate and instantly induce cell degranulation leading to a massive release of inflammatory preformed mediators from sensitized mast cells and basophils. Anaphylaxis therefore corresponds to the explosive clinical expression of the silent underlying sensitization and should be considered as an exaggerated inflammatory acute response to a designated foreign antigen. A very small dose of allergen is sufficient for the cells to react. The different target organs involved commonly include the skin, the mucous membranes, the cardiovascular and respiratory systems and the gastrointestinal tract.

In conclusion, anaphylaxis is an acute inflammatory IgE-mediated reaction which is mostly unanticipated in onset and potentially life-threatening.

## 11.3 Epidemiology

### *11.3.1 Immediate Reactions Following Iodinated Contrast Agents*

Large epidemiological studies (retrospective and prospective) on immediate reactions following iodinated contrast media (ICM) have been published in different countries. The common point of these studies is the absence of an etiological diagnosis performed in order to distinguish the pathophysiological mechanisms and identify the culprit agent. Therefore, data on immediate reactions and deaths following ICM correspond to their incidence regardless of the mechanisms involved.

#### 11.3.1.1 Hyperosmolar Ionic Iodinated Contrast Media

In 1975 and 1980, two prospective multicenter surveys on immediate adverse reactions following hyperosmolar ionic ICM administration involving 30 teaching hospitals from the USA, Canada, Europe and Australia, and including more than 112,000 and 300,000 procedures respectively, found an overall incidence of adverse reactions of 5% [6, 7]. A 1-year prospective multicenter survey in the United Kingdom among more than 150,000 patients who had intravenous urography found an incidence of severe reactions of 0.02% [8].

#### 11.3.1.2 Comparison Between Ionic and Non-ionic Contrast Media

In Australia, the overall incidences of reactions (1.2% vs 3.8%) and of severe reactions (0.02% versus 0.09%) were significantly lower with non-ionic ICM than with ionic ICM, respectively [9]. The largest multicenter prospective study included more than 330,000 patients and was carried out in Japan over 22 months [10]. In this study, where 50.1% of the patients received high-osmolar ionic

ICM and 49.9% low-osmolar non-ionic, the overall incidence of adverse reactions was 12.7% with ionic and 3.1% with non-ionic ICM. Severe reactions occurred in 0.22% of the patients who received ionic ICM and 0.04% of the patients who received non-ionic. Thereafter, a quantitative meta-analysis carried out by collecting relevant data reported between 1980 and 1989 demonstrated that the risk of severe, non-fatal reactions with high-osmolar ionic ICM was estimated at 1,570 per million uses compared to 310 per million for low-osmolar ionic and non-ionic ICM, suggesting that 80% of severe reactions could be prevented by using low-osmolar ICM [11].

Lasser published a comparison of adverse reactions following ICM reported to the US Food and Drug Administration and to the manufacturers between 1990 and 1994 [12]. The incidence per million procedures was higher with high-osmolar ionic ICM than with low-osmolar non-ionic ICM for all reported reactions (193.8 vs 44.4), for severe reactions (37.4 vs 10.5) and for deaths (3.9 vs 2.1). A higher overall incidence of total reactions was also found for high-osmolar ionic ICM compared with low-osmolar ionic ICM (193.8 vs 142.5 per million examinations), whereas the incidence of severe reactions was similar (37.4 versus 33.6). In older studies, the mean incidence of deaths with high-osmolar ICM was 100 per million uses before 1975 [6]. It was reduced 16-fold (six deaths per million uses) 15 years later, the number of deaths being the same for ionic and for non-ionic ICM [10]. Conversely, Lasser [12] demonstrated that the highest incidence of deaths was observed with low-osmolar ionic ICM (6.4 per million procedures), followed by high-osmolar ionic ICM (3.9 per million) and by low-osmolar non-ionic monomers (2.1 per million). The highest incidence of deaths with low-osmolar ionic ICM when compared to high-osmolar was probably due to the moving from high-osmolar to low-osmolar ICM. In France, in a study carried out in 1996 in public hospitals, the incidence of deaths following ICM was estimated at 3–6 per million uses [13]. In the United States, between 1967 and 1994, 1,078 deaths related to ICM have been reported to the *US Food and Drug Administration*, 850 occurring during the period 1978–1994 [14]. This retrospective analysis showed an increase of 42% in the number of deaths each year from 1987 to 1994, compared with the previous period 1978–1986. Most of this increase was associated with the use of non-ionic ICM, whereas during the same period, a decrease of 32% in the number of deaths was annually reported with the use of ionic ICM. Thus, and in contrast to older studies, this analysis demonstrated that the number of deaths increased significantly with non-ionic ICM. This trend reflected the increase of procedures involving ICM as well as the evolution of the market share moving from ionic to non-ionic ICM.

Finally, different criteria for grading ICM reactions have been proposed by Shehadi [6, 7], Ansell [8], Palmer [9] and Katayama [10], based on the necessity to initiate a treatment and/or a hospitalization. Clinical signs were described in only two studies [6, 7, 10], and death was not considered in the classification of Palmer [9]. Therefore, the comparison of these surveys is made difficult by the differences in the severity scales used and the absence of a documented diagnosis.

In summary, all non-ionic and ionic ICM may induce immediate reactions including anaphylaxis, sometimes being fatal.

### 11.3.2 Immediate Reactions to Gadolinium-Containing Contrast Agents

No prospective multicenter study investigating patients having presented immediate reactions following gadolinium chelates has been published. Acute adverse reactions to gadolinium chelates were recorded in one center between 1999 and 2004 and retrospectively analyzed according to the severity of the reaction. They were subdivided into mild, moderate and severe based on presentation and the requirement for treatment [15]. The adverse reaction rate was considered to be at 0.48% and the incidence of severe *anaphylactoid* reactions was 0.01%. In a post-marketing surveillance study, adverse effects following gadoterate meglumine were considered to be at 0.4% among more than

24,000 procedures performed in 61 institutions, most of these considered to be mild [16]. However, no investigation of the different pathophysiological mechanisms involved was performed in these studies [15, 16]. Anaphylaxis to gadolinium chelates has been reported [17–21], including deaths (unpublished personal data). Moreover, immediate hypersensitivity reactions may occur with each commercially available gadolinium chelates [22].

Finally, in the absence of systematic follow-up and investigation of patients experiencing immediate reactions following ICM and gadolinium chelates, the incidence of anaphylaxis and its associated mortality remain unknown. However, the potential allergic risk involving these agents should not be underestimated.

### *11.3.3 Immediate Reactions in the Perioperative Setting*

In contrast to the data provided on immediate reactions to contrast agents, the epidemiology on perioperative immediate reactions is more accurate even if underreported. Indeed, many prospective multicenter studies have been performed in Australia [23–25], New Zealand [26], the United Kingdom [27–31] and France [32–34] for many decades. Moreover, other follow-up studies have been reported more recently in Scandinavia [35, 36] and Spain [37].

By promoting an allergological assessment linked to the clinical history, some studies have provided data on the incidence of perioperative immediate reactions and anaphylaxis, on the different pathophysiological mechanisms involved, on the causes and on the risk factors. Thus, the overall incidence of perioperative immediate hypersensitivity reactions was estimated in the early 1980s to be at one in 5,000–13,000 anesthetic procedures in Australia [23], one in 1,250–5,000 in New Zealand [26, 38], one in 3,500 in the United Kingdom [27], and one in 4,600 in France [39].

While the overall incidence of perioperative anaphylaxis is estimated to be one in 10,000–20,000 anesthetic procedures in Australia [40] and one in 13,000 in France [41], the incidence of perioperative anaphylaxis to neuromuscular blocking agents (NMBAs) is estimated to be one in 6,500 administrations of NMBAs in France [41] and one in 5,200 in a single-center follow up study in Norway [36]. The morbidity of perioperative anaphylaxis remains unknown, likely underreported, probably due to medicolegal concerns. In the early 1990s, the mortality was estimated to be 3% of anesthesia-related immediate reactions in Australia [42] and 5% in Japan [43]. More recently, 3% of the deaths partially or completely related to anesthesia in France were related to anaphylaxis [44] and 10% of anesthesia-related immediate hypersensitivity reactions reported to the United Kingdom Medicines Control Agency and occurring between January 1995 and June 2001 were fatal [45]. However, the data provided by this British report should be interpreted cautiously as less-severe reactions were probably underreported [2].

Finally, the exact incidence of perioperative anaphylaxis and their associated morbidity and mortality remain underestimated because not all cases are explored, published, reported to the Drug Safety Monitoring Authorities, or included in a national register.

## 11.4 How to Diagnose Anaphylaxis

The etiological diagnosis of immediate reactions occurring in the radiological and perioperative settings is linked to a triad including clinical, biological and allergological elements. The interpretation of the allergological assessment *should always* be correlated to the careful and complete review of the clinical history. The joint analysis of these elements helps to ensure an accurate diagnosis, i.e., to determine the pathophysiological mechanism involved, to identify the culprit agent and to provide subsequent recommendations for further anesthetic or radiological procedures.

### 11.4.1 The Clinical History Should Always Be Known for an Appropriate Diagnosis

The initial diagnosis of anaphylaxis is only presumptive but needs to be promptly made because anaphylaxis may be life-threatening within a few minutes even in previously healthy patients [46]. The first element for the diagnosis of anaphylaxis includes the timing between the introduction of the suspected allergen and the onset of symptoms, and the description of the features and severity of clinical signs. The epinephrine total dosage requirement is likely to help estimating the severity level of the reaction [47]. Anaphylaxis is a clinical syndrome that varies in severity and is associated with clinical features which may include cardiovascular symptoms (tachycardia, bradycardia, cardiac arrythmia, hypotension, cardiovascular collapse, cardiac arrest), bronchospasm and mucocutaneous signs (erythema, urticaria, angioedema) [2, 46–49]. The clinical signs are described according to the Ring and Messmer four-step grading scale [50] which was adapted for perioperative immediate reactions (Table 11.2) [47, 48, 51]. This clinical scale also helps to guide care accordingly to the severity of the reaction. Grade I reactions involve mucocutaneous signs and grade II reactions correspond to moderate clinical features which may be associated with mucocutaneous, cardiovascular and respiratory signs. While the cardinal sign of grade III reactions is cardiovascular collapse which may be associated with mucocutaneous signs and bronchospasm, cardiac arrest is associated with grade IV reactions. Thus, grades I and II reactions are not usually life-threatening conditions, whereas grades III and IV reactions correspond to emergency situations requiring prompt resuscitation.

Multisystem involvement is usually present but not always observed. Anaphylaxis consists of cardiovascular homeostasis disturbances usually associated with mucocutaneous signs, and which may be associated with respiratory signs. Bronchospasm is usually present in patients with asthma and chronic obstructive pulmonary disease [2, 47]. Cardiovascular symptoms often include hypotension and tachycardia, but may rapidly evolve into severe arrhythmias and cardiovascular collapse if not recognized and treated promptly [47]. Moreover, cardiovascular collapse or cardiac arrest may be the presenting feature [2, 46–48]. Consequently, for severe reactions (Grade III and IV), the prognosis relies on the hemodynamic response to the initial treatment.

Some singular cardiovascular events are also reported with the occurrence of allergic hypersensitivity. Acute coronary syndromes *(Kounis syndrome)* associated with mast cell activation, also called *allergic angina* or *allergic myocardial infarction,* have been recently reported [52]. Patients without predisposing factors for coronary artery disease in whom the allergic reaction triggers either coronary artery spasm without cardiac enzymes increase, or coronary artery spasm evolving to myocardial infarction belong to the variant I of this entity. This variant might represent a clinical manifestation of underlying endothelial dysfunction [52]. Conversely, variant II occurs in patients with predisposing factors where the allergic reaction induces plaque erosion or rupture and consequently myocardial infarction.

**Table 11.2** Clinical severity scale of immediate reactions adapted from [46]

| Grades | Clinical signs |
|---|---|
| I | *Cutaneous-mucous signs:* erythema, urticaria with or without angioedema |
| II | *Moderate multivisceral signs:* cutaneous-mucous signs ± hypotension ± tachycardia ± dyspnea ± gastrointestinal disturbances |
| III | *Life-threatening mono or multivisceral signs:* cardiovascular collapse, tachycardia or bradycardia ± cardiac dysrythmia ± bronchospasm ± cutaneous-mucous signs ± gastrointestinal disturbances |
| IV | *Cardiac arrest* |

Apical ballooning syndrome also called *Tako-Tsubo syndrome* or stress cardiomyopathy has been reported following perioperative anaphylaxis [53, 54] or anaphylaxis outside the perioperative period [55–58]. This cardiac syndrome is characterized by an acute but rapidly reversible left ventricular systolic dysfunction. The diagnosis is supported by four criteria: (1) ST-segment changes or T-wave inversions on the electrocardiogram; (2) transient wall motion abnormalities; (3) normal coronary anatomy; (4) absence of any underlying pathology which may explain the myocardial dysfunction (head trauma, intracranial hemorrhage, pheochromocytoma) [57]. Three variants have been described where the common denominator is midventricular akinesis. These include the *apical ballooning variant* (apical and midventricular akinesis with preserved base), the *midventricular ballooning variant* (midventricular akinesis with preserved apex and base), and the *basal ballooning variant* (midventricular and basal akinesis with preserved apex) [59]. The pathophysiology of Tako-Tsubo syndrome remains unclear and different triggers may be involved including emotional, physical, non-cardiac surgery, severe pain or cocaine abuse. Nevertheless, it has been suggested that the administration of epinephrine and other catecholamines at pharmacologic or supra-pharmacologic doses can be sufficient to induce one of the three variants of Tako-Tsubo cardiomyopathy. However, the role of endogenous catecholamines in response to anaphylaxis cannot be ruled out [54]. In the few reported cases following anaphylaxis, inappropriate doses of epinephrine seem to be the common trigger of this cardiomyopathy [53–58]. The various distribution of cardiac β(beta)-receptors in the general population might explain the different anatomic forms [57]. A complete resolution of stress cardiomyopathy is usually the case [60]. Thus, it is important for practitioners to be aware of the potential harmful effects of the inappropriate use of epinephrine during anaphylaxis.

The clinical signs of anaphylaxis usually occur after a few minutes, especially after intravascular routes, but may be delayed up to an hour [2]. Anaphylaxis typically resolves in 2–8 h and resolution is usually complete except in cases of brain damage or disordered clotting [2]. *Biphasic anaphylaxis,* a potentially life-threatening recurrence of anaphylaxis, has been described with an onset of 8 h (ranges from 1 to 78 h) following initial presentation and an incidence of up to 20%, and has been described following contrast agents, antibiotics, other drugs and food [61]. However, no study concerning biphasic anaphylaxis occurring during the perioperative period has been published. Thus, its incidence during the perioperative period remains unknown. The severity of the second response varies indicating that patients should be followed carefully after apparent remission of anaphylaxis [61].

Some risk factors of anaphylaxis have been suggested but remain controversial. Although asthmatic patients or those receiving β(beta)-blockers have been considered to be at-risk of anaphylaxis, no epidemiologic study indicates that anaphylaxis is more frequent in either of these patients[2, 4] during the perioperative or radiological settings. Asthma, especially if not optimally controlled, is an important risk factor for death from anaphylaxis [62]. Concurrent administration of β(beta)-blockers, angiotensin-converting enzyme blockers and to a lesser extent angiotensin II blockers might interfere with the hemodynamic response to treatment [2, 62], requiring higher than usual doses of epinephrine. Moreover, concurrent underlying cardiovascular disease might be aggravated by the occurrence of anaphylaxis [2, 62]. Thus, all of these factors should be considered comorbid rather than at-risk factors [62].

In contrast, risk factors for subsequent anaphylaxis include uninvestigated patients experiencing clinical signs that suggest an allergic reaction during a previous anesthetic or radiological procedure, and patients having experienced clinical manifestations of allergy when exposed to latex or following tropical fruits ingestion (e.g., avocado, banana, papaya or kiwi); this latter entity known as Latex-Fruit Syndrome [63]. In addition, there is cross-reactivity of latex with chestnuts, hazelnuts, walnuts, and peanuts [63].

In contrast, atopic patients (except for latex due to the high prevalence of latex sensitization in these patients) or those who are allergic to a medication (except for antibiotics) that is not likely to be used during the perioperative period are not to be considered at risk for anaphylaxis [48].

## 11.4.2 Predictive Criteria of Anaphylaxis Severity

Three predictive criteria have been identified to be associated with the severity of the anaphylactic reaction [51]: (1) The speed of onset of the anaphylactic reaction after allergen exposure: the fastest the onset, the more likely is the reaction to be severe and life-threatening [4]; (2) The occurrence of urticaria and angioedema: although these are the most common cutaneous manifestations of anaphylaxis, they might be delayed or absent in a rapidly progressive anaphylaxis as the subcutaneous vascular bed is susceptible to *vasoconstrictive* influences especially when circulatory homeostasis is threatened [4]. The usual cutaneous signs of *vasodilatation* may only appear following normalization of the blood pressure. Although rare, the clinician should be aware of its possibility, as the absence of an initial cutaneous vasodilation should not preclude the diagnosis of anaphylaxis; (3) Paradoxical sinus bradycardia, a relatively infrequent hemodynamic sign observed in major hypovolemic states, can also be seen in severe anaphylaxis. This paradoxical bradycardia is a result of massive hypovolemia and has been reported to be as high as 10% of patients with anaphylaxis during anesthesia [2]. Under this circumstance, bradycardia should be considered as a life-saving adaptative mechanism. A sudden decrease in peripheral resistance along with decreased venous return triggers bradycardia probably in order to preserve cardiac filling despite profound hypovolemia. This cardio-inhibitory reflex, knows as *Bezold-Jarisch reflex,* is originating in sensory receptors of the left ventricle and is transmitted by unmyelinated vagal C-fibers. Thus, it is now understood that some inhibitory reflexes originating from cardiac sensory receptors play a role in cardiovascular homeostasis [64]. Physicians should be aware of this possibility since the administration of atropine is contraindicated in this clinical setting, as it would oppose this reflex and lead to cardiac arrest [51]. The adequate treatment in this clinical setting is a large volume expansion followed by epinephrine [51].

## 11.4.3 Are There Any Clinical Differences Between Anaphylaxis Occurring During the Perioperative and the Radiological Setting?

### 11.4.3.1 In the Perioperative Setting

Reactions occur mostly immediately after the induction of anesthesia and usually involve NMBAs or antibiotics [46]. However, anaphylaxis may also occur at any time during the perioperative period with all drugs or substances used during anesthesia or surgery being potentially allergenic [47, 48]. The clinical symptoms usually appear within minutes, even within 1 min, after intravascular routes but anaphylaxis may also occur following other routes, i.e., cutaneous, mucosal or intra-articular [2]. Latex-induced reactions, which account for the second most common cause of anaphylaxis under anesthesia behind NMBAs [33], are usually described as occurring 30–60 min after the beginning of the surgical procedure [2]. However, they may occur relatively soon after the induction, likely correlated to the higher level of sensitization to latex of high-risk patients [65, 66].

The reported clinical features are cardiovascular symptoms (tachycardia, cardiac arrhythmias, hypotension, cardiovascular collapse, cardiac arrest), bronchospasm and mucocutaneous signs (erythema, urticaria, angioedema) [46]. However, during severe perioperative anaphylaxis, the most common reported initial clinical features are pulselessness, desaturation and lung insufflation difficulty due to severe bronchospasm [40]. Cutaneous signs seem to be more frequently observed than angioedema during the perioperative period [33, 36]. In contrast, gastrointestinal signs are usually not present under anesthesia. Accordingly, in three recent studies on perioperative anaphylaxis, cardiovascular, respiratory and mucocutaneous signs were predominant. In the latest French multicenter study including 491 perioperative anaphylaxis cases, the majority of reactions were severe (60% grade III and 6% grade IV). Grade I reactions accounted for 11% of all reactions and Grade II reactions for 23%. Whereas cardiovascular signs, including cardiac arrest, were involved in 79% of the cases, respiratory and cutaneous manifestations were present in 40% and 66% of cases respectively [34]. In a single-center follow-up Norwegian study of 83 patients, only 1% of perioperative anaphylaxis cases were grade I, 30% grade II, 63% grade III and 6% grade IV. The most frequent reported clinical feature was bronchospasm (78%), followed by cardiovascular signs (63%) and mucocutaneous signs (70%) [36]. More recently, in a Spanish study investigating 48 less severe perioperative anaphylaxis cases (primarily grade I and II reactions), cardiovascular and respiratory signs and symptoms were present in 27% and 23% of patients respectively, while cutaneous signs were present in 83% of cases [37].

#### 11.4.3.2 In the Radiological Setting

As early as 1940, severe immediate reactions attributed to anaphylaxis were reported with a di-iodinated contrast medium *iodopyracet* (Diodrast) [67–71]. Clinical signs consistent with an immediate allergic reaction including cyanosis, bronchospasm, seizures, cardiovascular collapse and cardiac arrest, occurring within 10 min of the ICM injection, were reported. Some of these reactions were triggered by a very small dose of contrast agent.

More recently, anaphylaxis following intravascular ICM or gadolinium chelates was supported by an allergological assessment including biochemical measurements and/or skin testing [19–21, 72–76]. *General signs* reported during these immediate reactions involved shivering, hypothermia and hyperthermia, while pruritus, nausea, dyspnea, and weakness constituted *functional signs. Objective signs* included mucocutaneous (erythema, urticaria, angioedema), cardiovascular (tachycardia, supraventricular or ventricular arrhythmias, arterial hypotension, cardiovascular collapse, cardiac arrest), respiratory (dyspnea, bronchospasm), digestive (vomiting) and neurologic (consciousness impairment). Documented anaphylaxis following ICM has also been reported following ureteropyelography [77], and gastric band adjustment [78]. Angioedema seems to be relatively frequent during immediate hypersensitivity reactions following ICM. In a small series of patients following ICM, angioedema was observed in 25% of the cases, urticaria in 33% and erythema in 11% [79].

Clinical signs following contrast agents usually occur within minutes following intravascular ICM injection [19–21, 72–76]. However, the reported onset delay can be as late as 30 min [75].

A recent multicenter prospective study including 26 Canadian and American university-affiliated radiology departments demonstrated that although radiologists should be able to manage ICM-induced allergic reactions in the acute setting, they have a poor knowledge of epinephrine administration for severe contrast agent-induced anaphylaxis [80]. Thus, since the hallmark of anaphylaxis in the perioperative period or following radiological procedures are sustained cardiovascular homeostasis disturbances, their care management should be taught regularly in order to compensate for the relative low frequency with which the average practitioner would encounter anaphylaxis in routine clinical care.

### *11.4.4 Which Tools to Prove the Diagnosis?*

In vivo and in vitro procedures can be used to differentiate between allergic and non-allergic (i.e., anaphylactoid) hypersensitivity reactions.

#### 11.4.4.1 Biological Assessment Is a Contributive Tool to the Appropriate Diagnosis

In vivo Biochemical Tests

Histamine is a preformed mediator produced by basophils and mast cells. An increased concentration of plasma histamine indicates in vivo release and is observed during both allergic and non-allergic reactions. The peak of plasma histamine is immediate; its plasma half-life is around 15–20 min [81], and can be measured by radio-immunoassay [82]. Following an immediate hypersensitivity reaction, blood should be withdrawn for histamine measurement within a short time (15 min after the reaction) for grade I reactions, within 30 min for grade II reactions and within 30 and 120 min for more severe reactions [48, 81]. Moreover, histamine and its metabolite (N-methylhistamine) may also be measured in a 24-h urine sample [83].

Tryptase is a neutral serine protease contained predominantly in mast-cells. Human basophils also contain tryptase, but their levels are 300- to 700-fold lower than in skin or lung mast cells [84]. Tryptases secreted by these inflammatory cells may enter into the circulation. Three forms of tryptase including α(alpha)-, β(beta)- and γ(gamma)-tryptases are described. At present, there is no evidence that δ(delta) tryptase appears in serum or that it plays a biologic role. β(beta)-tryptases, processed by removal of the propeptide (β(beta)-protryptase), are assembled into tetramers, stored within the mast-cells and released into the bloodstream during anaphylaxis [84, 85]. α(alpha)-tryptases, which have a mutation preventing removal of the propeptide, are secreted constitutively by mast cells along with residual pro-β(beta) tryptase. However, α(alpha)-tryptases are not stored in secretory granules and thus will not contribute either to an increase in tryptase levels following mast cell degranulation or to mast cell burden [85] γ(gamma)-tryptase, activated by propeptide removal, remains tethered to the membrane of mast cells when released from the granules [85]. While mature β(beta)-tryptase reflects mast cell activation, pro-β(beta)-tryptase secreted constitutively serves as a measure of total body mast cell content [84]. The total tryptase level, measured in serum by fluoro-immunoassay, consists primarily of the sum of pro- α(alpha) and pro-β(beta)-tryptases, the latter being the major contributor [2, 85]. A higher specificity in the diagnosis of anaphylaxis might be obtained by measuring mature β(beta)-tryptase in addition to total tryptase (pro- β(beta) and pro- α(alpha)-tryptases) [85].

Following allergic reactions, tryptase concentration reaches a peak between 15 min and 1 h and decreases slowly, with a half-life of 90–120 min [2, 47, 48]. Tryptase increase is specific for mast cell activation, as occurring during anaphylaxis[2, 47, 48, 84]. However, less pronounced rise of tryptase may be observed during non-immunological reactions [2]. While an increase in tryptase can be measured 30–60 min after onset of symptoms in cases of mild reactions, sampling is recommended within 30 min and 2 h in cases of grades III or IV reactions [47, 48, 84]. A new sample of tryptase should be collected more than 24 h after the reaction or at the time of the consultation in order to compare the concentrations at the time of the reaction with baseline levels [47, 48, 84].

Thus, in cases of immediate non-allergic reactions (e.g., *histamine release*), histamine may be increased while tryptase usually remains normal. However, the absence of histamine increase does not preclude a histamine-release mechanism, as histamine has a short half-life. Conversely, histamine and tryptase concentrations correlate with the severity of the allergic reaction [86].

Combined histamine and tryptase measurements are recommended for the diagnosis of allergic reactions during anesthesia in France [48]. In contrast, the British and Scandinavian Societies of Anesthesia only recommend tryptase [2, 47]. Finally, whereas measurement of methyl histamine is still recommended in the United States [4, 83], it is no longer recommended in Europe [2, 47, 48, 84, 87] because the sensitivity of this test is lower than that of plasma histamine and tryptase [88].

In conclusion, histamine and tryptase measurement constitute the second element in the diagnosis of anaphylaxis.

In vitro Biochemical Tests

*Anesthetics* In vitro tests available in clinical practice detect the presence of IgE-antibodies by binding the allergen onto a solid phase (Radio-Allergo Sorbent Test or RAST) and using radioactive system detection or by binding the allergen onto a sponge matrix (CAP) while using fluorescent detection [2, 48]. RAST is now rarely used but its name has persisted in clinical practice. Currently, only the suxamethonium-specific assay is available among the different commercialized NMBAs, but its sensitivity is relatively low around 30–60% [84]. The use of a quaternary ammonium (choline chloride), by coupling an analogue of choline onto a polysaccharide support sepharose (SAQ) [89] or p-aminophenylphosphoryl-choline on agarose (PAPPC) [90] has been proposed. Their sensitivity and specificity approximate 90% in some studies [84]. More recently, a morphine-based solid phase IgE was proposed, as the tertiary methylamino group belonging to the chemical structure of morphine cross-reacts strongly in vitro with NMBAs [91, 92]. These in vitro tests may be used to evaluate sensitization to quaternary ammoniums of NMBAs [84]. They may also help to confirm the diagnosis in patients experiencing an anaphylactic reaction to a NMBA [2, 47, 48].

IgE-antibody testing is commercially available for very few drugs used during anesthesia (thiopental, propofol, morphine), antibiotics (amoxicillin, penicillin G, penicillin V, cefaclor), chlorhexidine and latex but is not available everywhere [2, 47, 48]. The RAST test available for latex is less sensitive than the skin prick test, being positive only in 50–70% of the cases [4]. Finally, serum specific IgEs measurement may be performed at the time of the reaction or later [47, 48]. Nevertheless, the interpretation of specific IgEs and specific IgE-inhibition assays should be performed cautiously, as it might only correspond to in vitro cross-reactivity between NMBAs without any clinical relevance [84].

Several other tests have been proposed for indirect detection of specific IgEs to anesthetic drugs. The basophile histamine release test is reliable for NMBAs with a sensitivity of about 40–100%, and a specificity of 98–100% [88]. This technique may be helpful when cross-reactivity among NMBAs is investigated prior to reintroduction in patients having already presented a documented anaphylactic reaction to a particular NMBA [48, 84]. The study of basophil activation using a flow-cytometry test, in the presence of the allergen, is assessed by the expression of CD63 coupled to CD203c on the plasma membrane. Its sensitivity and specificity are around 60–85% and 60–100%, respectively, according to different studies [93–96]. The technique might help in the assessment of cross-reactivity and identification of safe alternatives [84]. Nevertheless, further investigations are needed to assess the value of this method in the diagnosis of anaphylaxis to NMBAs.

*Contrast Agents* Specific IgE-assays have not been validated for ICM. When compared to control patients, Laroche found a significant increase of ICM-IgEs in patients experiencing severe reactions following ICM [86]. Mita demonstrated the presence of ioxaglate-specific IgEs in a series of reactors along with tryptase release [97]. Furthermore, in addition to the clinical history and skin tests, basophil activation analysis by flow cytometry may be a useful tool in cases of anaphylaxis to ICM [98].

Serum-IgEs provide a possible explanation of the mechanism but do not constitute a proof that the drug or agent is responsible for the reaction [2]. Methods, such as flow cytometry-based basophil activation, need to be validated before being proposed in clinical practice.

In conclusion, biological assessment is a useful tool in order to investigate immediate reactions occurring during the perioperative or radiological settings, but should never be interpreted without the support of a rigorous clinical history linked to the results of skin tests.

#### 11.4.4.2 Skin Testing Is Essential to Prove the Diagnosis and Prevent Further Recurrences

Following an immediate hypersensitivity reaction, skin tests are required in order to identify the culprit agent, prove the pathophysiological mechanism of the reaction (non-allergic versus allergic), suggest a safe alternative drug for future exposures and thus provide advice regarding subsequent anesthetics or radiological procedures.

Skin tests are meant to reproduce the reaction by challenging the skin mast cells in vivo with the culprit drug or agent. A very small amount of the drug is used in order to avoid direct toxic effects and non-specific response. However, skin testing should be preferentially performed after a delay of 4–6 weeks after the reaction in order to avoid false negative tests because of mast cell depletion following an immediate hypersensitivity reaction [47, 48]. Conversely, preoperative screening in the absence of a clinical history should not be performed as the positive and negative predictive values of skin tests for the occurrence of perioperative anaphylaxis remain unknown [48, 84].

### General Considerations: How to Perform Skin Testing?

Cutaneous reactivity needs to be assessed prior to skin testing by a negative (saline) and a positive control (extract of 9% codeine phosphate solution and/or 10 mg·mL$^{-1}$ solution of histamine) [2, 47, 48, 84, 87]. $H_1$-antihistamines and antidepressants should be stopped a few days before the skin challenge in order to avoid false negative tests [47, 48]. $H_1$-antihistamines inhibit the cutaneous reactivity whereas antidepressants may induce a modified cutaneous response to the challenge. Conversely, there is no need to discontinue oral or inhaled steroids [2]. While dialysis and tobacco smoking may induce a decreased response to the skin challenge due to cutaneous vasoconstriction [46], cutaneous reactivity may be increased in case of dermographism [87]. Moreover, patients should be free of infectious diseases, fever or inflammatory reactions at the time of skin testing [99]. All drugs to which the patient was exposed prior (1 h before) to the reaction, as well as latex, must be skin-tested [47, 48]. Investigation of anesthetics is performed by prick-tests (PTs) followed by intradermal tests (IDTs) using commercial solutions undiluted or freshly diluted without exceeding the maximum recommended concentrations (Table 11.3) [2, 47, 48, 84]. PTs are usually performed on the anterior part of the forearm, whereas IDTs are performed on the forearm or the back. PTs may produce false negative results whereas IDTs are more sensitive but less specific than PTs [47, 87]. However, IDTs are more likely to trigger a systemic allergic reaction and, thus, should only be performed if PTs are negative [87]. Diagnostic criteria for a positive skin test (PT and IDT) have been defined in France [48] and recommended in Scandinavia [47]. The different concentrations of normally non-reactive anesthetic drugs have been strictly defined in France [48] (Table 11.3), have been approved in Scandinavia and the United Kingdom [2, 47] and have been adapted by others [84].

### Skin Testing with Drugs or Agent Used During the Perioperative Setting?

NMBAs, latex and antibiotics are the substances most likely to be involved during the perioperative setting.

*Neuromuscular Blocking Agents* NMBAs are the most common cause of anaphylaxis occurring during anesthesia accounting for 50–70% of cases. All NMBAs have been reported to trigger anaphylaxis [46, 84]. Documented anaphylactic reactions to NMBAs have been reported in patients without previous exposure to a NMBA [2, 33, 37] and previous safe injections do not rule out an anaphylactic reaction in case of repeated injections [2, 100]. The sensitivity of skin tests for patients having experienced anaphylaxis following a NMBA injection is excellent [101]. Cross-reactivity between NMBAs is around 60–70% [47, 49, 84, 92]. Thus, cross-reactivity with other NMBAs should be assessed through skin tests in order to propose a safe alternative for further procedures when anaphylaxis to a definite NMBA has been documented [47, 48]. As PTs are less sensitive than IDTs, cross-reactivity is performed by PTs followed by IDTs without exceeding the maximal

**Table 11.3** Normal nonreactive ncentrations of anesthetic agents during skin tests (Reproduced with authorization from [48])

| | | Prick-tests | | Intradermal tests | |
|---|---|---|---|---|---|
| Drugs | Concentration ($mg \cdot mL^{-1}$) | Dilution | Maximal concentration ($mg \cdot mL^{-1}$) | Dilution | Maximal concentration ($\mu g \cdot mL^{-1}$) |
| *NMBAs* | | | | | |
| Suxamethonium | 50 | 1/5 | 10 | 1/500 | 100 |
| Atracurium | 10 | 1/10 | 1 | 1/1,000 | 10 |
| Cis-atracurium | 2 | Undiluted | 2 | 1/100 | 20 |
| Mivacurium | 2 | 1/10 | 0.2 | 1/1,000 | 2 |
| Pancuronium | 2 | Undiluted | 2 | 1/10 | 200 |
| Rocuronium | 10 | Undiluted | 10 | 1/100 | 100 |
| Vecuronium | 4 | Undiluted | 4 | 1/10 | 400 |
| *Hypnotics* | | | | | |
| Etomidate | 2 | Undiluted | 2 | 1/10 | 200 |
| Midazolam | 5 | Undiluted | 5 | 1/10 | 500 |
| Propofol | 10 | Undiluted | 10 | 1/10 | 1,000 |
| Thiopental | 25 | Undiluted | 25 | 1/10 | 2,500 |
| *Opioids* | | | | | |
| Alfentanil | 0.5 | Undiluted | 0.5 | 1/10 | 50 |
| Fentanyl | 0.05 | Undiluted | 0.05 | 1/10 | 5 |
| Morphine | 10 | 1/10 | 1 | 1/1,000 | 10 |
| Remifentanil | 0.05 | Undiluted | 0.05 | 1/10 | 5 |
| Sufentanil | 0.005 | Undiluted | 0.005 | 1/10 | 0.5 |
| *Local Anesthetics* | | | | | |
| Bupivacaine | 2.5 | Undiluted | 2.5 | 1/10 | 250 |
| Lidocaine | 10 | Undiluted | 10 | 1/10 | 1,000 |
| Mepivacaine | 10 | Undiluted | 10 | 1/10 | 1,000 |
| Ropivacaine | 2 | Undiluted | 2 | 1/10 | 200 |

*NMBAs* neuromuscular blocking agents

recommended concentrations [48] (Table 11.3). Recently, some have recommended to perform only PTs [2]. However, cross-reactivity with NMBAs should be assessed through PTs followed by IDTs in order to reduce false-negative tests.

Succinylcholine is the NMBA most likely to produce anaphylaxis [2, 49]. While reports in France and Norway suggest an increased frequency of anaphylaxis to rocuronium [33, 102], this remains controversial as this trend has not been observed in Australia [103] or in the United States [104]. Further epidemiological studies are therefore required and the apparent excess of anaphylaxis to rocuronium should be interpreted with caution [2, 49].

*Latex* In Europe, investigation of latex is performed by PTs using commercial extracts, which are not available in the United States [2, 47–49]. Their sensitivity is around 75–90% [2]. Conversely, in the United States, the diagnosis relies essentially on in vitro tests as no commercial skin test reagents are currently available [63]. Latex gloves extracts are often used but their amount of latex proteins are not standardized and, therefore, not recommended [4].

*Antibiotics* All types of antibiotics may induce anaphylaxis [47], and it may occur at first exposure in cases of cross-sensitization [47, 87]. However, penicillins and cephalosporins, which share a β(beta)-lactam ring, are responsible for approximately 70% of antibiotic-induced anaphylaxis [2, 84]. The specificity of skin testing with β(beta)-lactams is between 97% and 99%, whereas the sensitivity is around 50% [46]. The maximum concentrations of antibiotics for skin testing proposed by the European Network Drug Allergy interest group on drug hypersensitivity are as follows: amoxicillin 20–25 $mg{\cdot}ml^{-1}$, ampicillin 20–25 $mg{\cdot}ml^{-1}$ and for most cephalosporins 1–2 $mg{\cdot}mL^{-1}$ [105]. The structure of the side chains attached to the β(beta)-lactam ring is also important in determining the allergenicity of the molecule. First generation cephalosporins and cefamandole share a similar side chain with penicillin and amoxicillin [2]. A meta-analysis suggested that patients allergic to penicillins or amoxicillin have a higher incidence of allergic reactions to first generation cephalosporins and cefamandole (or: 4%, 79%, 95% CI = 3.71 to 6.17). Conversely, second and third generation cephalosporins have different side chains from penicillin and amoxicillin and were not associated with a risk of cross-reactivity with penicillin [106]. Anaphylaxis with vancomycin remains rare but, if necessary, IDT should be performed with a concentration below 10 $\mu g{\cdot}mL^{-1}$ [84]. It should be distinguished from Red Man Syndrome, a clinical entity resulting from non-specific histamine release and observed when the drug is rapidly injected [4, 84]. Teicoplanin may also induce Red Man Syndrome [84]. Skin tests with quinolones may be difficult to interpret due to histamine release.

*Hypnotics* Anaphylaxis to thiopental or propofol is uncommon whereas anaphylaxis to etomidate and ketamine remains extremely rare [2, 47, 49]. Hypnotics may be skin tested according to Table 11.3 [47, 48, 84].

*Opioids* Anaphylaxis to opioids is extremely rare when compared to their wider use [2, 47, 49, 84]. The sensitivity of IDT with morphine is good, while specificity is not because morphine induces histamine release. Maximum concentrations should not be exceeded (Table 11.3). Phenylpiperidines (alfentanil, fentanyl, remifentanil, sufentanil) may be skin tested undiluted by PTs, followed by IDTs if negative (Table 11.3) [47–49, 84].

*Local Anesthetics* Anaphylaxis to local anesthetics is very uncommon [47–49, 84]. The metabolism of amide local anesthetics is primarily in the liver, while that of esters is via plasma cholinesterases. Para-aminobenzoic acid (PABA) is the common metabolite of ester local anesthetics responsible for causing allergic reactions. Preservatives or antioxidants such as methylparaben and propylparaben (both metabolized to PABA), and metabisulfite are often added to multiple-dose vials of local anesthetics. These preservatives may also lead to allergic reactions. However, most reactions are vasovagal or toxic reactions from inadvertent intravascular injection of a local anesthetic or the systemic absorption of epinephrine [2, 47]. Thus, while cross-reactivity is the rule among esters due to PABA, it is rare in the amide group and absent between amide and ester local anesthetics [49]. Local anesthetics may be skin tested with preservative-free solutions according to Table 11.3 [47, 48, 84].

*Colloids* The frequency of anaphylaxis with colloids is very low, but higher with gelatins (0.35%) when compared to hydroxyethylstarch (HES) (0.06%) [107]. Skin tests begin with PTs (1/10 dilution) followed by IDTs in case of negativity [47, 48, 84].

*Aprotinin* While aprotinin was previously used to reduce blood loss and the need for blood transfusion during surgery, it was recently withdrawn from the worldwide market. However, some fibrin glue products still contain aprotinin. Skin tests begin with PTs (1/10 or pure dilution) and are followed by IDTs (up to 1/10 dilution) in case of negativity [48, 84].

*Dyes* While the incidence of anaphylaxis to isosulfan or patent blue is less than 2% [49, 108], documented anaphylaxis with methylene blue has been reported only once [109]. Dyes may be skin tested by PTs followed by IDTs (up to 1/100 for methylene blue because it is a histamine-releaser and up to 1/10 dilution for isosulfan/patent blue).

*Other Drugs* Protamine and antiseptics (chlorhexidine, povidone iodine) may also induce anaphylaxis. Skin testing may be performed to prove the diagnosis [47, 49].

#### Skin Testing with Contrast Agents

Each ICM or gadolinium chelate may induce anaphylaxis. Contrast agents may be skin tested by PTs followed by IDTs in case of negativity. The sensitivity of PTs with ICM seems to be low whereas sensitivity and specificity seem to be very good with IDTs. Gadolinium chelates may also be skin-tested by PTs followed by IDTs. In case of a documented anaphylaxis to an ICM, cross-reactivity with the others commercialized ICM should be performed in order to propose a non-reactive ICM for further procedures. Cross-reactivity is also assessed with gadolinium chelates in case of a documented anaphylaxis to a gadolinium chelate. No cross-reactivity has been observed between ICM and gadolinium chelates.

### 11.4.4.3 The Allergenic Determinant Is Not Iodine for Iodinated Contrast Agents

The part of the molecule causing immediate hypersensitivity reactions following ICM is not known but is not the iodine atom itself [68, 70, 75, 110]. Even though the tri-iodobenzenic ring is common to all ICMs, there is no cross-reactivity among all of them, or with other iodinated drugs such as povidone iodine or lugol solution, indicating that the iodine atom is not the allergenic sequence involved [72, 74, 76, 98]. The allergenic determinant responsible for patient sensitization to povidone iodine is likely due to the povidone [111–114]. The major allergen is the protein M in fish [115, 116], whereas tropomyosin is the cross-reactive allergen among crustaceans and molluscs [117]. Therefore, since the iodine atom has never been demonstrated to be involved during allergic hypersensitivity reactions due to iodinated drugs or seafood [118], the concept of *iodine allergy* should be abandoned. Moreover, the allergenic sequence has not been identified for gadolinium chelates.

A detailed description of all drugs administered and the chronology of the clinical event is fundamental in cases of immediate hypersensitivity reactions during the radiological procedure in order to identify the offending drug or substance and to perform the appropriate skin tests. This is particularly important given the fact that not every reaction is related to ICM but may also be related to latex or other given drugs.

Finally, the interpretation of skin tests should always be linked to the clinical event and, when performed, to the results of the tryptase measurement in order to provide a pertinent diagnosis.

## 11.5 Management of Anaphylaxis

Management of anaphylaxis occurring in the perioperative or radiological settings consists of: (1) immediate withdrawal of the culprit drug if known; (2) discontinuation of anesthetic drugs; (3) shortening of the surgical/radiological procedure when occurring during perioperative/radiological procedure; (4) 100% oxygen with airway support; (5) early administration of epinephrine especially during severe reactions (Grades III and IV); (6) massive vascular loading especially for severe reactions; (7) supine with Trendelenburg position; and (8) a call for help especially for severe reactions.

### *11.5.1 Epinephrine: When and How?*

Epinephrine remains the key-drug in the treatment of anaphylaxis [2, 47, 48, 119]. The beneficial effects of epinephrine during anaphylaxis are mediated by the $\alpha_1$-adrenergic receptors which increase the left ventricular preload by reducing venous capacitance, and the $\beta_1$- and $\beta_2$-adrenergic receptors. These receptors increase cardiac inotropy and chronotropy, and reverse bronchoconstriction, respectively. Epinephrine also reduces the release of inflammatory mediators such as histamine [47, 48]. Poor outcomes, including deaths, have been associated with late administration, inadequate or excessive doses of epinephrine during anaphylaxis emphasizing the role of early epinephrine during severe reactions (Grade III or IV) and the need for careful titration [47, 120]. Thus, there is no contraindication to epinephrine when required (Grade III and IV) [4] and early intravenous administration should be the rule. Accordingly, the Ring and Messmer four-step grading scale may help to stratify care management [50] (Table 11.2). Thus, although epinephrine should not be injected during grade I reactions, titrated intravenous bolus (10–20 μg) of epinephrine may sometimes be necessary during grade II reactions. Conversely, titrated intravenous bolus administration of epinephrine (100–200 μg) are required in grade III reactions, renewed every 1 or 2 min as necessary according to the hemodynamic response and followed by a continuous infusion (1–4 $\mu g{\cdot}min^{-1}$) to prevent the need for repeated injections [2, 47, 48, 119]. Grade IV reactions (cardiac arrest) require cardiopulmonary resuscitation and high doses of epinephrine [48, 119]. A commonly used sequence is to administer 1 to 3 mg intravenously (over 3 min), then 3–5 mg intravenously (over 3 min), if necessary, followed by a continuous infusion (4–10 $\mu g{\cdot}min^{-1}$) [119].

### *11.5.2 Fluid Therapy: When and How?*

Fluid therapy may be initiated at a high rate with crystalloids (saline 0.9% or lactated Ringer's solution) [2, 119] and replaced by colloids when their volume exceeds 30 $mL{\cdot}kg^{-1}$ [2, 47, 48]. While hydroxyethylstarch (HES) is usually preferred due to the low frequency of anaphylaxis following HES [48, 107], others recommend gelatin-based colloid [2].

### *11.5.3 Bronchospasm*

Isolated bronchospasm is initially treated with inhaled $\beta$(beta)$_2$-agonists (salbutamol, albuterol) [2, 47, 48, 119]. If a breathing-system connector is available, an inhaler may be appropriate [2, 48]. In cases of persistent bronchospasm, intravenous injection of β(beta)-agonist (salbutamol, 100–200 μg) is recommended and a continuous infusion (5–25 $\mu g{\cdot}min^{-1}$) should be considered [2, 48, 119].

Conversely, when cardiovascular collapse and bronchospasm occur together, epinephrine remains the first-line therapy to correct the cardiovascular homeostasis while often resolving hypotension and bronchospasm together [48, 119]. Moreover, the administration of high-dose intravenous corticosteroids early in the course of therapy is recommended because of their anti-inflammatory effects on the airway. Their beneficial effects are delayed at least 4–6 h [47, 48, 119].

### *11.5.4 Additional Therapy*

Corticosteroids and/or $H_1$-receptor antagonists are often recommended in the management of anaphylaxis [2, 47, 48, 119] but their effects have never been evaluated [4, 83]. However, corticosteroids are useful for angioedema as detailed above [51].

### *11.5.5 Anaphylaxis and Catecholamine Failure*

Anaphylaxis is sometimes refractory to catecholamines. This clinical entity is called *anaphylactic shock refractory to catecholamines,* and it remains undefined in the literature. Its pathophysiology remains unknown. Norepinephrine, metaraminol and glucagon for patients taking β(beta)-blockers are recommended in this clinical setting [2, 47, 48]. Nevertheless, as desensitization of adrenergic receptors might be one of the contributing factors of catecholamine failure occurring during anaphylaxis, arginine vasopressin (AVP) may be an alternative through its vasoconstrictive effects mediated by non-adrenergic vascular AVP $V_1$-receptors. Thus, 12 patients experiencing anaphylaxis in the pre-hospital or perioperative settings refractory either to epinephrine and/or norepinephrine and/or phenylephrine were successfully treated with AVP injected at least 10–40 min following anaphylactic shock onset [121–126] (Table 11.4). Therefore, AVP has been suggested as an alternative in cases where there is a lack of response to epinephrine [47, 119]. Further studies are necessary in order to clarify the role of AVP during anaphylaxis.

## 11.6 Premedication

### *11.6.1 Anesthetic Drugs*

No prospective randomized study evaluating the use of a specific protocol of premedication on the prevention of perioperative anaphylaxis has been published. Furthermore, many clinical cases of perioperative anaphylaxis have been reported despite premedication [49, 127]. Therefore, it has been agreed that the use of antihistamines $H_1$ and/or $H_2$, and/or corticosteroids will not prevent anaphylaxis [47–49].

### *11.6.2 Iodinated Contrast Agents*

Several studies have been published over the past 20 years underlining the prevention of ICM-induced immediate reactions [128–132]. However, most of these studies were not randomized [128, 130, 132], used different protocols of premedication including corticosteroids, $H_1$ and $H_2$ antihistamines

**Table 11.4** Anaphylactic shock refractory to either epinephrine and/or norepinephrine and/or phenylephrine and successfully treated with arginine vasopressin (AVP) injected at least 10–40 min after anaphylactic shock onset

| Reference | Age gender | Suspected allergen | Inaugural clinical signs | First-line treatment (drugs used and cumulative dosages) | Delay between shock onset and AVP (min) | Cumulative i.v AVP dosage (IU) | Reported delay between AVP and hemodynamic restoration |
|---|---|---|---|---|---|---|---|
| Kill 2004 [121] | 42, M | Hornet | HR: 135 b·min$^{-1}$<br>AP not measurable | Epinephrine: 1 mg | 15–20 | 10+40<br>Over 60 min | Immediately After 10 IU Bolus |
| | 47, M | Wasp | Deep cyanosis<br>HR: 140 b·min$^{-1}$<br>AP not measurable<br>Expiratory stridor | None | 15–20 | 40 | Immediately |
| Schummer 2004 [122] | 59, F | Gelatin | HR: 90 b·min$^{-1}$<br>AP: 50/25 mm Hg | Epinephrine: 1.5 mg<br>Norepinephrine: up to 1 μg·kg$^{-1}$·min$^{-1}$ for 40 min | 20 | 2 | 5 min |
| Williams 2004 [123] | 57, F | Aprotinin | HR: 115 b·min$^{-1}$<br>SAP: 50 mmHg<br>Bronchospasm | Phenylephrine 20 mg | 10–15 | 5+5 | Rapidly |
| Hussain 2008 [124] | 24, F | Atracurium | HR: 140 b·min$^{-1}$<br>AP not measurable<br>Bronchospasm<br>Cyanosis | Epinephrine: 2 mg<br>Phenylephrine: 4 mg<br>Epinephrine and Norepinephrine: up to 0.5 μg·kg$^{-1}$·min$^{-1}$ for 2 h | 40 | 2 | Immediately |
| Meng 2008 [125] | 17, F | Rocuronium | HR: 119–138 b·min$^{-1}$<br>AP: 62/38 mmHg<br>Erythema | Phenylephrine: 200 μg<br>Epinephrine: 1.2 mg | 15 | 2 | 2 min |
| Schummer 2008 [126] | 63, F | Aprotinin | HR: 130 b·min$^{-1}$<br>MAP: 30 mmHg | Epinephrine: 1 mg<br>Norepinephrine: 0.44 μg·kg$^{-1}$·min$^{-1}$ | ? | 2 | Quickly |

(continued)

**Table 11.4** (continued)

| Reference | Age gender | Suspected allergen | Inaugural clinical signs | First-line treatment (drugs used and cumulative dosages) | Delay between shock onset and AVP (min) | Cumulative i.v AVP dosage (IU) | Reported delay between AVP and hemodynamic restoration |
|---|---|---|---|---|---|---|---|
| | 53, M | Aprotinin | HR: 160 b·min$^{-1}$<br>MAP: 30 mmHg | Epinephrine: 1 mg<br>Norepinephrine: 0.5 μg·kg$^{-1}$·min$^{-1}$ | ? | 2 | Subsequently |
| | 58, M | Metamizol | HR: 160 b·min$^{-1}$<br>MAP: 30 mmHg<br>Bronchospasm | Epinephrine: 1.4 mg<br>Norepinephrine: 0.4 μg·kg$^{-1}$·min$^{-1}$ | ? | 5 | Immediately |
| | 47, M | Metamizol | Cardiac arrest<br>Bronchospasm | Epinephrine: 3 mg<br>Norepinephrine: 0.75 μg·kg$^{-1}$·min$^{-1}$ | ? | 5+5+5 | ? |
| | 73, M | Metamizol | | Epinephrine: 1.6 mg<br>Norepinephrine: 0.8 μg·kg$^{-1}$·min$^{-1}$ | ? | 8 | ? |
| | 43, F | Gelatin | HR: 95 b·min$^{-1}$<br>MAP: 30 mmHg | Epinephrine: 0.3 mg<br>Norepinephrine: 1.2 μg·kg$^{-1}$·min$^{-1}$ | ? | 2 | Quickly |

*AVP* arginine vasopressin, *HR* heart rate, *AP* arterial pressure, *SAP* systolic arterial pressure, *MAP* mean arterial pressure and ephedrine, [128–132] and did not investigate the pathomechanisms of immediate reactions [128–132]. Moreover, in patients having presented a previous reaction with an ICM, it has never been clarified whether the same ICM (as those which induced the previous reaction) was reinjected; this constitutes a significant bias, as the injection of a structurally-different ICM may by itself avoid the recurrence of the reaction [128–131].

There are many cases reporting the occurrence of anaphylactic reactions following contrast agents despite premedication with steroids and/or antihistamines [71, 72, 75, 76, 133–142]. In addition, in a retrospective study reviewing breakthrough adverse reactions, recurrent reactions occurred with a similar severity in 85% of the patients despite premedication with steroids and use of low-osmolar contrast agents. Moreover, severe or life-threatening reactions were observed in 24% of these patients [143]. A recent meta-analysis of nine trials testing the efficacy of antihistamines and corticosteroids confirmed that a premedication may not be helpful in preventing serious anaphylaxis following ICM [144].

Whereas recommendations are still in order for the use of prophylactic steroids and antihistamines for contrast agents anaphylaxis in the United States [4], their use has been questioned by the European Academy of Allergology and Clinical Immunology interest group on drug hypersensitivity [145]. Prophylactic antihistamines or steroids prior to contrast agent reintroduction in patients with a history of anaphylaxis is not currently recommended in France [146].

Finally, as no preemptive therapeutic strategies have been proven to prevent anaphylaxis during the perioperative or radiological settings, an allergological follow-up in patients having presented an immediate reaction following ICM or anesthetics drugs is highly recommended in order to prevent further recurrences. Moreover, severe or life-threatening reactions were observed in 24% of these patients [143].

## 11.7 Conclusion

Anaphylaxis occurring during the perioperative or radiological settings may be a life-threatening condition even in previously healthy patients. The different clinical symptoms heralding anaphylaxis must be known by the practitioner in order to provide the appropriate care management according to the severity of the reaction. Allergological follow-up including tryptase measurement at the time of the reaction and skin testing later should be emphasized in order to prove the diagnosis, prevent further recurrences and provide a safe alternative for future procedures. Although anaphylaxis is an adverse effect of drugs or substances commonly used in the perioperative or radiological settings, its occurrence is relatively rare. Therefore, teaching of the care management, including in an anesthesia simulator, of this peculiar clinical entity should be encouraged. Treatment protocols for anaphylaxis are based on understanding its cellular mechanism and clinical presentation. Immediate discontinuation of the offending agent, and early epinephrine administration along with vascular loading are the cornerstones of treating anaphylaxis.

## References


1. Johansson SG, Hourihane JO, Bousquet J, et al. A revised nomenclature for allergy. An EAACI position statement from the EAACI nomenclature task force. *Allergy.* 2001;56:813–824.
2. Harper NJ, Dixon T, Dugue P, et al. Suspected anaphylactic reactions associated with anaesthesia. *Anaesthesia* 2009;64:199–211.
3. Johansson SG, Bieber T, Dahl R, et al. Revised nomenclature for allergy for global use: Report of the Nomenclature Review Committee of the World Allergy Organization, October 2003. *J Allergy Clin Immunol* 2004; 113: 832–836.
4. Liberman P, Nicklas RA, Oppenheimer J, et al. The diagnosis and management of anaphylaxis practice parameter: 2010 update. *J Allergy Clin Immunol* 2010;126:477–480.

5. Sampson HA, Munoz-Furlong A, Campbell RL, et al. Second symposium on the definition and management of anaphylaxis: Summary Report-Second National Institute of Allergy and Infectious Disease/Food Allergy and Anaphylaxis Network symposium. *J Allergy Clin Immunol* 2006;117:391–397.
6. Shehadi WH. Adverse reactions to intravascularly administered contrast media. A comprehensive study based on a prospective survey. *Am J Roentgenol Radium Ther Nucl Med* 1975;124:145–152.
7. Shehadi WH, Toniolo G. Adverse reactions to contrast media: a report from the Committee on Safety of Contrast Media of the International Society of Radiology. *Radiology* 1980;137:299–302.
8. Ansell G, Tweedie MC, West CR, et al. The current status of reactions to intravenous contrast media. *Invest Radiol* 1980;15(Suppl):S32–S39.
9. Palmer FJ. The RACR survey of intravenous contrast media reactions. Final report. *Australas Radil.* 1988;32:426–428.
10. Katayama H, Yamaguchi K, Kozuka T, et al. Adverse reactions to ionic and nonionic contrast media. A Report from the Japanese Committee on the Safety of Contrast Media. *Radiology* 1990;175:621–628.
11. Caro JJ, Trindade E, McGregor M. The risks of death and of severe nonfatal reactions with high- vs low-osmolality contrast media: a meta-analysis. *AJR Am J Roentgenol* 1991;156:825–832.
12. Lasser EC, Lyon SG, Berry CC. Reports on contrast media reactions: analysis of data from reports to the U.S. Food and Drug Administration. *Radiology* 1997;203:605–610.
13. Agence Nationale pour le Développement de l'Évaluation Médicale. *Eléments d'Evaluation pour le Choix et l'Emploi des Différentes Classes de Produits de Contraste Iodés Hydrosolubles lors des Examens Tomodensitométriques et Urographiques.* Paris: ANDEM; 1994.
14. Spring DB, Bettmann MA, Barkan HE. Deaths related to iodinated contrast media reported spontaneously to the U.S. Food and Drug Administration, 1978-1994: effect of the availability of low-osmolality contrast media. *Radiology* 1997;204:333–337.
15. Li A, Wong CS, Wong MK, et al. Acute adverse reactions to magnetic resonance contrast media-gadolinium chelates. *Br J Radiol* 2006;79:368–371.
16. Herborn CU, Honold E, Wolf M, et al. Clinical safety and diagnostic value of the gadolinium chelate gadoterate meglumine (Gd-DOTA). *Invest Radiol* 2007;42:58–62.
17. Tardy B, Guy C, Barral G, et al. Anaphylactic shock induced by intravenous gadopentetate dimeglumine. *Lancet* 1992;339:494.
18. Meuli RA, Maeder P. Life-threatening anaphylactoid reaction after i.v. injection of gadoterate meglumine. *AJR Am J Roentgenol* 1996;166:729.
19. Beaudouin E, Kanny G, Blanloeil Y, et al. Anaphylactic shock induced by gadoterate meglumine (Dotarem). *Eur Ann Allergy Clin Immunol* 2003;35:382–385.
20. Kalogeromitros DC, Makris MP, Aggelides XS, et al. Anaphylaxis to gadobenate dimeglumine (Multihance): a case report. *Int Arch Allergy Immunol* 2007;144:150–154.
21. Hasdenteufel F, Luyasu S, Renaudin JM, et al. Anaphylactic shock after first exposure to gadoterate meglumine: two case reports documented by positive allergy assessment. *J Allergy Clin Immunol* 2008;121:527–528.
22. Runge VM. Allergic reactions to gadolinium chelates. *AJR Am J Roentgenol* 2001;177:944–945.
23. Fisher MM, More DG. The epidemiology and clinical features of anaphylactic reactions in anaesthesia. *Anaesth Intensive Care* 1981;9:226–234.
24. Fisher MM. The epidemiology of anaesthetic anaphylactoid reactions in Australasia. *Klin Wochenschr* 1982;60:1017–1020.
25. Fisher MM, Baldo BA. The incidence and clinical features of anaphylactic reactions during anesthesia in Australia. *Ann Fr Anesth Reanim* 1993;12:97–104.
26. Galletly DC, Treuren BC. Anaphylactoid reactions during anaesthesia. Seven years' experience of intradermal testing. *Anaesthesia* 1985;40:329–333.
27. Watkins J. Adverse anaesthetic reactions. An update from a proposed national reporting and advisory service. *Anaesthesia* 1985;40:797–800.
28. Watkins J. Allergic and pseudoallergic mechanisms in anesthesia. *Int Anesthesiol Clin* 1985;23:17–40.
29. Watkins J. The allergic reaction to intravenous induction agents. *Br J Hosp Med* 1986;36:45–48.
30. Watkins J. Investigation of allergic and hypersensitivity reactions to anaesthetic agents. *Br J Anaesth* 1987;59:104–111.
31. Pepys J, Pepys EO, Baldo BA, et al. Anaphylactic/anaphylactoid reactions to anaesthetic and associated agents. Skin prick tests in aetiological diagnosis. *Anaesthesia* 1994;49:470–475.
32. Laxenaire MC, Mertes PM. Anaphylaxis during anaesthesia. Results of a two-year survey in France. *Br J Anaesth* 2001;87:549–558.
33. Mertes PM, Laxenaire MC, Alla F. Anaphylactic and anaphylactoid reactions occurring during anesthesia in France in 1999–2000. *Anesthesiology* 2003;99:536–545.
34. Mertes PM, Laxenaire MC. Épidémiologie des réactions anaphylactiques et anaphylactoïdes peranesthésiques en France. Septième enquête multicentrique (Janvier 2001–Décembre 2002). *Ann Fr Anesth Reanim* 2004;23:1133–1143.

35. Garvey LH, Roed-Petersen J, Menne T, et al. Danish Anaesthesia Allergy Centre: preliminary results. *Acta Anaesthesiol Scand* 2001;45:1204–1209.
36. Harboe T, Guttormsen AB, Irgens A, et al. Anaphylaxis during anesthesia in Norway: a 6-year single-center follow-up study. *Anesthesiology* 2005;102:897–903.
37. Lobera T, Audicana MT, Pozo MD, et al. Study of hypersensitivity reactions and anaphylaxis during anesthesia in Spain. *J Investig Allergol Clin Immunol* 2008;18:350–356.
38. Youngman PR, Taylor KM, Wilson JD. Anaphylactoid reactions to neuromuscular blocking agents: a commonly undiagnosed condition? *Lancet* 1983;2:597–599.
39. Hatton F, Tiret L, Maujol L, et al. Enquête épidémiologique sur les anesthésies. *Ann Fr Anesth Reanim* 1983;2:333–385.
40. Whittington T. Anaphylactic and anaphylactoid reactions. *Baillières Clin Anaesthesiol* 1998;12:301–323.
41. Laxenaire MC. Épidémiologie des réactions anaphylactoïdes peranesthésiques. Quatrième enquête multicentrique (Juillet 1994 - Décembre 1996). *Ann Fr Anesth Reanim* 1999;18:796–809.
42. Currie M, Webb RK, Williamson JA, et al. The Australian Incident Monitoring Study. Clinical anaphylaxis: An analysis of 2000 incident reports. *Anaesth Intensive Care* 1993;21:621–625.
43. Mitsuhata H, Hasegawa J, Matsumoto S, et al. The epidemiology and clinical features of anaphylactic and anaphylactoid reactions in the perioperative period in Japan: A survey with a questionnaire of 529 hospitals approved by Japan Society of Anesthesiology. *Masu.* 1992;41:1825–1831.
44. Lienhart A, Auroy Y, Pequignot F, et al. Survey of anesthesia-related mortality in France. *Anesthesiology* 2006;105:1087–1097.
45. The Association of Anaesthetists of Great-Britain and Ireland and British Society for Allergy and Clinical Immunology. Suspected anaphylactic reactions associated with anaesthesia. Revised Edition 2003. http://www.aagbi.org/publications/guidelines/docs/anaphylaxis03.pdf. Accessed December 14, 2009.
46. Dewachter P, Mouton-Faivre C. What investigation after an anaphylactic reaction during anaesthesia? *Curr Opin Anaesthesiol.* 2008;21:363–368.
47. Kroigaard M, Garvey LH, Gillberg L, et al. Scandinavian Clinical Practice Guidelines on the diagnosis, management and follow-up of anaphylaxis during anaesthesia. *Acta Anaesthesiol Scand* 2007;51:655–670.
48. French Society of Anesthesiology and Intensive Care Medicine. Reducing the risk of anaphylaxis during anaesthesia. Abbreviated text. *Ann Fr Anesth Reanim* 2002;21(Suppl 1):7–23.
49. Hepner DL, Castells MC. Anaphylaxis during the perioperative period. *Anesth Analg* 2003;97:1381–1395.
50. Ring J, Messmer K. Incidence and severity of anaphylactoid reactions to colloid volume substitutes. *Lancet* 1977;1:466–469.
51. Dewachter P, Mouton-Faivre C, Emala CW. Anaphylaxis and anesthesia: controversies and new insights. *Anesthesiology* 2009;111:1141–1150.
52. Kounis NG. Kounis syndrome (allergic angina and allergic myocardial infarction): a natural paradigm? *Int J Cardiol* 2006;110:7–14.
53. Cabaton J, Rondelet B, Gergele L, et al. Un syndrome de Tako-Tsubo secondaire à un choc anaphylactique à la succinylcholine lors d'une anesthésie génerale. *Ann Fr Anesth Reanim* 2008;27:854–857.
54. Suk E, Kim D, Kweon T, et al. Stress-induced cardiomyopathy following cephalosporin-induced anaphylactic shock during general anesthesia. *Can J Anaesth* 2009;56:432–436.
55. Han Y, Yeon S. Midventricular hypokinesis as a cardiac manifestation of anaphylaxis: a case report. *J Am Soc Echocardiogr* 2006;19:1529 e9–e11.
56. Zubrinich C, Farouque H, Rochford S, et al. Tako-tsubo-like cardiomyopathy after EpiPen administration. *Intern Med J* 2008;38:862–865.
57. Litvinov I, Kotowycz M, Wassmann S. Iatrogenic epinephrine-induced reverse Takotsubo cardiomyopathy: direct evidence supporting the role of catecholamines in the pathophysiology of the "broken heart syndrome." *Clin Res Cardiol* 2009;98:457–462.
58. Manivannan V, Li J, Prasad A, et al. Apical ballooning syndrome after administration of intravenous epinephrine during an anaphylactic reaction. *Mayo Clin Proc* 2009;84:845–846.
59. Abraham J, Mudd JO, Kapur N, et al. Stress cardiomyopathy after intravenous administration of catecholamines and beta-receptor agonists. *J Am Coll Cardiol* 2009;53:1320–1325.
60. Prasad A, Lerman A, Rihal CS. Apical ballooning syndrome (Tako-Tsubo or stress cardiomyopathy): A mimic of acute myocardial infarction. *Am Heart J* 2008;155:408–417.
61. Tole JW, Lieberman P. Biphasic anaphylaxis: review of incidence, clinical predictors, and observation recommendations. *Immunol Allergy Clin N Am* 2007;27:309–326.
62. Simons FER. Anaphylaxis, killer-allergy: long term management in the community. *J Allergy Clin Immunol* 2006;117:367–377.
63. Hepner DL, Castells MC. Latex allergy: an update. *Anesth Analg* 2003;96:1219–1229.
64. Campagna J, A, Carter C. Clinical relevance of the Bezold-Jarisch reflex. *Anesthesiology* 2003;98:1250–1260.
65. Delaunay F, Blasco V. Choc anaphylactique au latex en cours de césarienne: a propos de deux cas survenus en Guadeloupe. *Ann Fr Anesth Reanim* 2008;27:1023–1025.

66. Turillazzi E, Greco P, Neri M, et al. Anaphylactic latex reaction during anaesthesia: the silent culprit in a fatal case. *Forensic Sci Int* 2008;179:e5–e8.
67. Dolan LP, Toledo MD. Allergic death due to intravenous use of Diodrast. *JAMA* 1940;114:138–139.
68. Goldburgh H, Baer S. Death following the intravenous administration of Diodrast. *JAMA* 1942;118:1051–1052.
69. Naterman HL. Cutaneous test with Diodrast to predict allergic systemic reactions. *JAMA* 1942;119:491–493.
70. Alyea EP, Haines CE. Intradermal test for sensitivity to iodopyracet injection or Diodrast. *JAMA* 1947;135:25–27.
71. Crepea SB, Allanson JC, Delambre L. The failure of antihistaminic drugs to inhibit Diodrast reactions. *N Y State J Med* 1949;49:2556–2558.
72. Kanny G, Maria Y, Mentre B, et al. Case report: recurrent anaphylactic shock to radiographic contrast media. Evidence supporting an exceptional IgE-mediated reaction. *Allerg Immunol.* 1993;25:425–430.
73. Brockow K, Vieluf D, Puschel K, et al. Increased postmortem serum mast cell tryptase in a fatal anaphylactoid reaction to nonionic radiocontrast medium. *J Allergy Clin Immunol* 1999;104:237–238.
74. Alvarez-Fernandez JA, Valero AM, Pulido Z, et al. Hypersensitivity reaction to ioversol. *Allergy.* 2000;55:581–582.
75. Dewachter P, Mouton-Faivre C, Felden F. Allergy and contrast media. *Allergy* 2001;56:250–251.
76. Valfrey J, Newinger G, Arbogast R, et al. Choc à l'ioxaglate (Hexabrix 320) lors de coronarographies. A propos de 2 cas. *Rev Fr Allergol Immunol Clin* 2002;42:157–162.
77. Dewachter P, Nicaise-Roland P, Kalaboka S, et al. Anaphylaxis to amidotrizoate proved by skin testing and flow cytometry-based basophil activation test. *Allergy* 2009;64:501–502.
78. Dewachter P, Mouton-Faivre C. Allergic reaction to contrast medium following gastric band adjustment. *Obes Surg* 2007;17:1413–1415.
79. Brockow K, Romano A, Aberer W, et al. Skin testing in patients with hypersensitivity reactions to iodinated contrast media: A European multicenter study. *Allergy* 2009;64:234–241.
80. Lightfoot C, Abraham R, Mammen T, et al. Survey of Radiologists' kwowledge regarding the management of severe contrast material-induced allergic reactions. *Radiology* 2009;251:691–696.
81. Laroche D, Vergnaud MC, Sillard B, et al. Biochemical markers of anaphylactoid reactions to drugs. Comparison of plasma histamine and tryptase. *Anesthesiology* 1991;75:945–949.
82. Morel A, Delaage M. Immunoanalysis of histamine through a novel chemical derivatization. *J Allergy Clin Immunol* 1988;82:646–654.
83. Simons FER. Anaphylaxis: recent advances in assessment and treatment. *J Allergy Clin Immunol* 2009;124:625–636.
84. Ebo DG, Fisher MM, Hagendorens MM, et al. Anaphylaxis during anaesthesia: diagnostic approach. *Allergy* 2007;62:471–487.
85. Caughey GH. Tryptase genetics and anaphylaxis. *J Allergy Clin Immunol* 2006;117:1411–1414.
86. Laroche D, Aimone-Gastin I, Dubois F, et al. Mechanisms of severe, immediate reactions to iodinated contrast material. *Radiology* 1998;209:183–190.
87. Mirakian R, Ewan PW, Durham SR, et al. BSACI guidelines for the management of drug allergy. *Clin Exp Allergy* 2009;39:43–61.
88. Laroche D, Guilloux L, Gueant JL. Comment rapporter à l'anaphylaxie l'accident observé ? Tests diagnostiques in vitro. *Ann Fr Anesth Reanim* 2002;21(Suppl 1):73s–96s.
89. Gueant JL, Mata E, Monin B, et al. Evaluation of a new reactive solid phase for radioimmunoassay of serum specific IgE against muscle relaxant drugs. *Allergy* 1991;46:452–458.
90. Guilloux L, Ricard-Blum S, Ville G, et al. A new radioimmunoassay using a commercially available solid support for the detection of IgE antibodies against muscle relaxants. *J Allergy Clin Immunol* 1992;90:153–159.
91. Fisher MM, Baldo BA. Immunoassays in the diagnosis of anaphylaxis to neuromuscular blocking drugs: The value of morphine for the detection of IgE antibodies in allergic subjects. *Anaesth Intensive Care* 2000;28:167–170.
92. Baldo BA, Fisher MM, Pham NH. On the origin and specificity of antibodies to neuromuscular blocking (muscle relaxant) drugs: an immunochemical perspective. *Clin Exp Allergy* 2009;39:325–344.
93. Abuaf N, Rajoely B, Ghazouani E, et al. Validation of a flow cytometric assay detecting in vitro basophil activation for the diagnosis of muscle relaxant allergy. *J Allergy Clin Immunol* 1999;104(2Pt1):411–418.
94. Monneret G, Benoit Y, Debard AL, et al. Monitoring of basophil activation using CD63 and CCR3 in allergy to muscle relaxant drugs. *Clin Immunol* 2002;102:192–199.
95. Sudheer PS, Hall JE, Read GF, et al. Flow cytometric investigation of peri-anaesthetic anaphylaxis using CD63 and CD203c. *Anaesthesia* 2005;60:251–256.
96. Kvedariene V, Kamey S, Ryckwaert Y, et al. Diagnosis of neuromuscular blocking agent hypersensitivity reactions using cytofluorimetric analysis of basophils. *Allergy* 2006;61:311–315.
97. Mita H, Tadokoro K, Akiyama K. Detection of IgE antibody to a radiocontrast medium. *Allergy* 1998;53:1133–1140.
98. Dewachter P, Mouton-Faivre C, Laroche D, et al. Allergie immédiate aux produits de contraste iodés et prévention des réactions. *Rev Med Interne* 2009;30:872–881.
99. Brockow K, Romano A, Blanca M, et al. General considerations for skin test procedures in the diagnosis of drug hypersensitivity. *Allergy* 2002;57:45–51.

100. Cottenceau V, Dewachter P, Nouette-Gaulain K, et al. Previous safe administrations of neuromuscular blocking agents do not exonerate from the risk of anaphylactic shock. *Ann Fr Anesth Reanim* 2008;27:509 e1–e3.
101. Moneret-Vautrin DA. Tests cutanés pour le diagnostic d'allergie aux curares. *Ann Fr Anesth Reanim* 2002;21(Suppl 1):97s–107s.
102. Guttormsen AB. Allergic reactions during anaesthesia: increased attention to the problem in Denmark and Norway. *Acta Anaesthesiol Scand* 2001;45:1189–1190.
103. Rose M, Fisher M. Rocuronium: high risk for anaphylaxis? *Br J Anaesth* 2001;86:678–682.
104. Bhananker S, O'Donnell J, Salemi J, et al. The risk of anaphylactic reactions to rocuronium in the United States is comparable to that of vecuronium: an analysis of food and drug administration reporting of adverse events. *Anesth Analg* 2005;101:819–822.
105. Torres MJ, Blanca M, Fernandez J, et al. Diagnosis of immediate allergic reactions to beta-lactam antibiotics. *Allergy* 2003;58:961–972.
106. Pichichero ME, Casey JR. Safe use of selected cephalosporins in penicillin-allergic patients: a meta-analysis. *Otolaryngol Head Neck Surg* 2007;136:340–347.
107. Laxenaire MC, Charpentier C, Feldman L. Réactions anaphylactoïdes aux substituts colloïdaux du plasma: incidence, facteurs de risque, mécanismes. Enquête prospective multicentrique française. *Ann Fr Anesth Reanim* 1994;13:301–310.
108. Mertes PM, Malinovsky JM, Mouton-Faivre C, et al. Anaphylaxis to dyes during the perioperative period: reports of 14 clinical cases. *J Allergy Clin Immunol* 2008;122:348–352.
109. Dewachter P, Mouton-Faivre C, Trechot P, et al. Severe anaphylactic shock with methylene blue instillation. *Anesth Analg* 2005;101:149–150.
110. Coakley FV, Panicek DM. Iodine allergy: an oyster without a pearl? *AJR Am J Roentgenol* 1997;169:951–952.
111. Lopez Saez MP, de Barrio M, Zubeldia JM, et al. Acute IgE-mediated generalized urticaria-angioedema after topical application of povidone-iodine. *Allergol Immunopathol* 1998;26:23–26.
112. Adachi A, Fukunaga A, Hayashi K, et al. Anaphylaxis to polyvinylpyrrolidone after vaginal application of povidone-iodine. *Contact Dermatitis* 2003;48:133–136.
113. Le Pabic F, Sainte-Laudy J, Blanchard N. First case of anaphylaxis to iodinated povidone. *Allergy* 2003;58:826–827.
114. Palobart C, Cros J, Orsel I, et al. Choc anaphylactique à la povidone iodée. *Ann Fr Anesth Reanim* 2009;28:168–170.
115. Aas K, Jebsen J. Studies of hypersensitivity to fish. Partial purification and crystallization of a major allergenic component of cod. *Int Arch Allergy Immunol* 1967;32:1–20.
116. Elsayed S, Bennich H. The primary structure of allergen M from cod. *Scand J Immunol* 1975;4:203–208.
117. Hoffman D. Major heat stable allergen of shrimp. *Ann Allergy Asthma Immunol* 1981;47:127–132.
118. Dewachter P, Trechot P, Mouton-Faivre C. "Allergie à l'iode": le point sur la question. *Ann Fr Anesth Reanim* 2005;24:40–52.
119. American Heart Association. Guidelines for cardiopulmonary resuscitation and emergency cardiovascular care: Part 10.6: anaphylaxis. *Circulation* 2005;112:IV143–IV145. http://circ.ahajournals.org/cgi/reprint/112/24_suppl/IV-143.
120. Pumphrey RS. Lessons for management of anaphylaxis from a study of fatal reactions. *Clin Exp Allergy* 2000;30:1144–1150.
121. Kill C, Wranze E, Wulf H. Successful treatment of severe anaphylactic shock with vasopressin. Two case reports. *Int Arch Allergy Immunol* 2004;134:260–261.
122. Schummer W, Schummer C, Wippermann J, et al. Anaphylactic shock: is vasopressin the drug of choice? *Anesthesiology* 2004;101:1025–1027.
123. Williams SR, Denault AY, Pellerin M, et al. Vasopressin for treatment of shock following aprotinin administration. *Can J Anaesth* 2004;51:169–172.
124. Hussain AM, Yousuf B, Khan MA, et al. Vasopressin for the management of catecholamine-resistant anaphylactic shock. *Singapore Med J* 2008;49:e225–e228.
125. Meng L, Williams EL. Case report: treatment of rocuronium-induced anaphylactic shock with vasopressin. *Can J Anaesth* 2008;55:437–440.
126. Schummer C, Wirsing M, Schummer W. The pivotal role of vasopressin in refractory anaphylactic shock. *Anesth Analg* 2008;107:620–624.
127. Dewachter P. La prévention du risque allergique peut-elle être assurée par une médication préanesthésique? *Ann Fr Anesth Reanim* 2002;21(Suppl 1):151s–167s.
128. Greenberger PA, Patterson R, Tapio CM. Prophylaxis against repeated radiocontrast media reactions in 857 cases. Adverse experience with cimetidine and safety of beta-adrenergic antagonists. *Arch Intern Med* 1985;145:2197–2200.
129. Lasser EC, Berry CC, Talner LB, et al. Pretreatment with corticosteroids to alleviate reactions to intravenous contrast material. *N Engl J Med* 1987;317:845–849.
130. Marshall GD Jr, Lieberman PL. Comparison of three pretreatment protocols to prevent anaphylactoid reactions to radiocontrast media. *Ann Allergy* 1991;67:70–74.

131. Bertrand PR, Soyer PM, Rouleau PJ, et al. Comparative randomized double-blind study of hydroxyzine versus placebo as premedication before injection of iodinated contrast media. *Radiology* 1992;184:383–384.
132. Nilsson S, Bergstrand L, Erikson U, et al. Allergic reactions at repeat femoral angiography with ioxaglate. *Acta Radiol* 2001;42:608–611.
133. Finby N, Evans JA, Steinberg I. Reactions from intravenous organic iodide compounds: pretesting and prophylaxis. *Radiology* 1958;71:15–17.
134. Madowitz J, Schweiger M. Severe anaphylactoid reaction to radiographic contrast media. Recurrence despite premedication with diphenylhydramine and prednisone. *JAMA* 1979;241:2813–2815.
135. Mohan JC, Reddy KS, Bhatia ML. Anaphylactoid reaction to angiographic contrast media: recurrence despite pretreatment with corticosteroids. *Cathet Cardiovasc Diagn* 1984;10:465–469.
136. Roberts M, Fisher M. Anaphylactoid reaction to iopamiron after pretreatment. *Australas Radiol* 1992;36:144–146.
137. Ketkar M, Shrier D. An allergic reaction to intraarterial nonionic contrast material. *AJNR Am J Neuroradiol* 2003;24:292.
138. Armstrong PA, Pazona JF, Schaeffer AJ. Anaphylactoid reaction after retrograde pyelography despite preoperative steroid preparation. *Urology* 2005;66:880,e1–e2.
139. Worthley DL, Gillis D, Kette F, et al. Radiocontrast anaphylaxis with failure of premedication. *Intern Med J* 2005;35:58–60.
140. Williams AN, Kelso JM. Radiocontrast-induced anaphylaxis despite pretreatment and use of iso-osmolar contrast. *Ann Allergy Asthma Immunol* 2007;99:467–468.
141. Chengot T, Goncalves J, Marzo K. Back from irreversibility: use of percutaneous cardiopulmonary bypass for treatment of shock from refractory anaphylaxis during coronary intervention. *J Invasive Cardiol* 2009;21:e97–e100.
142. Dewachter P, Laroche D, Mouton-Faivre C, et al. Immediate reactions following iodinated contrast media injection: A study of 38 cases. *Eur J Radiol* 2009; Dewachter P, Laroche D, Mouton-Faivre C, etal. Immediate reactions following iodinated contrast media injection: A study of 38 cases. Eur J Radiol(2009), doi:10.1016/j.ejrad.2009.09.019.
143. Freed KS, Leder RA, Alexander C, et al. Breakthrough adverse reactions to low-osmolar contrast media after steroid premedication. *AJR Am J Roentgenol* 2001;176:1389–1392.
144. Tramèr M, von Elm E, Loubeyre P, Hauser C. Pharmacological prevention of serious anaphylactic reactions due to iodinated contrast media: systematic review. *BMJ*.2006;333:675.
145. Brockow K, Christiansen C, Kanny G, et al. Management of hypersensitivity reactions to iodinated contrast media. *Allergy* 2005;60:150–158.
146. Société Française de Radiologie. Comité Interdisciplinaire de Recherche et de Travail sur les Agents de Contraste en Imagerie (CIRTACI). Produits de contraste et allergie: hypersensibilité de type immédiat. Fiche de Recommandations pour la Pratique Clinique. http://www.sfrnet.org/Data/upload/documents/CIRTACI/Fiche%20Allergie%2029%2009%202009.pdf. Accessed December 14, 2009.

# Chapter 12
# Hymenoptera-Induced Hypersensitivity Reactions and Anaphylaxis

**Mitja Kosnik and Peter Korosec**

**Abstract** Most Hymenoptera (honeybees, bumblebees, yellow jackets, hornets, wasps and fire ants) stings lead to a local reaction. Up to 7% of population develops systemic allergic reaction to the constituents of venom. Up to 0.5 per one million people die per year due to Hymenoptera venom allergy. Risk factors for the most severe reactions are advanced age, concomitant cardiovascular diseases, concomitant treatment with beta-blockers or angiotensin-converting enzyme inhibitors, mastocytosis, and European hornet *(V. crabro)* allergy. In a patient presenting with a history of Hymenoptera-induced reactions, the severity of the reaction should be assessed, and responsible insect should be identified. Both answers are critical when specific venom immunotherapy (VIT) is considered for treatment. VIT is the only effective treatment for the prevention of serious allergic reactions to Hymenoptera stings in sensitized individuals. Contraindications for VIT are not as strict as they are for respiratory allergic diseases. In patients at high risk for anaphylaxis, VIT should be done under careful supervision even if it is not possible to take the patient off beta-blockers. VIT is safe and effective in patients with a malignant disease in remission and in autoimmune diseases. The optimal duration of VIT is 5 years. Longer or even lifelong treatment should be considered in patients with systemic mastocytosis, near death anaphylaxis, patients with systemic allergic reactions to immunotherapy injections or stings during VIT and highly exposed patients, such as beekeepers. Nearly complete tolerance is established after only a few days of rush immunotherapy. Long-term effectiveness after stopping immunotherapy is less reliable. In patients with venom induced anaphylaxis, mastocytosis should be actively investigated by testing the baseline serum tryptase level and by a clinical examination searching for characteristic skin lesions. VIT in those patients is associated with a higher rate of severe side effects. VIT is recommended for life because there are some case reports of fatal reactions after stopping venom immunotherapy.

**Keywords** Hymenoptera venom allergy • Anaphylaxis • Venom crossreactivity • Basophil activation test • Immunotherapy • Mastocytosis

## 12.1 Introduction

Hymenoptera insects can sting and inject venom into a victim. They sting to protect themselves and their nests. Most Hymenoptera stings lead to a local reaction, namely redness, swelling, itching and pain. In a minority of people, an allergic reaction to the constituents of venom can develop.

M. Kosnik(✉)
University Clinic of Respiratory and Allergic Diseases, Golnik, Slovenia
e-mail: mitja.kosnik@klinika-golnik.si

M.C. Castells (ed.), *Anaphylaxis and Hypersensitivity Reactions*,
DOI 10.1007/978-1-60327-951-2_12, 

## 12.2 Taxonomy of Hymenoptera Insects

The order of Hymenoptera insects consists of the families Apidae, Vespidae, Myrmicinae and Formicinae [1]. The honeybee (*Apis mellifera*) and the bumblebee (*Bombus*) belong to the family of Apidae. The family Vespidae divides into subfamilies Polistinae, with *Polistes* species, and Vespinae, with *Vespula*, *Dolichovespula* and *Vespa* species. The common names for species of the Vespidae family are different in Europe than in the United States. The American names for *Vespula*, *Dolichovespula*, *Vespa crabro* and *Polistes* are yellow jacket, hornet, European hornet and wasp, whereas the British names are wasp (for both *Vespula* and *Dolichovespula*), hornet and paper wasp, respectively. In the USA, many allergic reactions are due to stings of fire ants (*Solenopsis*) belonging to the Myrmicinae family.

The allergenic components of the Hymenoptera venoms are shown in Table 12.1 [2, 3].

There is extensive allergic cross-reactivity among the venoms of species in the same family, but only a weak cross-reactivity among the venoms of insects from different families. Because of biogene amines and kinins found in all Hymenoptera venoms, the sting is always painful. Venoms from fire ants contain oily, strongly basic, water-insoluble *N*-alkyl and alkenyl-piperidines. These alkaloids generate the characteristically sterile pustule that develops at the site of imported fire ant stings.

**Table 12.1** Protein and peptide components of the Hymenoptera venoms [2, 3]

| Insect | Components of the venom (allergen name) | MW (kDa) | Action |
|---|---|---|---|
| Honeybee | Phospholipase $A_2$ (Api m 1) | 16 | Transforms phospholipids to lysophospholipids, which are strong surfactants and therefore cytotoxic |
| | Hyaluronidase (Api m 2) | 39 | Splits mucopolysaccharides, allowing deeper penetration of other venom constituents |
| | Acid phosphatase (Api m 3) | 43 | Unknown |
| | Melittin (Api m 4) | 3 | Increases membrane permeability, liberation of enzymes from lysosomes, liberation of mediators from mast cells/basophils/thrombocytes, and interruption of oxidative phosphorylation |
| | Protease (Api m 5) | 28 | Serine protease |
| | Api m 6 | 8 | Unknown |
| | Allergen C | 105 | Unknown |
| | MCD peptide | 2, 5 | Mast cell degranulation |
| Yellow jacket | Phospholipase $A_1$ (Ves v 1) | 34 | Transforms phospholipids to lysophospholipids, which are strong surfactants and therefore cytotoxic |
| | Hyaluronidase (Ves v 2) | 39 | Splits mucopolysaccharides, allowing deeper penetration of other venom constituents |
| | Antigen 5 (Ves v 5) | 23 | Unknown |
| Fire ant | Phospholipase $A_1$ (Sol i 1) | 34 | Transforms phospholipids to lysophospholipids, which are strong surfactants and therefore cytotoxic |
| | (Sol i 2) | | Unknown |
| | Antigen 5 (Sol i 3) | 23 | Unknown |
| | (Sol i 4) | | Unknown |

## 12.3 Epidemiology of Hymenoptera Venom Allergy

The prevalence of reactions to Hymenoptera stings is reported to be between 2% and 26% for local reactions and between 0.3% and 7% for systemic reactions and is largely dependent on the exposure rate, namely, the probability of receiving repeated stings from Hymenoptera insects of the same family [4]. The prevalence is higher in rural than urban areas and higher in males than females. The prevalence is highest in beekeepers, in whom it can exceed 30% [5]. Up to 75% of the patients with a history of systemic anaphylactic sting reactions following bee stings and a much lower proportion of wasp-allergic patients develop systemic symptoms once again when re-stung [6]. The majority of the repeated reactions are of the same severity or milder than the first reaction [7]. Risk factors for the most severe reactions are advanced age, concomitant cardiovascular diseases, concomitant treatment with beta-blockers or angiotensin-converting enzyme (ACE) inhibitors, and mastocytosis [8]. Reactions caused by the European hornet *(V. crabro)* stings are likely to be severe: the relative risk for life-threatening reactions after a *V. crabro* sting is about three times higher than it is for a honeybee or yellow jacket sting [9]. Golden et al. studied the outcome of childhood venom allergy in 1,033 patients followed 10–20 years [10]. Systemic reactions occurred in 3% of patients who had received venom immunotherapy and in 17% of untreated patients. The risk was 32% in the group of untreated patients with a history of moderate-to-severe reactions.

## 12.4 Reactions to Hymenoptera Venom Stings

**A normal reaction** of a non-allergic person to a Hymenoptera sting is a painful erythematous swelling with a diameter of up to 10 cm at the site of sting, which resolves in a few hours. In fire ant stings, pustulous necrosis follows the immediate wheal reaction.

**A large local reaction** is defined as a local swelling larger than 10 cm lasting over 24 h. It can be accompanied by malaise, fever and lymphadenopathy. The majority of these patients have IgE against Hymenoptera venom.

**Systemic reactions** of the anaphylactic type start a few minutes after the sting. Mueller classified reactions according to severity and leading symptoms: **Grade I** reactions present as generalized urticaria, itching, tachycardia, malaise and anxiety. For **grade II**, angio-oedema, chest constriction, nausea, vomiting, diarrhoea, abdominal pain and dizziness are characteristic symptoms. In **grade III**, respiratory symptoms predominate: dyspnea, wheezing, stridor, dysphagia, dysarthria, hoarseness, and confusion. **Grade IV** is anaphylactic shock with hypotension, collapse, loss of consciousness, incontinence, and cyanosis [11].

Symptoms of myocardial ischemia or even myocardial infarction may occur during an episode of anaphylaxis due to histamine- or leukotriene-induced contraction of coronary arteries (Kounis syndrome or allergic angina/myocardial infarction) [12, 13].

**Delayed reactions**, such as serum sickness-like syndrome, vasculitis, and nephritis, are rare and appear typically 5–7 days after the sting or few hours after the sting if the patient is already sensitized.

**Toxic reactions** are due to cytotoxic effects of venoms and occur only after stings of many insects (more than 100).

**Psychogenic reactions**, such as vasovagal syncope and hyperventilation syndrome, are quite common following insect stings. They mimic severe systemic allergic reactions and complicate differential diagnostics and decisions about immunotherapy.

### 12.4.1 Fatalities from Anaphylaxis to Hymenoptera Stings

Up to 0.5 per one million people die per year due to Hymenoptera venom allergy [4]. The majority of fatalities occur during the first ever Hymenoptera-induced anaphylactic reaction, without previous exposure [14]. Most of the patients have a history or autopsy evidence of preexisting cardiovascular or pulmonary disease. At least 75% of fatal reactions occur in males over 50 years of age, however children under 10 years are also at higher risk of dying [15, 16]. In eastern half of United States 75% of fatal reactions are due to vespid stings, 15% due to honey bee stings and the rest due to imported fire ant stings [17]. Among victims with previously known hymenoptera sting allergy, none had a suitable emergency kit available when stung [14]. Only few fatalities were described in patients treated with immunotherapy [18]. Patients with systemic mastocytosis are at a particular risk for fatal outcome [19].

## 12.5 Diagnosis of Venom Hypersensitivity

In a patient presenting with a history of Hymenoptera-induced reactions, two questions should be answered. First, the severity of the reaction, and second, the identity of the stinging insect. Both answers are critical when specific immunotherapy is considered for treatment. The first question is easier to answer, particularly if the symptoms and emergency treatment are well documented upon discharge from the emergency room visit. Without objective measurements of blood pressure and medical examination during the episode, it is impossible to differentiate between subjective chest tightness and dyspnea with wheezing and between dizziness and hypotension. This differentiation is important, as patients with grades III or IV are offered immunotherapy, but patients with grade II are not. Further confusion is caused by psychogenic reactions, which might resemble allergic reactions, or in the case of an objectively mild allergic reaction, where the perception of a more severe reaction is given through the patient's history.

The second question is the insect responsible. Many patients do not firmly recognize the insect. Some circumstances might help to clarify which was the culprit insect [1]. After a bee sting, the stinger most often remains in the skin. Other Hymenoptera insects, including bumblebees, do not normally lose the stinger. Bee stings can occur all year round, as the entire beehive survives the winter. On the other hand, in vespids, only the queen survives the winter and the majority of vespid stings occur in late summer and autumn.

Skin tests and venom-specific IgE are used to confirm the diagnosis of venom allergy and to help identify the responsible insect. However, there are many problems in the interpretation of diagnostic tests with venoms. Skin prick tests in concentrations of up to 100 μg/mL have quite poor sensitivity, even below 60% [20]. Intradermal tests at the concentration of 1 μ(mu)g/mL are quite often falsely positive [21, 22]. Specific IgEs have higher sensitivity; however, they are often falsely positive due to cross-reactivity. They are positive in up to 30% of subjects with no history of venom allergy, particularly in patients with high total IgE, most probably due to the presence of clinically irrelevant IgEs against carbohydrate epitopes (CCDs). These antibodies are particularly frequent in patients sensitized with pollens [23]. Out of 81 apparently healthy subjects with detectable IgEs specific to bee and wasp venom by the CAP system, only four patients reacted to a sting challenge with a mild systemic reaction, and large local reactions occurred in about one third of subjects [21].

The flow cytometry-based basophil activation test (BAT) offers higher sensitivity with comparable positive predictive value compared to skin tests and specific IgEs in detecting Hymenoptera venom sensitization [24]. Namely, basophils are not activated by clinically unimportant sIgE antibodies against CCD. However, the test is expensive and available only in a few clinical settings [21].

**Table 12.2** Diagnostic values of commonly used diagnostic tests for venom allergy

| Test | Sensitivity | Specificity |
|---|---|---|
| Skin prick test (100 μg/mL) | 60–90% [20, 22] | 62% [22] |
| Intradermal test (0.1 μg/mL) | 69–89% [22] | 96% [24] |
| Intradermal test (1 μg/mL) | 83–96% [22] | 54–85% [22] |
| Specific IgE (Uni CAP) | 76% [24] | 70% [23] |
| Basophil activation test | 90% [24] | 92% [43] |
| Sting challenge | 85% [27] | 100% |

The CAST-ELISA test, which measures the release of sulphidoleukotrienes from leukocytes after in vitro provocation with allergens, is sensitive and specific but is less widely used [25]. Diagnostic values of commonly used diagnostic tests for venom allergy are shown in Table 12.2.

Sting challenges with a living insect are not used any more for diagnostic purposes in untreated venom allergic patients for ethical reasons [26]. Moreover, their negative predictive value is not absolute [27].

### *12.5.1 Patients with Positive Allergy Tests to Both Honeybee and Wasp Venom*

Up to 50% of patients with sting reactions have positive skin tests and/or specific IgE to both honeybee and wasp venom. True double sensitization and cross-reactivity must be considered as a cause of the double positivity [28]. Cross-reactivity is possible on the protein level, most often through venom hyaluronidases and cross-reactivity between Api m5 and Ves v3, or through carbohydrates epitopes [29, 30].

Distinguishing between double sensitization and cross-reactivity can help make recommendations for specific immunotherapy in patients who do not recognize the culprit insect [31]. Specifically, patients should be treated with the venom that induces sensitization. Immunotherapy with venom to which a patient is not primarily sensitized can lead to an incomplete protection and treatment failure. On the other hand, treatment with a cross-reactive venom only or a mixture of venoms can lead to the formation of sIgE against epitopes to which the patient was not sensitized prior to immunotherapy [32, 33].

If double sensitization is proven in a patient who did not recognize the culprit insect, immunotherapy should be performed with both venoms; RAST inhibition assays, immunoblotting or the basophil activation test can help to distinguish between cross-reactivity and double sensitization. Using specific IgE inhibition tests, Straumann et al. were able to identify the insect that caused sensitization in four out of 24 double-positive patients [28]. Using BATs in bee and wasp double-positive patients (sIgE and/or skin tests), it was possible to characterize primary sensitization in one third of them (nearly all were found to be wasp-allergic) [24]. The BAT has an advantage over inhibition tests as BAT is also feasible in patients with very low levels of sIgE in whom inhibition tests were not possible.

Approximately one half of double-positive patients have IgE antibodies against CCD [34]. Hausmann et al. showed that some patients with double positivity and sIgE against CCDs remain double-positive, even with the BAT assay [35].

Interestingly, even in patients in whom cross-reactivity between wasp and honeybee hyaluronidases is proven, the majority cross-react because of anti-CCD antibodies. In fact, IgE antibodies directed against protein epitopes of hyaluronidase were detected only in 1/31 of single wasp-positive patients, in 24% of single honeybee venom-positive patients and in 35% of double-positive patients [36]. The majority of double-positive patients can be characterized as bee, wasp or double sensitized using measurements of sIgE against the recombinant major epitopes of honeybee and wasp venoms, namely Api m1 and Ves v5; however, at the moment the test is not commercially available [37].

## 12.6 Anaphylaxis in Patients with Negative Allergy Tests

Although sIgE is believed to be the cause of allergic reactions after Hymenoptera insect stings, there are some patients with repeated systemic reactions and no detectable IgE [38, 39]. Current guidelines for VIT suggest that immunotherapy should be performed only in patients with an IgE-mediated systemic reaction [31], but there are differences in the management of patients with systemic reactions without demonstrated IgE [40]. A negative skin test and no specific IgE may indicate a non-allergic reaction, a limited diagnostic sensitivity of the test used or an alternative mechanism of mast cell activation through complement and anaphylatoxins C3a and C5a [41, 42]. However, at least two thirds of sIgE- and skin prick test-negative patients have a positive reaction in the flow cytometry-based basophil activation test BAT [43, 44]. The limitation of those studies is that due to ethical reasons, the clinical history and not a sting challenge was used as a gold standard [26]. The BAT is shown to give a very low rate of false positive results [45].

## 12.7 Treatment of Venom Hypersensitivity

Large local reactions are treated with cooling with ice or cold water, local glucocorticoides and/or systemic antihistamines [31]. Systemic reactions are treated according to the general principles for treatment of anaphylaxis. Much effort should be directed towards prevention of further stings and further reactions [31]. Patients should avoid walking barefoot, gardening, picking fruit, outdoor sporting and eating, staying close to beehives, and removing vespid nests from attic or windows. Patients should also carry an emergency medical kit consisting of two antihistamine tablets (terfenadine, loratadine, cetirizine, desloratadine, levocetirizine, etc.), glucocorticoide tablets [methylprednisolone]), and adrenaline autoinjectors (Fastjekt, Epipen, Anapen, Anapen Jr, and Epipen Jr). Tablets should be swallowed immediately after the sting. Intramuscular adrenaline should be injected in the case of severe reactions (dyspnea, dizziness). Patients should be informed that medical supervision should be sought after using the emergency kit.

### *12.7.1 Venom Immunotherapy*

VIT is the only effective treatment for the prevention of serious allergic reactions to Hymenoptera stings in sensitized individuals.

### *12.7.2 Selection of Patients Requiring Venom Immunotherapy*

VIT is the therapy of choice for patients who have experienced a severe sting reaction (Mueller grades III (dyspnea) and IV (hypotension)), particularly if there is a substantial risk of further sings [31]. Although VIT is generally not advocated in patients with non-life-threatening systemic reactions, it is considered in selected patients with frequent reactions, such as occupations and/or hobbies in which the risk of exposure is high, in patients with concomitant cardiovascular diseases who are prone to serious side effects of adrenaline, in patients with mastocytosis, and in very anxious patients who have a seriously impaired quality of life. North American guidelines recommend VIT for all adult patients with systemic reactions of any kind [46].

VIT is not indicated when tests for immediate hypersensitivity are negative or for unusual reactions, such as vasculitis, nephrosis, fever, and thrombocytopenia. VIT is not indicated for large local reactions.

### 12.7.3 Contraindications for VIT

Contraindications for immunotherapy are not as strict as they are for respiratory allergic diseases. In relation to the use of beta-blockers, the decision must always consider the risk of cardiac disease if the beta-blocker treatment is stopped. If the cardiac risk is high and the risk of re-sting is minimal, VIT should not be started in patients receiving beta-blockers. In patients at high risk for anaphylaxis, VIT should be done even if it is not possible to take the patient off beta-blockers, but under careful supervision, including monitoring of blood pressure and electrocardiograms during the dose-increase phase. [47, 48].

Although a few case reports on particularly severe systemic reactions while taking ACE inhibitors have been published [49], the frequency of systemic reactions during VIT is not increased in patients taking ACE inhibitors [50, 51].

Although autoimmune and malignant diseases are considered as contraindications for allergen-specific immunotherapy, it has been shown that VIT was safe and effective in patients with a malignant disease in remission. On the other hand, discontinuation of VIT should be seriously considered if cancer progresses or therapeutic priorities have changed (e.g., oncological treatment). Additionally, VIT was safe, effective and did not induce any progression of underlying diseases in autoimmune diseases, such as rheumatoid arthritis, Crohn's disease, and autoimmune thyroiditis. However, data on the long-term safety of VIT in those patients are lacking [52].

Due to the risk of systemic reactions, VIT should not be started during pregnancy. In well-tolerated VIT, it is safe to continue maintenance injections during pregnancy [53].

### 12.7.4 Selection of Venom To Be Used in Immunotherapy

As honeybee and bumblebee venoms show marked cross-reactivity, VIT with honeybee venom alone is sufficient in bumblebee-allergic patients who most likely react based on cross-reactivity in the presence of primary sensitization to bee venom. Cross-reactivity exists between the major venom components of several vespids, particularly between *Vespula, Dolichovespula*, and *Vespa* venoms, but less so between *Vespula* and *Polistes* venoms. Using cross-inhibition tests in 24 consecutive patients who experienced anaphylactic reactions after European hornet stings, it was shown that 17/24 patients were sensitized only with wasp *(Vespula germanica)* venom, 2/24 with completely cross-reactive epitopes, one with only European hornet venom and four with separate epitopes of both venoms [54]. Although *V. germanica* venom remains the most appropriate immunotherapeutic agent for the majority of those patients, some patients may fail with this approach. In particular, patients with reactions after a European hornet sting who do not remember previous yellow jacket stings should be tested for the possibility of primary European hornet sensitization [55].

Cross-reactivity is very limited between Apidae and Vespidae. In the cases of double-positive tests to honeybee and *Vespula* and in which identification of the insect responsible is not possible, treatment with both venoms is indicated. It is not recommended to mix venoms together (e.g., wasp or honeybee with yellow jacket), even though yellow jacket and hornet venom are available premixed as a mixed vespid extract, but to perform separate immunotherapies using a single allergen [46]. Fire ant-allergic patients are effectively treated with the whole body extract [56].

### 12.7.5 Treatment Protocols

The time required to reach the generally adequate maintenance dose of 100 μg (equivalent to approximately two bee stings and a much higher number of *Vespula* stings) with slow protocols is several weeks to months, while rush and ultra-rapid (ultra-rush) protocols take several days or only a few hours, respectively [57, 58]. The starting dose is 0.01 μg and is approximately doubled in weekly intervals (in slow conventional protocols) or 15 min intervals (in ultra-rush protocols). An example of the ultra-rush protocol is presented in Table 12.3.

Dose-increasing phases of rush and ultra-rush VIT should be performed in the hospital. Maintenance injections are given in the outpatient department of the hospital. After an injection, patients have to be observed for at least 30 min. The maintenance interval should be kept at 4 weeks for the first year and then extended for 2 weeks each year up to 3 months [59].

**Table 12.3** Ultra-rush treatment protocol for VIT

| DAY | Flask | Concentration (μ(mu)g/mL) | Volume (mL) | Antihistamine tablets |
|---|---|---|---|---|
| Day 1[a] | | | | 2 tbls |
| | I. | 0.1 μ(mu)g/ml | 0.3 | |
| | | | 0.7 | |
| | II. | 1μ(mu)g/ml | 0.3 | |
| | | | 0.7 | |
| | III. | 10 μ(mu)g/ml | 0.2 | |
| | | | 0.3 | |
| | | | 0.5 | |
| | IV. | 100μ(mu)g/ml | 0.1 | |
| | | | 0.2 | |
| | | | 0.3 | |
| | | | 0.4 | |
| Day 2[a] | IV. | | | 2 tbls |
| | | 100μ(mu)g/ml | 0.5 | |
| | | | 0.5 | |
| Day 5[a] | IV. | | | 2 tbls |
| | | 100μ(mu)g/ml | 1.0 | |
| Day 11 | IV. | 100μ(mu)g/ml | 1.0 | 2 tbl |
| Week 4 | IV. | 100μ(mu)g/ml | 1.0 | 1 tbl |
| Week 7 | IV. | 100μ(mu)g/ml | 1.0 | 1 tbl |
| Week 11 | IV. | 100μ(mu)g/ml | 1.0 | 1 tbl |
| Every 4 weeks | IV. | 100μ(mu)g/ml | 1.0 | No premedication |

Each year, the interval between maintenance doses is extended for 2 weeks (maximum interval between injections is 12 weeks in patients on prolonged VIT)

[a]Injections are given every 20 min

### *12.7.6 Duration of Venom Immunotherapy*

VIT should be performed for at least 3 years; the optimal duration is 5 years. Longer or even lifelong treatment should be considered in high risk patients:

1. Patients with a higher risk of very severe sting reactions (e.g., Systemic Mastocytosis, near death anaphylaxis)
2. Patients with systemic allergic reactions to immunotherapy injections or stings during VIT
3. Highly exposed patients, such as beekeepers

In those patients, it is recommended to increase the maintenance dose to 200 μ(mu)g [60].

### *12.7.7 Safety of Venom Immunotherapy*

In venom immunotherapy, the risk of systemic reaction is high. For that reason, VIT should be performed only in clinical settings in which knowledge and equipment are ready for treatment of severe anaphylaxis. Before starting VIT, concomitant internal diseases should be treated. Substitution of drugs, such as beta-blockers or ACE inhibitors, should be considered.

Up to 20% of patients exhibit systemic allergic reactions during the dose-increase phase of VIT. Side effects are much more frequent in honeybee- than in wasp-allergic patients An EAACI multicenter study collected data from 840 patients (71% were wasp-allergic), totalling 26,601 injections, with a variety of treatment regimens. A total of 20% of patients had systemic reactions, corresponding to 1.9% of injections during the dose-increase phase and 0.5% during the maintenance phase. The vast majority of the 280 reported reactions was mild, and only one third required medical treatment. Childhood does not seem to represent an increased risk with such regimens or, in general, with any stage of VIT [61, 62]. It should be kept in mind that very severe reactions are occurring in the maintenance phase of the VIT, even in patients with a well-tolerated dose-increase phase [63]. In fire ant whole body immunotherapy, 9.1% of patients experienced mild systemic reactions [64]. It has been shown that patients prone to systemic reaction during immunotherapy could be identified, as their basophils show higher sensitivity to allergens [65, 66]. There was no correlation between the risk of side effects of VIT and the severity of reaction before immunotherapy. In the same study, it was shown that an elevated basal tryptase level was not a predicting factor for side effects of VIT [65].

Pre-treatment with antihistamines reduces the number and severity of large local reactions and mild systemic reactions, such as urticaria and angio-edema. It is advised that antihistamines are prescribed 1 h before injection until the maintenance dose has been well tolerated at least three times [62, 67, 68].

Depot extracts seem to be associated with somewhat fewer side effects than aqueous preparations and have comparable efficacy [69]. Depot extracts are of course not recommended for rush or ultra-rush protocols, but many allergists switch to depot preparations after the up-dosing phase.

To improve the tolerability of VIT, removal of toxic non-allergenic peptides from the venom extract is being attempted [70]. Melittin is a major toxic peptide in honeybee venom responsible for local side effects; however, it is of marginal importance as an IgE inducer. Modification of the venom with potassium cyanate strongly inhibits the enzymatic activity of phospholipase$A_2$ and hyaluronidase, as evidenced by assays of determination of their specific enzymatic activity, while preserving their immunogenic effect.

Pre-treatment with humanized anti-IgE antibodies (omalizumab) is efficient in patients with repeated systemic reactions while receiving immunotherapy injections [71].

## 12.7.8 Efficacy of Venom Immunotherapy

Nearly complete tolerance after only a few days of rush immunotherapy was confirmed in a sting challenge-controlled study performed by Hunt [72]. Only one bee venom treated patient out of 19 reacted with a mild systemic reaction to a sting challenge compared to 14 out of 23 placebo- or whole body extract-treated patients who reacted with a severe reaction. This is the only double-blind study in Hymenoptera venom immunotherapy, and even this study was terminated prematurely after clear evidence of the effectiveness of venom over whole body extract was obtained. Recently, Goldberg performed a larger study submitting 67 bee-allergic patients to a sting challenge just after reaching the maintenance dose of 100 μ(mu)g. In total, 6.6% of patients developed a systemic reaction, and those patients continued VIT on a maintenance dose of 200 μ(mu)g [73].

Long-term effectiveness after stopping immunotherapy is less reliable [74]. In a Swiss study, 16% of bee-allergic patients and 7.5% of wasp-allergic patients treated for 3–7 years developed systemic reactions after stopping immunotherapy. Most reactions are mild, but there is a tendency for an increase in the severity of reactions after repeated re-stinging [75]. The risk of reaction was the same in patients who were skin test-positive and skin test-negative at the moment of stopping immunotherapy. Moreover, a fatal reaction 9 years after the discontinuation of immunotherapy was recently described [17].

In a follow-up study of 229 patients (108 treated with honeybee, 100 with yellow jacket and 20 with both venoms), 55% of the VIT-treated patients were stung after the treatment [76]. A total of 60% of those patients were stung once, 15% twice, 9% had three stings and 16% had four or more stings. In patients treated more than 3 years after the first sting, 8% had a systemic reaction. In patients with more than one sting, the second systemic reaction was more severe than the first one in 2.5%, and a systemic reaction occurred after the first sting was well tolerated in 17%. Other patients had no allergic reactions even after repeated stings. All patients reported that their reactions after ending VIT were milder than before treatment. The likelihood of systemic reactions to stings was almost identical in patients treated for either more than or less than 3 years with VIT. Furthermore, patients who reacted after discontinuation of immunotherapy were found to have higher basophil sensitivity (the sensitivity was comparable to a group of patients without immunotherapy) compared to a group of protected patients [77].

The failure rate for venom-allergic children is similar to that observed in adults. Immunotherapy is associated with an improved quality of life [78, 79]. The efficacy of VIT has also been demonstrated by assessing health-related quality of life (HRQL). In a cross-sectional study, about one third of venom-allergic patients held self-imposed debilitating beliefs with impairment of their HRQL [80].

A randomised prospective study compared the effects of VIT versus Epipen as an emergency medication on HRQL. The group randomized to VIT showed a statistically significant improvement in their HRQL scores, while in those randomized to the Epipen, HQRL scores were unchanged or even deteriorated [81].

Some risk factors for relapse after immunotherapy are recognized [61]:

- Bee venom allergy
- Severe pre-treatment reaction
- Reaction to VIT injection
- Reaction during VIT
- Duration of VIT <5 years
- Repeated re-stings after stopping VIT

Patients with reactions during immunotherapy are encouraged to receive immunotherapy indefinitely.

## 12.8 Anaphylaxis After Hymenoptera Sting and Mastocytosis

The baseline serum level of tryptase is an indicator of the whole body mast cell load. Potier et al. found elevated basal cell tryptase in 10.7% of patients on venom immunotherapy, and one third of them were eventually diagnosed with mastocytosis [82]. Similarly, systemic mastocytosis was diagnosed in 5.8% of 379 consecutive patients with Hymenoptera sting anaphylaxis in a study by Bonadonna [83]. Patients with mastocytosis are at a highly increased risk of developing anaphylaxis. Those patients sustained significantly more severe reactions (mostly cardiovascular anaphylactic sting reactions) than those with normal basal tryptase. Cutaneous symptoms present predominantly as a flush and rarely as urticaria and angio-edema [84]. These patients are also at a higher risk of dying during anaphylaxis [18].

In patients with anaphylaxis, mastocytosis should be actively investigated by testing the baseline serum tryptase level and by a clinical examination searching for characteristic skin lesions. If a patient has characteristic skin signs and a basal tryptase level over 11.4 ng/mL or if the basal tryptase level is over 20 ng/mL, a bone marrow biopsy is indicated [85]. Patients who fulfil only one or two minor diagnostic criteria for the diagnosis of systemic mastocytosis seem to have a comparable risk for Hymenoptera venom allergy as patients with mastocytosis [86].

Patients with anaphylaxis and elevated basal tryptase levels with or without documented mastocytosis should be instructed carefully on how to avoid further allergen exposure.

VIT in those patients is associated with a higher rate of severe side effects. However, in the majority of patients, it is possible to achieve tolerance [87]. Although VIT is effective in the latter patients, it may be necessary to use an elevated maintenance dose to protect individual patients [88]. VIT is recommended for life in venom allergic patients with mastocytosis because there are some case reports of fatal reactions after stopping venom immunotherapy [19].

## References

1. Mueller UR. *Insect sting allergy.* Stuttgart: Gustav Fisher; 1990.
2. Winningham KM, Fitch CD, Schmidt M, et al. Hymenoptera venom protease allergens. *J Allergy Clin Immunol.* 2004;114:928–33.
3. Hoffman DR. Hymenoptera venom allergens. *Clin Rev Allergy Immunol.* 2006;30:109–128.
4. Bilo` BM, Bonifazi F. Epidemiology of insect-venom anaphylaxis. *Curr Opinion Allergy Clin Immunol.* 2008;8:330–337.
5. Münstedt K, Hellner M, Winter D, et al. Allergy to bee venom in beekeepers in Germany. *J Investig Allergol Clin Immunol.* 2008;18:100–105.
6. Kampelmacher MJ, van der Zwan JC. Provocation test with a living insect as a diagnostic tool in systemic reactions to bee and wasp venom: a prospective study with emphasis on the clinical aspects. *Clin Allergy.* 1987;17:317–327.
7. Settipane GA, Chafee FH. Natural history of allergy to Hymenoptera. *Clin Allergy.* 1979;9:385–390.
8. Ruëff F, Przybilla B, Biló MB, et al. Predictors of severe systemic anaphylactic reactions in patients with Hymenoptera venom allergy: importance of baseline serum tryptase-a study of the European Academy of Allergology and Clinical Immunology Interest Group on Insect Venom Hypersensitivity. *J Allergy Clin Immunol.* 2009;124:1047–1054.
9. Antonicelli L, Bilò MB, Napoli G, et al. European hornet (Vespa crabro) sting: a new risk factor for life-threatening reaction in hymenoptera allergic patients? *Eur Ann Allergy Clin Immunol.* 2003;35:199–203.
10. Golden DB, Kagey-Sobotka A, Norman PS, et al. Outcomes of allergy to insect stings in children, with and without venom immunotherapy. *N Engl J Med.* 2004;351:668–674.
11. Mueller HL. Diagnosis and treatment of insect sensitivity. *J Asthma Res.* 1966;3:331–333.
12. Rekik S, Andrieu S, Aboukhoudir F, et al. ST elevation myocardial infarction with no structural lesions after a wasp sting. *J Emerg Med.* 2009 Mar 26;doi:10.1016/j.jemermed.2009.02.019 DOI:dx.doi.org .
13. Sinkiewicz W, Sobański P, Bartuzi Z. Allergic myocardial infarction. *Cardiol J.* 2008;15:220–225.
14. Sasvary T, Müller U. Fatalities from insect stings in Switzerland 1978 to 1987. *Schweiz Med Wochenschr.* 1994;124:1887–1894.

15. Müller UR. Cardiovascular disease and insect sting anaphylaxis. Handouts of EAACI Congress, Warsaw; 2009.
16. Prado M, Quirós D, Lomonte B. Mortality due to Hymenoptera stings in Costa Rica, 1985-2006. *Rev Panam Salud Publica.* 2009;25:389–393.
17. Hoffman DR. Fatal Reactions to Hymenoptera Stings. *Allergy Asthma Proc.* 2003;24:123–127.
18. Light WC. Insect sting fatality 9 years after venom treatment. *J Allergy Clin Immunol.* 2001;107:925.
19. CD Oude Elberink JNG, de Monchy JGR, Kors JW, et al. Fatal anaphylaxis after a yellow jacket sting in two patients with mastocytosis. *J Allergy Clin Immunol.* 1997;99:153–154.
20. Korosec P, Silar M, Kopac P, et al. Low sensitivity of venom skin prick tests in patients with severe anaphylactic reactions to hymenoptera stings. *Allergy.* 2009;64(Suppl. 90):341.
21. Sturm G, Kranzelbinder B, Schuster C, et al. Correlation of the basophil activation test (BAT) and routine diagnostic tools with the outcome of sting challenges in asymptomatically sensitised subjects to hymenoptera venom. *Allergy.* 2009;64(Suppl.90):39.
22. Jeep S, Reiprich G, Kunkel G. Comparison of skin prick tests and intradermal tests with three diflerent yellow jacket venom extracts. *Allergy.* 1992;47:35–40.
23. Mari A, Iacovacci P, Afferni C. et al. Specific IgE to cross-reactive carbohydrate determinants strongly affect the in vitro diagnosis of allergic diseases. *J Allergy Clin Immunol.* 1999;103:1005–1011.
24. Peternelj A, Silar M, Bajrovic N, et al. Diagnostic value of the basophil activation test in evaluating Hymenoptera venom sensitisation. *Wien Klin Wochenschr.* 2009;121:344–348.
25. Scherer K, Weber JM, Jermann TM, et al. Cellular in vitro assays in the diagnosis of Hymenoptera venom allergy. *Int Arch Allergy Immunol.* 2008;146:122–132.
26. Ruëff F, Przybilla B, Müller U, et al. The sting challenge test in Hymenoptera venom allergy. Position paper of the Subcommittee on Insect Venom Allergy of the European Academy of Allergology and Clinical Immunology. *Allergy.* 1996;51:216–225.
27. Franken HH, Dubois AE, Minkema HJ, et al. Lack of reproducibility of a single negative sting challenge response in the assessment of anaphylactic risk in patients with suspected yellow jacket hypersensitivity. *J Allergy Clin Immunol.* 1994;93:431–436.
28. Straumann F, Bucher C, Wütrich B. Double sensitization to honeybee and wasp venom: immunotherapy with one or with both venoms? Value of FEIA inhibition for the identification of the cross-reacting IgE antibodies in double-sensitized patients to honeybee and wasp venom. *Int Arch Allergy Immunol.* 2000;123:268–274.
29. Wypych JI, Abeyounis CJ, Reisman RE (1989) Analysis of differing patterns of cross-reactivity of honeybee and yellow jacket venom-specific IgE: use of purified venom fractions. *Int Arch Allergy Appl Immunol.* 89:60–6.
30. Hemmer W, Focke M, Kolarich D et al. Identification by immunoblot of venom glycoproteins displaying immunoglobulin E-binding N-glycans as cross-reactive allergens in honeybee and yellow jacket venom. *Clin Exp Allergy.* 2004;34:460–9.
31. Bonifazi F, Jutel M, Biló BM et al. Prevention and treatment of hymenoptera venom allergy: guidelines for clinical practice. *Allergy.* 2005;60:1459–70.
32. Modrzyński M, Zawisza E. Possible induction of oral allergy syndrome during specific immunotherapy in patients sensitive to tree pollen. *Med Sci Monit.* 2005;11: 351–5.
33. Juarez C, Blanca M, Miranda A et al. Specific IgE antibodies to vespids in the course of immunotherpay with Vespula germanica administered to patients sensitized to Polistes dominulus. *Allergy.* 1992;47:299–302.
34. Erzen R, Korosec P, Silar M et al. Carbohydrate epitopes as a cause of cross-reactivity in patients allergic to Hymenoptera venom. *Wien Klin Wochenschr.* 2009;121:349–52.
35. Hausmann O, Gentinetta T, Schneider M et al. Double positivity in insect venom allergy – diagnostic approach with basophil activation test. *Allergy.* 2009;64 (Suppl. 90):140.
36. Jin C, Focke M, Léonard R, HJarisch R, Altmann F, Hemmer W. Reassessing the role of hyaluronidase in yellow jacket venom allergy. *J Allergy Clin Immunol.* 2010;125:184–90.
37. Müller UR, Johansen N, Petersen AB et al. Hymenoptera venom allergy: analysis of double positivity to honey bee and Vespula venom by estimation of IgE antibodies to species-specific major allergens Api m1 and Ves v5. *Allergy.* 2009;64:543–48.
38. Kosnik M. Anaphylaxis to venom without IgE antibody. *Allergy.* 2000;55:676–7.
39. Zidarn M, Kosnik M, Drinovec I. Anaphylaxis after Hymenoptera sting without detectable specific IgE. *Acta Dermatovenerol Alp Panonica Adriat.* 2007;16:31–3.
40. Diwakar L, Noorani S, Huissoon AP et al. Practice of venom immunotherapy in the United Kingdom: a national audit and review of literature. *Clin Exp Allergy.* 2008;38:1651–8.
41. Van der Linden PWG, Hack CE, van der Zwan et al. Preliminary report: complement activation in wasp-sting anaphylaxis. *Lancet.* 1990;336:904–6.
42. Oettgen HC, Martin TR, Drazen JM et al. Active anaphylaxis in IgE-deficient mouse. *Nature.* 1994;370:367–70.
43. Korosec P, Erzen R, Silar M et al. Basophil responsiveness in patients with insect sting allergies and negative venom-specific immunoglobulin E and skin prick test results. *Clin Exp Allergy.* 2009;39:1730–7.

44. Ebo DG, Hagendorens MM, Bridts CH et al. Hymenoptera venom allergy: taking the sting out of difficult cases. *J Investig Allergol Clin Immunol.* 2007;17:357–60.
45. Erdmann SM, Sachs B, Kwiecien R et al. The basophil activation test in wasp venom allergy: sensitivity, specificity and monitoring specific immunotherapy. *Allergy.* 2004;59:1102–9.
46. Joint Task Force on Practice Parameters; American Academy of Allergy. Asthma and Immunology; American College of Allergy, Asthma and Immunology; Joint Council of Allergy, Asthma and Immunology. Allergen immunotherapy: a practice parameter second update. *J Allergy Clin Immunol.* 2007;120(Suppl 3):25–85.
47. Müller UR, Haeberli G. Use of beta-blockers during immunotherapy for Hymenoptera venom allergy. *J Allergy Clin Immunol.* 2005;115:606–10.
48. Hepner MJ, Ownby DR, Anderson JA et al. Risk of systemic reactions in patients taking beta-blocker drugs receiving allergy immunotherapy injections. *J Allergy Clin Immunol.* 1990;85:407–11.
49. Ober AI, MacLean JA, Hannaway PJ. Life-threatening anaphylaxis to venom immunotherapy in a patient taking an angiotensin-converting enzyme inhibitor. *J Allergy Clin Immunol.* 2003;112:1008–9.
50. Tunon-de-Lara JM, Villanueva P, Marcos M et al. Ace inhibitors and anaphylactoid reactions during venom immunotherapy. *Lancet.* 1992;340:908.
51. White KM, England RW. Safety of angiotensin-converting enzyme inhibitors while receiving venom immunotherapy. *Ann Allergy Asthma Immunol.* 2008;101:426–30.
52. Bilo BM. Venom immunotherapy in hymenoptera venom allergic patients with immunologic diseases and neoplasms. Handouts of EAACI congress, Warsaw 2009.
53. Schwartz HJ, Golden DBK, Lockey RF. Venom immunotherapy in the Hymenoptera-allergic pregnant patient. *J Allergy Clin Immunol.* 1990;85:709–712.
54. Kosnik M, Korosec P, Silar M et al. Wasp venom is appropriate for immunotherapy of patients with allergic reaction to the European hornet sting. *Croat Med J.* 2002;43:25–7.
55. Erzen R, Bajrovic N, Music E et al. Efficiency of wasp venom specific immunotherapy in patients with allergic reactions to European hornet sting. *Allergy.* 2009;64 (Suppl. 90): 457.
56. Freeman TM, Hylander R, Ortiz A et al. Imported fire ant immunotherapy: effectiveness of whole body extracts. *J Allergy Clin Immunol.* 1992;90:210–5.
57. Brehler R, Wolf H, Kutting B, Schnitker J et al. Safety of a two-day ultrarush insect venom immunotherapy protocol in comparison with protocols of longer duration and involving a larger number of injections. *J Allergy Clin Immunol.* 2000;105:1231–5.
58. Steiss JO, Jödicke B, Lindemann H. A modified ultrarush insect venom immunotherapy protocol for children. *Allergy Asthma Proc.* 2006;27:148–50.
59. Goldberg A, Confino-Cohen R. Maintenance venom immunotherapy administered at 3-month intervals is both safe and efficacious. *J Allergy Clin Immunol.* 2001;107:902–6.
60. Rueff F, Wenderoth A, Przybilla B. Patients still reacting to a sting challenge while receiving conventional Hymenoptera venom immunotherapy are protected by increased venom doses. *J Allergy Clin Immunol.* 2001;108:1027–32.
61. Mosbech H, Mueller U. Side-effects of insect venom immunotherapy: results from an EAACI multicenter study. European Academy of Allergology and Clinical Immunology. *Allergy.* 2000;55:1005–10.
62. Gorska L, Chelminska M, Kuziemski K et al. Analysis of safety, risk factors and pretreatment methods during rush hymenoptera venom immunotherapy. *Int Arch Allergy Immunol.* 2008;147:241–5.
63. Adamic K, Zidarn M, Bajrovic N et al. The local and systemic side-effects of venom and inhaled-allergen subcutaneous immunotherapy. *Wien Klin Wochenschr.* 2009;121:357–60.
64. La Shell MS, Calabria CW, Quinn JM. Imported fire ant field reaction and immunotherapy safety characteristics: the IFACS study. *J Allergy Clin Immunol.* 2010;125:1294–9.
65. Kosnik M , Silar M, Bajrovic N et al. High sensitivity of basophils predicts side-effects in venom immunotherapy. *Allergy.* 2005;60:1401–6.
66. Zitnik S, Glavnik V, Avcin T et al. High sensitivity of basophils predict side effect in bee venom immunotherapy in children. *Allergy.* 2008;63(Suppl 88):642.
67. Jutel M, Watanabe T, Klunker S et al. Histamine regulates T-cell and antibody responses by differential expression of H1 and H2 receptors. *Nature.* 2001;413: 420–5.
68. Müller U, Hari Y, Berchtold E. Premedication with antihistamines may enhance efficacy of specific-allergen immunotherapy. *J Allergy Clin Immunol.* 2001;107:81–6.
69. Rueff F, Wolf H, Schnitker J et al. Specific immunotherapy in honey bee venom allergy: a comparative study using aqueous and aluminium adsorbed preparations. *Allergy.* 2004;59:589–95.
70. Bilo B, Roncarolo D, Falagiani P et al. A new potential candidate for ITS of bee venom allergic patients. *Allergy.* 2009;64 (Suppl. 90):140.
71. Kontou-Fili K, Filis CI. Prolonged high-dose omalizumab is required to control reactions to venom immunotherapy in mastocytosis. *Allergy.* 2009;64:1384–5.
72. Hunt KJ, Valentine MD, Sobotka AK et al. A controlled trial of immunotherapy in insect hypersensitivity. *N Engl J Med.* 1978;299:157–61.

73. Goldberg A, Confino-Cohen R. Bee venom immunotherapy – How early is it effective. *Allergy*. 2010;65:391–5.
74. Golden DB, Kagey-Sobotka A, Lichtenstein LM. Survey of patients after discontinuing venom immunotherapy. *J Allergy Clin Immunol*. 2000;105:385–90.
75. Lerch E, Müller UR. Long-term protection after stopping venom immunotherapy: results of re-stings in 200 patients. *J Allergy Clin Immunol*. 1998;101:606–12.
76. Hafner T, DuBuske L, Kosnik M. Long-term efficacy of venom immunotherapy. *Ann Allergy Asthma Immunol*. 2008;100:162–5.
77. Peternelj A. Silar M, Erzen R et al. Basophil sensitivity in patients not responding to venom immunotherapy. *Int Arch Allergy Immunol*. 2008;146:248–54.
78. Joanne NG, Elberink O, Monchy JGR et al. Venom immunotherapy improves health related quality of life in patients allergic to yellow jacket venom. *J Allergy Clin Immunol*. 2002;110:174–82.
79. Roesch A, Boerzsoenyi J, Babilas P et al. Outcome survey of insect venom allergic patients with venom immunotherapy in a rural population. *J Dtsch Dermatol Ges*. 2008;6:292–7.
80. Confino-Cohen R, Melamed S, Goldberg A. Debilitating beliefs, emotional distress and quality of life in patients given immunotherapy for insect sting allergy. *Clin Exp Allergy*. 1999;29:1626–31.
81. Oude Elberink J, de Monchy J, van der Heide S et al. Venom immunotherapy improves health related quality of life in patients allergic to yellow jacket venom. *J Allergy Clin Immunol*. 2002;110:174–82.
82. Potier A, Lavigne C, Chappard D et al. Cutaneus manifestations of Hymenoptera and Diptera anaphylaxis: relationship to basal serum tryptase. *Clin Exp Allergy*. 2009;39:717–25.
83. Bonadonna P, Zanotti R, Caruso B et al. Allergen specific immunotherapy is safe and effective in patients with systemic mastocytosis and Hymenoptera allergy. *J Allergy Clin Immunol*. 2008;121:256–257.
84. Brockow K, Jofer C, Behrendt H et al. Anaphylaxis in patients with mastocytosis: a study on history, clinical features and risk factors in 120 patients. *Allergy*. 2008;63:226–32.
85. Müller U. Elevated baseline serum tryptase, mastocytosis and anaphylaxis. *Clin Exp Allergy*. 2009;39:620–2.
86. Bonadonna P, Perbellini O, Passalacqua G et al. Clonal mast cell disorders in patients with systemic reactions to Hymenoptera stings and increased serum tryptase levels. *J Allergy Clin Immunol*. 2009;123:680–686.
87. Fricker M, Helbling A, Schwartz L et al. Hymenoptera sting anaphylaxis and urticaria pigmentosa: Clinical findings and results of venom immunotherapy in ten patients. *J Allergy Clin Immunol*. 1997;100:11–15.
88. Rueff F, Wenderoth A, Przybilla B. Patients still reacting to a sting challenge while receiving Hymenoptera venom immunotherapy are protected by increased venom doses. *J Allergy Clin Immunol*. 2001;108:1027–1032.

# Chapter 13
# Idiopathic Anaphylaxis

**Karen Hsu Blatman and Leslie C. Grammer**

**Abstract** When anaphylaxis occurs in the absence of an identifiable trigger, the anaphylactic reaction is termed idiopathic. It is a well-described type of anaphylaxis with treatment that is associated with good prognosis. Episodes may be reduced with prophylactic corticosteroids and antihistamines. There is no definitive diagnostic test for idiopathic anaphylaxis. By definition, it is a diagnosis of exclusion after eliminating other causes. Disorders that may mimic anaphylaxis should be considered for evaluation. The cause of idiopathic anaphylaxis remains uncertain.

**Keywords** Idiopathic anaphylaxis • Clonal mast cell • Urticaria • Angioedema • Anaphylaxis • Mast cells • Mastocytosis • Tryptase • Histamine • Corticosteroids • Histamine-releasing factor • Scrombroidosis • Exercise-induced anaphylaxis • Aspirin • Latex hypersensitivity • Carcinoid • Vocal cord dysfunction • Undifferentiated somatoform anaphylaxis • Oral cromolyn • Montelukast • Leukotriene D4 • Progesterone • C-kit • Mite-contaminated flour • Bee pollen • Hydatid cyst disease • Pheochromocytoma • Munchausen stridor • Oral albuterol • Ketotifen • Omalizumab • Doxepin

## 13.1 Introduction

Anaphylaxis is often associated with an identifiable precipitant, such as food, medication or insect sting. When anaphylaxis occurs in the absence of an identifiable trigger, after an extensive diagnostic evaluation, the anaphylactic reaction is termed idiopathic. Despite the fact that much is still unknown regarding the etiology of this disease, it is a well-described type of anaphylaxis with treatment that is associated with a good prognosis. Unlike antigen-induced anaphylaxis, idiopathic anaphylaxis episodes may be reduced with prophylactic treatment of oral glucocorticosteroids [1, 2]. Despite the frequency of the diagnosis, fatalities are rare [3, 4].

Idiopathic anaphylaxis was first described more than 30 years ago by Bacal, Patterson and Zeiss in a series of 21 patients with anaphylaxis, 11 of whom had no causal explanation [5]. The series was expanded to include more than 335 patients who had been followed without an external allergen being implicated [6].

The prevalence of idiopathic anaphylaxis in 1995 was estimated to be approximately 1 in 10,000 patients from a survey of 75 US allergists [7]. In the same year, Kemp et al. published a study of 266 sequential cases of anaphylaxis noting that 37% were unexplained [8]. Since then, the series has been updated to include 601 cases of anaphylaxis; more than 50% were unexplained. However,

K. Hsu Blatman (✉)
Northwestern University, Feinberg School of Medicine, Chicago, IL, USA
e-mail: khsublatman@partners.org

M.C. Castells (ed.), *Anaphylaxis and Hypersensitivity Reactions*,
DOI 10.1007/978-1-60327-951-2_13, © Springer Science+Business Media, LLC 2011

**Table 13.1** Age distribution of 335 patients with idiopathic anaphylaxis [6]

| Age | Number | % of 335 |
|---|---|---|
| 0–9 | 4 | 1.2 |
| 10–19 | 28 | 8.4 |
| 20–29 | 88 | 26.3 |
| 30–39 | 94 | 28.1 |
| 40–49 | 55 | 16.4 |
| 50–59 | 39 | 11.6 |
| 60–69 | 16 | 4.8 |
| >70 | 11 | 3.3 |

the study excluded anaphylaxis caused by hymenoptera stings and tightened its criteria for diagnosis of food-induced anaphylaxis; if skin prick test was negative, then the patient was diagnosed as idiopathic [9]. In a retrospective study of patients from Olmstead County, Minneapolis, 32% were found to have idiopathic anaphylaxis [10].

It has been reported that idiopathic anaphylaxis is more common in women, with several studies reporting more than 60% of affected patients were women [6, 9, 11]. Approximately 50% of these patients were atopic [6, 11]. Patients with idiopathic anaphylaxis may also have separate episodes of anaphylaxis caused by known triggers [6].

Although idiopathic anaphylaxis was first reported in adults, subsequently the disease has been reported in the pediatric population. Idiopathic anaphylaxis has been reported across the entire age spectrum (Table 13.1) Pediatric patients have been treated with the same protocol as adults, adjusting for pediatric doses, and their response has been similar [12–15].

Idiopathic anaphylaxis, by definition, is a diagnosis of exclusio. There is no definitive diagnostic test for idiopathic anaphylaxis. In some cases, an episode of anaphylaxis can be confirmed by acute measurement of histamine and tryptase, indicating mast cell activation [16]. The symptoms of idiopathic anaphylaxis are identical to known cases of anaphylaxis. Moro and colleagues reported 435 patients diagnosed with anaphylaxis in 2004–2005; those diagnosed with idiopathic anaphylaxis were more frequently had lower respiratory symptoms [17].

Currently, there is not a universally accepted definition of anaphylaxis, and it is often used to describe non-IgE mediated or "anaphylactoid" events. There have been two symposia sponsored by the National Institutes of Health and the Food Allergy and Anaphylaxis Network, where panels of experts were unable to agree on a "true" definition of anaphylaxis. There was an agreement of signs and symptoms defining the necessity for epinephrine treatment [18].

## 13.2 Pathogenesis

While the pathogenesis of idiopathic anaphylaxis is still unknown, several theories have been proposed over the years. Idiopathic anaphylaxis is associated with increased activation of mast cells, as is anaphylaxis with a known trigger [16].

One theory evaluated two decades ago was the possibility of increased mast cell numbers. Mast cell numbers in the skin and the bone marrow of idiopathic anaphylaxis patients were studied; no clinically significant increase in the number of mast cells in patients with idiopathic anaphylaxis were noted. In normal individuals, each square millimeter of cutaneous tissue contained approximately 38 mast cells, while patients with idiopathic anaphylaxis averaged 72. In contrast, patients with urticaria pigmentosa averaged 697 mast cells and those with systemic mastocytosis averaged 721 mast cells. The slightly higher number of mast cells reported in patients with idiopathic anaphylaxis compared to normals was not considered to be clinically significant when compared to those patients with diagnoses such as systemic mastocytosis and urticaria pigmentosa [19].

Another study also revealed that in vitro studies on peripheral blood basophils from patients with idiopathic anaphylaxis did not demonstrate increased histamine release upon stimulation with anti-IgE. Furthermore, Keffer and colleagues demonstrated that there were no differences between normal patients and patients with idiopathic anaphylaxis in terms of cutaneous response to intradermal morphine [20].

Not only have studies shown that mast cells from patients with idiopathic anaphylaxis do not release more histamine upon stimulation with anti-IgE, but there are also reports that patients with idiopathic anaphylaxis had the same threshold cutaneous response upon exposure to increasing dilutions of various mediators such as histamine, platelet activating factor and leukotriene D4 when compared with patients with asthma, allergic rhinitis and chronic idiopathic urticaria. Patients with idiopathic anaphylaxis actually had slightly less cutaneous sensitivity compared to patients with allergic rhinitis or asthma [21]. However, Tejedor et al. evaluated mast cell releasibility in patients with idiopathic anaphylaxis and found those patients showed a higher cutaneous response to codeine than did atopic patients without anaphylaxis [22, 23]. In contrast, in a study of 18 patients with idiopathic anaphylaxis, Reed and colleagues could not confirm an increased cutaneous sensitivity to codeine. The control group included both atopic and non-atopic patients without anaphylaxis [24].

Other studies also tried to identify possible "hidden" allergens causing proposed idiopathic anaphylaxis. Sonin and Patterson evaluated the possible role of metabisulfite, a common food additive/preservative. They challenged 12 idiopathic anaphylaxis patients with the compound, however there were no positive responses [25].

Progesterone sensitivity was also proposed as a possible explanation for idiopathic anaphylaxis. Endogenous progesterone sensitivity was reported in three women whose episode of idiopathic anaphylaxis improved after surgical or pharmacological castration [26]. However, the episodes of anaphylaxis had no correlation with the sharp rise in progesterone during the luteal phase of the menstrual cycle. In addition peripheral blood samples did not display histamine release that would correlate with progesterone stimulation [27].

Autoimmune activation of mast cells via anti-IgE antibodies, which have been described as playing a role in chronic idiopathic urticaria [28], have also been proposed as a possible cause of idiopathic anaphylaxis. Preliminary studies at Northwestern of ten samples were unable to confirm this link (unpublished results).

Investigators have also proposed dysregulation of histamine-releasing factors (HRFs) and histamine-releasing inhibitory factors as an underlying cause of patients with idiopathic anaphylaxis [29]. The success of corticosteroids in treating idiopathic anaphylaxis could be explained by its suppressive effects on activated cells producing such factors. Two known HRFs have subsequently been studied at Northwestern, monocyte chemoattractant protein type 1 (MCP-1) and macrophage-inflammatory protein type 1a (MIP-1a). Levels of MCP-1 and MIP-1a were measured in the serum of normal atopic individuals and idiopathic anaphylaxis patients and no significant differences were found [30].

Patients with mastocytosis have continued elevation of serum total tryptase after resolution of an acute anaphylactic episode. In a study by Akin, a subset of patients with idiopathic anaphylaxis was identified that had a clonal mast cell population secondary to a mutation in *c-kit*, which codes for KIT, a receptor for stem cell factor. The mutation appears in a hyperresponsive mast cell phenotype [31, 32]. Case reports also exist of patients with idiopathic anaphylaxis having elevated tryptase levels, and Shanmugam reported one patient in whom the tryptase was still elevated 26 h after onset of symtpoms [33, 34].

Koterba and Akin found that the baseline tryptase level was more elevated in 15 patients with indolent systemic mastocytosis versus idiopathic anaphylaxis (71.5 versus 7.6 ng/mL), and those with idiopathic anaphylaxis had higher IgE levels (109.6 versus 43.3 IU/mL). The 15 patients diagnosed with systemic indolent mastocytosis all displayed markers of clonal mast cell disease (CD25+, c-kit D816V mutation). In addition, no patient with indolent systemic mastocytosis experienced urticaria during the anaphylactic episodes, while urticaria was frequently reported in patients with idiopathic anaphylaxis [35] (Table 13.2).

In a study by Grammer et al., patients with idiopathic anaphylaxis were found to have an increased percentage of activated T cells in their peripheral blood during acute episodes compared to during remission. In addition, they have more activated B cells, regardless of whether idiopathic anaphylaxis patients were in an acute episode or in remission, than in the general population or in patients with chronic idiopathic urticaria [36].

Howell et al. compared nine patients with idiopathic anaphylaxis with five non-atopic controls and investigated their gene expression profiles of mononuclear cells. Howell found 53 genes predicting idiopathic anaphylaxis from controls and among these found genes that correlate with the level of cd203c, a marker of basophil activation [37].

## 13.3 Differential Diagnosis

There is no definitive diagnostic test for idiopathic anaphylaxis. Patients suspected of having idiopathic anaphylaxis should be referred to an allergist for work-up of known triggers for anaphylaxis. In addition, disorders that may mimic anaphylaxis should be considered for evaluation before diagnosing a patient with idiopathic anaphylaxis. Physicians should obtain a meticulous history from patients to exclude causes of anaphylaxis.

Some of these causes of anaphylaxis include exercise-induced anaphylaxis, and food-associated exercise-induced anaphylaxis. Exercise-induced anaphylaxis is a result of mast cell activation and can be difficult to distinguish from idiopathic anaphylaxis, since the intensity and duration of exercise required to induce anaphylaxis can vary significantly. In some cases, exercised-induced anaphylaxis has been reported to occur after 10 min of slow jogging or dancing, but did not occur the previous week even though the patient participated in a triathalon [38–40].

If the anaphylaxis seems to be related to food ingestion, but the typical foods have been ruled out, then the possibility of a spice causing anaphylaxis should be entertained [41]. However, positive skin test to foods in the absence of correlation to anaphylactic episodes has been found to be of no use in identifying a cause of idiopathic anaphylaxis [42]. Undeclared or unsuspected food allergens could also be a trigger, such as peanut butter in egg rolls [43]. Food dyes, such as carmine, have also been implicated [44]. In rare cases, aeroallergens can be added to or contaminate foods. An example is that "bee pollen" can be added to various health food drinks; bee pollen often contains ragweed pollen. Therefore, in a ragweed-sensitized patient, anaphylaxis can result from ingestion of a fruit smoothie or other beverage to which bee pollen may be added [45]. Another example of anaphylaxis that might seem idiopathic when a patient is not known to have food allergies is anaphylaxis caused by mite-contaminated flour [46, 47]. In 2009, Commins et al. reported a novel food allergy related to IgE antibodies to the carbohydrate galactose-α(alpha)-1,3-galactose (alpha-gal) from patients who experience delayed symptoms of anaphylaxis, angioedema or urticaria 3–6 h after ingestion of beef, pork or lamb [66]. Of 60 patients from Tennessee, Virginia and Western Australia initially diagnosed with idiopathic anaphylaxis, Commins found 25 with elevated IgE antibodies to galactose-α(alpha)-1,3-galactose [67].

Symptoms of scrombroidosis, which is histamine poisoning from spoiled fish such as tuna, may resemble an IgE-mediated allergic reaction [48]. This diagnosis should be considered in patients who have had a suspected episode of anaphylaxis after ingestion of fish, but a thorough workup for fish allergy is negative and serum tryptase levels are normal.

**Table 13.2** Symptoms of patients with idiopathic anaphylaxis compared to clonal mast cell activation disorder [6]

| | Ditto et al. [6] | Tejedor Alonso M et al. [23] | Koterba and Akin [35] | Koterba and Akin [35] |
|---|---|---|---|---|
| | Idiopathic anaphylaxis | Idiopathic anaphylaxis | Idiopathic anaphylaxis | Clonal mast cell activation disorder |
| | *N*=335 | *N*=81 | *N*=15 | *N*=15 |
| Gender M:F | 118:217 | 26:55 (68%F) | 7:8 | 3:12 |
| Urticaria | 335[a] (100%) | 74 (91%) | 5 (33%) | 0 |
| Angioedema | 335[a] (100%) | 70 (86%) | 4 (27%) | 2 (13%) |
| Upper airway obstruction | 210 (63%) | 67 (83%) | ND | ND |
| Bronchospasm | 132 (39%) | (Lower airway sx) 43 (53%) | 3 (20%) | 4 (27%) |
| Syncope | 78[b] (23%) | 7 (9%) | 10 (67%) | 10 (67%) |
| Hypotension | 78[b] (23%) | ND | 7 (47%) | 6 (40%) |
| Gastrointestinal symptoms | 75 (23%) | 26 (32%) | 11(73%) | 9 (60%) |
| Flushing | ND | ND | 10 (67%) | 12 (80%) |

[a]In original publication by Ditto et al. [6], listed 100% urticaria or angioedema. Of 98 patients between 1991 and 1994, 61 (62%) IA patients presented with urticaria. Of 98 patients, 72 (73%) patients presented with angioedema. This likely represented a large referral patient base

[b]In original publication by Ditto et al. [6], listed 23% syncope or hypotension

Medication is one of the most common triggers that should be considered before labeling a patient with idiopathic anaphylaxis. Sometimes patients do not recognize certain ingredients in medications, such as aspirin in Alka-Seltzer or Goody's Powder. Consequently, a thorough medication history, including over the counter medications and supplements should be obtained from the patient.

Other triggers can include hydatid cyst disease, a parasitic infestation of humans endemic in the Mediterranean region. Initial infection with the tapeworm *Echinococcus* is usually asymptomatic, so anaphylactic reactions can be the first manifestations of the disease, occurring due to cyst rupture [49]. Latex hypersensitivity has become well-known, however causes of anaphylaxis can also include "hidden" latex products such as hair bonding "glue" for hair extensions [50].

There are several disorders characterized by excessive endogenous production of histamine that should be considered before diagnosis of idiopathic anaphylaxis is assigned. Mastocytosis is one of them because it can present as idiopathic anaphylaxis. In systemic mastocytosis, the total tryptase level can be elevated when the patient is asymptomatic, while in idiopathic anaphylaxis, it is usually normal. The total (beta) β(beta)-tryptase ratio in systemic mastocytosis is usually more than 20, compared to ten or less in idiopathic anaphylaxis [51]. Most patients with systemic mastocytosis have urticaria pigmentosa, salmon-colored macules that develop into urticaria upon stroking (Darier's sign). Some leukemias can also have overproduction of histamine-containing cells (e.g., acute promyelocytic leukemia, basophilic leukemia) [52]. Patients with systemic mastocytosis or leukemias consequently have abnormal bone scans and abnormal bone marrow biopsies, which is the definitive test [53, 54].

Hereditary angioedema can mimic idiopathic anaphylaxis, but hives and other anaphylactic symptoms are not usually present, and the angioedema in this disorder tends to progress slowly and without pruritis. Episodes may be provoked by dental procedures or local trauma. The gastrointestinal tract may also be involved, and produce symptoms of cramping or abdominal pain. This disorder can be differentiated from anaphylaxis by laboratory findings and lack of other symptoms of anaphylaxis. Laboratory findings consist of decreased levels of C4, CH50 and C1 esterase inhibitor concentration or function [54]. There are also two forms of acquired C1 esterase inhibitor deficiency; one occurs in association with autoimmune diseases and the other with lymphoproliferative malignancy.

Carcinoid syndrome also produces symptoms similar to anaphylaxis: carcinoid tumors secrete histamine, kallikerin, neuropeptides and prostaglandins in addition to serotonin. Patients with pheochromocytoma can also present with symptoms that are similar to those in patients with idiopathic anaphylaxis. They often experience flushing as a result of the release of vasoactive substances (epinephrine, norepinephrine, and vanillylmandelic acid in pheochromocytoma and 5-HIAA in carcinoid). The laboratory detection of these mediators, however, differentiates these two disorders from idiopathic anaphylaxis [53, 55, 56]. Medullary carcinoma of the thyroid usually presents a single thyroid nodule; however, it may present with facial flushing. Gastrointestinal tumors producing vasoactive intestinal polypeptide (VIPomas) or substance P are rare. Measurement of serum VIP or substance P can be helpful [53].

A severe asthma attack may also be mistaken for an anaphylactic reaction. Patients may present with severe bronchoconstriction leading to wheezing and shortness of breath which may also occur in patients with idiopathic anaphylaxis [18]. However, the limitation of symptoms to the lungs or a previous history of hospitalizations for asthma would make idiopathic anaphylaxis less likely.

Vocal cord dyfunction, panic attacks, or undifferentiated somatoform anaphylaxis can also mimic idiopathic anaphylaxis. Panic attacks are accompanied by tachycardia, flushing and shortness of breath. Vocal cord dysfunction is involuntary adduction of the true vocal cords. There may also be bunching of the false vocal cords, which can produce obstruction in both inspiration and expiration [57].

Episodes of vocal cord adduction may also be self-induced, such as Munchausen stridor [58]. Patients will complain of shortness of breath and imitate stridorous sounds over the neck region. They are also likely to overuse Epi-pens, emergency phone numbers, and have frequent visits to emergency departments. Patients with Munchausen stridor also fail to respond to antihistamines and steroids. This disease can be distinguished from vocal cord dysfunction by laryngoscopy during an acute episode. Patients with Munchausen stridor can be distracted from their vocal cord adduction by asking them to perform maneuvers such as coughing [59].

Undifferentiated somatoform anaphylaxis is a term used to describe patients who present with manifestations that mimic idiopathic anaphylaxis but who lack objective confirmatory findings, do not respond to therapy and exhibit psychological signs of an undifferentiated somatoform disorder [60].

## 13.4 Classification of Idiopathic Anaphylaxis

Classification of idiopathic anaphylaxis is based on both manifestations and frequency [2]. Patients are classified as having either frequent (F) or infrequent episodes (I). Frequent is defined as more than six episodes per year or two or more episodes within 2 months.

Patients are also categorized as idiopathic anaphylaxis-generalized (IA-G) or idiopathic anaphylaxis-angioedema (IA-A) based on spectrum of symptoms. Patients with IA-A experience urticaria or angioedema with upper airway compromise such as laryngeal edema, severe pharyngeal edema or massive tongue swelling without other signs of systemic anaphylaxis. Patients with IA-G suffer from urticaria or angioedema with bronchospasm, hypotension, syncope, or gastrointestinal symptoms with or without upper airway compromise. Some patients have recurrent episodes of anaphylaxis if steroids are reduced below a certain threshold; these patients suffer from corticosteroid-dependent idiopathic anaphylaxis.

Some cases are unclear and cannot be classified as either general or angioedema. These last three categories were created to help identify patients who have atypical presentation for IA. These cases are categorized as either idiopathic anaphylaxis-questionable (IA-Q), idiopathic-variant, or undifferentiated somatoform IA (USIA). IA-Q is applied to patients who possibly have idiopathic anaphylaxis but have no documentation of objective findings, response to appropriate doses of prednisone dose do not occur, and consequently the diagnosis of idiopathic anaphylaxis becomes unclear. IA-V is used when symptoms and clinical findings differ from classic IA. IA-V may also be subsequently classified as IA-Q, IA-A, IA-G or USIA. The term USIA is applied to patients who describe symptoms consistent with IA but have no organic disease or objective findings that are documented. Moreover, symptoms are not responsive to the regimen for idiopathic anaphylaxis. These patients may be treated excessively with unnecessary corticosteroids without resolution. Many of these patients have an underlying psychiatric illness and should be referred to a psychiatrist [60].

## 13.5 Treatment

Treatment regimens for idiopathic anaphylaxis are implemented on an individual basis based on the frequency and severity of the patient's symptoms (Fig. 13.1). The medical regimen was derived initially from experience in the treatment of anaphylaxis secondary to radiocontrast media administration [61]. All patients should be instructed on the management of an acute episode. At the first sign of anaphylaxis, patients should self-administer 0.3 mL (1:1,000) aqueous epinephrine intramuscularly, 60 mg prednisone orally and a H1 antihistamine. Although only first-generation antihistamines

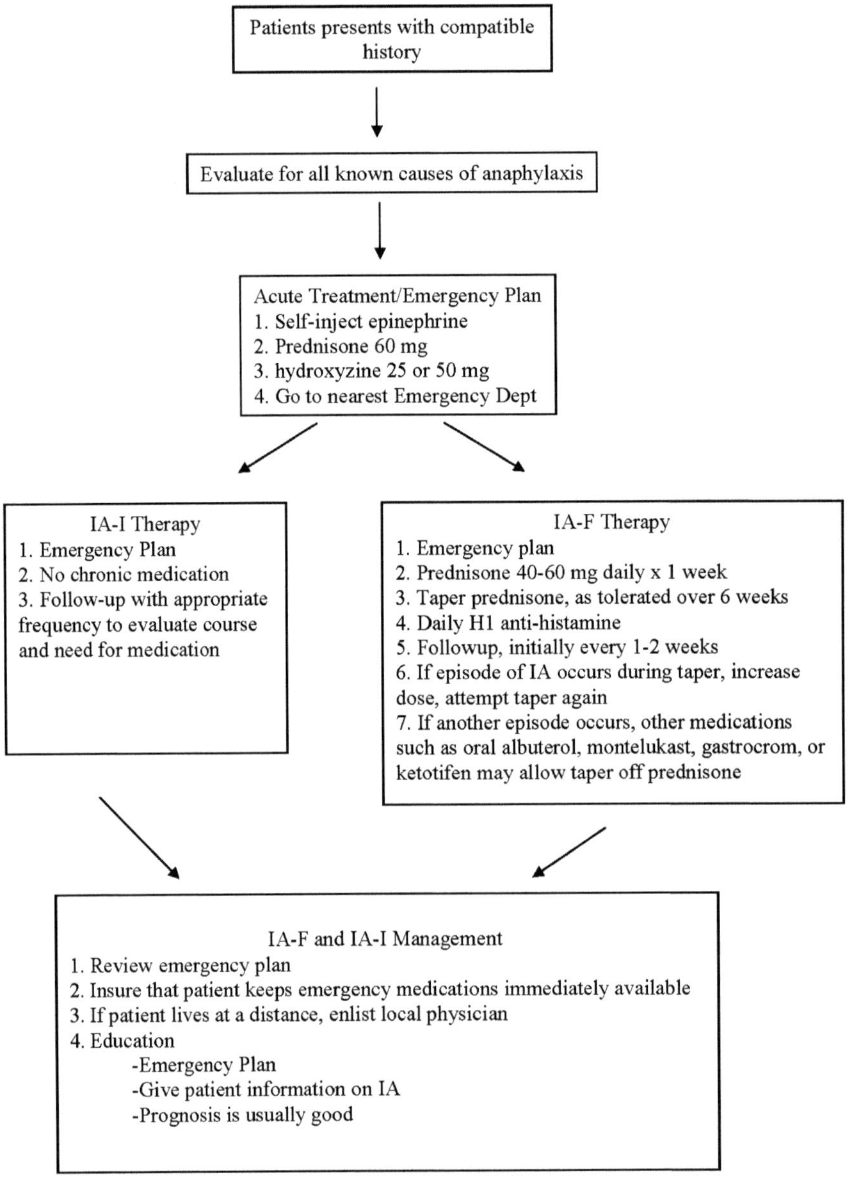


**Fig. 13.1** Algorithm for the management of idiopathic anaphylaxis (Adapted and Reprinted from [2]. With permission)

have been studied for the treatment of idiopathic anaphylaxis, second-generation antihistamines, such as cetirizine are preferred as first-line treatment due to their more favorable benefit-to-risk ratio. Patients should then proceed to the nearest emergency room [1].

Patients with infrequent episodes (IA-I) do not require any maintenance therapy unless the most recent episodes were considered extremely severe or life-threatening. Patients with frequent episodes are placed on prednisone and an antihistamine; an oral sympathomimetic (e.g. albuterol 2 mg three times daily) may also be prescribed. The usual starting dose of prednisone is 40–60 mg daily for 1 week or until symptoms are controlled. Increased dosages may be necessary. Daily dosing may be required for 1–6 weeks for symptoms to be controlled. If longer daily prednisone is required, then the diagnosis of idiopathic anaphylaxis becomes questionable. Once the patient is stable, the

**Table 13.3** Medications for long-term treatment to help reduce need for prednisone

| | |
|---|---|
| Cetirizine | 1 tablet qhs to bid |
| Fexofenadine | 1 tablet qam to bid |
| Doxepin | 25–50 mg qhs |
| Oral albuterol | 2 mg daily to bid |
| Montelukast | 10 mg qhs |
| Oral cromolyn | 200 mg every 6 h |
| Ketotifen | 2 mg every 8 h |
| Omalizumab | SQ monthly or twice monthly |

The sequence in which the medications should be prescribed varies with multiple considerations including co-morbidities and insurance co-pays

prednisone dose may be converted to alternate day dosing. The prednisone should then be carefully tapered (5–10 mg per dose per month). Following successful tapering of prednisone, the antihistamine and sympathomimetic agent can be gradually discontinued [1, 63]. Patients who are unable to discontinue prednisone because of recurrent symptoms are considered corticosteroid dependent (CSD-IA). Patients with CSD-IA may be given a trial of a mast cell stabilizer, either oral cromolyn (Gastrocrom) 200 mg every 6 h, or ketotifen (Zaditen) 2 mg orally two or three times a day. The oral formulation of ketotifen has never been approved for use in the United States or many other countries. It may have significant sedative effects [62]. Other medications that may be useful include oral albuterol or montelukast (Singulair). This may allow a further reduction and possible discontinuation of steroids, achieving a remission. If the prednisone requirement does not change once the additional therapy is added, then the additional therapy should be discontinued. (Table 13.3).

There have been a couple of case reports of successful anti-IgE therapy with omalizumab for idiopathic anaphylaxis [64, 65].

Patients who have experienced an anaphylactic episode should wear a Medic Alert bracelet or carry identification cards that include their diagnosis of anaphylaxis. A major goal in the prevention and management of patients with idiopathic anaphylaxis is education. Patients, family members and primary care physicians should be educated regarding their diagnosis, the symptomatology, the consequences of the disease, the importance of the treatment, and the complications of the treatment. Most importantly, patients should be educated regarding the emergency treatment plan for an acute episode consisting of injectable epinephrine, prednisone, antihistamine and proceeding to the nearest emergency department. Finally, patients with recurrent episodes of idiopathic anaphylaxis are often seeking an etiology. They should be educated that their disease is idiopathic and that there is no external agent.

## References


1. Wong S, Yarnold PR, Yango C, et al. Outcome of prophylactic therapy for idiopathic anaphylaxis. *Ann Intern Med.* 1991; 114:133–136.
2. Patterson R, Stoloff RS, Greenberger PA, Grammer LC, Harris KE. Algorithms for the diagnosis and management of idiopathic anaphylaxis. *Ann Allergy* 1993; 71:40–44.
3. Patterson R, Clayton D, Booth B, et al. Fatal and near fatal idiopathic anaphylaxis. *Allergy Proc.* 1995; 16:103–108.
4. Krasnick J, Patterson R, Meyers G. A fatality from idiopathic anaphylaxis, *Ann Allergy Asthma Immunol* 1996 76: 376–379.
5. Bacal E, Patterson, R, Zeiss CR. Evaluation of severe (anaphylactic) reactions. *Clinical Allergy* 1978; 8: 295–304.
6. Ditto AM, Harris KE, Karsnick J, et al. Idiopathic anaphylaxis: a series of 335 cases. *Ann Allergy Asthma Immunol* 1996; 77:285–291.

7. Patterson R, Hogan M, Yarnold P, et al: Idiopathic anaphylaxis. An attempt to estimate the incidence in the United States, *Arch Intern Med* 1995; 155: 869–871.
8. Kemp SF, Lockey RF, Lieberman P, et al: Anaphylaxis, a review of 266 cases. *Arch Intern Med* 1995;155: 1749–1954.
9. Webb LM, Lieberman P. Anaphylaxis: a review of 601 cases. *Ann Allergy Asthma Immunol* 2006; 97: 39–43.
10. Yocum MW, Butterfield J, Klein J, et al. Epidemiology of anaphylaxis in Olmstead County, a population-based study. *J Allergy Clin Immunol* 1999; 104:452–456.
11. Tejedor Alonso M, Dominguez J, Sanchez-Hernandez J, Frances C, Caballer B. Idiopathic anaphylaxis: a descriptive study of 81 patients in Spain. *Ann Allergy Asthma Immunol* 2002; 88:313–318.
12. Ditto AM, Patterson R, Sider L. Allergic bronchopulmonary aspergillosis, idiopathic anaphylaxis and cystic fibrosis in a 9 year old: a case report. *Pediatr Asthma Allergy Immunol* 1995; 9:107–115.
13. Dykewicz MS, Blaser M, Evans R, Patterson R. Pediatric idiopathic anaphylaxis: A report of 3 cases with recommendations for evaluation and management. *Pediatr Asthma Allergy Immunol* 1990; 4:217–223.
14. Patterson R, Ditto A, Dykewicz MS, Greenberger PA, Harris KE, Kelly KJ, et al. Pediatric idiopathic anaphylaxis: additional cases and extended observations. *Pediatr Asthma Allergy Immunol* 1995; 9:107–115.
15. Ditto AM, Krasnick J, Greenberger PA, et al. Pediatric idiopathic anaphylaxis: experience with 22 patients. *J Allergy Clin Immunol* 1997; 100:320–326.
16. Schwartz LB, Metcalfee DD, Miller JS, Earl H, Sullivan T. Tryptase levels as an indicator of mast-cell activation in systemic anaphylaxis and mastocytosis. *N Engl J Med* 1987; 316:1622–1626.
17. Moro M, Tejedor MA, Esteban J et al. Severity of Anaphylaxis According to Causes and Demographic Characteristics [abstract]. *J Allergy Clin Immunol* 2008; 121:S24.
18. Sampson HA, Munoz-Furlong A, Campbell RL, et al. Second symposium on the definition and management of anaphylaxis: summary report – Second National Institute of Allergy and Infectious Disease/Food Allergy and Anaphylaxis Network symposium. *J Allergy Clin Immunol* 2006; 117:391–397.
19. Garriga MM, Friedman MM, Metcalfe DD. A survey of the number and distribution of mast cells in the skin of patients with mast cell disorders. *J Allergy Clin Immunol* 1988; 82: 425–432.
20. Keffer J, Bressler RB, Wright R, Kaliner MA, Metcalfe DD. Analysis of the wheal and flare reactions that follow the intradermal injection of histamine and morphine in adults with recurrent, unexplained anaphylaxis and systemic mastocytosis. *J Allergy Clin Immunol* 1989; 83: 595–601.
21. Greenberger PA, Smith LJ, Patteron R. Comparison of cutaneous and bronchial reactivity to leukotriene D4 in humans. *J Lab Clin Med* 1986; 108:70–75.
22. Tejedor MA, Perez C, Sastre et al. Mast cell releasibility in idiopathic anaphylaxis subtypes [abstract]. *J Allergy Clin Immunol* 2000; 105: S348.
23. Tejedor Alonso MA. Sastre Dominguez J, Sanchez-Hernandez JJ, PerezFrances C., Hoz de la Caballer B. Clinical and functional differences among patients with idiopathic anaphylaxis. *J Invest Allergol Clin Immunol* 2004; 14:177–186.
24. Reed J, Yedulapuram M, Lieberman P, et al. Differences in cytokine production between idiopathic anaphylaxis (IA) subjects and controls [abstract]. *J Allergy Clin Immunol* 2006; 117: S305.
25. Sonin L, Patterson R. Metbisulfite challenge in patients with idiopathic anaphylaxis. *J Allergy Clin Immunol* 1985; 75:67–69.
26. Slater JE, Raphael G, Cutler GB. Recurrent anaphylaxis in menstruating women: treatment with luteinizing hormone releasing hormone – a preliminary report. *Obstet Gynecol* 1987; 70:542–546.
27. Slater JE, Kaliner M. Effects of sex hormones on histamine release in recurrent idiopathic anaphylaxis. *J Allergy Clin Immunol* 1987; 80: 285–290.
28. Gruber BL, Baeza ML, Marchese MJ, Agnello V, Kaplan AP. Prevalence and functional role of anti-IgE autoantibodies in urticarial syndromes. *J Invest Dermatol* 1988; 90:213.
29. Grant JA, Alam R, Lett-Brown MA. Histamine-releasing factors and inhibitors: historical perspectives and possible implications in human illness. *J Allergy Clin Immunol* 1991; 88:683–693.
30. Mozelsio N, Grammer L. Quantitation of monocyte chemoattractant protein-1 in patients with idiopathic anaphylaxis [abstract]. *J Allergy Clin Immunol* 2001; 107:S80.
31. Akin C, Scott LM, Kocabas CN, Kushnir-Sukjov N, Brittain E, Noel P, Metcalfe DD. Demonstration of an aberrant mast-cell population with clonal markers in a subset of patients with "idiopathic" anaphylaxis. *Blood.* 2007; 110:2331–2333.
32. Metcalfe DD, Schwartz L. Assessing anaphylactic risk? Consider mast cell clonality. *J Allergy Clin Immunol* 2009; 123: 687–688.
33. Tanus T, Mines D, Atkins PC, Levinson AI. Serum tryptase in idiopathic anaphylaxis a case report and review of the literature. *Ann Emerg Med* 1994; 24: 104–107.
34. Shanmugam G, Schwartz LB, Khan DA. Prolonged elevation of serum tryptase in indiopathic anaphylaxis. *J Allergy Clin Immunol* 2006 117: 950–951.

35. Koterba AP, Akin C. Differences in the Clinical Presentation of Anaphylaxis in Patients with indolent Systemic Mastocytosis (ISM) versus Idiopathic Anaphylaxis (IA) [abstract]. *J Allergy Clin Immunol* 2008; 121: S68–S69.
36. Grammer LC, Shaughnessy MA, Harris KE, Goolsby CL. Lymphocyte subsets and activation markers in patients with acute episodes of idiopathic anaphylaxis. *Ann Allergy Asthma Immunol* 2000; 85:368–371.
37. Howell DL, Jacobs C, Metz G et al. Molecular Profiling Distinguishes Patients with Active Idiopathic Anaphylaxis from Normal Volunteers and Reveals Novel Aspects of Disease Biology [abstract]. *J Allergy Clin Immunol* 2009; 123:S150.
38. Munoz MF, Lopez Cazana JM, Villas F, et al. Exercise-induced anaphylactic reaction to hazelnut. *Allergy* 1994; 49:314.
39. Sheffer AL, Soter NA, McFadden ER Jr, et al. Exercise-induced anaphylaxis: a distinct form of physical allergy. *J Allergy Clin Immunol* 1983: 71:311.
40. Romano A, Di Fonso M, Giuffreda F, et al. Food-dependent exercise-induced anaphylaxis: clinical and laboratory findings in 54 subjects. *Int Arch Allergy Immunol* 2001; 125:264–272.
41. Moneret-Vautrin DA, Morisset M, Lemerdy M, et al. Food allergy and IgE sensitization caused by spices: CICBAA data (based on 589 cases of food allergy). *Allerg Immunol* (Paris) 2002; 34:135–140.
42. Stricker WE, Anorve-Lopez E, Reed CE. Food skin testing in patients with idiopathic anaphylaxis. *J Allergy Clin Immunol* 1986; 77: 516–519.
43. Furlong TJ, DeSimone J, Sicherer SH. Peanut and tree nut allergic reactions in restaurants and other food establishments. *J Allergy Clin Immunol* 2001; 108:867–870.
44. DiCello MC, MycA, Baker JR Jr. Baldwin JL. Anaphylaxis after ingestion of carmine colored foods: two case reports and a review of the literature. *Allergy Asthma Proc* 1999; 20:377.
45. Greenberger PA, Flais MJ. Bee pollen-induced anaphylactic reaction in an unknowingly sensitized subject. *Ann Allergy Asthma Immunol* 2001; 86:239.
46. Blanco C, Quiralte J, Castillo R et al. Anaphylaxis after ingestion of wheat flour contaminated with mites. *J Allergy Clin Immunol* 1997; 99:308–313.
47. Sanchez-Borges M, Suarez-Chacon R, Capriles-HulettA, Caballero-Fonseca F. An update on oral anaphylaxis from mite ingestion. *Ann Allergy Asthma Immunol* 2005; 94:216.
48. Becker K, Southwick K, Readon J. Histamine poisoning associated with eating tuna burgers. *JAMA* 2001; 285:1327.
49. Gelincik A, Ozseker F, BuyukozturkS et al. Recurrent anaphylaxis due to non-ruptured hepatic hydatid cysts. *Int Arch Allergy Immunol* 2007; 143:296.
50. Cogen FC, Beezhold D. Hair glue anaphylaxis: a hidden latex allergy *Ann Allergy Asthma Immunol* 2002; 88:61–63.
51. Schwartz LB, Irani AM. Serum tryptase in the laboratory diagnosis of systemic mastocytosis. *Hematol Oncol Clin North Am* 2000; 14: 641–657.
52. Lieberman P. Anaphylaxis. Middleton: Allergy: Principles and Practice, 7th ed. St Louis, Mosby; 2009:1027–1049.
53. Lieberman P, Kemp S, Oppenheimer J, et al. The diagnosis and management of anaphylaxis: an updated practice parameter. *J Allergy Clin Immunol* 2005; 115:S483–S523.
54. Saltoun CA. Urticaria, Angioedema and Hereditary Angioedema. In: Grammer LC, Greenberger PA, eds. Allergic Diseases, Diagnosis and Management, 7th ed. Lippincott Williams & Wilkins, Philadephia, PA; 2009:539–553.
55. Erem C, Kocak M, Onder Ersoz H et al. Epinephrine-secreting cystic pheochromocytoma presenting with an incidental adrenal mass: a case report and a review of the literature. *Endocrine* 2005; 28: 225–230.
56. Ueda T, Oka N, Matsumoto A et al. Pheochromocytoma presenting as recurrent hypotension and syncope. *Intern Med* 2005; 44:222–227.
57. Bahrainwala AH, Simon MR. Wheezing and vocal cord dysfunction mimicking asthma. *Curr Opin Pulm Med* 2001; 7:8–13.
58. Patterson R, Schatz M, Harton M. Munchausen's stridor: non-organic laryngeal obstruction. *Clin Allergy* 1974; 4:307–310.
59. McGrath K. Anaphylaxis. In: Grammer LC and Greenberger PA, eds. Allergic Diseases, Diagnosis and Management, 7th ed. Lippincott Williams & Wilkins, Philadelphia, PA; 2009:197–219.
60. Choy AC, Patterson R, Patterson DR et al. Undifferentiated somatoform idiopathic anaphylaxis: non-organic symptoms mimicking idiopathic anaphylaxis. *J Allergy Clin Immunol* 1995; 96:893–900.
61. Greenberger PA, Patterson R. The prevention of immediate generalized reaction to radiocontrast media in high-risk patients. *J Allergy Clin Immunol* 1991; 87: 867–872.
62. Patterson R, Fitzsimons EJ, Choy AC, Harris KE. Malignant and corticosteroid-dependent idiopathic anaphylaxis: successful responses to ketotifen. *Ann Allergy Asthma Immunol* 1997; 79:138.
63. Boxer MR, Greenberger PA, Patterson R. The impact of prednisone in life-threatening idiopathic anaphylaxis: reduction in acute episodes and medical costs. *Ann Allergy* 1989; 62:201.

64. Warrier P, Casale TB. Omalizumab in idiopathic anaphylaxis. *Ann Allergy Asthma Immunol.* 2009 Mar;102(3):257–258.
65. Jones JD, Marney SR Jr, Fahrenholz JM. Idiopathic anaphylaxis successfully treated with omalizumab. *Ann Allergy Asthma Immunol.* 2008 Nov;101(5):550–551.
66. Commins SP, Satinover SM, Hosen J, Mozena J, Borish L, Lewis BD et al. Delayed anaphylaxis, angioedema, or urticaria after consumption of red meat in patients with IgE antibodies specific for galactose-α(alpha)-1,3-galactose. *J Allergy Clin Immunol* 2009; 123:426–433.
67. Commins SP, James H, Tran N, Kelly RE, Liberman P, Platts-Mills T. Testing for IgE antibody to the carbohydrate galactose-α(alpha)-1,3-galactose (alpha-gal) in patients with recurrent, idiopathic anaphylaxis: how many cases are we missing? [Abstract] *J Allergy Clin Immunol* 2009; 125: S119.

# Chapter 14
# Exercise-Induced Anaphylaxis and Food-Dependent Exercise-Induced Anaphylaxis

**Anna M. Feldweg and Albert L. Sheffer**

**Abstract** Exercise-induced anaphylaxis (EIAn) is characterized by symptoms of anaphylaxis in the setting of significant physical exertion. A food-dependent form of exercise-induced anaphylaxis also exists, in which symptoms develop only if the patient has eaten in the hours immediately preceding exercise. In most patients with the food-dependent form, only a specific food(s) will elicit symptoms when combined with exercise, and patients usually have demonstrable IgE to this food. Attacks of exercise-induced anaphylaxis are unpredictable. Management of these disorders involves teaching the patient to stop exercise immediately at the first sign of symptoms and preparing them to self-administer intramuscular epinephrine if needed. Depending on the role of food, patients may need to avoid the culprit food for 4–6 h before exercise, remove the food from their diet altogether, or avoid ingesting any food for several hours before exercise. Pharmacotherapy to prevent attacks has been generally disappointing, although some patients with the food-dependent form may be helped by oral cromolyn, taken before meals. Most patients report fewer attacks over time.

**Keywords** Anaphylaxis • Athletes • Epinephrine • Exercise-induced anaphylaxis • Exercise • Food allergy • Food-dependent exercise-induced anaphylaxis • Food-induced anaphylaxis • Histamine • IgE-mediated food allergy • Mast cell degranulation • Serum tryptase concentration • Wheat allergy

## 14.1 Introduction and Definition

Exercise-induced anaphylaxis (EIAn) is characterized by symptoms of anaphylaxis in the setting of significant physical exertion. Food-dependent, exercise-induced anaphylaxis (FD-EIAn) is a related disorder, in which symptoms develop only if the patient has eaten in the hours immediately preceding exercise. In most patients with FD-EIAn, only a specific food(s), to which the patient has demonstrable IgE, will elicit symptoms when combined with exercise. In both EIAn and FD-EIAn, exercise/physical exertion is the immediate eliciting factor for symptoms.

A.M. Feldweg (✉)
Harvard Medical School, Brigham and Women's Hospital, Boston, MA, USA
e-mail: Afeldweg@partners.org

M.C. Castells (ed.), *Anaphylaxis and Hypersensitivity Reactions*,
DOI 10.1007/978-1-60327-951-2_14, © Springer Science+Business Media, LLC 2011 

## 14.2 Clinical Manifestations

### *14.2.1 Triggering Activities*

The symptoms of EIAn and FD-EIAn are unpredictable, and patients typically report that a given activity elicited symptoms on one occasion, but not at other times. Vigorous exercises, such as jogging, racquet sports, dancing, and aerobics, most consistently elicit symptoms, although lower levels of exertion such as brisk walking or yard work are capable of triggering attacks in some patients (Table 14.1) [1]. Cessation of exercise consistently results in prompt improvement.

### *14.2.2 Signs and Symptoms*

Typical early symptoms include diffuse warmth, flushing, pruritus, urticaria, and extreme fatigue [2, 3]. These may begin at any point during exercise. If exertion continues, there may be progression to anaphylaxis, with angioedema of the face and extremities, gastrointestinal symptoms, laryngeal edema, hypotension, or collapse. Wheezing may occur, although it is less common than other symptoms. A few patients experience headache that may persist after an episode (Table 14.2) [1, 3].

Many patients instinctively cease all activity when they first experience symptoms and quickly realize that resting accelerates resolution of symptoms. However, others may try to run for help, and

**Table 14.1** Activities associated with symptoms of EIA in 279 subjects [1]

| Activity | Number of subjects (%) |
|---|---|
| Jogging | 219 (78) |
| Walking | 117 (42) |
| Tennis/racquetball | 78 (28) |
| Dancing | 73 (26) |
| Bicycling | 68 (24) |
| Downhill skiing | 18 (6) |
| Yard work | 17 (6) |
| Basketball | 12 (4) |
| Stairmaster | 5 (2) |

**Table 14.2** Frequency of symptoms during episodes of Exercise-induced anaphylaxis (EIAn) in 279 subjects [1]

| Symptom | Number of subjects (%) |
|---|---|
| Pruritus | 257 (92) |
| Urticaria | 241 (86) |
| Angioedema | 201 (72) |
| Flushing | 194 (70) |
| Shortness of breath | 141 (51) |
| Dysphagia | 94 (34) |
| Chest tightness | 92 (33) |
| Loss of consciousness | 90 (32) |
| Diaphoresis | 90 (32) |
| Headache | 78 (28) |
| Nausea/diarrhea/colic | 77 (28) |
| Choking/throat constriction/hoarseness | 71 (25) |

this can precipitate a dramatic worsening of symptoms. Patients may also try to "push through" mild early symptoms, and this also leads to more severe symptoms. Educating patients about the need to stop the exercise activity immediately at the first sign of symptoms is critical to successful management (see Management below).

### 14.2.3 Co-triggers

Many patients require the presence of one or more other factors or "co-triggers" to develop symptoms on exercise. In FD-EIAn, the critical co-trigger is the ingestion of specific foods in FD-EIAn, as mentioned previously. In a small percentage of patients with FD-EIAn, the ingestion of any solid food prior to exercise is sufficient to precipitate symptoms [4].

Other co-triggers include ingestion of nonsteroidal anti-inflammatory drugs (NSAIDs) [1, 5] or narcotic medications, extremes of temperature and high humidity, alcoholic beverages, seasonal pollen exposure [1] in pollen-sensitized patients, or certain stages of the menstrual cycle (Table 14.3) [6, 7]. These co-triggers are tolerated if there is no association with exercise, e.g., patients with NSAID ingestion as a co-trigger can take these medications without symptoms or exercise without symptoms, although they cannot do both in close proximity.

In most cases, exposure to the co-trigger occurs first, followed by exercise, with the latter triggering symptoms. Ingestion of NSAIDs may precede exercise by hours to a day, whereas food or alcohol ingestion typically has occurred within the 4–6 h before exercise. Occasional reports have described cases of FD-EIAn in which the food was ingested shortly after exercise, although this is rare [5]. Accordingly, it may be unclear how to categorize some cases. For example, exercise may exacerbate some episodes of food-induced or NSAID-induced anaphylaxis, or alternatively, food and NSAIDs may be co-triggers in exercise-induced anaphylaxis. However, the term exercise-induced anaphylaxis is the most appropriate diagnosis in cases in which the exercise is the immediate stimulus for symptoms, regardless of the presence or absence of co-triggers.

### 14.2.4 Causative Foods in FD-EIAn

The foods most commonly implicated in FD-EIAn are wheat, other grains, and nuts in Western populations, and wheat and seafood in Asian populations [8], although a wide variety of foods have been reported [6, 8–13]. In some cases, the amount of food ingested or the processing of the food is also important [14, 15].

**Table 14.3** Possible co-triggers in exercise-induced anaphylaxis

- The ingestion of one or more foods to which specific IgE is demonstrable (i.e., food-dependent exercise-induced anaphylaxis)
- High humidity
- Extremes of temperature (either hot or cold)
- Nonsteroidal anti-inflammatory drugs (NSAIDs)
- Peak pollen season in pollen-sensitized individuals
- Alcoholic beverages
- Narcotic medications
- The ingestion of any solid food (i.e., the postprandial state) (specific IgE to food is not demonstrable)
- Specific stages of the menstrual cycle in women

Patients should be questioned about each of these possible co-triggers. Some patients identify several of these factors as relevant to their attacks. Avoidance of co-triggers in association with exercise is an important aspect of management

## 14.3 Prevalence

EIAn and FD-EIAn are rare disorders that have been reported around the world. The only study to systematically estimate prevalence polled all school nurses in a single prefecture of Japan, asking about cases that were suggestive of EIAn or FD-EIAn [16]. Each possible case was then investigated and confirmed or disproved. The prevalence of EIAn and FD-EIAn among Japanese adolescents was approximately 0.03% and 0.017%, respectively, with no clear gender preference [16]. Rare familial cases have been reported [17, 18].

## 14.4 Pathophysiology

The pathophysiology of EIAn is not well understood, although there is evidence that it is a mast cell-mediated disorder, similar to anaphylaxis from other causes. Skin biopsies demonstrate degranulation of dermal mast cells following attacks [19], *with ultrastuctural events similar to those observed in other types of anaphylaxis*. Transient elevations in plasma histamine [20, 21] and serum tryptase [22] have been documented in case reports. However, the mechanisms for mast cell activation have not been identified, and the events during exercise that may alter the activity of mast cells or other leukocytes have not been defined.

One area of investigation has identified omega-5 gliadin as a specific allergen responsible for wheat-dependent EIAn [23]. This allergen appears to be distinct from the wheat allergens causing other forms of immediate allergy [24]. In addition, tissue transglutaminase, an intestinal enzyme that is capable of binding and aggregating gliadin moieties to form large complexes, may be upregulated during exercise [25].

Other workers have demonstrated enhanced gastric permeability with exercise and NSAIDs, and proposed that increased levels of allergens or incompletely digested allergens are able to enter the circulation, possibly contributing to the disorder in patients with FD-EIAn [26]. In the field of exercise physiology, some researchers have postulated that exercise mobilizes and activates immune cells from gut-associated depots, stimulating pro-inflammatory responses that are then normally countered by anti-inflammatory responses [27]. Dysregulation of this process in patients with food-sensitized leukocytes could result in exercise-induced reactions.

## 14.5 Evaluation and Diagnosis

The diagnosis of exercise-induced anaphylaxis is based on a meticulous clinical history, occasionally supported by studies documenting mast cell activation if these can be obtained in the minutes or hours immediately following an attack. As part of the history, each episode that can be recounted by the patient should be reviewed in detail to discern if any co-triggers were present. A careful skin examination for lesions of urticaria pigmentosa should be performed. Patients with any symptoms to suggest mastocytosis should have a baseline serum tryptase level measured.

Ideally, the diagnosis of EIAn is confirmed by eliciting symptoms with exercise testing combined with assessment of lung function. This procedure could also be used to assess the importance of various co-triggers by demonstrating that the patient tolerates exercise in the absence of that co-trigger. The Bruce treadmill protocol has been used in this setting with variable success [16, 28].

The utility of exercise testing in the clinical setting is limited by the observation that symptoms are difficult to reproduce [9, 21]. Hanakawa et al. published a case and literature review in which 234 reports of FD-EIAn were identified, of which 81 had been evaluated with food/exercise challenges [14]. Symptoms were elicited by challenge in 55%. Thus, a positive challenge can confirm the diagnosis, but a negative challenge does not exclude the diagnosis. There are currently no consensus guidelines concerning the use of exercise testing in the diagnosis of EIAn. We do not routinely perform exercise tests in our clinic, relying instead on the patient's clinical history.

A thorough evaluation for co-triggers involves skin testing for sensitization to foods and environmental allergens, to identify each patient's potential co-triggers. Patients with possible FD-EIAn should be evaluated for specific IgE to the suspect food, as this is usually demonstrable, either through skin testing or in vitro immunoassays. If testing for food sensitization is negative but the history is strongly suggestive of a food co-trigger, then repeat testing at yearly intervals may subsequently demonstrate sensitization. The authors have observed a small number of patients with histories that were highly suggestive of FD-EIAn to wheat, in which skin tests and in vitro tests were initially negative, but became positive within a year.

## 14.6 Differential Diagnosis

The differential diagnosis includes primary food allergy exacerbated by exercise, arrhythmias and other cardiovascular events, exercise-induced bronchoconstriction, exercise-induced gastroesophageal reflux, cholinergic urticaria with systemic symptoms, and mastocytosis. Most of these disorders can be distinguished from exercise-induced anaphylaxis by a careful clinical history.

Primary food allergy exacerbated by exercise is in the differential diagnosis of the patient with apparent FD-EIAn. Patients with primary food allergy should have symptoms following ingestion of the food, even in the absence of exertion. Arrhythmias and cardiovascular events do not involve pruritus, urticaria, angioedema, or upper airway obstruction. Exercise-induced bronchoconstriction presents with symptoms that are limited to the airways. Exercise-associated gastroesophageal reflux could mimic mild symptoms of EIAn, although again, urticaria and pruritus are not observed.

Cholinergic urticaria, a physical urticaria usually limited to the skin, can mimic the early cutaneous symptoms of EIAn. Cholinergic urticaria is characterized by initially punctate (1–3 mm in diameter) wheals with surrounding erythema of the affected skin. Cholinergic urticaria is elicited by raising the core body temperature, such as with a sauna or hot bath, very strong emotion, or very spicy food and can be discerned with a careful history and confirmed with passive warming. In contrast, the wheals of EIAn are usually larger (10–15 mm in diameter), although this is not universal and patients with EIAn can demonstrate punctate urticaria [29]. Exercise is critical to eliciting the symptoms of EIAn; passively raising the core body temperature should not cause symptoms, and this difference distinguishes EIAn from cholinergic urticaria with systemic symptoms [30].

Mastocytosis, a group of disorders characterized by excessive mast cell accumulation in one or multiple tissues, can involve anaphylaxis triggered by a wide array of factors, both allergic and physical, but rarely identify exercise or exertion as the only trigger for their symptoms. In addition, this condition can usually be distinguished by persistent elevations in baseline serum tryptase, which are not seen with EIAn or FD-EIAn.

## 14.7 Management

The management of EIAn and FD-EIAn must be individualized for each patient, depending on the severity of symptoms, the presence of co-triggers, and the patient's desire to continue regular exercise. The fundamentals of management are the following:

- Any co-triggers should be identified and avoided prior to exercise. Specifically, in patients with FD-EIAn, the culprit food(s) should be avoided for at least 4–6 h prior to exercise. Exercising in the mornings is a simple way to comply with this restriction. It may be more effective to eliminate the food from the diet altogether in children, who cannot avoid exertion in their daily activities, and in adults in whom low levels of exertion precipitate attacks. It is also helpful to plan specific replacement foods that the patient can safely eat prior to exercise, so these can be kept on hand. Patients with NSAIDs as a co-trigger should avoid these medications completely, or refrain from exercise for 24 h after taking them. Pollen-sensitive patients should exercise indoors during pollen season.
- Patients must be vigilant for early symptoms of EIAn (e.g., extreme fatigue, flushing, pruritus) and stop exercise *immediately* if these develop.
- Patients should be counseled *never* to "push through" symptoms, as this will only lead to escalation of the attack.
- Patients must carry an epinephrine autoinjector or have immediate access to one whenever they engage in exercise or vigorous physical exertion. The clinician should discuss with the patient how this will be accomplished, as some patients are reluctant to carry things during exercise (especially runners) and will be tempted to leave their autoinjector behind unless specifically counseled against doing this. Epinephrine should be injected intramuscularly in the anterolateral thigh if lightheadedness, upper airway edema, chest tightness, or severe urticaria develops. The patient should then lie down to maximize blood flow to the vital organs and brain (provided they are in a safe setting).
- Patients with EIAn should exercise with a companion or in a supervised setting at all times. The companion or supervisor (e.g., coach) should be educated about the condition and trained to administer epinephrine. It is also prudent for patients to carry a cell phone when exercising, in case emergency medical services are required.

The authors have encountered rare patients who report that if they exercise again the day after a significant attack, they can do so without developing symptoms and thereafter continue daily exercise without attacks [31]. This suggests that some type of hyposensitization is possible in a subset of individuals. Most clearly cannot do this, however. Until the safety and effectiveness of this approach is better understood, we do not recommend that patients experiment to determine if this applies to them.

Most patients have a strong desire to keep exercising, and we make every attempt to construct a management plan that allows them to do so, because of the many mental and physical benefits of regular exercise. For patients with identifiable co-triggers, avoidance of these factors should allow them to resume exercise safely. We advise such patients to begin exercising slowly, gradually building back up to their previous level. This approach has proved successful for all but the most severely affected individuals.

We have also administered subcutaneous allergen immunotherapy to patients with pollen-induced respiratory allergies, for the purposes of reducing the impact of pollen as a co-trigger. The effectiveness of this has not been studied systematically.

If patients have no identifiable co-triggers, we still advise avoidance of eating any solid food for 4 h before exercise initially. If, over time, food-ingestion does not appear to be a co-trigger, then the period of fasting before exercise can be gradually shortened and then eliminated.

Several case reports describe successful treatment of FD-EIAn with oral cromolyn, taken 20 min before a meal, in patients who were unable to avoid exertion in the hours after eating [32–35]. However, further studies are needed to determine whether this intervention is successful in the majority of patients. Until more information is available, caution is advised.

Pharmacologic therapy with H1 antihistamines for EIAn is not consistently effective, and should not be relied on to prevent future episodes. However, if patients are taking H1 antihistamines for other reasons (e.g., allergic rhinitis), we do not stop them. The utility of other therapies, such as oral corticosteroids, H2 antihistamines, or omalizumab has either not been evaluated in controlled studies and/or have not been consistently effective. We specifically avoid the use of H2 antihistamines in patients with FD-EIAn, because of preliminary evidence that these medications may interfere with normal digestion of food allergens [36–38].

## 14.8 Prognosis

Most patients with EIAn report fewer attacks over time [1]. Much of this improvement may be attributable to modifications in exercise habits and recognition of co-triggers, such that patients simply learn to avoid situations that are most likely to elicit symptoms. Shadick et al. [1] administered a questionnaire to 279 patients with EIAn for more than a decade and found that the average number of episodes per year decreased from 14 at the time of diagnosis to 8 in the year of the study. Patients reported avoiding exercise during extremely hot, cold, or humid weather conditions, during pollen season (pollen-allergic patients), after eating, and after taking NSAIDs.

It is not known how often EIAn or FDEIAn result in fatal anaphylaxis, although this outcome appears to be rare. There are a small number of convincing reports describing fatalities [39–41]. Two of these victims had not been formally diagnosed or counseled about how to manage attacks at the time of their deaths [39, 41], and a third was in a remote location and did not have an epinephrine autoinjector available [40].

## 14.9 Summary

EIAn is a heterogeneous form of anaphylaxis in which exercise is the immediate trigger for the development of symptoms. Typical symptoms include extreme fatigue, warmth, flushing, pruritus, and urticaria, progressing to angioedema, wheezing, upper airway obstruction, and collapse.

Some patients experience symptoms only if other co-triggers are present in association with exercise. These co-triggers include specific foods, ingestion of any food, extremes of temperature, NSAIDs, narcotics, high pollen levels (if pollen-allergic), and menstrual status in some women. The clinical history should focus on identification of these possible co-triggers.

The diagnosis is usually made based on history and exclusion of other disorders. Treadmill exercise testing does not consistently reproduce symptoms, but if positive, does confirm the diagnosis. Evaluation for sensitization to food allergens, particularly grains and seafood, should be performed in patients suspected of having a food co-trigger.

All patients with exercise-induced anaphylaxis must be advised to stop exercising immediately at the first sign of symptoms because continued exertion causes the attacks to worsen. In addition, all patients should carry an epinephrine autoinjector and exercise with a companion who can recognize symptoms and administer epinephrine if necessary.

Prophylactic antihistamines or other medications do not appear to prevent attacks in the majority of patients.

The prognosis of patients with exercise-induced anaphylaxis is generally favorable, with most patients experiencing fewer and less severe attacks over time.

## References


1. Shadick NA, Liang MH, Partridge AJ, et al. The natural history of exercise-induced anaphylaxis: survey results from a 10-year follow-up study. *J Allergy Clin Immunol.* 1999;104:123.
2. Maulitz RM, Pratt DS, Schocket AL. Exercise-induced anaphylactic reaction to shellfish. *J Allergy Clin Immunol.* 1979;63:433.
3. Sheffer AL, Austen KF. Exercise-induced anaphylaxis. *J Allergy Clin Immunol.* 1980;66:106.
4. Kidd JM 3rd, Cohen SH, Sosman AJ, Fink JN. Food-dependent exercise-induced anaphylaxis. *J Allergy Clin Immunol.* 1983;71:407.
5. Harada S, Horikawa T, Ashida M, et al. Aspirin enhances the induction of type I allergic symptoms when combined with food and exercise in patients with food-dependent exercise-induced anaphylaxis. *Br J Dermatol.* 2001;145:336.
6. Bito T, Kanda E, Tanaka M, et al. Cow's milk-dependent exercise-induced anaphylaxis under the condition of a premenstrual or ovulatory phase following skin sensitization. *Allergol Int.* 2008;57:437.
7. Wade JP, Liang MH, Sheffer AL. Exercise-induced anaphylaxis: epidemiologic observations. *Prog Clin Biol Res.* 1989;297:175.
8. Dohi M, Suko M, Sugiyama H, et al. Food-dependent, exercise-induced anaphylaxis: a study on 11 Japanese cases. *J Allergy Clin Immunol.* 1991;87:34.
9. Romano A, Di Fonso M, Giuffreda F, et al. Food-dependent exercise-induced anaphylaxis: clinical and laboratory findings in 54 subjects. *Int Arch Allergy Immunol.* 2001;125:264.
10. Kano H, Juji F, Shibuya N, et al. [Clinical courses of 18 cases with food-dependent exercise-induced anaphylaxis]. *Arerugi.* 2000;49:472.
11. Orhan F, Karakas T. Food-dependent exercise-induced anaphylaxis to lentil and anaphylaxis to chickpea in a 17-year-old boy. *J Invest Allergol Clin Immunol.* 2008;18:465.
12. Sanchez-Borges M, Iraola V, Fernandez-Caldas E, et al. Dust mite ingestion-associated, exercise-induced anaphylaxis. *J Allergy Clin Immunol.* 2007;120:714.
13. Beaudouin E, Renaudin JM, Morisset, M et al. Food-dependent exercise-induced anaphylaxis – update and current data. *Eur Ann Allergy Clin Immunol.* 2006;38:45.
14. Hanakawa Y, Tohyama M, Shirakata Y, et al. Food-dependent exercise-induced anaphylaxis: a case related to the amount of food allergen ingested. *Br J Dermatol.* 1998;138:898.
15. Adachi A, Horikawa T, Shimizu H, et al. Soybean beta-conglycinin as the main allergen in a patient with food-dependent exercise-induced anaphylaxis by tofu: food processing alters pepsin resistance. *Clin Exp Allergy.* 2009;39:167.
16. Aihara Y, Takahashi Y, Kotoyori T, et al. Frequency of food-dependent, exercise-induced anaphylaxis in Japanese junior-high-school students. *J Allergy Clin Immunol.* 2001;108:1035.
17. Longley S, Panush RS. Familial exercise-induced anaphylaxis. *Ann Allergy.* 1987;58:257.
18. Grant JA, Farmnam J, Lord RA, et al. Familial exercise-induced anaphylaxis. *Ann Allergy.* 1985;54:35.
19. Sheffer, AL, Tong, AK, Murphy, GF, et al. Exercise-induced anaphylaxis: a serious form of physical allergy associated with mast cell degranulation. *J Allergy Clin Immunol.* 1985; 75:479.
20. Lewis J, Lieberman P, Treadwell G, Erffmeyer J. Exercise-induced urticaria, angioedema, and anaphylactoid episodes. *J Allergy Clin Immunol.* 1981;68:432.
21. Sheffer AL, Soter NA, McFadden ER Jr, Austen KF. Exercise-induced anaphylaxis: a distinct form of physical allergy. *J Allergy Clin Immunol.* 1983;71:311.
22. Schwartz HJ. Elevated serum tryptase in exercise-induced anaphylaxis. *J Allergy Clin Immunol.* 1995;95:917.
23. Palosuo K, Alenius H, Varjonen E, et al. A novel wheat gliadin as a cause of exercise-induced anaphylaxis. *J Allergy Clin Immunol.* 1999;103:912.
24. Lauriere M, Pecquet C, Boulenc E, et al. Genetic differences in omega-gliadins involved in two different immediate food hypersensitivities to wheat. *Allergy.* 2007;62:890.
25. Palosuo, K, Varjonen E, Nurkkala J, et al. Transglutaminase-mediated cross-linking of a peptic fraction of omega-5 gliadin enhances IgE reactivity in wheat-dependent, exercise-induced anaphylaxis. *J Allergy Clin Immunol.* 2003;111:1386.
26. Matsuo H, Morimoto K, Akaki T, et al. Exercise and aspirin increase levels of circulating gliadin peptides in patients with wheat-dependent exercise-induced anaphylaxis. *Clin Exp Allergy.* 2005;35:461.
27. Cooper DM, Radom-Aizik S, Schwindt C, Zaldivar F Jr. Dangerous exercise: lessons learned from dysregulated inflammatory responses to physical activity. *J Appl Physiol.* 2007;103:700.
28. Aihara M, Miyazawa M, Osuna H, et al. Food-dependent exercise-induced anaphylaxis: influence of concurrent aspirin administration on skin testing and provocation. *Br J Dermatol.* 2002;146:466.
29. Sheffer AL, Austen KF. Exercise-induced anaphylaxis. *J Allergy Clin Immunol.* 1984;73:699.
30. Casale TB, Keahey TM, Kaliner M. Exercise-induced anaphylactic syndromes. Insights into diagnostic and pathophysiologic features. *JAMA.* 1986;255:2049.

31. Anna Feldweg, MD, Unpublished observation.
32. Juji F, Suko M. Effectiveness of disodium cromoglycate in food-dependent, exercise-induced anaphylaxis: a case report. *Ann Allergy.* 1994;72:452.
33. Sugimura T, Tananari Y, Ozaki Y, et al. Effect of oral sodium cromoglycate in 2 children with food-dependent exercise-induced anaphylaxis (FDEIA). *Clin Pediatr.* 2009;48:945.
34. Aihara Y, Kotoyori T, Takahashi Y, et al. The necessity for dual food intake to provoke food-dependent exercise-induced anaphylaxis (FEIAn): a case report of FEIAn with simultaneous intake of wheat and umeboshi. *J Allergy Clin Immunol.* 2001;107:1100.
35. Ueno M, Adachi A, Shimoura S, et al. A case of wheat-dependent exercise-induced anaphylaxis controlled by sodium chromoglycate, but not controlled by misoprostol. *J Environ Dermatol Cutan Allergol.* 2008;2:118.
36. Untersmayr E, Scholl I, Swoboda I, et al. Antacid medication inhibits digestion of dietary proteins and causes food allergy: a fish allergy model in BALB/c mice. *J Allergy Clin Immunol.* 2003;112:616.
37. Scholl I, Untersmayr E, Bakos N, et al. Antiulcer drugs promote oral sensitization and hypersensitivity to hazelnut allergens in BALB/c mice and humans. *Am J Clin Nutr.* 2005;81:154.
38. Untersmayr E, Bakos N, Scholl I, et al. Anti-ulcer drugs promote IgE formation toward dietary antigens in adult patients. *FASEB J.* 2005;19:656.
39. Ausdenmoore, RW. Fatality in a teenager secondary to exercise-induced anaphylaxis. *Pediatr Asthma Allergy Immunol.* 1991;5:21.
40. Drouet M, Sabbah A, Le Sellin J, et al. Fatal anaphylaxis after eating wild boar meat in a patient with pork-cat syndrome. *Allerg Immunol* (Paris). 2001;33:163.
41. Flannagan LM, Wolf BC. Sudden death associated with food and exercise. *J Forensic Sci.* 2004;49:543.

# Chapter 15
# Mastocytosis and Mast Cell Activation Syndromes Presenting as Anaphylaxis*

**Cem Akin and Dean D. Metcalfe**

**Abstract** Anaphylaxis results from mast cell degranulation induced by allergen-specific IgE as well as various non-IgE-mediated mechanisms. It has been recently demonstrated that intrinsic abnormalities in mast cells, such as presence of activating D816V c-kit mutation, may influence susceptibility to anaphylaxis, especially in patients with "idiopathic" or hymenoptera-induced anaphylaxis. However, despite an improved understanding of the role of clonal mast cell disease in susceptibility to anaphylaxis, the basis of an apparent increase in susceptibility in the majority of patients remains poorly understood. In this chapter, we will review the potential mechanisms of mast cell activation as well as the range of symptoms and the differential diagnosis of patients suspected of having a disease caused by mast cell activation. In addition, we offer a global classification for disorders involving mast cells.

**Keywords** Anaphylaxis • Mast cells • Mastocytosis • Mast cell activation disorders • C-kit

## 15.1 Introduction

Mast cells are central effector cells of allergic disorders [1]. Mast cell proliferation and activation also contribute to the symptoms and pathogenesis of many nonallergic inflammatory and neoplastic diseases [2]. Activation of mast cells by IgE- and non-IgE-mediated mechanisms leads to release of mediators affecting multiple tissues including those of the respiratory, cardiovascular, cutaneous, gastrointestinal, and central nervous systems. Disease states caused by IgE-mediated mast cell activation including anaphylaxis as well as diseases of neoplastic proliferation have been fairly well characterized and have well-accepted diagnostic criteria. In contrast, existence of a clinical disease associated with intrinsic defects in mast cell activation resulting in mast cell hyperreactivity has long been debated, but not scientifically proven. No current diagnostic guidelines or algorithms are available for patients presenting with symptoms strictly from mast cell activation, i.e., a mast cell activation syndrome. In this chapter, we will review the potential mechanisms of mast cell activation as well as the range of symptoms and differential diagnosis of patients suspected of having a disease caused by mast cell activation. In addition, we offer a global classification for disorders involving mast cells.

---

*This work was in part supported by the Division of Intramural Research of the NIH/NIAID.

C. Akin (✉)
Harvard Medical School, Brigham and Women's Hospital, Boston, MA, USA
e-mail: dmetcalfe@niaid.nih.gov

M.C. Castells (ed.), *Anaphylaxis and Hypersensitivity Reactions*,
DOI 10.1007/978-1-60327-951-2_15, © Springer Science+Business Media, LLC 2011

## 15.2 Mechanisms of Mast Cell Activation

Mast cells are derived from hematopoietic stem cells and undergo terminal differentiation in tissues [3]. They are found concentrated in locations such as mucosal and endothelial surfaces where tissues interface with the external environment. This is consistent with the current understanding of the roles of mast cells as sentinels of the innate and adaptive immune systems [4]. While the exact role of mast cells in maintaining the healthy homeostatic state is yet to be understood, mast cells most often come to clinical attention because of their involvement in allergic diseases.

Mast cell activation in allergic diseases results from crosslinking of high-affinity IgE receptors by allergen-bound IgE. Mast cells may also be activated through non-IgE-mediated mechanisms including IgG, complement, microbial components, drugs, hormones, physical and emotional stimuli, hormones, and cytokines (Table 15.1). IFN-γ(gamma) can induce human mast cells to upregulate high-affinity IgG receptors, crosslinking of which is followed by mast cell degranulation comparable to the levels achieved by allergen--IgE interaction [5]. This mechanism of mast cell activation may be operational in IFN-γ(gamma)-rich autoimmune disease states such as psoriasis and inflammatory bowel disease. C3a and C5a, activation products of the complement pathway, are capable of activating certain mast cell types (e.g., skin mast cells, mast cells in rheumatoid arthritis) [6] by directly binding to their respective receptors on the mast cell surface [7,8]. Complement-induced mast cell activation may thus contribute to disease symptoms in infectious, autoimmune, and neoplastic diseases.

Infectious agents stimulate mast cells directly via toll-like receptors recognizing patterns common to microbial or viral pathogens. In this regard, human mast cells have been shown to carry TLR1-7 and 9 and respond to TLR stimulation by release of cytokines and LTC4 [9].

Drugs such as opioid analgesics [10], adenosine [11], and vancomycin induce pruritus, flushing, and bronchoconstriction in part by directly activating mast cells. Hypersensitivity reactions to nonsteroidal anti-inflammatory drugs inhibiting cyclooxygenase pathway have been attributed to shifting of arachidonic acid metabolism to the 5-lipoxygenase pathway in mast cells, causing symptoms due to overproduction of leukotrienes.

**Table 15.1** Mast cell activators of clinical relevance

| |
|---|
| *IgE-dependent* |
| Allergen |
| *IgE-independent* |
| IgG via Fcγ(gamma)RI and III |
| Bacterial components |
| Peptidoglycan: TLR2/6 |
| LPS: TLR4 |
| fMLP |
| C3a, C5a |
| Cysteinyl leukotrienes |
| Cytokines/chemokines |
| SCF, NGF |
| Neuropeptides |
| Drugs |
| Opioids, muscle relaxants, radiocontrast material, adenosine |
| Physical stimuli |
| Heat, cold, pressure, exercise |
| Hormones |
| Estrogen, progesterone, CRH, α(alpha)-MSH |

Physical stimuli such as cold, heat, and pressure in some instances activate mast cells directly, contributing to clinical presentations of physical urticarias (Table 15.1). Cytokines have variable effects on mast cells. Stem cell factor, the major cytokine involved in mast cell growth and differentiation from hematopoietic progenitor cells, also enhances IgE-mediated mast cell degranulation and acts as a chemotactic factor [12]. IL-4 enhances human mast cell maturation by upregulating IgE receptors [13] and chymase production [14], but downregulates mast cell differentiation from progenitors in some in vitro culture systems [13].

Regardless of the mechanism, activation of mast cells results in (1) degranulation with resulting release of preformed mediators stored in granules including histamine, heparin, proteases, and cytokines such as TNF-α(alpha), (2) de novo synthesis of arachidonic acid metabolites (most notably PGD2 and LTC4) from membrane lipids, and (3) synthesis and secretion of cytokines and chemokines [15].

Negative regulators of mast cell activation have also been described. Likewise, several drugs, such as glucocorticosteroids, and cyclosporine A, interfere with IgE-dependent mast cell (and basophil) activation. Glucocorticoids also reduce tissue numbers of mast cells by decreasing SCF in the microenvironment [16].

Fc-γ(gamma)RIIb receptor crosslinking has been shown to reduce IgE-mediated mast cell activation and therapeutic uses of this mechanism to reduce IgE receptor mediated mast cell activation have been explored [17]. Other inhibitory molecules such as gp41B1 have been described [18].

## 15.3 Clinical Manifestations of Mast Cell Activation

In clinical practice, patients are suspected of having a disease involving mast cell activation based on symptoms, physical examination findings, and results of diagnostic laboratory evaluations. It should be emphasized that there is no single symptom specific to mast cell activation; however, some consider the appropriate combination of multiple symptoms to be suggestive of systemic mast cell activation.

Some patients with mast cell activation symptoms are erroneously diagnosed as having systemic mastocytosis. Systemic mastocytosis is a clonal neoplastic disorder of the mast cell and should be diagnosed according to the World Health Organization's criteria and not based on symptoms alone [19]. Patients with systemic mastocytosis often have symptoms of mast cell activation, while the opposite is not true (Table 15.2). In other words, most patients with mast cell activation symptoms do not have systemic mastocytosis according to the WHO criteria, and should not be diagnosed as such. The following discussion provides a brief account of most common symptoms of mast cell activation with reference to findings in systemic mastocytosis.

### *15.3.1 Skin and Soft Tissues*

Mast cell activation is a critical event in acute and chronic urticarias. Mast cell-derived histamine, LTC4, PGD2, and platelet-activating factor cause wheal and flare reactions in skin. Acute urticaria

**Table 15.2** Symptoms commonly encountered in mastocytosis and clonal mast cell disorders

| |
|---|
| Skin: Flushing, pruritus |
| Cardiovascular: Tachycardia, hypotension, presyncope, syncope |
| Gastrointestinal: Abdominal pain, cramping, nausea, vomiting, diarrhea, acid reflux, dyspepsia |
| Musculoskeletal: Bone and/or muscle pain |
| General: Fatigue, lack of concentration |

is often caused by stimulation of mast cells by allergens, microbial pathogens, and drugs. An additional mechanism of mast cell activation in a subset of patients with chronic urticaria is through autoantibodies against IgE or IgE receptors. However, despite an extensive workup, the majority of cases of chronic urticaria remain idiopathic.

Urticaria accompanies systemic anaphylaxis in more than 80% of patients [20]. Mast cell activation in deeper dermis and subcutaneous tissues results in angioedema. Angioedema caused by mast cell activation should be differentiated from other causes of angioedema such as ACE-inhibitors or C1 esterase inhibitor deficiency, which presents without hives.

Acute urticaria lesions must be differentiated from lesions of urticaria pigmentosa seen in cutaneous and systemic mastocytosis. Urticaria pigmentosa skin lesions associated with mastocytosis are fixed hyperpigmented maculopapular lesions, in contrast to migratory and transient lesions of typical "hives." Interestingly, urticaria and angioedema are not common manifestations of systemic mastocytosis.

A mast cell disorder should not be diagnosed solely based on mild to moderate increases in the number of mast cells in a skin biopsy. This is because mast cell numbers in skin are increased in a number of inflammatory skin disorders including atopic dermatitis, contact dermatitis, and vasculitis. Likewise, skin biopsy of a telengiectatic lesion is likely to yield a report showing an increased density of mast cells around blood vessels. Such biopsy reports should always be interpreted in the context of clinical presentation of the patient and the physical appearance of the skin lesion [21]. Mast cells in psoriatic plaques have upregulated Fc-γ(gamma)RI receptors, which can potentially cause mast cell degranulation and pruritus after crosslinking by autoimmune IgG [5].

Mast cell activation in systemic allergic reactions may be accompanied by flushing caused by the vasodilatory effects of histamine and lipid-derived mast cell mediators. Episodic flushing induced by exercise, alcohol, temperature changes, and emotional stress is a common complaint in mastocytosis. Therefore, mast cell activation is often considered in the differential diagnosis of patients with recurrent unexplained flushing. Further, the differential diagnosis of flushing is extensive and includes hormonal, neurologic, and cardiovascular etiologies [22]. Flushing observed in the context of systemic mast cell activation usually occurs in the presence of other organ manifestations and, in our experience, patients presenting with flushing as the only complaint are unlikely to have a mast cell-related etiology to their symptoms.

### *15.3.2 Respiratory*

Mast cell-derived histamine, prostaglandin D2, and cysteinyl leukotrienes cause bronchoconstriction and contribute to the clinical symptoms of asthma. Moreover, cytokines and chemotactic factors released from mast cells promote the development of airway inflammation in asthma [23]. Bronchoconstriction resulting in shortness of breath and wheezing can be seen as a manifestation of systemic mast cell degranulation and anaphylaxis. Patients with pre-existing lung disease and asthma are more likely to have a fatal outcome in an anaphylactic reaction [24–26].

Mast cell activation in allergic rhinoconjunctivitis results in typical symptoms of this disease including rhinorrhea, congestion, sneezing, and nasal itching [27]. Angioedema of the upper airways can be life-threatening in systemic anaphylactic reactions.

In contrast to the frequent occurrence of upper and lower respiratory symptoms in anaphylaxis and mast cell activation, the prevalence of asthma, rhinitis, and structural lung disease does not appear to be more common in systemic mastocytosis than in general population. Moreover, local inflammatory reactions limited to a particular tissue site, such as the nose, alone logically are not sufficient to allow the assumption that the patient is suffering from generalized mast cell activation.

### 15.3.3 Cardiovascular

Systemic mast cell degranulation may lead to episodic hypotension with resultant lightheadedness and syncope in a subset of patients with recurrent anaphylaxis despite the etiology. A compensatory tachycardia is often associated with the hypotensive event. There may be associated rhythm abnormalities and life-threatening myocardial perfusion abnormalities superimposed. This is especially the case in patients with co-existing structural heart disease. Mast cell disease is thus appropriate to consider in the differential diagnosis of patients with unexplained recurrent syncope, especially those associated with other symptoms such as flushing and gastrointestinal complaints [28]. Localized activation of mast cells in coronary arteries has been implicated in rupture of atherosclerotic plaques [29].

### 15.3.4 Gastrointestinal

Systemic mast cell degranulation is frequently associated with gastrointestinal complaints such as heartburn, nausea, vomiting, diarrhea, and abdominal cramping [30]. Peptic complaints such as heartburn and nausea may be partially caused by gastric acid hypersecretion from parietal cells stimulated by histamine in patients with increased mast cell burden. However, the physiologic basis of diarrhea and abdominal pain in mast cell disorders is largely speculative.

In practice, we occasionally encounter patients diagnosed as having a mast cell disorder (either systemic mastocytosis or "mast cell activation syndrome") based on increased numbers of mast cells in gastrointestinal tract biopsies. In these patients, we attempt to verify or rule out diagnostic criteria for systemic mastocytosis according to World Health Organization's criteria. Bone marrow is the preferred tissue to evaluate in applying WHO criteria.

One difficulty is that there are conflicting reports about the gastrointestinal mast cell density in patients with systemic mastocytosis. One study found decreased numbers of mast cells in gastric and duodenal biopsies of patients with systemic mastocytosis when compared to controls [31], while other studies reported increased numbers [32]. Considering that mast cell numbers can also be found increased in gastrointestinal track biopsies in patients with inflammatory bowel diseases, or bacterial and parasitic infections, diagnosis of a mast cell disease should not be based on demonstration of increased mast cells in gastrointestinal biopsy tissues unless mast cells form diagnostic large compact clusters of coherently packed atypical (CD25+ and KIT D816V+) mast cells and thus fulfill WHO criteria for systemic mastocytosis.

### 15.3.5 Musculoskeletal

Mast cells increase in number in synovial tissue in rheumatoid arthritis. Mast cell derived TNF-$\alpha$(alpha) has been implicated to play an important role in cartilage destruction [33]. Patients with mastocytosis often complain about generalized and vague musculoskeletal discomfort resembling fibromyalgia. Mastocytosis is also associated with accelerated osteoporosis in a subset of patients. However, joint swelling and effusion are rarely encountered in patients with mastocytosis unless there is an accompanying diagnosis of osteoarthritis or rheumatoid arthritis. Patients with aggressive and advanced variants of systemic mastocytosis may have bone pain resulting from red marrow expansion or from an accompanying osteopathy, and pathological fractures may occur.

### *15.3.6 Urinary*

Increased numbers of activated mast cells in bladder mucosa and detrusor muscle have been reported in bladder biopsies from patients with interstitial cystitis [34]. Whether mast cell activation represents the primary pathogenetic event or occurs in response to another yet-to-be-identified inflammatory stimulus in interstitial cystitis is unknown. Cystitis is not a feature of systemic mastocytosis.

### *15.3.7 Hematopoietic and Immune Systems*

Patients with systemic (often advanced) mastocytosis may have an associated non-mast cell lineage hematologic disorder, which commonly involves the myeloid lineage. Hematologic disorders in this variant of mastocytosis may thus include myeloproliferative or myelodysplastic syndromes, acute or chronic myeloid leukemias, and less commonly lymphoproliferative disorders [35]. Patients with mastocytosis and an associated hematologic disorder more often than not do not present with mast cell activation symptoms. Their diagnosis is often and almost always established by a bone marrow examination following concern of an evolving hematologic disorder because of easy bruisability, a bleeding tendency, or abnormalities on a peripheral blood count such as an unexplained thrombocytopenia. Mast cell disease or activation is not typically associated with clinically significant immune suppression or susceptibility to infection, unless patients have severe neutropenia or immune suppression as a result of bone marrow replacement by mast cells or myelosuppressive chemotherapy regimens used in treatment of aggressive mastocytosis or mast cell leukemia.

### *15.3.8 Constitutional*

Unexplained fevers have been described in patients with advanced categories of mastocytosis and may be explained by release of cytokines such as TNF-$\alpha$(alpha), IL-1, and IL-6 from activated mast cells, but are rare in episodic mast cell activation events. Fatigue, lack of concentration, and mild cognitive problems are frequent complaints in patients with allergic disorders as well as mastocytosis and patients with other symptoms of ongoing mast cell activation. These symptoms may be due to the effects of mast cell mediators, medications, or psychosomatic effects of having a chronic illness.

## 15.4 Disorders of MC Activation

Disorders involving mast cell activation and mediator release are represented within two major categories (Table 15.3). Clonal mast cell disorders are those where the basis of the disease (based on available information) is associated with intrinsic defects in mast cells affecting proliferation or activation pathways. These include clonal disorders of mast cells and idiopathic syndromes where mast cells are implicated. In nonclonal mast cell activation disorders, normal mast cells react to an external stimulus such as allergen, autoantibody, drug, or complement activation. Some examples of disease states causing mast cell activation are listed in Table 15.3.

Currently, there are two well-characterized molecular defects resulting in increased numbers of mast cells in tissues. The first involves a point mutation (D816V) in KIT associated with mastocytosis. The second molecular defect is a translocation involving PDGFRA (FIP1L1-PDGFRA) associated

**Table 15.3** Systemic mast cell activation disorders

| |
|---|
| 1. Clonal |
| (a) Mastocytosis |
| (b) Monoclonal mast cell activation syndrome |
| (c) Idiopathic anaphylaxis with associated clonal mast cell disorder |
| 2. Nonclonal, IgE, and/or immune-mediated |
| (a) Anaphylaxis induced by IgE and known antigen |
| (b) Mast cell activation associated with chronic inflammatory or neoplastic disorders |
| (c) Idiopathic systemic mast cell activation disorder |

with chronic eosinophilic leukemia with increased mast cells. The latter molecular defect results in a disease primarily manifested by symptoms attributable to eosinophilic proliferation and will not be reviewed here.

D816V KIT mutation is the only well-characterized molecular defect associated not only with increased mast cell numbers in tissues (systemic mastocytosis), but also with a clinical syndrome manifesting itself primarily as mast cell activation. KIT is a transmembrane receptor encoded by the proto-oncogene c-kit, which has intrinsic tyrosine kinase activity. KIT is activated when it is crosslinked by its ligand, stem cell factor. Stem cell factor binding to KIT is critical for mast cell growth and differentiation from hematopoietic progenitors, as well as survival and chemotaxis. Activation of KIT has also been shown to enhance IgE-mediated mast cell activation. The D816V point mutation results in constitutive activation of the tyrosine kinase domain of KIT and leads to SCF-independent autophosphorylation of the molecule. While there is no direct in vitro evidence that D816V mutation causes mast cell activation, identification of the mutation in patients with systemic mastocytosis as well as a subset of patients presenting with recurrent anaphylactic episodes makes it a likely possibility that the mutation is involved in the pathogenesis of mast cell activation or in the increased responsiveness of mast cells observed in these diseases. Because some patients with mastocytosis who carry the KIT D816V mutation do not develop mediator-related symptoms, it is clear that other prorelease mechanisms or a relative lack of inhibitory influences must exist.

## 15.5 Systemic Mastocytosis

Patients with systemic mastocytosis frequently have episodic symptoms attributable to mast cell activation, such as flushing, lightheadedness, and gastrointestinal cramping [28]. The D816V KIT gain-of-function point mutation has been shown to be associated with more than 90% of adults with systemic mastocytosis [36]. Since the original description of mastocytosis, its primary diagnostic feature has been the demonstration of multifocal mast cell clusters of atypical morphology in a bone marrow biopsy specimen. This characteristic finding has been repeatedly validated as the major diagnostic criterion for mast cell disease in consensus meetings on diagnostic criteria and classification of mastocytosis [19]. The minor diagnostic criteria for the disease include a tryptase level consistently greater than 20 ng/mL, atypical (spindle shaped, hypogranulated) mast cell morphology, aberrant expression of CD2 and CD25 on KIT+ mast cells, and detection of a codon 816 mutation in *KIT*. According to WHO guidelines, the major plus one minor or three minor criteria are needed for the diagnosis of mastocytosis. Typical skin lesions of cutaneous mastocytosis, where the most frequent pattern is that of urticaria pigmentosa, are present in approximately 80% of patients with mastocytosis, although they are not a diagnostic criteria for systemic disease.

## 15.6 Monoclonal Mast Cell Activation Syndrome

A group of patients with recurrent anaphylaxis have been described that have clonal mast cells as demonstrated by aberrant CD25 expression and/or a *KIT* D816V point mutation. Such patients thus fulfill one or two minor diagnostic criteria for mastocytosis [37–39]. These patients usually do not have urticaria pigmentosa, nor the characteristic bone marrow mast cell clusters typical of mastocytosis, and often have normal or only slightly elevated serum tryptase levels. The D816V *KIT* mutation may be only detectable in a bone marrow sample enriched for mast cells and not in peripheral blood or unfractionated bone marrow. A careful morphologic examination of bone marrow mast cells in Wright--Giemsa-stained aspirates or in tryptase-stained biopsy sections may reveal hypogranulated and spindle-shaped aberrant mast cell morphology, which may form small clusters and display blood vessel or bone tropism [40]. These patients thus have a disease process manifesting itself primarily as mast cell activation rather than mast cell proliferation, although they share some similar pathologic features with systemic mastocytosis. Limited follow-up of this patient population has not suggested thus far progression of the extent of bone marrow mast cell infiltration, arguing against the possibility that these findings represent an early form of systemic mastocytosis.

The characteristic clinical presentation of these patients includes episodic symptoms attributable to mast cell degranulation, most commonly involving flushing, lightheadedness, and abdominal symptoms such as cramping, nausea, and diarrhea. Symptoms may progress to loss of consciousness and life-threatening hypotension (shock). The episodes usually last for a few minutes to several hours. There are no identifiable precipitating events in most patients, although some events have followed eating and exercise with no food-specific IgE identified. Some of these patients may have been formerly diagnosed as having idiopathic anaphylaxis or exercise-induced anaphylaxis.

There is convincing evidence that a significant number of patients who experience anaphylaxis with hypotension after hymenoptera stings have elevated baseline tryptase levels and underlying clonal mast cell disease [41,42]. Therefore, patients with idiopathic, exercise-, or hymenoptera-induced anaphylaxis may be candidates for an evaluation to determine if a clonal mast cell disorder is present. Specialized techniques are required to demonstrate the small abnormal mast cell population including mast cell flow cytometry [43] and mutational analysis of the mast cell enriched bone marrow samples [36].

## 15.7 Mast Cell Activation Syndrome

The presence of a disease due to an intrinsic defect within the mast cell compartment has long been debated, but has not been universally accepted. Despite the absence of objective diagnostic guidelines for such a disorder, this diagnosis is assigned to some patients with symptoms of mast cell activation discussed above with an otherwise negative diagnostic workup.

Patients referred to our clinic with a presumptive diagnosis of "mast cell activation syndrome" generally have at least two or more of the organ manifestations of mast cell activation such as flushing, urticaria, diarrhea, wheezing, and a variety of constitutional symptoms such as fatigue, and musculoskeletal pain. Some patients may have elevated mast cell mediators such as serum tryptase, 24-h *N*-methylhistamine, and 11β(beta)PGF2 with a negative workup for systemic mastocytosis or clonal mast cell disease in bone marrow biopsies [44]. It is important to rule out diseases associated with secondary mast cell activation in this patient population. It is also helpful to obtain a biochemical proof of mast cell mediator release during symptomatic periods to establish that the symptoms are indeed related to mast cell activation. This is of importance in order to avoid missing a diagnosis of a disorder unrelated to mast cell pathology but presenting with similar symptoms in the absence of a robust biochemical proof of mast cell activation. Some patients with gastrointestinal or urinary symptoms may have increased numbers of degranulated mast cells in biopsies obtained from gut or bladder tissue, suggesting that mast cells contribute to some of the pathology of the disease process in these patients. In some patients, improvement of symptoms with drugs targeting mast cell mediators (such as H1 and H2 antihistamines, cromolyn, leukotriene antagonists) are considered as further supporting evidence of mast cell involvement in disease process. Our current practice, however, is not to assign a diagnosis of "mast cell activation disorder" to patients until a consensus opinion or evidence-based diagnostic guidelines become available.

Considering the well-established role mast cells play in urticaria, angioedema, and anaphylaxis, it should also be recognized that patients presenting with these disorders and no identifiable etiology could be considered under the term mast cell activation syndrome. It is not known whether mast cell activation in these situations results from an intrinsic mast cell defect or from a yet-to-be-identified endogenous or environmental stimulus.

## 15.8 Diagnostic Approach to Mast Cell Activation Disorders

In a patient presenting with symptoms of mast cell activation, it is reasonable to start with an allergy evaluation to search for IgE-mediated etiologies such as food or drug allergies. If the allergy workup does not satisfactorily identify a trigger accounting for the patient's symptoms, systemic mastocytosis or clonal mast cell disease should be considered in the differential diagnosis. A careful skin examination should be performed for urticaria pigmentosa. A serum tryptase level greater than 20 ng/mL is a minor diagnostic criterion of systemic mastocytosis, and should generally prompt consideration of a workup for systemic mastocytosis in patients who have mast cell activation symptoms [45]. It should be kept in mind that tryptase can be elevated in other hematologic disorders such as chronic eosinophilic leukemia, myelodysplastic syndromes, and acute leukemias. These disorders can generally be readily diagnosed based on peripheral blood and bone marrow findings. A normal tryptase level, on the other hand, does not rule out clonal mast cell disease. The likelihood of diagnosing mast cell disease by observing characteristic multifocal bone marrow aggregates diminishes significantly in those with tryptase levels less than 20 ng/mL, and these patients should be considered for referral to a center capable of specialized testing including mast cell flow cytometry and mutational analysis on bone marrow sorted cells.

Patients with recurrent flushing should also be considered for neurologic and endocrinologic evaluations including estrogen or testosterone deficiency, carcinoid, pheochromocytoma, and medullary thyroid cancer [22]. The diagnosis of systemic mast cell disease based on biopsies other than bone marrow should generally be avoided. Documentation of mast cell mediator release during and after episodes provides valuable information about whether the symptoms are due to mast cell activation. These tests include serum tryptase (which should be obtained within 4 h after the onset of symptoms), and 24 urine collections for *N*-methylhistamine and 11β(beta) PGF2. Levels of these mediators during symptomatic periods should be compared with patient's baseline values. Patients with elevated mast cell mediator levels should be carefully evaluated for secondary causes of mast cell activation (Table 15.4). The diagnosis of idiopathic anaphylaxis should be considered in those with recurrent anaphylaxis and no identifiable allergic or clonal mast cell etiology [46].

In light of the discussion above, we propose that the evidence suggesting a disorder caused by mast cell activation should require all of the following three criteria providing primary (clonal) and secondary disorders of mast cell activation (Table 15.4) are ruled out:

1. Episodic symptoms consistent with mast cell mediator release affecting two or more organ systems evidenced as follows:

   (a) Skin: urticaria, angioedema, flushing.

**Table 15.4** Clinical conditions with mast cell participation

| Disease | Activation attributed to |
|---|---|
| Atopic diseases | Allergen-specific IgE |
| Chronic autoimmune urticaria | Anti-IgE or anti-Fcε(epsilon)RI autoantibodies |
| Autoimmunity | IgG, complement |
| Chronic infections | TLR ligands, IgG, complement |
| Drug allergy | Direct activation, complement, IgE |
| Physical stimuli | Direct/indirect mast cell activation |
| Neoplasms | Cytokines, IgG/IgE, complement |

(b) Gastrointestinal: nausea, vomiting, diarrhea, abdominal cramping.
(c) Cardiovascular: hypotensive syncope or near syncope, tachycardia.
(d) Respiratory: wheezing.
(e) Naso-ocular: conjunctival injection, pruritus, nasal stuffiness.

2. A decrease in the frequency or severity; or resolution of symptoms with antimediator therapy: H1 and H2 histamine receptor antagonists, antileukotriene medications (cysLT receptor blocker or 5-LO inhibitor), or mast cell stabilizers (cromolyn sodium). The list of medications may be expanded in the future as more medications targeting mast cell mediated processes become available.
3. Evidence of an elevation in a validated urinary or serum marker of mast cell activation: Documentation of elevation of the marker above the patient's baseline during a symptomatic period on at least two occasions; or if baseline tryptase levels are persistently >15 ng, documentation of elevation of the tryptase above baseline on one occasion. Total serum tryptase is recommended as the markers of choice; less specific (also from basophils) 24h urine histamine metabolites, or 11-β-prostaglandin F2.

If clonal markers of mast cell disease are found (i.e., *KIT* mutation or aberrant CD25 expression), the patient should be assigned a diagnosis of systemic mastocytosis or Monoclonal Mast Cell Activation Syndrome (MMAS) depending on the presence or absence of other WHO diagnostic criteria, regardless of the presence of a secondary diagnosis, which may cause mast cell activation. The evaluation should also include a repeat serum tryptase test after complete resolution of symptoms to see whether basal tryptase is elevated (exceeding 20 ng/mL) as a minor SM criterion.

If clonal markers are absent and a concurrent diagnosis of allergic, inflammatory, infectious, or neoplastic disease is established, then the patient should be considered to have a secondary mast cell activation disorder due to the concurrent illness. If neither clonal markers nor a secondary diagnosis is detectable, it would be reasonable to entertain a diagnosis of primary idiopathic mast cell activation syndrome. We believe that these recommendations form a starting point for the diagnosis of mast cell activation syndrome, which can be validated or modified by prospective multicenter clinical trials.

## References


1. Williams CM, Galli SJ. The diverse potential effector and immunoregulatory roles of mast cells in allergic disease. *J Allergy Clin Immunol.* 2000;105:847.
2. Bachelet I, Levi-Schaffer F, Mekori YA. Mast cells: not only in allergy. *Immunol Allergy Clin North.* 2006;26:407.
3. Kitamura Y, Oboki K, Ito A. Molecular mechanisms of mast cell development. *Immunol Allergy Clin North Am.* 2006;26:387.
4. Galli SJ, Maurer M, Lantz CS. Mast cells as sentinels of innate immunity. *Curr Opin Immunol.* 1999;11:53.

5. Okayama Y, Kirshenbaum AS, Metcalfe DD. Expression of a functional high-affinity IgG receptor, Fc gamma RI, on human mast cells: Up-regulation by IFN-gamma. *J Immunol.* 2000;164:4332.
6. Kiener HP, Baghestanian M, Dominkus M, et al. Expression of the C5a receptor (CD88) on synovial mast cells in patients with rheumatoid arthritis. *Arthritis Rheum.* 1998;41:233.
7. el-Lati SG, Dahinden CA, Church MK. Complement peptides C3a- and C5a-induced mediator release from dissociated human skin mast cells. *J Invest Dermatol.* 1994;102:803.
8. Fureder W, Agis H, Willheim M, et al. Differential expression of complement receptors on human basophils and mast cells. Evidence for mast cell heterogeneity and CD88/C5aR expression on skin mast cells. *J Immunol.* 1995;155:3152.
9. Kulka M, Alexopoulou L, Flavell RA, Metcalfe DD. Activation of mast cells by double-stranded RNA: evidence for activation through Toll-like receptor 3. *J Allergy Clin Immunol.* 2004;114:174.
10. Hermens JM, Ebertz JM, Hanifin JM, Hirshman CA. Comparison of histamine release in human skin mast cells induced by morphine, fentanyl, and oxymorphone. *Anesthesiology.* 1985;62:124.
11. Spicuzza L, Di Maria G, Polosa R. Adenosine in the airways: implications and applications. *Eur J Pharmacol.* 2006;533:77.
12. Galli SJ, Tsai M, Wershil BK, et al. Regulation of mouse and human mast cell development, survival and function by stem cell factor, the ligand for the c-kit receptor. *Int Arch Allergy Immunol.* 1995;107:51.
13. Xia HZ, Du Z, Craig S, et al. Effect of recombinant human IL-4 on tryptase, chymase, and Fc epsilon receptor type I expression in recombinant human stem cell factor- dependent fetal liver-derived human mast cells. *J Immunol.* 1997; 159:2911.
14. Ahn, K, Takai, S, Pawankar, R, et al. Regulation of chymase production in human mast cell progenitors. *J Allergy Clin Immunol.* 2000;106:321
15. Castells M. Mast cell mediators in allergic inflammation and mastocytosis. *Immunol Allergy Clin North Am.* 2006;26:465.
16. Finotto S, Mekori YA, Metcalfe DD. Glucocorticoids decrease tissue mast cell number by reducing the production of the c-kit ligand, stem cell factor, by resident cells: in vitro and in vivo evidence in murine systems. *J Clin Invest.* 1997;99:1721.
17. Zhu D, Kepley CL, Zhang K, et al. A chimeric human-cat fusion protein blocks cat-induced allergy. *Nat Med.* 2005;11:446.
18. Katz HR, Vivier E, Castells MC, et al. Mouse mast cell gp49B1 contains two immunoreceptor tyrosine-based inhibition motifs and suppresses mast cell activation when coligated with the high-affinity Fc receptor for IgE. *Proc Natl Acad Sci USA.* 1996;93:10809.
19. Valent P, Horny H, Escribano L, et al. Diagnostic criteria and classification of mastocytosis: a consensus proposal. *Leuk Res.* 2001;25:603.
20. Webb LM, Lieberman P. Anaphylaxis: a review of 601 cases. *Ann Allergy Asthma Immunol.* 2006;97:39.
21. Valent P, Akin C, Escribano L, et al. Standards and standardization in mastocytosis: Consensus statements on diagnostics, treatment recommendations, and response criteria. *Eur J Clin Invest.* 2007;37:435.
22. Metcalfe DD. Differential diagnosis of the patient with unexplained flushing/anaphylaxis. *Allergy Asthma Proc.* 2000;21:21.
23. Bradding P, Walls AF, Holgate ST. The role of the mast cell in the pathophysiology of asthma. *J Allergy Clin Immunol.* 2006;117:1277.
24. Pumphrey RS. Lessons for management of anaphylaxis from a study of fatal reactions. *Clin Exp Allergy.* 2000;30:1144.
25. Sampson HA, Mendelson L, Rosen JP. Fatal and near-fatal anaphylactic reactions to food in children and adolescents. *N Engl J Med.* 1992;327:380.
26. Amin HS, Liss GM, Bernstein DI. Evaluation of near-fatal reactions to allergen immunotherapy injections. *J Allergy Clin Immunol.* 2006;117:169.
27. Parikh SA, Cho SH, Oh CK. Preformed enzymes in mast cell granules and their potential role in allergic rhinitis. *Curr Allergy Asthma Rep.* 2003;3:266.
28. Akin C, Metcalfe DD. Systemic mastocytosis. *Annu Rev Med.* 2004;55:419.
29. Lindstedt KA, Kovanen PT. Mast cells in vulnerable coronary plaques: potential mechanisms linking mast cell activation to plaque erosion and rupture. *Curr Opin Lipidol.* 2004;15:567.
30. Jensen RT. Gastrointestinal abnormalities and involvement in systemic mastocytosis. *Hematol Oncol Clin North Am.* 2000;14:579.
31. Siegert SI, Diebold J, Ludolph-Hauser D, Lohrs U. Are gastrointestinal mucosal mast cells increased in patients with systemic mastocytosis? *Am J Clin Pathol.* 2004;122:560.
32. Ferguson J, Thompson RP, Greaves MW. Intestinal mucosal mast cells: enumeration in urticaria pigmentosa and systemic mastocytosis. *Br J Dermatol.* 1988;119:573.
33. Tetlow LC, Woolley DE. Mast cells, cytokines, and metalloproteinases at the rheumatoid lesion: dual immunolocalisation studies. *Ann Rheum Dis.* 1995;54:896.

34. Theoharides TC, Kempuraj D, Sant GR. Mast cell involvement in interstitial cystitis: a review of human and experimental evidence. *Urology.* 2001;57:47.
35. Parker RI. Hematologic aspects of mastocytosis: I: Bone marrow pathology in adult and pediatric systemic mast cell disease. *J Invest Dermatol.* 1991;96:47S.
36. Akin C. Molecular diagnosis of mast cell disorders: a paper from the 2005 William Beaumont Hospital Symposium on Molecular Pathology. *J Mol Diagn.* 2006;8:412.
37. Akin C, Metcalfe DD. Occult bone marrow mastocytosis presenting as recurrent systemic anaphylaxis [abstract]. *J Allergy Clin Immunol.* 2003;111:S206.
38. Akin C, Scott LM, Kocabas CN, et al. Demonstration of an aberrant mast-cell population with clonal markers in a subset of patients with "idiopathic" anaphylaxis. *Blood.* 2007;110:2331.
39. Sonneck K, Florian S, Mullauer L, et al. Diagnostic and subdiagnostic accumulation of mast cells in the bone marrow of patients with anaphylaxis: monoclonal mast cell activation syndrome. *Int Arch Allergy Immunol.* 2007;142:158.
40. Hungness SI, Singer AM, Akin C. Food-dependent exercise-induced anaphylaxis associated with clonal mast cells carrying an activating c-kit mutation. *J Allergy Clin Immunol.* 2007;119:S29.
41. Haeberli G, Bronnimann M, Hunziker T, Muller U. Elevated basal serum tryptase and hymenoptera venom allergy: relation to severity of sting reactions and to safety and efficacy of venom immunotherapy. *Clin Exp Allergy.* 2003;33:1216.
42. Ludolph-Hauser D, Rueff F, Fries C, et al. Constitutively raised serum concentrations of mast-cell tryptase and severe anaphylactic reactions to Hymenoptera stings. *Lancet.* 2001;357:361.
43. Akin C, Valent P, Escribano L. Urticaria pigmentosa and mastocytosis: the role of immunophenotyping in diagnosis and determining response to treatment. *Curr Allergy Asthma Rep.* 2006;6:282.
44. Kassab D, Koterba A, Jiang Y, Akin C. Elevated baseline tryptase levels in patients with mast cell activation syndromes without evidence mastocytosis. *J Allergy Clin Immunol.* 2008;121:S67.
45. Schwartz LB. Diagnostic value of tryptase in anaphylaxis and mastocytosis. *Immunol Allergy Clin North Am.* 2006;26:451.
46. Ditto AM, Harris KE, Krasnick J, et al. Idiopathic anaphylaxis: a series of 335 cases. *Ann Allergy Asthma Immunol.* 1996;77:285.

# Chapter 16
# Anaphylaxis in Mastocytosis*

**Luis Escribano and Alberto Orfao**

**Abstract** An increase in anaphylaxis has been reported in mastocytosis, with a predominance of males. Recurrent idiopathic anaphylaxis and either hymenoptera-venom or drug-induced anaphylaxis are the most frequent types of anaphylaxis, no correlation being found between the signs and symptoms of anaphylaxis and MC burden or serum tryptase levels. Less frequently, anaphylaxis can occur during general anesthesia, and other invasive and therapeutic procedures, indicating that appropriate management of SM patients before, during, and after these procedures is required. Venom immunotherapy (VIT) has proved to be effective in mastocytosis, but adverse reactions have also been reported in 10–15% of the patients and fatal reactions have been described after discontinuation of venom immunotherapy.

Therapeutic measures of anaphylaxis in mastocytosis should include: (1) adequate information and training of patients, their relatives, and care providers, (2) availability of individual emergency kits, (3) avoidance of triggering factors, and (4) administration of preventive medication prior to anesthesia and other therapeutic procedures. Additionally, specific treatment of anaphylaxis should be carefully evaluated in each individual patient. Prompt recognition and appropriate control of the acute episodes together with a decrease in the frequency and intensity of chronic symptoms should be attempted with antimediator therapy (e.g. sedating and nonsedating H1 antihistamines and other NSAIDs, oral disodium cromolyn or, in selected cases, aspirin). Steroids should be used in selected cases. Interferon-alpha, hydroxyurea, cytoreductive therapy with cladribine, and omalizumab anti-IgE monoclonal antibody therapy might be of benefit in selected refractory cases.

**Keywords** Mast cell • Mastocytosis • Anaphylaxis • Treatment

## 16.1 Introduction

Mast cells (MC) are a key structural and functional component of the immune system, which are distributed throughout the human body, preferentially in the vicinity of blood vessels; from the functional point of view, they play a key role in inflammation and they are the major effector cells in allergic reactions including anaphylaxis. At present, it is well established that a wide variety of

---

*Sources of Funding
Supported by grants from the Ministerio de Sanidad y Consumo, Instituto de Salud Carlos III (REMA G03/007, FIS050769, FIS060529, FIS061377, PS09/00032, and RETICS RD06/0020/0035-FEDER); Junta de Castilla y León (Grant SAN196/SA10/07); Junta de Comunidades de Castilla La Mancha (FISCAM 2007/36).

L. Escribano (✉)
Centro de Estudios de Mastocitosis de Castilla La Mancha, Hospital Virgen del Valle, Toledo, Spain
e-mail: lescribanom@sescam.jccm.es

M.C. Castells (ed.), *Anaphylaxis and Hypersensitivity Reactions*,
DOI 10.1007/978-1-60327-951-2_16, © Springer Science+Business Media, LLC 2011

stimuli can trigger activation of MC during inflammation as well as in allergic and nonallergic diseases (see Chap. 20). Cross-linking of high-affinity Fc receptors for IgE (Fcε(epsilon)RI) on the cytoplasmic membrane of normal/reactive MC elicits the release of inflammatory mediators from MC secretory granules (1–3) in IgE-sensitized MC. In addition, release of MC-mediators can also be induced through Fcγ(gamma) [4–6] and complement receptors [1–3] or aggregated IgG and C3a [7]. In turn, normal/reactive MC also express on their cell surface toll-like receptor (TLR) 4 and TLR2, CD48, and complement receptor 1 [8–11], which can activate MC without requirements for antibody or other immunological signaling [12].

Although important advances have been achieved in the understanding of the functionality of normal/reactive MC, little is known about the mechanisms of MC activation in systemic mastocytosis (SM). As normal/reactive MC, clonal MC from patients with SM also express a number of functionally relevant cell surface antigens related to MC activation including the stem cell factor receptor (c-kit or CD117), high-affinity receptors for IgE (Fcε(epsilon)RI), IgG receptors (Fcγ(gamma)R), LAMP molecules such as CD63 and complement-related receptors, among other molecules. Except for the so-called well-differentiated systemic mastocytosis (WDSM) [13], KIT mutations at exon 17, most frequently leading to the D816V single change in the kit protein, are present in the vast majority of SM [14]; as described, the D816V mutation as well as other "enzymatic pocket" type KIT mutations directly affect the enzymatic site at the TK2 activation loop and induce conformational changes associated with subsequent activation of kit in the absence of dimerization of the receptor [15]. This KIT mutation is viewed as a critical genetic change associated with constitutive activation of clonal MC in SM. Overexpression of several adhesion and activation-related antigens such as CD63 [16] and CD69 [17], as well as the CD35 (CR1) [18], CD11b, CD11c, and CD88/C5a complement receptors [3], and the CD59 complement-regulatory molecule [3] are constitutively found on BMMC from most patients with SM. These findings support the notion that MC from SM display a unique immunophenotypical profile with increased expression of activation-related molecules, reflecting a switch-on of MC activation pathways. Functional studies are required to determine the implications of the higher expression of these activation molecules in the constitutive and acute release of MC mediators in mastocytosis.

## 16.2 Mastocytosis

Mastocytosis is a heterogeneous group of disorders characterized by an abnormal expansion and accumulation of MC in one or multiple organs, which most frequently include the skin, bone marrow, and gastrointestinal tract among other tissues. Patients with mastocytosis have symptoms related to tissue responses to the release of MC mediators, infiltration of tissues by MC, or both.

Seven categories of mastocytosis have been identified, namely cutaneous mastocytosis (CM), extracutaneous mastocytoma, indolent SM (ISM), aggressive SM (ASM), SM associated with other hematological clonal non-MC lineage disease (SM-AHNMD), MC leukemia (MCL). and MC sarcoma [19–21]. The presence of multifocal dense aggregates of ≥15 MC in BM and/or other extracutaneous tissues is considered as the only major criterion for the diagnosis of SM; additional minor criteria include: (1) identification of morphologically atypical MC in smears or biopsy sections of BM or other extracutaneous organs, (2) aberrant expression of CD25 and/or CD2 by BM MC, (3) detection of the D816V KIT mutation in BM, blood, or other extracutaneous organs, and, (4) serum tryptase levels over 20 μ(mu)g/L. One major and one minor or three minor criteria are currently required for the diagnosis of SM according to the World Health Organization (WHO) [19–21].

Despite its great utility and its wide acceptation, the efficiency of the WHO criteria for the diagnosis of nonaggressive categories of SM at onset may be difficult, particularly in cases with very low BM MC numbers (i.e., $<10^{-3}$ BM MC), because such cases lack BM MC aggregates. In a recent report where the WHO criteria for SM were prospectively applied to the diagnosis and classification of 59 patients [22], only 53 (90%) strictly met the diagnostic criteria for SM; among the six cases who did not meet the WHO criteria for SM, one had mast cell spleen involvement. The authors concluded that their study supports the value of the WHO criteria for the diagnosis of SM but that the BM examination using the WHO criteria is neither completely specific nor sensitive for every patient with SM. The failure of the WHO criteria for the diagnosis of some SM cases could be due to the specific variants of the disease. In particular, patients with well-differentiated SM (WDSM) who present morphologically mature, round-shaped MC in the absence of an aberrant phenotype and the D816V KIT mutation (with or without increased serum tryptase), and patients where clinical symptoms may develop at very early phases of the disease – e.g., clonal MC activation disorders (cMCAD) including ISM without skin lesions (ISMs–). This is of particular relevance because 90% of all mastocytosis correspond to good-prognosis categories and in the cases with low MC burden, symptoms are related to the release of MC mediators rather than to tissue infiltration by MC (reviewed in references [23, 24]). Highly sensitive and specific methods for cytology, immunophenotyping, and analysis of KIT mutational status are thus required to detect low burden cases. We have found a higher frequency of KIT mutation among ISM cases who have aberrant BM MC [14] compared to others [25–27], probably related to the analysis of FACS-purified BM MC enriched with anti-CD25 monoclonal antibodies. The increased sensitivity of the assay allows for the detection of KIT mutations in some ISM patients who do not have skin lesions (ISMs–), in which the disease manifests with severe, life-threatening anaphylactic episodes and very low MC numbers at onset [28]. In patients with recurrent anaphylaxis, who present with syncopal or near-syncopal episodes [29, 30] without associated hives or angioedema [31], mastocytosis needs to be ruled out. Anaphylaxis can be the presenting symptom in ISM with and without skin lesions, and in clonal and nonclonal MCAD (described in Chap. 15).

## 16.3 Allergy in Mastocytosis

Few studies have addressed the comorbidity between allergic conditions and mastocytosis. In two small studies, the prevalence of atopy in adults and children with mastocytosis has been reported to be similar to that observed in the general population, ranging from 31% [32] to 36% [33]. In two other studies in large series of cases including 210 [34] and 120 [35] patients with mastocytosis, the percentage of allergy among adult patients and children was of 23.9% and 28%, and of 17% and 11%, respectively [34, 35]. Interestingly, in our series, 26% of cases showed similar symptoms in the absence of specific IgE against the suspected trigger(s), and thus, they were classified as nonallergic cases [34]. When compared to the overall prevalence of IgE-mediated allergy among the general population-range: 17.9[36]–21.6% [37] – no significant differences were found, supporting the notion that the prevalence of IgE-mediated allergy in patients with mastocytosis does not differ from that of the general population without mastocytosis.

## 16.4 Anaphylaxis in Mastocytosis

The first case of fatal anaphylaxis in a patient suffering from ASM was described in 1979 [38]. Since then, both case reports and large series of patients have been described in the literature (reviewed in references [31, 39, 40]). Interestingly, anaphylaxis is the presenting symptom in a variable percentage of adult mastocytosis, mainly among patients who do not have skin lesions [27, 30, 34, 41, 42], with a clear predominance of hymenoptera-venom anaphylaxis (HVA) [27, 34].

Interestingly, in our series we did not observe a clear relationship between the occurrence of anaphylaxis and the overall MC burden as assessed by histology, percentage of bone marrow MC by flow cytometry, and baseline serum tryptase levels [34]. Nevertheless, there are two specific situations in which massive MC-mediator release is directly related to a high MC burden, namely diffuse cutaneous mastocytosis in children and adult MCL; in both, cases a marked increase in serum tryptase levels (often >1,000 μ(mu)g/L) [43–45] and life-threatening systemic symptoms including hypotension and cardiovascular collapse are frequently observed; such patients need aggressive antimediator treatment and in some adult cases, cytoreductive therapy [43, 44]. The indications for cytoreductive therapy in children are extremely rare due to the overall benign nature of the disease.

The prevalence of anaphylaxis in the general population is estimated to be of between 1 and 3 [46] to 10.5 cases per 100,000 individuals/year [47–49]. The prevalence of anaphylaxis in adult mastocytosis is much higher than that described for subjects who do not have mastocytosis varying from 8/40 (20%) [29] and 36/163 (22%) [34] to 36/74 patients (49%) [35] (Table 16.1) with clear predominance in males. Of note, caution should be made when applying such data in an epidemiological basis. Accordingly, in our series, the percentage of anaphylaxis in ISM with skin lesions

**Table 16.1** Anaphylaxis in adults and children with mastocytosis

| | Brockow et al. [34] | | González de Olano et al. [33] | |
|---|---|---|---|---|
| Disease features | Adults | Children | Adults | Children |
| *Anaphylaxis* | 36/74 (49) | 4/46 (9) | 36/163 (22) | 3/47 (6) |
| *Male gender* | ND | ND | 26 (72%) | 3 (100%) |
| *Diagnostic subtype* | | | | |
| CM | 13 | 46[a] | 1 (2.7%) | 47[a] |
| ISM | 59 | NA | 16 (44.4%) | NA |
| ISMs– | ND | NA | 16 (44.4%) | NA |
| SM-AHNMD | 1 | NA | 2 (5.5%) | NA |
| WDSM | 0 | NA | 1 (2.7%) | NA |
| ASM | 1 (%) | NA | 0 (0%) | NA |
| Tryptase >11.4 (mu)g/L | ND | ND | 32 (88.8%) | 3 (100%) |
| Tryptase >20 (mu)g/L | ND | ND | 30 (83.3%) | 3 (100%) |
| Serum Tryptase[b] | 25.5 (3–200) | 6 (1–46) | 38.3 (4.15–193) | 3 (100%) |
| Serum IgE (kU/L) | NA | NA | 26 (5–550) | 269 (30–440) |
| CAP or SPT positive | NA | NA | 9 (25%) | 1 (33%) |
| *Etiology*[c] | | | | |
| Idiophatic | 9 (25%) | 4 (100%) | 15 (41.6%) | 2 (66%) |
| Mosquito | 0 | 0 | 1 (2.7%) | 0 |
| Hymenoptera | 9 (25%) | 0 | 8 (22.2%) | 0 |
| Specific IgE | NA | NA | 6 (75%) | NA |
| Anisakis simplex | 0 | 0 | 2 (5.5%) | 0 |
| Food | 6 (17%) | 2 (50%) | 1 (2.7%) | 1 (33.3%) |
| Drugs | 8 (22%) | 1 | 8 (22.2%) | 0 |
| Anesthesia | 0 | 0 | 1 (2.7%) | 0 |
| Vaccine | 0 | 1 (25%) | 0 | 0 |
| Mixed | 8 (22%) | 2 (50%) | ND | ND |

Reactions occurred only after a combination of several factors, especially alcohol and foods.

*CM* cutaneous mastocytosis, *ISM* indolent systemic mastocytosis, *SM-AHNMD* systemic mastocytosis associated with a hematological nonmast cell disorder, *WDSM* well-differentiated systemic mastocytosis, *ASM* aggressive systemic mastocytosis

[a]Bone marrow study was not performed.

Results expressed as number of cases and percentage between brackets, [b]as mean values (range) or [c]as number (percentage) of anaphylaxis episodes.

(ISMs+) was of 15.4%, while this percentage was of 67% in cases lacking skin lesions (ISMs–) [34]; furthermore, among ISMs– patients anaphylaxis was the presenting symptom in all cases, supporting the notion that the prevalence of anaphylaxis in SM is overestimated. Among children, a significantly lower percentage of anaphylaxis has been reported ranging from 6% [34] to 9% [35] (Table 16.1).

### *16.4.1 Idiopathic Anaphylaxis and Triggers for Anaphylaxis in Mastocytosis*

Diagnosis of idiopathic anaphylaxis is typically reached after all potential triggers have been excluded [50] and its exact incidence remains unknown. Several studies estimate that nearly 20% of cases of anaphylaxis are idiopathic (reviewed in references [51–52]), but it is much more common in our Mastocytosis series [25, 33, 51] accounting for 42% of the cases [34]. Anaphylaxis can occur at night and in our series one death was attributed to nocturnal anaphylaxis [50]. A summary of the most frequent triggers for anaphylaxis in mastocytosis is depicted in Table 16.2.

### *16.4.2 Hymenoptera Venom Anaphylaxis in Mastocytosis*

One of the most frequent triggers for anaphylaxis in SM is insect venom from hymenoptera (HVA) [27, 53–59] and fatalities have been described [54, 59] even after venom immunotherapy (VIT) [54]. Association between HVA and mastocytosis has been documented in large series of patients

**Table 16.2** Triggers in mastocytosis associated to anaphylaxis [1, 2]

| |
|---|
| *Emotional factors* |
| Stress, anxiety |
| *Drugs* |
| Aspirin and NSAIDS[a] |
| Anesthesia drugs[b] (– succinylcholine, D-tubocurarine, gallamine, decamethonium) |
| Morphine and derivatives |
| Radiocontrast dyes [b, c] |
| *Venoms* |
| Hymenoptera |
| Ants |
| *Physical stimuli* |
| Heat/cold |
| Changes of temperature |
| Friction of skin lesions (Darier's sign in mastocytomas) |
| *Food* |
| *Vaccines* |
| *Therapeutic agents* |
| Interferon alpha |

1. Responses greatly vary from patient to patient. For references, see text
2. Patients with known sensitivities must wear a Medic Alert bracelet or necklace

[a]Aspirin and other nonsteroidal anti-inflammatory drugs (NSAIDS) may induce mast cell degranulation in some patients and have proven to be effective as a treatment for others. If patients have not taken these drugs before, provocation tests and treatment must be administered under close medical supervision.

[b]Patients should be premedicated with H1 and H2 antihistamines, leukotriene antagonists, and adequate sedation (For information on REMA's protocol, see text).

[c]If x-ray studies are necessary low molecular weight dyes should be used.

**Table 16.3** Indications for mastocytosis work up in the absence of skin lesions in patients with anaphylaxis[a]

| |
|---|
| 1. Recurrent idiopathic anaphylaxis, regardless of baseline serum tryptase |
| 2. Hymenoptera sting anaphylaxis in the absence of venom specific IgE, regardless of baseline serum tryptase |
| 3. Hymenoptera sting anaphylaxis with specific venom IgE and increased baseline serum tryptase[b] or anaphylaxis during Venom Immunotherapy, regardless of baseline serum tryptase |
| 4. IgE-mediated anaphylaxis with increased baseline serum tryptase[b] |

[a]Mastocytosis should be suspected in patients with recurrent anaphylaxis lacking skin mastocytosis, who present with syncopal or near-syncopal episodes [28, 29] without associated hives or angioedema [30].
[b]Normal baseline serum tryptase does not exclude the diagnosis of mastocytosis.

[27, 34, 60] and mastocytosis is a risk factor for severe reactions in HVA patients [35, 61]. A common initial presentation for patients with ISM without skin lesions (ISMs−) is anaphylaxis induced by hymenoptera venom (Table 16.3).

### 16.4.3 Anaphylaxis and Venom Immunotherapy in Mastocytosis

Adverse reactions to venom immunotherapy (VIT), including anaphylaxis, in 12% of the cases have been reported [62] (reviewed in reference [63]). In a study including 10 patients with urticaria pigmentosa, no side effects during VIT were described and only one patient presented a mild systemic reaction after re-sting or sting challenge [64]. Venom immunotherapy in mastocytosis has been reported to be effective [57, 64, 65] and proposed as a treatment for life [57, 61, 64], because cases of fatal reactions after VIT have been described after discontinuation [54, 66]. The risk of discontinuing VIT for mastocytosis patients with a history of anaphylaxis is high and should only be considered if the side effects are severe and recurrent [67].

In mastocytosis patients, systemic reactions to VIT have been reported, ranging from 18% [67] to 24% of the cases [61]. In our own experience [61], 6/21 patients suffered from an adverse reaction during VIT injection, and immunotherapy had to be discontinued in 2 of them. Among these 6 patients, another 2 required a change in the VIT extract administered with good tolerance to a different extract. Although no fatalities were observed in our study, VIT should be considered as a high-risk procedure in patients with mastocytosis and HVA. Premedication prior to VIT should be considered in all patients and in reactors changes in the VIT regime, dose, or extract.

### 16.4.4 Anaphylaxis During Surgical Procedures and General Anesthesia

Safe anesthetic procedures in the absence of adverse reactions have been reported both in adults [68–73] and children with mastocytosis [70, 74–76], using different premedication protocols and recommendations [24, 77–80]. The prevalence of anaphylaxis during general anesthesia is largely unknown, but many cases have been documented both in adult [81–83] and pediatric mastocytosis patients [84, 85], indicating that acute mast cell activation is a risk during general anesthesia. Management of mastocytosis patients before, during, and after surgical procedures requires close communication between anesthesiologists, surgeons, and intensivists. Premedication of all patients is recommended and monitoring serum tryptase, histamine levels [86, 87], and blood coagulation parameters perioperatively and during anesthesia should be done if mast cell degranulation events occur.

In addition to general anesthesia, many triggers have been described for anaphylaxis in patients with Mastocytosis such as iodinated contrast media administration [88], endoscopic procedures [71], manipulation of the gastrointestinal tract during surgery (Escribano, unpublished data), and administration of hydroxyurea (Escribano, unpublished data). Because of the unpredictability of each patient reactivity during anesthesia, diagnostic procedures and surgery, premedication and aggressive treatment of the reactions is recommended in all patients.

## *16.4.5 Treatment of Patients with Mastocytosis Associated to Anaphylaxis*

### 16.4.5.1 General Considerations

Adequate information and training should be given to the patients, their relatives, and care providers and an action plan for the treatment of acute episodes should be in place. Self-administered epinephrine, antihistamines anti-H1 and anti-H2, and corticosteroids should be administered at the time of the acute episode (see Chap. 20). Patients should carry a medi-alert identification bracelet and should avoid triggering factors (Tables 16.3 and 16.4). Patients and healthcare provides are encouraged to contact centers with expertise in the diagnosis and treatment of mastocytosis.

### 16.4.5.2 Anesthesia

Premedication with anti-histamines H1 and H2 and leukotriene receptor blockade with montelukast, 1 h before the procedure is recommended. Adequate sedation prior to surgery is also recommended in order to prevent stress-induced MC-mediator release. A protocol currently used at a large mastocytosis referral center (REMA) includes the use of etomidate, propophol or ketamine, inhalants of the flurane family (sevoflurane) and vecuronium as muscle relaxant, and midazolam. As analgesics, fentanyl, sufentanil, and remifentanil together with NSAIDs can be considered if they have been used before and no adverse reaction has been reported. In a retrospective study by the REMA (Spanish Network on Mastocytosis) referral center in 148 anesthetic procedures (73 general anesthesia, 40 epidural anesthesia, 27 local anesthesia, and 6 with sedation) adverse reactions occurred in 1 patient (flushing) out of 22 cases (4.5%) managed with the above medications and in 14 (2 severe coagulopathy, 2 ardiac arrest, 1 anaphylaxis, 9 generalized erythema and hives, 1 flushing,

**Table 16.4** Treatment of anaphylaxis in mastocytosis (for references, see text)

| |
|---|
| *Strict avoidance of triggers* (see Table 16.2) |
| *Acute life-threatening events* |
| Epinephrine and vasopressors |
| Intravenous fluid resuscitation |
| H1 and H2 antihistamines |
| Corticosteroids |
| *Maintenance in recurrent episodes* |
| Self-administration of epinephrine |
| Scheduled sedating and nonsedating H1 antihistamines + H2 antihistamines |
| Cromolyn sodium |
| Leukotriene antagonists |
| Low doses of corticosteroids (frequent episodes, urticaria, and/or angioedema) |
| Consider doxepin in stress-induced MC-mediator release |
| Consider psychiatric work-up and adequate sedation |
| *Treatment of episodes unresponsive to intensive antimediator therapy* |
| Consider interferon-alpha, hydroxyurea, or cladribine |
| Consider anti-IgE monoclonal antibody |

1 generalized pruritus) out of 126 patients (11%) managed with conventional anesthetic procedures (Matito, Escribano June 2009).

Anesthesia-associated events are less frequent in children with mastocytosis [75], but anxiety may induce irritability, pruritus, and flushing, and premedication is also recommended.

#### 16.4.5.3 Systemic Therapy

Mastocytosis associated with recurrent episodes of cardiovascular collapse during anaphylaxis represents a therapeutic challenge (Table 16.4). To decrease the frequency and intensity of the episodes, avoidance of triggers and antimediator therapy are recommended therapeutic challenge (Table 16.4). Acute or impending episodes of cardiovascular collapse should be treated with epinephrine (see Chap. 20). Preventive treatment includes: (1) combined use of sedating and nonsedating H1 antihistamines which has been shown to be effective in controlling MC mediator-related symptoms [89–92] (reviewed in reference [93]); (2) oral disodium cromolyn (effective at controlling diarrhea, abdominal pain, nausea, and vomiting) [93–96], (3) although aspirin and other NSAIDs may cause MC degranulation, high dose of aspirin has been used in selected patients, to treat flushing associated with elevated prostaglandin levels [97, 98]. Since high doses may lead to gastric irritation, low doses of aspirin have been reported to be effective and to overcome gastric toxicity [99, 100]. Aspirin should be started in a controlled setting with H1 and H2 antihistamine blockers [101, 102]. Other NSAIDs, such as ibuprofen, can be effective and may be better tolerated than aspirin (reviewed in references [24, 27, 34, 61, 103]).

Steroids are effective in cases associated with urticaria and/or angioedema and abdominal cramping with diarrhea unresponsive to sodium cromolyn. Oral budesonide has proved to be effective in eosinophilic ileitis with mastocytosis [104]. Ketotifen has been described to be beneficial in isolated cases with idiopathic anaphylaxis [105].

A psychiatric work-up, psychological support, and specific training in relaxation techniques has been shown to be helpful in a subset of patients with anxiety disorders.

### *16.4.6 Treatment of Refractory Cases*

Life-threatening anaphylactic events unresponsive to antimediator therapy in an acute or chronic basis require chemotherapy treatment.

#### 16.4.6.1 Interferon Alpha

Interferon-alpha has been reported to be effective in controlling clinical symptoms in a percentage of SM patients [106] (reviewed in reference [107]). Low doses Interferon-alpha have been used by the authors in 4 ISM patients and 1 patient with MCL with effective reduction in anaphylactic episodes in 2/4 ISM and 1 MCL [43, 44].

#### 16.4.6.2 Cladribine

Cladribine has been proven to induce response in a subset of SM [108–110] including ISM and ISM associated to clonal lymphoid disorders [109], with a decreased percentage of CD25-expressing MC [109]. Thus, use of cladribine in SM associated to anaphylaxis could also be considered in refractory cases.

#### 16.4.6.3 Omalizumab

Omalizumab, a humanized monoclonal antibody that complexes with free IgE in the serum [111], has been used in the treatment of idiopathic anaphylaxis [112, 113] and VIT-induced anaphylaxis [114–116]. Omalizumab has proven to be effective in the treatment of three patients with mastocytosis, elevated total and specific IgE and recurrent anaphylaxis refractory to intensive antimediator therapy [117]. Downregulation of FCεRI receptors was observed, indicating an increased threshold for degranulation. Omalizumab may be considered in the treatment of Mastocytosis patients with recurrent anaphylaxis and increased serum IgE.

## 16.5 Concluding Remarks

Mast cells from mastocytosis patients present a constitutively altered activation-associated immunophenotype, which is reflected by an increased serum tryptase level and symptoms related to the effect of mediators in tissues. Anaphylaxis is observed in a proportion of SM patients, typically with low MC burden and in the absence of skin lesions (ISMs–). Although the prevalence of IgE-mediated allergic conditions in mastocytosis appears to be similar to that of the general population, there is a predominance of males with Mastocytosis and increased anaphylactic episodes, including hymenopter-venom anaphylaxis (HVA), with no correlation with MC burden or elevated serum tryptase levels. VIT has proved to be effective in mastocytosis, but adverse reactions have been reported in 10–15% of the patients and fatal reactions have been described. Anaphylaxis can occur during general anesthesia, and other invasive or therapeutical procedures, and appropriate management of SM patients before, during, and after these procedures is necessary.

The treatment of anaphylaxis in mastocytosis should include adequate information and training of patients, their relatives and care providers, the availability of individual emergency kits, the avoidance of triggering factors, and the administration of preventive medication prior to anesthesia and other therapeutic procedures. Specific treatment of anaphylaxis should be carefully evaluated in each individual patient. Prompt recognition and appropriate control of the acute episodes and decrease frequency and intensity of chronic symptoms should be attempted with antimediator therapy (e.g., sedating and nonsedating H1 antihistamines and other NSAIDs, oral disodium cromolyn, or, in selected cases, aspirin). Steroids should be used in selected cases. Interferon-alpha, cytoreductive therapy with cladribine, and omalizumab anti-IgE monoclonal antibody therapy might be of benefit in selected refractory cases.

## References

1. Galli SJ, Dvorak AM, Dvorak HF. Basophils and mast cells: morphologic insights into their biology, secretory patterns, and function. *Prog Allergy.* 1984;34:1–141.
2. Fukuoka Y, Xia HZ, Sanchez-Munoz LB, Dellinger AL, Escribano L, Schwartz LB. Generation of anaphylatoxins by human β(beta)-tryptase from C3, C4, and C5. *J Immunol.* 2008;180:6307–6316.
3. Nuñez R, Escribano L, Schernthaner G, et al. Overexpression of complement receptors and related antigens on the surface of bone marrow mast cells in patients with systemic mastocytosis. *Br J Haematol.* 2002;120:257–265.
4. Katz HR, Raizman MB, Gartner CS, Scott HC, Benson AC, Austen KF. Secretory granule mediator release and generation of oxidative metabolites of arachidonic acid via Fc-IgG receptor bridging in mouse mast cells. *J Immunol.* 1991;148:868–871.
5. Lobell RB, Arm JP, Raizman MB, Austen KF, Katz HR. Intracellular degradation of Fc gamma RIII in mouse bone marrow culture-derived progenitor mast cells prevents its surface expression and associated function. *J Biol Chem.* 1993;268:1207–1212.

6. Lobell RB, Austen KF, Katz HR. FcgammaR-mediated endocytosis and expression of cell surface FcgammaRIIb1 and FcgammaRIIb2 by mouse bone marrow culture- derived progenitor mast cells. *J Immunol.* 1994;152:811–818.
7. Woolhiser MR, Brockow K, Metcalfe DD. Activation of human mast cells by aggregated IgG through FcgammaRI: additive effects of C3a. *Clin Immunol.* 2004;110:172–180.
8. Malaviya R, Gao ZM, Thankavel K, Van der Merwe PA, Abraham SN. The mast cell tumor necrosis factor alpha response to FimH-expressing *Escherichia coli* is mediated by the glycosylphosphatidylinositol-anchored molecule CD48. *Proc Natl Acad Sci USA.* 1999;96:8110–8115.
9. Gommerman JL, Oh DY, Zhou XN, et al. A role for CD21/CD35 and CD19 in responses to acute septic peritonitis: a potential mechanism for mast cell activation. *J Immunol.* 2000;165:6915–6921.
10. Supajatura V, Ushio H, Nakao A, Okumura K, Ra C, Ogawa H. Protective roles of mast cells against enterobacterial infection are mediated by Toll-like receptor 4. *J Immunol.* 2001;167:2250–2256.
11. Varadaradjalou S, Féger F, Thieblemont N, et al. Toll-like receptor 2 (TLR2) and TLR4 differentially activate human mast cells. *Eur J Immunol.* 2003;33:899–906.
12. Boyce JA. Mast cells: beyond IgE. *J Allergy Clin Immunol.* 2003;111:24–33.
13. Akin C, Fumo G, Yavuz AS, Lipsky PE, Neckers L, Metcalfe DD. A novel form of mastocytosis associated with a transmembrane c-kit mutation and response to imatinib. *Blood.* 2004;103:3222–3225.
14. Garcia-Montero AC, Jara-Acevedo M, Teodosio C, et al. KIT mutation in mast cells and other bone marrow haematopoietic cell lineages in systemic mast cell disorders. A prospective study of the Spanish Network on Mastocytosis (REMA) in a series of 113 patients. *Blood.* 2006;108:2366–2372.
15. Longley BJ, Reguera MJ, Ma Y. Classes of c-KIT activating mutations: proposed mechanisms of action and implications for disease classification and therapy. *Leuk Res.* 2001;25:571–576.
16. Escribano L, Orfao A, Díaz Agustín B, et al. Human bone marrow mast cells from indolent systemic mast cell disease constitutively express increased amounts of the CD63 protein on their surface. *Cytometry.* 1998;34:223–228.
17. Diaz-Agustin B, Escribano L, Bravo P, et al. The CD69 early activation molecule is overexpressed in human bone marrow mast cells from adults with indolent systemic mast cell disease. *Br J Haematol.* 1999;106:400–405.
18. Escribano L, Orfao A, Diaz-Agustin B, et al. Indolent systemic mast cell disease in adults: immunophenotypic characterization of bone marrow mast cells and its diagnostic implications. *Blood.* 1998;91:2731–2736.
19. Valent P, Horny HP, Escribano L, et al. Diagnostic Criteria and Classification of Mastocytosis: a consensus proposal. *Leuk Res.* 2001;25:603–625.
20. Valent P, Horny HP, Li CY, et al. Mastocytosis (Mast cell disease). In: Jaffe ES, Harris NL, Stein H, Vardiman JW, eds. *World Health Organization (WHO) Classification of Tumours. Pathology & Genetics. Tumours of Haematopoietic and Lymphoid Tissues.* Lyon, France: IARC Press; 2001:291–302.
21. Horny HP, Metcalfe DD, Bennet JM, et al. Mastocytosis. In: Swerdlow SH, Campo E, Harris NL, Jaffe ES, eds. *WHO Classification of Tumours of Haematopoietic and Lymphoid Tissues.* 4th ed. Lyon: IARC; 2008:54–63.
22. Johnson MR, Verstovsek S, Jorgensen JL, et al. Utility of the World Heath Organization classification criteria for the diagnosis of systemic mastocytosis in bone marrow. *Mod Pathol.* 2009;22:50–57.
23. Worobec AS. Treatment of systemic mast cell disorders. *Hematol Oncol Clin North Am.* 2000;14:659–687.
24. Escribano L, Akin C, Castells M, Orfao A, Metcalfe D. Mastocytosis: current concepts in diagnosis and treatment. *Ann Hematol.* 2002;81:677–690.
25. Akin C, Metcalfe DD. Occult bone marrow mastocytosis presenting as recurrent anaphylaxis. *J Allergy Clin Immunol.* 2003;111[2]:S206.
26. Akin C, Scott LM, Kocabas CN, et al. Demonstration of an aberrant mast cell population with clonal markers in a subset of patients with "idiopathic" anaphylaxis. *Blood.* 2007;110:2331–2333.
27. Bonadonna P, Perbellini O, Passalacqua G, et al. Clonal mast cell disorders in patients with systemic reactions to Hymenoptera stings and increased serum tryptase levels. *J Allergy Clin Immunol.* 2009;123:680–686.
28. Metcalfe DD. Classification and diagnosis of mastocytosis: current status. *J Invest Dermatol.* 1991;96:2 S-4 S.
29. Florian S, Krauth MT, Simonitsch-Klupp I, et al. Indolent systemic mastocytosis with elevated serum tryptase, absence of skin lesions, and recurrent severe anaphylactoid episodes. *Int Arch Allergy Immunol.* 2005;136:273–280.
30. Sonneck K, Florian S, Mullauer L, et al. Diagnostic and subdiagnostic accumulation of mast cells in the bone marrow of patients with anaphylaxis: monoclonal mast cell activation syndrome. *Int Arch Allergy Immunol.* 2006;142:158–164.
31. Greenhawt M, Akin C. Mastocytosis and allergy. *Curr Opin Allergy Clin Immunol.* 2007;7:387–392.
32. Brockow K, Akin C, Huber M, Metcalfe DD. Assessment of the extent of cutaneous involvement in children and adults with mastocytosis: relationship to symptomatology, tryptase levels, and bone marrow pathology. *J Am Acad Dermatol.* 2003;48:508–516.

33. Muller U, Helbling A, Hunziker T, et al. Mastocytosis and atopy: a study of 33 patients with urticaria pigmentosa. *Allergy.* 1990;45:597–603.
34. Gonzalez de Olano D, de la Hoz B, Nunez-Lopez R, et al. Prevalence of allergy and anaphylactic symptoms in 210 adult and pediatric patients with mastocytosis in Spain: a study of the Spanish network on mastocytosis (REMA). *Clin Exp Allergy.* 2007;37:1547–1555.
35. Brockow K, Jofer C, Behrendt H, Ring J. Anaphylaxis in patients with mastocytosis: a study on history, clinical features and risk factors in 120 patients. *Allergy.* 2008;63:226–232.
36. La alergia en la práctica clínica diaria del Médico de Asistencia Primaria y en la Farmacia. Patologías alérgicas de mayor alcance social. In: *Programa Zyrterigon-Data 2000, Gabinete estudios sociológicos.* Bernard Krief, UCB Pharma, SEAIC, eds. Madrid: Libro Blanco; 1999.
37. Gaig P, Muñoz-Lejarazu D, Lleonart R, et al. Prevalencia de alergia en la población adulta española. *Alergol Inmunol Clin.* 2004;19:68–74.
38. Dodd NJ, Bond MG. Fatal anaphylaxis in systemic mastocytosis. *J Clin Pathol.* 1979;32:31–34.
39. Muller UR, Haeberli G. The problem of anaphylaxis and mastocytosis. *Curr Allergy Asthma Rep.* 2009;9:64–70.
40. Niedoszytko M, de MJ, Van Doormaal JJ, Jassem E, Oude Elberink JN. Mastocytosis and insect venom allergy: diagnosis, safety and efficacy of venom immunotherapy. *Allergy.* 2009.
41. Kors JW, Van Doormaal JJ, De Monchy JGR. Anaphylactoid shock following Hymenoptera sting as a presenting symptom of systemic mastocytosis. *J Intern Med.* 1993;233:255–258.
42. Koenig M, Morel J, Reynaud J, Varvat C, Cathebras P. An unusual cause of spontaneous bleeding in the intensive care unit – mastocytosis: a case report. *Cases J.* 2008;1:100.
43. Escribano L, Orfao A, Villarrubia J, et al. Expression of lymphoid-associated antigens in mast cells: report of a case of systemic mast cell disease. *Br J Haematol.* 1995;91:941–943.
44. Escribano L, Orfao A, Villarrubia J, et al. Sequential immunophenotypic analysis of mast cells in a case of systemic mast cell disease evolving to a mast cell leukemia. *Cytometry.* 1997;30:98–102.
45. Escribano L, García-Belmonte D, Hernández-González A, et al. Successful management of a case of diffuse cutaneous mastocytosis with recurrent anaphylactoid episodes and hypertension. *J Allergy Clin Immunol.* 2004;113[2]:S335.
46. Bohlke K, Davis RL, DeStefano F, Marcy SM, Braun MM, Thompson RS. Epidemiology of anaphylaxis among children and adolescents enrolled in a health maintenance organization. *J Allergy Clin Immunol.* 2004;113:536–542.
47. Mullins RJ. Anaphylaxis: risk factors for recurrence. *Clin Exp Allergy.* 2003;33:1033–1040.
48. Peng MM, Jick H. A population-based study of the incidence, cause, and severity of anaphylaxis in the United Kingdom. *Arch Intern Med.* 2004;164:317–319.
49. Moneret-Vautrin DA, Morisset M, Flabbee J, Beaudouin E, Kanny G. Epidemiology of life-threatening and lethal anaphylaxis: a review. *Allergy.* 2005;60:443–451.
50. Ring J, Darsow U. Idiopathic anaphylaxis. *Curr Allergy Asthma Rep.* 2002;2:40–45.
51. Sampson HA, Munoz-Furlong A, Campbell RL, et al. Second symposium on the definition and management of anaphylaxis: summary report. Second National Institute of Allergy and Infectious Disease/Food Allergy and Anaphylaxis Network symposium. *J Allergy Clin Immunol.* 2006;117:391–397.
52. Metcalfe DD. Differential diagnosis of the patient with unexplained flushing/anaphylaxis. *Allergy Asthma Proc.* 2000;21:21–24.
53. Muller UR, Horat W, Wuthrich B, Conroy M, Reisman RE. Anaphylaxis after Hymenoptera stings in three patients with urticaria pigmentosa. *J Allergy Clin Immunol.* 1983;72:685–689.
54. Elberink JNGO, De Monchy JGR, Kors JW, Van Doormaal JJ, Dubois AEJ. Fatal anaphylaxis after a yellow jacket sting, despite venom immunotherapy, in two patients with mastocytosis. *J Allergy Clin Immunol.* 1997;99:153–154.
55. Biedermann T, Ruëff F, Sander CA, Przybilla B. Mastocytosis associated with severe wasp sting anaphylaxis detected by elevated serum mast cell tryptase levels. *Br J Dermatol.* 1999;141:1110–1112.
56. Ludolph-Hauser D, Ruëff F, Fries C, Schöpf P, Przybilla B. Constitutively raised serum concentrations of mast-cell tryptase and severe anaphylactic reactions to *Hymenoptera* stings. *Lancet.* 2001;357:361–362.
57. Haeberli G, Brönnimann M, Hunziker T, Müller U. Elevated basal serum tryptase and hymenoptera venom allergy: relation to severity of sting reactions and to safety and efficacy of venom immunotherapy. *Clin Exp Allergy.* 2003;33:1216–1220.
58. Kim DC, Horan R. Anaphylaxis to insect sting associated with urticaria pigmentosa. *Allergy Asthma Proc.* 2003;24:175–178.
59. Wagner N, Fritze D, Przybilla B, Hagedorn M, Rueff F. Fatal Anaphylactic Sting Reaction in a Patient with Mastocytosis. *Int Arch Allergy Immunol.* 2008;146:162–163.
60. Bonadonna P, Zanotti R, Pagani M, et al. How much specific is the association between hymenoptera venom allergy and mastocytosis? *Allergy.* 2009.

61. Gonzalez de Olano D, varez-Twose I, Esteban-Lopez MI, et al. Safety and effectiveness of immunotherapy in patients with indolent systemic mastocytosis presenting with Hymenoptera venom anaphylaxis. *J Allergy Clin Immunol.* 2008;121:519–526.
62. Lockey RF, Turkeltaub PC, Olive ES, Hubbard JM, Baird-Warren IA, Bukantz SC. The Hymenoptera venom study. III: safety of venom immunotherapy. *J Allergy Clin Immunol.* 1990;86:775–780.
63. Cox L, Li JT, Nelson H, Lockey R. Allergen immunotherapy: a practice parameter second update. *J Allergy Clin Immunol.* 2007;120:S25–S85.
64. Fricker M, Helbling A, Schwartz L, Müller U. Hymenoptera sting anaphylaxis and urticaria pigmentosa: clinical findings and results of venom immunotherapy in ten patients. *J Allergy Clin Immunol.* 1997;100:11–15.
65. Engler RJ, Davis WS. Rush Hymenoptera venom immunotherapy: successful treatment in a patient with systemic mast cell disease. *J Allergy Clin Immunol.* 1994;94:556–559.
66. Dubois AE. Mastocytosis and Hymenoptera allergy. *Curr Opin Allergy Clin. Immunol.* 2004;4:291–295.
67. Rueff F, Placzek M, Przybilla B. Mastocytosis and Hymenoptera venom allergy. *Curr Opin Allergy Clin Immunol.* 2006;6:284–288.
68. Scott HW Jr, Parris WC, Sandidge PC, Oates JA, Roberts LJ. Hazards in operative management of patients with systemic mastocytosis. *Ann Surg.* 1983;197:507–514.
69. Smith GB, Gusberg RJ, Jordan RH, Kim B. Histamine levels and cardiovascular responses during splenectomy and splenorenal shunt formation in a patient with systemic mastocytosis. *Anaesthesia.* 1987;42:861–867.
70. Borgeat A, Ruetsch YA. Anesthesia in a patient with malignant systemic mastocytosis using a total intravenous anesthetic technique. *Anesth Analg.* 1998;86:442–444.
71. Schwab D, Raithel M, Ell C, Hahn EG. Severe shock during upper GI endoscopy in a patient with systemic mastocytosis. *Gastrointest Endosc.* 1999;50:264–267.
72. Nelson LP, Savelli-Castillo I. Dental management of a pediatric patient with mastocytosis: a case report. *Pediatr Dent.* 2002;24:343–346.
73. Villeneuve V, Kaufman I, Weeks S, Deschamps A. Anesthetic management of a labouring parturient with urticaria pigmentosa. *Can J Anaesth.* 2006;53:380–384.
74. James PD, Krafchik BR, Johnston AE. Cutaneous mastocytosis in children: anaesthetic considerations. *Can J Anaesth.* 1987;34:522–524.
75. Carter MC, Uzzaman A, Scott LM, Metcalfe DD, Quezado Z. Pediatric mastocytosis: routine anesthetic management for a complex disease. *Anesth Analg.* 2008;107:422–427.
76. Ahmad N, Evans P, Lloyd-Thomas AR. Anesthesia in children with mastocytosis--a case based review. *Paediatr Anaesth.* 2009;19:97–107.
77. Lerno G, Slaats G, Coenen E, Herregods L, Rolly G. Anaesthetic management of systemic mastocytosis. *Br J Anaesth.* 1990;65:254–257.
78. Escribano L, Akin C, Castells M, Schwartz LB. Current options in the treatment of mast cell mediator-related symptoms in mastocytosis. *Inflamm Allergy Drug Targets.* 2006;5:61–77.
79. Dewachter P, Mouton-Faivre C, Cazalaa JB, Carli P, Lortholary O, Hermine O. Mastocytosis and anaesthesia. *Ann Fr Anesth Reanim.* 2009;28:61–73.
80. Konrad FM, Schroeder TH. Anaesthesia in patients with mastocytosis. *Acta Anaesthesiol Scand.* 2009;53:270–271.
81. Desborough JP, Taylor I, Hattersley A, et al. Massive histamine release in a patient with systemic mastocytosis. *Br J Anaesth.* 1990;65:833–836.
82. Vaughan STA, Jones GN. Systemic mastocytosis presenting as profound cardiovascular collapse during anaesthesia. *Anaesthesia.* 1998;53:804–807.
83. Russell WJ, Smith WB. Pseudoanaphylaxis. *Anaesth Intensive Care.* 2006;34:801–803.
84. Tirel O, Chaumont A, Ecoffey C. Circulatory arrest in the course of anesthesia for a child with mastocytosis. *Ann Fr Anesth Reanim.* 2001;20:874–875.
85. Macksey LF, White B. Anesthetic management in a pediatric patient with Noonan syndrome, mastocytosis, and von Willebrand disease: a case report. *AANA J.* 2007;75:261–264.
86. Fisher MM, Baldo BA. Mast cell tryptase in anaesthetic anaphylactoid reactions. *Br J Anaesth.* 1998;80:26–29.
87. Lorenzi P, Filoni M, Manetta G, Bonechi ML, Salvati G, Tanini A. Reazione anafilattica al tiopentale. Un caso documentato dalla positivita della triptasi sierica e del RAST. [Anaphylactic reaction to thiopental. A case documented by tryptase values and RAST]. *Minerva Anestesiol.* 1999;65:659–663.
88. Weingarten TN, Volcheck GW, Sprung J. Anaphylactoid reaction to intravenous contrast in patient with systemic mastocytosis. *Anaesth Intensive Care.* 2009;37:646–649.
89. Fenske NA, Lober CW, Pautler SE. Congenital bullous urticaria pigmentosa. Treatment with concomitant use of H1- and H2-receptor antagonists. *Arch Dermatol.* 1985;121:115–118.

90. Frieri M, Alling DW, Metcalfe DD. Comparison of the therapeutic efficacy of cromolyn sodium with that of combined chlorpheniramine and cimetidine in systemic mastocytosis. Results of a double-blind clinical trial. *Am J Med.* 1985;78:9–14.
91. Gasior-Chrzan B, Falk ES. Systemic mastocytosis treated with histamine $H_1$ and $H_2$ receptor antagonists. *Dermatologica.* 1992;184:149–152.
92. Zhang MQ. Chemistry underlying the cardiotoxicity of antihistamines. *Curr Med Chem.* 1997;4:171–184.
93. Dolovich J, Punthakee ND, MacMillan AB, Osbaldeston GJ. Systemic mastocytosis: control of lifelong diarrhea by ingested disodium cromoglycate. *Can Med Assoc J.* 1974;111:684–685.
94. Soter NA, Austen KF, Wasserman SI. Oral disodium cromoglycate in the treatment of systemic mastocytosis. *N Engl J Med.* 1979;301:465–469.
95. Horan RF, Sheffer AL, Austen KF. Cromolyn sodium in the management of systemic mastocytosis. *J Allergy Clin Immunol.* 1990;85:852–855.
96. Haustein UF, Bedri M. Bullous mastocytosis in a child. *Hautarzt.* 1997;48:127–129.
97. Crawhall JC, Wilkinson RD. Systemic mastocytosis: management of an unusual case with histamine (H1 and H2) antagonist and cyclooxygenase inhibition. *Clin Invest Med.* 1987;10:1–4.
98. Butterfield JH, Kao PC, Klee GG, Yocum MW. Aspirin idiosyncrasy in systemic mast cell disease: a new look at mediator release during aspirin desensitization. *Mayo Clin Proc.* 1995;70:481–487.
99. Butterfield JH, Weiler CR. Prevention of Mast Cell Activation Disorder-Associated Clinical Sequelae of Excessive Prostaglandin D(2) Production. *Int Arch Allergy Immunol. 2008*;147:338–343.
100. Butterfield JH. Survey of aspirin administration in systemic mastocytosis. *Prostaglandins Other Lipid Mediat.* 2009;88:122–124.
101. Metcalfe DD. Clinical advances in mastocytosis: an interdisciplinary roundtable discussion. *J Invest Dermatol.* 1991;96:suppl:1 S-65 S.
102. Austen KF. Systemic mastocytosis. *N Engl J Med.* 1992;326:639–640.
103. Bonadonna P, Zanotti R, Caruso B, et al. Allergen specific immunotherapy is safe and effective in patients with systemic mastocytosis and Hymenoptera allergy. *J Allergy Clin Immunol.* 2008;121:256–257.
104. Lombardi C, Salmi A, Savio A, Passalacqua G. Localized eosinophilic ileitis with mastocytosis successfully treated with oral budesonide. *Allergy.* 2007;62:1343–1345.
105. Patterson R, Fitzsimons EJ, Choy AC, Harris KE. Malignant and corticosteroid-dependent idiopathic anaphylaxis: successful responses to ketotifen. *Ann Allergy Asthma Immunol.* 1997;79:138–144.
106. Kluin-Nelemans HC, Jansen JH, Breukelman H, et al. Response to interferon ALFA-2b in a patient with systemic mastocytosis. *N Engl J Med.* 1992;326:619–623.
107. Hauswirth AW, Simonitsch-Klupp I, Uffmann M, et al. Response to therapy with interferon alpha-2b and prednisolone in aggressive systemic mastocytosis: report of five cases and review of the literature. *Leuk Res.* 2004;28:249–257.
108. Tefferi A, Li CY, Butterfield JH, Hoagland HC. Treatment of systemic mast-cell disease with cladribine. *N Engl J Med.* 2001;344:307–309.
109. Escribano L, Pérez de Oteyza J, Núñez R, Orfao A. Cladribine induces Immunophenotypical changes in Bone marrow mast cells from mastocytosis. Report of a Case of Mastocytosis Associated with a Lymphoplasmacytic Lymphoma. *Leuk Res.* 2002;26:1043–1046.
110. Kluin-Nelemans HC, Oldhoff JM, Van Doormaal JJ, et al. Cladribine therapy for systemic mastocytosis. *Blood.* 2003;102:4270–4276.
111. Milgrom H, Fick RB Jr, Su JQ, et al. Treatment of allergic asthma with monoclonal anti-IgE antibody. rhuMAb-E25 Study Group. *N Engl J Med.* 1999;341:1966–1973.
112. Jones JD, Marney SR Jr, Fahrenholz JM. Idiopathic anaphylaxis successfully treated with omalizumab. *Ann Allergy Asthma Immunol.* 2008;101:550–551.
113. Warrier P, Casale TB. Omalizumab in idiopathic anaphylaxis. *Ann Allergy Asthma Immunol.* 2009;102:257–258.
114. Schulze J, Rose M, Zielen S. Beekeepers anaphylaxis: successful immunotherapy covered by omalizumab. *Allergy.* 2007;62:963–964.
115. Kontou-Fili K, Filis CI. Prolonged high-dose omalizumab is required to control reactions to venom immunotherapy in mastocytosis. *Allergy.* 2009.
116. Galera C, Soohun N, Zankar N, Caimmi S, Gallen C, Demoly P. Severe anaphylaxis to bee venom immunotherapy: efficacy of pretreatment and concurrent treatment with omalizumab. *J Investig Allergol Clin Immunol.* 2009;19:225–229.
117. Carter MC, Robyn JA, Bressler PB, Walker JC, Shapiro GG, Metcalfe DD. Omalizumab for the treatment of unprovoked anaphylaxis in patients with systemic mastocytosis. *J Allergy Clin Immunol.* 2007;119:1550–1551.

# Chapter 17
# Flushing and Urticarial Syndromes Presenting as Anaphylaxis

**Joseph H. Butterfield**

**Abstract** Flushing, urticaria, and angioedema are clinical findings that are commonly associated with anaphylaxis. Flushing can be quite dramatic but is less common in anaphylaxis than are urticaria and angioedema, symptoms that are commonly mentioned together as a single symptom,"urticaria/angioedema." Differentiation of "dry flushing," due to circulating agents acting directly on smooth muscle, from "wet flushing," due to neurogenic triggers from the shared autonomic innervation of blood vessels and sweat glands, can be helpful in sorting out causes of flushing. Flushing may be idiopathic, but may also occur in conditions such as carcinoid syndrome (CS), mastocytosis, mast cell activation disorder (MCAD), pheochromocytoma, medullary carcinoma of the thyroid (MCT), icthyotoxicosis, and other conditions with symptoms that overlap those of anaphylaxis. Chronic urticaria can exist as an independent syndrome that does not commonly have anaphylactic features or signs. However, urticaria can also occur as one of the symptoms of an anaphylactic response. Cholinergic urticaria and cold urticaria are the two physical urticarias that are associated with anaphylaxis.

**Keywords** Flushing • Urticaria • Angioedema • Blush distribution • Anaphylaxis • Carcinoid syndrome • Mastocytosis • Spells • Mast cell activation disorder • Prostaglandin $D_2$ • Pheochromocytoma • Medullary carcinoma of the thyroid • Icthyotoxicosis • Physical urticarias • Cold urticaria • Cholinergic urticaria

## 17.1 Flushing and Urticaria

### *17.1.1 Introduction*

Flushing is a common finding that can occur in many disorders. Flushing can be a cutaneous sign in cases of idiopathic anaphylaxis in children [1], in adults with idiopathic [2, 3] or malignant idiopathic anaphylaxis [4] as well as in non-IgE anaphylaxis responses following oral provocation challenges [5]. However, flushing is not an invariable sign in anaphylaxis, is not listed in grading systems designed to define anaphylaxis severity [6], and in several large series of anaphylaxis cases was found less frequently than was urticaria or angioedema (25% vs 87%) [7], (48% vs 73–74%) [8]. Moreover, among patients with unexplained flushing, a high frequency of psychiatric diagnoses

J.H. Butterfield (✉)
Mayo Clinic, Rochester, MN, USA
e-mail: butterfield.Joseph@mato.edu

M.C. Castells (ed.), *Anaphylaxis and Hypersensitivity Reactions*,
DOI 10.1007/978-1-60327-951-2_17, © Springer Science+Business Media, LLC 2011

including mood and somatization disorders, and psychiatric hyperventilation has been reported [9]. For these reasons, the appearance of flushing cannot be regarded as a sine qua non for anaphylaxis.

The term "urticaria" has been utilized as a descriptive term for a constellation of conditions with wheals and angioedema, for example, idiopathic urticaria, cold-induced urticaria/angioedema, pressure urticaria/angioedema, urticarial vasculitis, and aquagenic urticaria [10, 11]. "Urticaria" is also utilized to indicate one of the component physical findings in cases of anaphylaxis [12] or non-IgE anaphylaxis reactions [5]. Angioedematous swelling occurs in deeper tissues than does urticaria [13]. Angioedema frequently, though not invariably, accompanies urticaria. In descriptions of anaphylaxis symptoms "urticaria" and "angioedema" are often mentioned together in the same phrase as a single symptom. Hence urticaria *or* angioedema is reported as a manifestation of anaphylaxis in 100% of cases in one series of 175 cases [12] and urticaria *and/or* angioedema is reported in 87% of another series of 601 cases [7].

### 17.1.2 Signs, Symptoms, and Pathophysiology of Flushing

Flushing is a symptom consisting of sudden onset of warmth and redness due to vasodilation of the skin. The involved areas include the skin of the face, neck, trunk, and upper limbs [14, 15]. The vasodilation can be due to (1) circulating vasodilator(s) that act on vascular smooth muscle, or (2) can be neurologically mediated. The "blush distribution" is explained in part by greater vascular capacitance in the visible, superficial cutaneous vasculature whether triggered, for example, by ingestion of nicotinic acid, which acts directly on vascular smooth muscle, or by ingestion of hot water, which triggers neural mediated flushing [16]. In addition, the anatomy of the facial cutaneous vasculature including an increased number of capillary loops per square millimeter of cutaneous surface [17], and the thinness of the facial skin, which makes the subpapillary plexus more visible [16, 18], contributes to the visibility of flushing. Chronic recurrent flushing can subsequently result in facial telangiectasia due to development of large cutaneous blood vessels containing slow-flowing deoxygenated blood [14].

Preganglionic sudomotor and vasomotor fibers supplying the eyelids, eyes, forehead, and cheeks leave the spinal cord at and below T1. Postganglionic sympathetic fibers project from the superior cervical ganglion and travel with blood vessels and peripheral cranial nerves to reach their final destinations [15, 19]. Cutaneous blood vessels possess $\beta$(beta)-adrenoceptors that mediate vasodilation, while small resistance vessels contain vasoconstrictor $\alpha$(alpha)$_2$-adrenoceptors [19–21]. The vessels in the areas involved in flushing are predominantly supplied by vasodilator rather than by vasoconstrictor fibers [22]. Because both $\alpha$(alpha)$_2$- and $\beta$(beta)-adrenoceptors lie outside the neuromuscular junction, circulating catecholamines, epinephrine, and norepinephrine, may, depending on the relative densities of the receptor types, either constrict or dilate cutaneous vessels [19, 23].

When triggered by circulating agents that act directly on smooth muscle, flushing is not accompanied by sweating and is termed a "dry flush"; however, when caused by neurogenic triggers, since cutaneous blood vessels and sweat glands share autonomic innervation, flushing can be accompanied by sweating and is termed a "wet flush" [15, 24, 25]. This distinction can be helpful when sorting out causes of flushing.

### 17.1.3 Flushing in Anaphylaxis and Disorders with Non-IgE Anaphylaxis Features

Population-based surveys suggest that anaphylaxis is uncommon, and though it can be a life-threatening event only 10% or so of patients with anaphylaxis symptoms require urgent treatment [2, 26]. Both cutaneous and additional multisystem organ involvement are generally required for a

**Table 17.1** Triggers of anaphylaxis that may be accompanied by flushing, urticaria, angioedema (A/E), or none of these dermatologic signs

| Trigger | Flush | Urticaria | A/E | Reference |
|---|---|---|---|---|
| Psyllium | N | Y | Y | [37, 38] |
| Chamomile-containing enema | N | Y | Y | [39] |
| Chamomile tea | N | N | N | [40] |
| Carboxymethyl cellulose | N | Y | N | [41] |
| Topical thrombin | Y | Y | N | [42] |
| Progesterone | Y | Y | Y | [43, 44] |
| Papain | N | Y | Y | [45] |

diagnosis of anaphylaxis [8, 27]. Among the cutaneous symptoms of anaphylaxis, flushing, urticaria, and angioedema are common both in idiopathic anaphylaxis [2] and anaphylaxis of determined cause [8] but, interestingly flushing is not reported in patients with systemic reactions to hymenoptera field stings [28]. Reports of fatal anaphylaxis among adults [29] and children (fatal food anaphylactic reactions), do not specifically mention flushing, although skin symptoms are mentioned in eight of 13 cases in one series [30].

Flushing is a prominent syndrome in exercise-induced anaphylaxis (EIA), a form of physical allergy precipitated by aerobic physical activities such as jogging, raking leaves, or shoveling snow, in which cutaneous symptoms are prominent [31, 32]. The frequency of flushing in EIA (70%) is nearly equivalent to that of angioedema (72%), but still less than that of urticaria (86%) or pruritus (92%) [32]. Interestingly, flushing was not found in cases of *food-dependent* exercise-induced anaphylaxis, in which disorder food ingestion within 2 h prior to exercise is a requirement of the anaphylaxis episodes [33–36]. Specific reported triggers of anaphylaxis may be accompanied by flushing, urticaria, angioedema (A/E), or none of these dermatologic signs (Table 17.1).

## *17.1.4 Specific Flushing Syndromes with Anaphylaxis Features*

### 17.1.4.1 Carcinoid Syndrome

Flushing is a prominent feature of the carcinoid syndrome (CS) and other symptoms common in this disorder such as diarrhea, abdominal pain, wheezing can suggest anaphylaxis. During "carcinoid crisis," flushing can be associated with a fall in blood pressure, further mimicking severe anaphylaxis. Carcinoid tumors arise from neuroendocrine cells (Kulchitsky cells) that can produce a large number of hormones and biogenic amines including corticotrophin [46], histamine [47], dopamine [48], substance P [49], neurotensin [50], prostaglandins [51], and kallikrein [52]. The contribution of each of these products to the individual manifestations of CS remains unknown.

CS-associated flushing patterns can differ depending on the site of origin of the tumor. For example, bronchial carcinoid tumors produce a prolonged bright red flush that can be accompanied by hypotension, facial edema, lacrimation, and sweating. The flushing from gastric carcinoid tumors has been described as erythematous/reddish brown in color with a geographic pattern involving the head and neck. Compare this pattern to ileal carcinoid flushing that may be more violaceous or darker red, involves the upper part of the body, and blush areas and recurs frequently though briefly throughout the day [53, 54]. Triggers for flushing in CS include foods (walnuts, plums, cheese, avocados, spices, chocolate), alcohol, exercise, and emotional stress associated with increased adrenergic activity [55, 56].

CS occurs in less than 10% of patients who have carcinoid tumors [57]. In order for a carcinoid tumor to cause CS, its secreted vasoactive substances must be able to reach the systemic circulation; hence carcinoid tumors of the intestine causing CS have metastasized to the liver in most cases while bronchial carcinoid tumors because they release their products directly into the systemic circulation, need not have metastasized [58]. The cause of flushing in CS remains unknown in most patients, save for gastric carcinoid tumors, which secrete histamine, and in whom prevention of flushing can be accomplished with H1 and H2 antihistamines [59, 60].

Clinical and laboratory features of CS can serve to differentiate it as a cause of flushing from patients with anaphylaxis: (1) The cardiac features of carcinoid syndrome, which are present in two-thirds of CS patients [61, 62], include plaquelike fibrous thickening with retraction and fixation of leaflets of the tricuspid and pulmonary valves. These cardiac findings do not occur in other disorders with non-IgE anaphylaxis features. (2) Production of serotonin from its precursor 5-hydroxytryptophan and subsequent excretion of the serotonin metabolite 5-hydroxyindoleacetic acid (5-HIAA) is widely used to screen for carcinoid tumors [61]. Although increased by ingestion of bananas, kiwi, plums, avocado, pineapples, walnuts, hickory and pecan nuts, caffeine, melphalan or flurouracil, the measurement of the 24-h excretion of 5-HIAA, the major urinary metabolite of serotonin, will generally reveal levels greater than 25 mg/24 h in CS. The excretion of 5-HIAA is normal in patients with mastocytosis, anaphylaxis, and idiopathic flushing [63]. (3) The diversion of tryptophan to serotonin synthesis plus associated diarrhea can result in nutritional deficiencies including hypoalbuminemia and pellagra [64] in some CS patients. Some of the symptomatic triggers such as flushing following ingestion of large meals can also be a tipoff to the presence of CS [55]. (4) Pentagastrin infusion can also be used as a provocative test to induce flushing and gastrointestinal symptoms in patients with carcinoid tumors with liver metastases or from gastric carcinoid tumors [59, 65]. (5) Phentolamine, an alpha-adrenergic blocking agent will block flushing triggered by intravenous infusion of adrenaline, noradrenaline, or dopamine in CS patients. However, propranolol, a beta-adrenergic blocking agent, does not block spontaneous or adrenaline-induced flushing in CS [66]. (6) The inhibition of CS-associated flushing, diarrhea, and wheezing by somatostatin analogs also serves to distinguish CS flushing syndromes from flushing associated with anaphylaxis, mastocytosis, and pheochromocytoma [57, 67].

#### 17.1.4.2 Systemic Mastocytosis

Mastocytosis Systemic mastocytosis (SM), with an estimated incidence of 0.000667% [68] is a very rare disorder of excessive mast cell proliferation. SM is diagnosed by the presence of the *major criterion* (presence of multifocal infiltrates of >15 mast cells/aggregate in tryptase stained bone marrow or an extracutaneous tissue biopsy) plus one of the *minor criteria:* (1) serum total tryptase of>20 ng/mL; (2) KIT D816V mutation in bone marrow mast cells; (3) KIT (+) bone marrow mast cells show abnormal phenotype with aberrant expression of CD2 and/or CD25; (4) more than 25% of bone marrow or extracutaneous mast cells show abnormal morphology such as spindle shape, hypogranulated cytoplasm, and oval decentralized nucleus. SM can also be diagnosed by the presence of three minor criteria [69]. Mast cells are factories for the production of preformed mediators such as histamine, eosinophil chemotactic factor, heparin, and enzymes (tryptase, chymase, peroxidase, superoxide dismutase, β(beta)-glucuronidase, hexosaminidase, and arylsulfatase). In addition, mast cells produce newly formed products of the cyclooxygenase, lipoxygenase, and leukotriene pathways, as well as chemokines, interleukins, and platelet-activating factor [69–71]. Mast cells are located in vascularized tissues in close relation to blood vessels and nerves, an ideal position to effect rapid delivery of mediators systemically [72, 73]. Because the mast cell release of mediators is of primary importance in anaphylaxis of diverse causes, episodic and constitutive release of mediators in SM patients can be expected to reproduce nearly perfectly the signs and symptoms of anaphylaxis.

Indeed, "spells" with symptoms from the remote or local release of mast cell mediators result in *skin* (flushing, pruritus, urticaria, angioedema), *cardiovascular* (tachycardia, hypotension), *respiratory* (shortness of breath, wheezing), *neurologic* (headache, impaired level of consciousness, sensation of impending doom), and *gastrointestinal* symptoms (abdominal cramps, diarrhea, nausea and vomiting) are one of the commonest presenting complaints of SM patients [74]. Understandably, these symptoms give the outward appearance of idiopathic anaphylaxis and lead initially to investigation for causes of collapse [75, 76].

Flushing in SM is bright red, and commonly affects the blush area. Frequent accompanying symptoms are pruritus or burning and end-organ symptoms of mast cell mediator release: wheezing, abdominal colic, diarrhea, headache, and lacrimation [55]. Flushing in SM, because it is mediated by (1) circulating mediator(s), and is not neurologically mediated, is a "dry flush" not accompanied by sweating.

One of the minor criteria for SM is a serum total tryptase value of greater than 20 ng/mL; however, during anaphylaxis sufficient to cause hypotension tryptase levels will also be elevated in serum [77]. For example, anaphylaxis to insect stings may be a presenting manifestation of SM [78, 79], hence the finding of an elevated serum tryptase value in a sample obtained between 15 and 120 min of the inciting event does *not* distinguish between SM and idiopathic anaphylaxis. Serum tryptase levels have also been used to investigate hypotension during surgery [80], drug reactions [81], and other diverse causes. To circumvent the problem of distinguishing between an elevation of tryptase due to an anaphylactic reaction from that due to SM, a *baseline tryptase* should be obtained no sooner than 24 h after complete subsidence of clinical signs and symptoms [82].

SM can be distinguished from CS and other causes of flushing and anaphylaxis by a combination of clinical and laboratory criteria: (1) The lesions of urticaria pigmentosa are present in over 90% of patients with indolent SM, though in less than 50% of patients with SM with an associated hematologic disorder [83]. These lesions and associated signs of pruritus, dermatographism, and elicitation of Darier's sign are not present in CS or other disorders of flushing with anaphylactic features. (2) Bone marrow biopsy findings in SM should clearly delineate this disorder from CS. The presence of either multifocal dense infiltrates of mast cells or tissue infiltration of mast cells showing >25% with abnormal morphology is seen only in SM. (3) Documentation of mediator release both constitutively and when sampled contemporaneously with symptoms can serve to distinguish several of the flushing disorders with anaphylaxis features: $PGD_2$, which is produced only by mast cells [84, 85], can be a valuable adjunct to distinguish SM from CS, in which $PGD_2$ release does not occur. Conversely, elevation of urinary 5-HIAA is found only in CS and not in SM [86]. (4) Flushing in CS, but not SM can be blocked by the somatostatin analog octreotide [63, 87]. (5) The response to adrenergic agonists and blockers can be used to distinguish SM from CS. Adrenergic agonists such as epinephrine will *inhibit* mast cell degranulation and improve flushing in patients with SM [88]. Conversely, triggers for flushing in CS commonly include emotional stress accompanied by increased adrenergic activity [55, 56]. Alpha-adrenergic blockade will prevent catecholamine-induced flushing in CS [89].

It potentially can be challenging to distinguish the flush of SM from that of gastric carcinoid tumors, which are quite rare. Not only is the appearance of the flush similar, but flushing in both conditions can be associated with excretion of increased levels of urinary histamine metabolites [90, 91]. Flushing from gastric carcinoid tumors often occurs postprandially. Clinically, these patients lack other cutaneous and biochemical characteristics of SM. Gastric carcinoid tumors can be detected by upper endoscopic examination, and are associated with elevated serum levels of chromogranin A [91]. Hence, the alert clinician can utilize both physical and biochemical features of SM to distinguish it from CS and other causes of flushing.

#### 17.1.4.3 Mast Cell Activation Disorder

Mast cell activation disorder (MCAD) can mimic many of the signs and symptoms of SM [92, 93]. In MCAD, episodic and profound release of one or more mast cell mediators occurs in patients who do not meet the criteria for SM. One series reported four MCAD patients who experienced either episodic or continual symptoms suggestive of mast cell mediator release including generalized pruritus, urticaria, flushing, abdominal cramps, diarrhea, pre-syncope, hypotension, and angioedema. Among these four patients, isolated release of $PGD_2$ occurred either constitutively or episodically in parallel with symptom occurrence; however, there was no accompanying increase in histamine excretion. Prevention of symptoms was associated with addition of aspirin to the therapeutic regimen and normalization of $PGD_2$ excretion [93].

#### 17.1.4.4 Pheochromocytomas

Pheochromocytomas most commonly originate from the adrenal medulla and produce, store, and secrete catecholamines. Paroxysmal release of catecholamines results in flushing or pallor, as well as many other symptoms that overlap with those of idiopathic anaphylaxis including breathlessness (67%), headaches (77%), sweating (60%), flushing (56%), palpitations (80%), a sense of apprehension/doom, chest or abdominal pain with nausea and vomiting [22, 63, 94]. Catecholamine stimulation of the predominant cutaneous β(beta)-adrenergic receptors in the face leads to vasodilation and flushing [19–22]. However, in addition to catecholamines, other flushing mediators including calcitonin gene-related peptide, vasoactive intestinal polypeptide, and adrenomedullin are produced by pheochromocytomas [95–98].

The diagnosis of pheochromocytoma entails quantitation of plasma-free metanephrines or urinary fractionated metanephrines [99], as well as imaging of the adrenal glands by CT or MRI scans [100]. Whole body scanning is indicated in cases of extra-adrenal pheochromocytomas. Radionuclear scintiscan with $^{131}$I-metallodibenzylguanidine (MBIG), which is concentrated by the amine uptake process can be especially useful in localizing extra-adrenal tumors [100]. Paroxysmal catecholamine release with hypertension, tachycardia, and flushing have also been described in autonomic epilepsy. Clonidine 0.2–0.4 mg/day suppressed basal catecholamine levels and greatly reduced levels during attacks as well as abolition of flushing in this disorder [101].

The occurrence of paroxysmal or sustained hypertension and general blood pressure lability can be helpful clinical signs to distinguish a patient with flushing due to a pheochromocytoma from a patient with flushing from CS, SM, or idiopathic anaphylaxis, where hypotension is the rule. Catecholamine-induced symptoms are prevented by sequential administration of alpha- and then beta-receptor blockers, and cured by surgical excision of the tumor, which procedure in skilled hands has a low mortality [63]. The improved response to catecholamine *blockade* in pheochromocytoma is also in direct contrast to the improvement in SM flushing when catecholamines such as epinephrine are administered [91].

#### 17.1.4.5 Medullary Carcinoma of the Thyroid

Medullary carcinoma of the thyroid (MCT), which is a malignant tumor of the parafollicular C cells, produces and secretes a large number of biologically active peptides and amines. Prolonged flushing of the face and upper extremities may occur. Measurement of elevated serum calcitonin levels after calcium or pentagastrin infusion, and fine needle aspiration of the thyroid mass are important diagnostic tools if MCT is suspected clinically [102]. Importantly, MCT can occur in the setting of multiple endocrine neoplasia type II (MEN II) syndrome, in which the additional presence of pheochromocytoma, and parathyroid hyperplasia or parathyroid adenoma (MEN IIA) [102, 103] can contribute additional clinical features that can overlap those of idiopathic anaphylaxis, and complicate diagnostic considerations and necessary tests. Treatment for MCT is thyroidectomy as this malignancy has not responded to chemotherapy or to external beam radiotherapy [102]. The presence of pheochromocytoma must also be excluded, and if present should be removed prior to thyroidectomy.

#### 17.1.4.6 Scombrotoxism

Flushing that follows ingestion of fish occurs in the syndrome of scombroid poisoning. In this condition, ingested histamine, produced via the enzyme histidine decarboxylase by bacteria in the eaten fish flesh, results in symptoms mimicking anaphylaxis or food allergy [104]. Both scombroid fish (tuna, mackerel, skipjack, bonito) as well as non-scombroid fish (mahi-mahi, bluefish, amberjack, herring, sardines, anchovies) have been implicated [105, 106] due to the presence in the tissue of large quantities of free histidine that can be decarboxylated to histamine [107]. Approximately 30–60 min after ingestion of spoiled fish flushing, sweating, nausea, vomiting, diarrhea, headache, palpitations, dizziness rash and occasionally swelling of the face and tongue, and rarely respiratory distress occur [104]. This constellation of symptoms closely mimics symptoms of anaphylaxis. Amelioration of symptoms occurs with administration of $H_1$ and $H_2$ receptor antagonists but rarely more aggressive treatment with epinephrine and corticosteroids is necessary [104].

#### 17.1.4.7 Medications

Adverse reactions to medications may be associated with prominent flushing symptoms [63]. In the recent reports of patients reacting adversely to heparin contaminated with oversulfated chondroitin sulfate multiple symptoms of anaphylaxis occurred. In this condition, flushing (23%) was a much more common symptom than was urticaria (3.3%) [108]. Flushing occurs with administration of cancer chemotherapeutic agents which, in the case of doxorubicin therapy can be accompanied by hypotension, hoarseness, palpitations, itching, shortness of breath swollen fingers, throat tightness, facial edema, nasal congestion, pruritus of the eyes and ears [109, 110]. Similarly, alcohol imbibed in combination with certain medications such as chlorpropamide or cephalosporins, or when imbibed alone, especially in people of Asian backgrounds, who may have a deficiency of aldehyde dehydrogenase-2, can cause flushing either directly via its vasodilator effects or via its metabolite, acetaldehyde [24, 111, 112].

## 17.2 Urticarial Syndromes Presenting as Anaphylaxis

### *17.2.1 Introduction*

In nearly every series of anaphylaxis cases reported the frequency of urticaria and/or angioedema invariably exceeds that of flushing as a clinical manifestation [6, 7, 12, 28, 113]. Emphasizing this distinction, Greenberger has divided idiopathic anaphylaxis into (1) those patients with acute severe bronchoconstriction or shock in association with urticaria and diarrhea/abdominal pain and

(2) those patients with severe tongue, pharyngeal, or laryngeal angioedema with or without urticaria. There is no mention of flushing in either subset [2].

### 17.2.2 Anaphylaxis Symptoms Associated with Specific Urticarial Syndromes

Symptoms of anaphylaxis are not common among patients with most types of chronic idiopathic urticaria [114–116]. Likewise, signs and symptoms of urticarial vasculitis are not those of anaphylaxis, but rather include diverse findings of pruritus, pain, burning, angioedema, livedo reticularis, dermatographism, arthralgias, arthritis, hematuria/proteinuria, abdominal or chest pain, COPD, uveitis/episcleritis, pseudotumor cerebri, nausea, vomiting, diarrhea, fever, Raynaud's phenomenon, and cardiac symptoms [117, 118].

### 17.2.3 Physical Urticarias

Physical urticarias are a subgroup of the chronic urticarias in which wheal formation and other symptoms are triggered by one or more physical stimuli such as heat, cold, pressure, vibration, or contact with water [119]. Two of the physical urticarias, however, may present with anaphylaxis.

#### 17.2.3.1 Cholinergic Urticaria

Cholinergic urticaria, which is estimated to occur in 5–7% of urticaria patients [120], is characterized by 2–4 mm pruritic wheals surrounded by bright macular erythema. Activities that increase the body's core temperature, such as exercise, hot showers, pyrexia, or emotional stress trigger attacks of cholinergic urticaria [121, 122]. Following exercise, systemic manifestations of confluent urticaria, angioedema, dizziness, pruritus, hypotension, wheezing, and gastrointestinal complaints (vomiting) have been reported in patients with cholinergic urticaria [123]. These symptoms were accompanied by a spike in the serum histamine levels between 20 and 30 min after exertion. In several respects, these patients' symptoms resembled exercise-induced anaphylaxis because in both conditions symptoms are precipitated after exercise-related release of mast cell mediators.

In other patients with cholinergic urticaria, exercise was followed by transient shortness of breath, wheezing, or both and statistically significant falls in $FEV_1$ and maximal midexpiratory flow (MMEF) rates, specific conductance (SGaw), and a rise in residual volume. These alterations were paralleled by increases in serum histamine concentration and eosinophil and neutrophil chemotactic activities [121]. Among these seven cases [121], three patients had additional forms of physical urticarias (cold-1, dermatographism-1, dermatographism + pressure urticaria-1).

Combined cold- and heat-induced cholinergic urticaria was reported in another patient who developed systemic symptoms after jumping into a heated pool [122]. Therapy includes avoidance of exogenous heat triggers, prompt cooling of affected patients, graded induction of tolerance by increasing stimuli, and possibly antihistamines [11]. In one report, combined $H_1$ and $H_2$ receptor antagonists completely prevented clinical symptoms or clinical response to intentional heat challenge in local heat urticaria [124].

### 17.2.4 Cold Urticaria Syndromes

Cold-induced systemic reactions can occur in acquired cold urticaria syndromes (ACU). ACU are nonfamilial disorders of cold-induced urticaria, angioedema, and occasionally hypotension [125].

Cold-induced systemic reactions after exposure to cold air or cold water among patients with ACU syndromes have been reported for over 70 years [126–129].

Aquatic activities are a leading cause of systemic reactions in this disorder [125] and should be avoided. Cold-induced release of histamine has been demonstrated in cold-induced urticaria both by in vivo cold water challenge with venous sampling of the challenged appendage [130] and by in vitro challenge of skin biopsies taken from patients with cold urticaria [131]. Histamine liberation occurs during rewarming rather than during cooling [131, 132]. In addition to histamine release during systematic reactions, tumor necrosis factor-α has also been detected in the blood of these patients 2 and 6 min after the end of cold immersion [133]. In other reports, cold challenges have released eosinophilic chemotactic factor and neutrophil chemotactic factor [134, 135]. Prevention of hypotension during hypothermic cardiopulmonary bypass was successfully achieved in a patient with ACU by the use of $H_1$ and $H_2$ receptor antagonists, but in the same patient premedication with hydrocortisone 100 mg IM did not prevent histamine release [132]. Although cyproheptadine, an agent with antihistamine and antiserotonin activity, has been the recommended agent for treatment of cold urticaria [136], subsequent studies have shown that sufficient doses of any standard antihistamine should be just as effective [137]. Repeated cold challenges have been reported to be an effective method to induce clinical tolerance in cold urticaria [138].

### *17.2.5 Urticaria and Angioedema in Systemic Reactions to Allergens, Vaccines, and Drugs*

#### 17.2.5.1 Vespids

In Muller's grading system that has been used to evaluate the severity of anaphylactic symptoms after insect stings Grade I symptoms are largely confined to skin manifestations including generalized urticaria/itching/erythema, while angioedema is included under the more severe, Grade 2 symptoms that also include gastrointestinal manifestations [139]. Grade I and Grade II anaphylaxis are each present in approximately 20% of patients reporting reactions to honeybee or yellow jacket stings [28]. These figures give an approximate frequency of urticaria and angioedema among sting-allergic patients.

#### 17.2.5.2 Vaccines

The incidence of anaphylactic reactions to vaccines is very low, less than one case per million vaccine doses [140]. The immunizing agent infrequently is the actual trigger for these responses. Rather, other components of the vaccine such as gelatin or antibiotics are the cause of these reactions especially if the reaction occurs upon the first administration of the vaccine [141]. Many adverse reactions to vaccines are cutaneous hypersensitivity responses that do not prevent subsequent administration of the vaccine [142].

#### 17.2.5.3 Drugs

The list of medications that have been reported to cause urticaria/angioedema is extensive [143]. Parenteral administration of medications is more likely to induce an anaphylactic response than oral or cutaneous routes [144]. Among allergic and anaphylactic responses to medications, reactions to penicillins have been studied most extensively. Patients experiencing allergic responses to penicillin have urticarial responses more often than angioedema [145]. In one series of 112 patients who had reacted a total of 143 times to penicillins (amoxicillin 66, bacampicillin 26, ampicillin 25, piperacillin 17, penicillin G benzathine 4, benzylpenicillin 5), anaphylactic shock was reported 89 times, urticaria 32 times, urticaria and angioedema 21 times, and angioedema once [146]. However, among autopsied cases of fatal anaphylaxis some of which were caused by injections of penicillin, angioedema of the upper airway was an important cause of death [147, 148].

## 17.3 Summary

Flushing is a common clinical symptom but is less frequently found in patients experiencing anaphylaxis syndromes than is urticaria or angioedema. Flushing can occur as a finding in carcinoid syndrome, systemic mastocytosis, pheochromocytoma, medullary carcinoma of the thyroid, scombroid poisoning, and as a component of reactions to certain drugs. Urticaria and angioedema occur more commonly than does flushing in anaphylaxis. Idiopathic clinical syndromes of urticaria and angioedema are generally not associated with anaphylaxis symptoms, nor is urticarial vasculitis. Physical urticarial syndromes with anaphylaxis features are limited to cholinergic urticaria and cold urticaria.

## References


1. Hogan MB, Kelly MA, Wilson NW. Idiopathic anaphylaxis in children. *Ann Allergy Asthma, Immunol.* 1998;81:140–142.
2. Greenberger PA, Idiopathic Anaphylaxis. *Immunol Allergy Clin N Am.* 2007;27:273–293.
3. Wiggins CA, Dykewicz MS, Patterson R. Idiopathic anaphylaxis: classification, evaluation, and treatment of 123 patients. *J Allergy Clin Immunol.* 1988;52:849–855.
4. Patterson R,Wong S, Dykewicz MS, Harris KE. Malignant idiopathic anaphylaxis. *J Allergy Clin Immunol.* 1990;85:86–88.
5. Hermann K, Rittweger R, Ring J. Urinary excretion of angiotensin I, II, arginine vasopressin and oxytocin in patients with anaphylactoid reactions. *Clin Expert Allergy.* 1992;22:845–853.
6. Brown SGA. Clinical features and severity grading of anaphylaxis. *J Allergy Clin Immunol.* 2004;114:371–376.
7. Webb LM, Lieberman P. Anaphylaxis: a review of 601 cases. *Ann Allergy Asthma Immunol.* 2006;97:39–43.
8. Yocum MW, Butterfield JH, Klein JS, Volcheck GW, Schoreder DR, Silverstein MD. Epidemiology of anaphylaxis in Olmsted County: a population-based study. *J Allergy Clin Immunol.* 1999;104:452–456.
9. Friedman BS, Germano P, Miletti J, Metcalfe DD. A clinicopathologic study of ten patients with recurrent unexplained flushing. *J Allergy Clin Immunol.* 1994;83;53–60.
10. Guin JD. Treatment of urticaria. *Med Clin NA.* 1982;66:831–849.
11. Mathews KP. Management of urticaria and angioedema. *J Allergy Clin Immunol.* 1980;66:347–357.
12. Wong S, Dykewicz MS, Patterson R. Idiopathic anaphylaxis. A clinical summary of 175 patients. *Arch Intern Med.* 1990;150:1323–1328.
13. Patterson R, Grammer LC, Greenberger PA, eds. *Allergic Diseases Diagnosis and Management.* 5th ed. Philadelphia, PA: Lippincott Williams & Wilkins; 1997:265–283.
14. Ray D, Williams G. Pathophysiological causes and clinical significance of flushing. *Br J Hosp Med.* 1993;50:594–598.
15. Greaves MW, Burova EP. Flushing: causes, investigation and clinical consequences. *J Euro Acad Dermatol Venereol.* 1997;8:91–100.
16. Wilkin JK. Why is flushing limited to a mostly facial cutaneous distribution? *J Am Acad Dermatol.* 1988;19:309–313.
17. Ryan TJ. Structure, pattern and shape of the blood vessels of the skin. In: Jarrett A, ed. *The Physiology and Pathophysiology of the Skin.* Vol 2. The nerves and blood vessels. New York: Academic; 1973:619.
18. Ryan TJ. Measurement of blood flow and other properties of the vessels of the skin. In: Jarret A, ed. *The Physiology and Pathophysiology of the Skin.* Vol 2. The nerves and blood vessels. New York: Academic; 1973:657.

19. Drummond PD. Sweating and vascular responses in the face: normal regulation and dysfunction in migraine, cluster headache and harlequin syndrome. *Clin Autonomic Res.* 1994;4:273–285.
20. Gustafsson D, Andersson L, Martensson L, Lundvall J. Microsphere analysis of $\beta_2$-adrenergic control of resistance in different vascular areas after hemorrhage. *Acta Physiol Scand.* 1984;121:119–126.
21. Nielson H, Thom SMcG, Hughes AD, Martin GN, Mulvany MJ, Sever PS. Postjunctional $\alpha_2$-adrenoceptors mediate vasoconstriction in human subcutaneous resistance vessels. *Br J Pharmacol.* 1989;97:829–834.
22. Fox RH, Goldsmith P, Kidd DJ. Cutaneous vasomotor control in human head, neck and upper chest. *J Physiol.* 1962;161:298–312.
23. Nielson CP, Vestal RE. In vivo methods for studying adrenergic receptors. In: Insel PA, ed. *Adrenergic Receptors in Man.* New York: Marcel Dekker; 1987:1–35.
24. Mohyi D, Tabassi K, Simon J. Differential diagnosis of hot flashes. *Maturitas.* 1997;27:203–214.
25. Gonzalez G, Onofrio BM, Kerr FWL. Vasodilator system for the face. *J Neurosurg.* 1975;42:696–703.
26. Peng MM, Jick H. A population-based study of the incidence, cause, and severity of anaphylaxis in the United Kingdom. *Arch Intern Med.* 2004;164:317–319.
27. Brown AFT, McKinnon D, Chu K. Emergency department anaphylaxis: a review of 142 patients in a single year. *J Allergy Clin Immunol.* 2001;108:861–866.
28. vanHalteren HK, van der Linden P-WG, Burgers SA, Bartelink AKM. Hymenoptera sting challenge of 348 patients: relation to subsequent field stings. *J Allergy Clin Immunol.* 1996;97:1058–1063.
29. Pumphrey RSH. Lessons for management of anaphylaxis from a study of fatal reactions. *Clin Expert Allergy.* 2000;30:1144–1150.
30. Sampson HA, Mendelson L, Rosen JP. Fatal and near-fatal anaphylactic reactions to food in children and adolescents. *New Engl J Med.* 1992;327:380–384.
31. Castells MC, Horan RF, Sheffer AL. Exercise-induced anaphylaxis. *Current Allergy Asthma Reports.* 2003;3:15–21.
32. Shadick NA, Liang MH, Partridge AJ, et al. The natural history of exercise-induced anaphylaxis: survey results from a 10-year follow-up study. *J Allergy Clin Immunol.* 1999;104:123–127.
33. Kidd JM III, Cohen SH, Sosman AJ, Fink JN. Food-dependent exercise-induced anaphylaxis. *J Allergy Clin Immunol.* 1983;71:407–411.
34. Maulitz RM, Pratt DS, Schocket AL. Exercise-induced anaphylactic reaction to shellfish. *J Allergy Clin Immunol.* 1979;63:433–434.
35. Novey HS, Fairshter RD, Salness K, Simon RA, Curd JG. Postprandial exercise-induced anaphylaxis. *J Allergy Clin Immunol.* 1983;71:498–504.
36. Buchbinder EM, Bloch KJ, Moss J, Guiney TE. Food-dependent, exercise-induced anaphylaxis. *JAMA.* 1983;21:2973–2974.
37. Lantner RR, Espiritu BR, Zumerchik P, Tobin MC. Anaphylaxis following ingestion of a psyllium-containing cereal. *JAMA.* 1990;264:2534–2536.
38. Zaloga GP, Hierlwimmer UR, Engler RJ. Anaphylaxis following psyllium ingestion. *J Allergy Clin Immunol.* 1984;74:79–80.
39. Jensen-Jarolim E, Reider N, Fritsch R, Breiteneder H. Fatal outcome of anaphylaxis to chamomile-containing enema during labor: a case study. *J Allergy Clin Immunol.* 1998;102:1041–1042.
40. Subiza J, Subiza JL, Hinojosa M, Garcia R, Jerez M, Valdivieso R, Subiza E. Anaphylactic reaction after the ingestion of chamomile tea: a study of cross-reactivity with other composite pollens. *J Allergy Clin Immunol.* 1989;84:353–358.
41. Muroi N, Nishibori M, Fujii T, et al. *New Eng J Med.* 1997;337:1275–1277.
42. Tadokoro K, Ohtoshi T, Takajuji S, et al. Topical thrombin-induced IgE-mediated anaphylaxis: RAST analysis and skin test studies. *J Allergy Clin Immunol.*1991;88:620–628.
43. Meggs WJ, Pescovitz OH, Metcalfe D, Loriaux DL, Cutler G, Kaliner M. Progesterone sensitivity as a cause of recurrent anaphylaxis. *New Engl J Med.* 1984;311:1236–1238.
44. Slater JE, Raphael G, Cutler GB Jr, Loriaux DL, Meggs WJ, Kaliner M. Recurrent anaphylaxis in menstruating women: treatment with a luteinizing hormone-releasing hormone agonist – a preliminary report. *Obstetrics Gynecol.* 1987;70:542–546.
45. Freye HB. Papain anaphlaxis: a case report. *Allergy Proc.*1988;9:571–574.
46. Limper AH, Carpenter PC, Scheithauer B, Staats BA. The Cushing syndrome induced by bronchial carcinoid tumors. *Ann Intern Med.* 1992;117:209–214.
47. Pernow B, Waldenstrom J. Determination of 5-hydroxytryptamine, 5-indole acetic acid, and histamine in thirty-three cases of carcinoid tumor (argentafinoma). *Am J Med.* 1957;23:16–25.
48. Feldman J. Increased dopamine production in patients with carcinoid tumors. *Metabolism.* 1985;34:255–260.
49. Skrabanek P, Cannon D, Kirrane J, Powell D. Substance P secretion by carcinoid tumours. *Ir J Med Sci.* 1978;147:47–49.
50. Feldman JM, O'Dorisio TM. Role of neuropeptides and serotonin in the diagnosis of carcinoid tumors. *Am J Med.* 1986;81(Suppl6B):41–48.

51. Sandler M, Karim SM, Williams ED. Prostaglandins in amine-peptide-secreting tumours. *Lancet.* 1968;2:1053–1054.
52. Lucas KJ, Feldman JM. Flushing in the carcinoid syndrome and plasma kallikrein. *Cancer.* 1986;58:2290–2293.
53. Maton PN. The carcinoid syndrome. *JAMA.* 1988;260:1602–1605.
54. Yale SH, Vasudeva S, Mazza JJ, et al. Disorders of flushing. *Compr Ther.* 2005;31:59–71.
55. Greaves MW, Burova EP. Flushing: causes, investigation and clinical consequences. *J Euro Acad Dermatol Venereol.* 1997;8:91–100.
56. Mohyi D, Tabassi K, Simon J. Differential diagnosis of hot flashes. *Maturitas.* 1997;27:203–214.
57. Vinik AI, Thompson N, Eckhauser F, Moattari AR. Clinical features of carcinoid syndrome and the use of somatostatin analogue in its management. *Acta Oncologica.* 1989;28:389–402.
58. Ricci C, Patrassi N, Massa R, Mineo C, Beneditti-Valentini FJ. Carcinoid syndrome in bronchial adenoma. *Am J Surg.* 1973;126:671–677.
59. Roberts LJ II, Bloomgarden ZT, Marney SR Jr, Rabin D, Oates JA. Histamine release from a gastric carcinoid: provocation by pentagastrin and inhibition by somatostatin. *Gastroenterology.* 1983;84:272–275.
60. Roberts LJ II, Marney SR Jr, Oates JA. Blockade of the flush associated with metastatic gastric carcinoid by combined histamine $H_1$ and $H_2$ receptor antagonists. Evidence for an important role of $H_2$ receptors in human vasculature. *New Engl J Med.* 1979;300:236–238.
61. Kulke MH, Mayer RJ. Carcinoid tumors. *New Engl J Med.* 1999;340:858–868.
62. Lundin L, Norheim I, Landelius J, Oberg K, Theodorsson-Norheim E. Carcinoid heart disease: relationship of circulating vasoactive substances to ultrasound-detectable cardiac abnormalities. *Circulation.* 1988;77:264–269.
63. Izikson L, English JC III, Zirwas MJ. The flushing patient: differential diagnosis, workup, and treatment. *J Am Acad Dermatol.* 2006;55:193–208.
64. Swain CP, Tavill AS, Neale G. Studies of tryptophan and albumin metabolism in a patient with carcinoid syndrome, pellagra, and hypoproteinemia. *Gastroenterology.* 1976;74:484–489.
65. Ahlman H, Dahlstrom A, Gronstad K, et al. The pentagastrin test in the diagnosis of the carcinoid syndrome. Blockade of gastrointestinal symptoms by ketanserin. *Ann Surg.* 1985;201:81–86.
66. Adamson AR, Grahame-Smith DG, Peart WS, Starr M. Pharmacological blockade of carcinoid flushing provoked by catecholamines and alcohol. *Lancet.* 1969;ii:293–297.
67. Kvols LK, Moertel CG, O'Connell MJ, Schutt AJ. Rubin J. Hahn RG. Treatment of the malignant carcinoid syndrome: evaluation of a long-acting somatostatin analogue. *New Engl J Med.* 1986;315:663–666.
68. Tharp MD. The spectrum of mastocytosis. *Am J Med Sci.* 1985;289:119–132.
69. Valent P, Horny H-P, Escribano L, et al. Diagnostic criteria and classification of mastocytosis: a consensus proposal. *Leukemia Res.* 2001;25:603–625.
70. Selvan RS, Butterfield JH, Krangel MS. Expression of multiple chemokine genes by a human mast cell leukemia. *J Biol Chem.* 1994;269:13893–13898.
71. Valent P, Akin C, Sperr WR, et al. Diagnosis and treatment of systemic mastocytosis: state of the art. *Br J Haematol.* 2003;122:695–717.
72. Galli SJ. New insights into "the riddle of the mast cells": microenvironmental regulation of mast cell development and phenotypic heterogenicity. *Lab Invest.* 1990;62:5–33.
73. Valent P, Sillaber C, Bettelheim P. The growth and differentiation of mast cells. *Prog Growth Factor Res.* 1991;3:27–41.
74. Castells M, Austen KF. Mastocytosis: mediator-related signs and symptoms. *Int Arch Allergy Immunol.* 2002;127:147–152.
75. Valabhji J, Robinson S, Johnson D, Bellamy M, Davies W, Bain B J . Unexplained loss of consciousness: systemic mastocytosis. *J R Soc Med.* 2000;93:141–142.
76. Dodd NJ, Bond MG. Fatal anaphylaxis in systemic mastocytosis. *J Clin Pathol.* 1979;32:31–34.
77. Schwartz LB, Metcalfe DD, Miller JS, Earl H, Sullivan T. Tryptase levels as an indicator of mast-cell activation in systemic anaphylaxis and mastocytosis. *New Engl J Med.* 1987;316:1622–1626.
78. Kors JW, van Doormaal JJ, deMonchy JGR. Anaphylactoid shock following hymenoptera sting as a presenting symptom of systemic mastocytosis. *J Intern Med.* 1993;233:255–258.
79. Fricker M, Helbling A, Schwartz L, Muller U. Hymenoptera sting anapylaxis and urticaria pigmentosa: clinical findings and results of venom immunotherapy in ten patients. *J Allergy Clin Immunol.* 1997;100:11–15.
80. Freiler JF, Steel KE, Hagan LL, Rathkopf MM, Roman-Gonzalez, J. Intraoperative anaphylaxis to bacitracin during pacemaker change and laser lead extraction. *Ann Allergy Asthma Immunol.* 2005;95:389–393.
81. Saito R, Moroi S, Okuno H, Ogawa O. Anaphylaxis following administration of intravenous methylprednisolone sodium succinate in a renal transplant recipient. *Int J Urol.* 2004;11:171–174.
82. Schwartz LB. Diagnostic value of tryptase in anaphylaxis and mastocytosis. *Immunol Allergy Clin NA.* 2006;26:451–463.
83. Soter NA. Mastocytosis and the skin. *Hematol/Oncol Clin NA.* 2000;14:537–555.

84. van der Donk EM, Blok W, Kok PT, Bruijnzeel PL. Leukotriene C4 formation by enriched human basophil preparations from normal and asthmatic subjects. *Prostaglandins Leukot Essent Fatty Acids.* 1991; 44(1):11–17.
85. Lewis RA, Soter NA, Diamond PT, Austen KF, Oates JA, Roberts LJ II. Prostaglandin $D_2$ generation after activation of rat and human mast cells with anti-IgE. *J Immunol.* 1982;129(4):1627–1631.
86. Butterfield JH. Systemic mastocytosis: clinical manifestations and differential diagnosis. *Immunol Allergy Clin NA.* 2006; 6:487–513.
87. Ray D, Williams G. Pathophysiological causes and clinical significance of flushing. *Br J Hosp Med.* 1993;50:594–598.
88. Turk J, Oates JA, Roberts LJ II. Intervention with epinephrine in hypotension associated with mastocytosis. *J Allergy Clin Immunol.* 1983;71:189–192.
89. Adamson AR, Peart WS, Grahame-Smith DG, Starr M. Pharmacological blockade of carcinoid flushing provoked by catecholamines and alcohol. *Lancet.*1969;ii:295–296.
90. Mallet AI, Norris P, Rendell NB, Wong E. Greaves MW. The effect of disodium cromoglycate and ketotifen on the excretion of histamine and N tau-methylimidazole acetic acid in urine of patients with mastocytosis. *Br J Clin Pharmacol.* 1989;27:88–91.
91. Bashir S, Gibril F, Ojeaburu JV, et al. Prospective study of the ability of histamine, serotonin or serum chromgranian A levels to identify gastric carcinoids in patients with gastrinomas. *Aliment Pharmacol Ther.* 2002;16:1367–1382.
92. Roberts LJ II. Carcinoid syndrome and disorders of systemic mast-cell activation including systemic mastocytosis. *Endocrinol Metabol Clin NA.* 1988;17:415–436.
93. Butterfield JH, Weiler CR. Prevention of mast cell activation disorder-associated clinical sequelae of excessive prostaglandin $D_2$ production. *Int Arch Allergy Immunol.* 2008;47:338–343.
94. Sharma N, Kumari S, Jain S, Varma S. Pheochromocytoma: a 10-year experience in a tertiary care North Indian Hospital. *Indian Heart J.* 2001;53:481–485.
95. Herrera MF, Stone E, Deitel M, Asa SL. Pheochromocytoma producing multiple vasoactive peptides. *Arch Surg.* 1992;127:105–108.
96. Smith SL, Slappy AL, Fox TP, Scolapio JS. Pheochromocytoma producing vasoactive intestinal peptide. *Mayo Clin Proc.* 2002;77:97–100.
97. Mouri T, Takahashi K, Sone M, et al. Calcitonin gene-related peptide-like immunoreactivities in pheochromocytomas. *Peptides.* 1989;10:210–214.
98. Letizia C, Rossi G, Cerci S. Adrenomedullin and endocrine disorders. *Panminerva Med.* 2003;45:241–251.
99. Lenders JW, Pacak K, Eisenhofer G. New advances in the biochemical diagnosis of pheochromocytoma: moving beyond catecholamines. *Ann N Y Acad Sci.* 2002;970:29–40.
100. Pacak K, Linehan WM, Eisenhofer G, Walther MM, Goldstein DS. Recent advances in genetics, diagnosis, localization, and treatment of pheochromocytoma. *Ann Intern Med.* 2001;134:315–329.
101. Metz SA, Halter JB, Porte D Jr, Robertson RP. Autonomic epilepsy: clonidine blockade of paroxysmal catecholamine release and flushing. *Ann Intern Med.* 1978;88:189–193.
102. Wells SA Jr, Franz C. Medullary carcinoma of the thyroid gland. *World J Surg.* 2000;24:952–956.
103. Bravo EL, Gifford RW Jr. Pheochromocytoma: diagnosis, localization and management. *New Engl J Med.* 1984;311:1289–1303.
104. Morrow JD, Margolies GR, Rowland J, Roberts LJ II. Evidence that histamine is the causative toxin of scomroid-fish poisoning. *New Engl J Med.* 1991;324;716–720.
105. Hughes JM, Merson MH. Fish and shellfish poisoning. *New Engl J Med.* 1976;295:1117–1129.
106. Taylor SL, Stratton JE, Nordlee JA. Histamine poisoning (scombroid fish poisoning): an allergy-like intoxication. *J Toxicol Clin Toxicol.* 1989;27:225–240.
107. Taylor SL. Histamine food poisoning: toxicology and clinical aspects. *CRC Crit Rev Toxicol.* 1986;17:91–128.
108. Blossom DB, Kallen AJ, Patel PR, et al. Outbreak of adverse reactions associated with contaminated heparin. *New Engl J Med.* 2008;359:2674–2684.
109. Wilkin JK. Flushing reactions in the cancer chemotherapy patient. *Arch Dermatol.* 1992;128:1387–1389.
110. Curran CF. Doxoubicin-associated facial flushing. *Arch Dermatol.* 1992;128:1408.
111. Pontiroli AE, DePasqua A, Colombo R, Ricordi C, Pozza G. Characterization of the chlorpropamide-alcohol-flush in patients with type 1 and type-2 diabetes. *Acta Diabetalogica Latina.* 1983;20:117–123.
112. Sticherling M, Brasch J. Alcohol: intolerance syndromes urticarial and anaphylactoid reactions. *Clin Dermatol.* 1999;17:417–422.
113. Ditto AM, Krasnick J, Greenberger PA, Kelly KJ, McGrath K, Patterson R. Pediatric idiopathic anaphylaxis: Experience with 22 patients. *J Allergy Clin Immunol.* 1997;100:320–326.
114. Poon E, Seed PT, Greaves MW, Kobza-Black A. The extent and nature of disability in different urticarial conditions. *Br J Dermatol.* 1999;140:667–671.
115. Greaves M. Chronic urticaria. *J Allergy Clin Immunol.* 2000;105:664–672.
116. Paul E, Greilich KD, Dominante G. Epidemiology of urticaria. *Monogr Allergy.* 1987;21:87–115.
117. Aboobaker J, Greaves MW. Urticarial vasculitis. *Clin Expert Dermatol.* 1986;11:436–444.

118. Sanchez NP, Winkelmann RK, Schroeter AL, Dicken CH. The clinical and histopathologic spectrums of urticarial vasculitis: study of forty cases. *J Am Acad Dermatol.* 1982;7:599–605.
119. Casale TB, Sampson HA, Hanifin J, et al. Guide to physical urticarias. *J Allergy Clin Immunol.* 1988;82:758–763.
120. Champion RH, Roberts SOB, Carpenter RG, Roger JH. Urticaria and angio-oedema: a review of 554 patients. *Br J Dermatol.* 1969;81:588–597.
121. Soter NA, Wasserman SI, Austen KF, McFadden ER Jr. Release of mast-cell mediators and alterations in lung function in patients with cholinergic urticaria. *New Engl J Med.* 1980;302:604–608.
122. Farnam J, Grant JA, Lett-Brown MA, Lord RA, Russell WL, Henry DP. Combined cold-and heat-induced cholinergic urticaria. *J Allergy Clin Immunol.* 1986;78:353–357.
123. Kaplan AP, Natbony SF, Tawil AP, Fruchter L, Foster M. Exercise-induced anaphylaxis as a manifestation of cholinergic urticaria. *J Allergy Clin Immunol.* 1981;68:319–324.
124. Irwin RB, Lieberman P, Friedman MM, et al. Mediator release in local heat urticaria: protection with combined H1 and H2 antagonists. *J Allergy Clin Immunol.* 1985;76:35–44.
125. Wanderer AA, Grandel KE, Wasserman SI, Farr RS. Clinical characteristics of cold-induced systemic reactions in acquired cold urticaria syndromes: recommendations for prevention of this complication and a proposal for a diagnostic classification of cold urticaria. *J Allergy Clin Immunol.* 1986;78:417–422.
126. Horton BT, Brown GE, Roth GM. Hypersensitiveness to cold with local and systemic manifestations of a histamine-like character: its amenability to treatment. *JAMA.* 1936;107:1263–1269.
127. Sigal C, Mitchell JC. Essential cold urticaria: a potential cause of death while swimming. *Can Med Assoc J.* 1964;91:609–611.
128. McGovern JP. An unusual case of hypersensitivity to cold complicated by paroxysmal diarrhea. *J Allergy.* 1948;19:408–410.
129. Juhlin L, Shelley WB. Role of mast cell and basophil in cold urticaria with associated systemic reactions. *JAMA.* 1961;177:371–377.
130. Kaplan AP, Gray L, Shaff RE, Horakova Z, Beaven MA. In vivo studies of mediator release in cold urticaria and cholinergic urticaria. *J Allergy Clin Immunol.* 1975;55:394–402.
131. Kaplan AP, Garofalo J, Sigler R, Hauber T. Idiopathic cold urticaria: in vitro demonstration of histamine release upon challenge of skin biopsies. *New Engl J Med.* 1981;305:1074–1078.
132. Johnston WE, Moss J, Philbin DM, et al. Management of cold urticaria during hypothermic cardiopulmonary bypass. *New Engl J Med.* 1982;306:219–221.
133. Tillie-Leblond I, Gosset P, Janin A, et al. Tumor necrosis factor-α release during systemic reaction in cold urticaria. *J Allergy Clin Immunol.* 1994;93:501–509.
134. Soter NA, Wasserman SI, Austen KF. Cold urticaria release into the circulation of histamine and eosinophil chemotactic factor of anaphylaxis during cold challenge. *New Engl J Med.* 1976;294:687–690.
135. Wasserman SE, Soter NA, Center DM, Austen KF. Cold urticaria recognition and characterization of a neutrophil chemotactic factor which appears in serum during experimental cold challenge. *J Clin Invest.* 1977;60:189–196.
136. Wanderer AA, St Pierre JP, Ellis EF. Primary acquired cold urticaria and double blind comparative study of treatment with cyproheptadine, chlorpheniramine, and placebo. *Arch Dermatol.* 1977;113:1375–1377.
137. Sigler RW, Evans R III, Horakova Z, Ottesen E, Kaplan AP. The role of cyproheptadine in the treatment of cold urticaria. *J Allergy Clin Immunol.* 1980;65:309–312.
138. Keahey TM, Indrisano J, Kaliner MA. A case study on the induction of clinical tolerance in cold urticaria. *J Allergy Clin Immunol.* 1988;82:256–261.
139. Muller HL. Diagnosis and treatment of insect sensitivity. *J Asthma Res.* 1966;3:331–333.
140. Nokleby H. Vaccination and Anaphylaxis. *Curr Allergy Asthma Rep.* 2006;6:9–16.
141. Nakayama T, Aizawa C, Kuno-Sakai H. A clinical analysis of gelatin allergy and a determination of its causal relationship to the previous administration of a gelatin-containing acellular pertussis vaccine combined with diphtheria and tetanus toxoids. *J Allergy Clin Immunol.* 1999;103:321–325.
142. Heidary N, Cohen DE. Hypersensitivity reactions to vaccine components. *Dermatitis.* 2005;16:115–120.
143. Mathelier-Fusade P. Drug-induced urticarias. *Clin Rev Allergy Immunol.* 2006;30:19–24.
144. Macy E. Drug allergies: what to expect, what to do. *J Respir Dis.* 2006;27:463–471.
145. Greenberger PA. Anaphylactic and anaphylactoid causes of angioedema. *Immunol Allergy Clin NA.* 2006;26:753–767.
146. Romano A, Viola M, Gueant-Rodriquez R-M, Gaeta F, Pettinato R, Gueant J-L. Imipenem in patients with immediate hypersensitivity to penicillins. *N Engl J Med.* 2006;354:2835–2837.
147. Delage C, Irey NS. Anaphylactic deaths: a clinicopathologic study of 43 cases. *J Forensic Sci.* 1972;17:525–540.
148. James LP, Austen KF. Fatal systemic anaphylaxis in man. *N Engl J Med.* 1964;270:597–603.

# Chapter 18
# Pharmacologic Management of Acute Anaphylaxis

**David I. Bernstein**

**Abstract** Prompt recognition and treatment of anaphylaxis are essential to assuring favorable clinical outcomes. Anaphylaxis has been defined as a serious allergic reaction that is rapid in onset and may cause death and is characterized by acute respiratory compromise and/or profound hypotension after injection or ingestion of an allergen. Once recognized, epinephrine is the treatment of choice and must be administered immediately, preferably via the intramuscular (IM) route in the anterolateral thigh and repeated every 5 min until clinical improvement. Other key measures include calling the emergency response team for assistance (i.e., 911); placing hypotensive patients in the supine position to improve cardiac output; maintenance of the airway; high flow oxygen; obtaining intravenous access; fluid resuscitation with crystalloid (i.e., normal saline) in the absence of a favorable response to IM epinephrine; and failing a response to all aforementioned interventions including IM epinephrine, intravenous administration of epinephrine, or a vasopressor agent (e.g., vasopressin). Glucocorticoids and antihistamines are generally recommended but considered secondary ancillary drugs. Following recovery, patients must be educated on future avoidance of causative agents and trained on self-administration of epinephrine with an auto-injector device, for future anaphylactic events after unforeseen allergen exposure.

**Keywords** Epinephrine • Anaphylaxis • Hypotension • Histamine • Vasopressin • Guidelines • Intravenous • Intramuscular • Fluids • Resuscitation

## 18.1 General Approach: Recognition of Anaphylaxis and Pharmacologic Management

Prompt recognition and timely administration of emergency drugs are essential for assuring favorable clinical outcomes in patients presenting with acute anaphylaxis. An algorithmic approach to management of acute anaphylaxis is shown in Fig. 18.1. Because clinical signs and symptoms vary from patient to patient, anaphylaxis can be difficult to differentiate from other conditions including vasovagal reactions, episodic vocal cord dysfunction, or panic attacks. In a recent 2006 NIAID sponsored symposium, an expert panel has defined anaphylaxis as "a serious allergic reaction that is rapid in onset and may cause death" [1]. Although simplistic, this operational definition is intended to facilitate rapid recognition and treatment by emergency responders and physicians. To further assist in rapid clinical assessment, the 2006 NIAID panel recommended three broadly

D.I. Bernstein (✉)
University of Cincinnati College of Medicine, Cincinnati, OH, USA
e-mail: bernstdd@ucmail.uc.edu

M.C. Castells (ed.), *Anaphylaxis and Hypersensitivity Reactions*,
DOI 10.1007/978-1-60327-951-2_18, © Springer Science+Business Media, LLC 2011

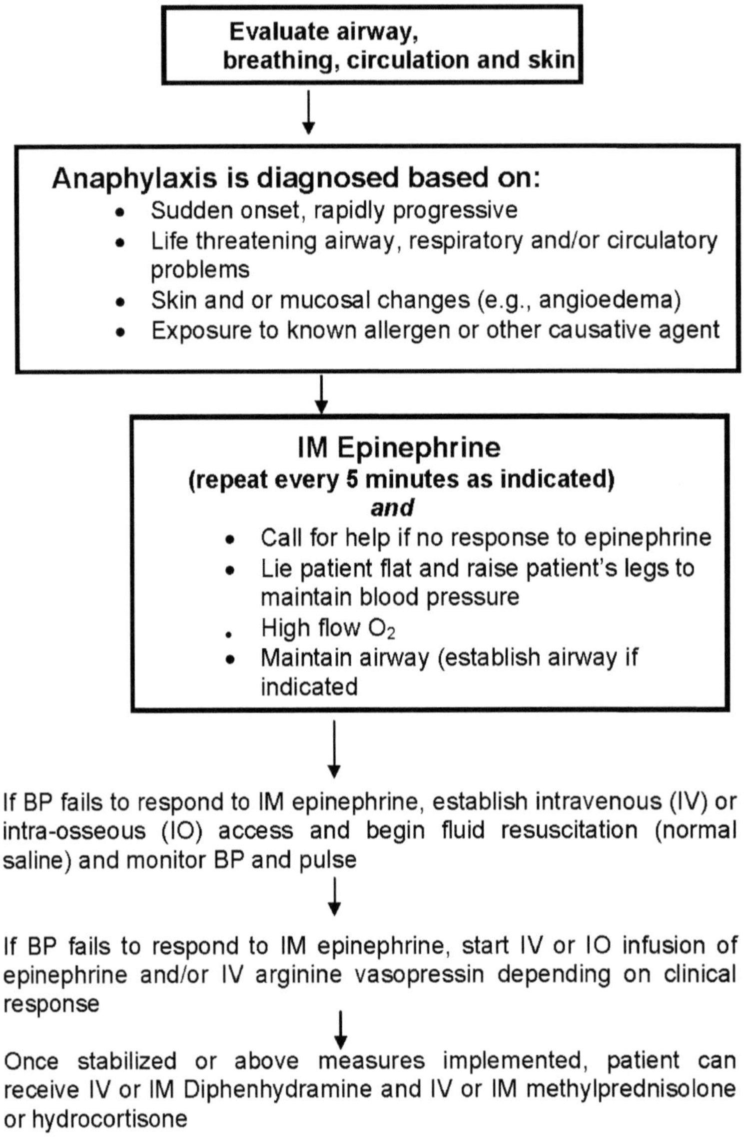


**Fig. 18.1** Algorithm for emergency treatment of anaphylaxis (Adapted from [2, 6])

defined criteria to diagnose acute anaphylaxis. The diagnosis is established by meeting ≥1 of the following criteria [1]:

1. Acute onset of skin eruptions or mucosal swelling combined with respiratory compromise and/or reduced blood pressure (BP) and symptoms associated with hypotension including syncope.
2. After exposure to a known allergen, rapid onset of ≥2 of the following: skin-mucosal manifestations, respiratory compromise, reduced blood pressure and symptoms associated with hypotension, and persistent gastrointestinal symptoms.
3. After exposure to a known allergen, rapid development of hypotension.

In a recently published guideline, Soar et al. suggest the following clinical criteria likely to correctly identify nearly all patients with an anaphylactic reaction [2]:

1. Sudden onset and rapid progression of symptoms (usually within minutes but rarely reactions may be slower in onset).
2. Life-threatening airway and/or breathing and/or circulatory problems.
3. Skin and/or mucosal changes (flushing, urticaria, angioedema).
4. Preceding exposure to a known allergen.

The aforementioned guideline emphasizes that skin or mucosal changes alone are not adequate to establish a diagnosis of anaphylaxis, that skin changes are absent in up to 20% of anaphylactic reactions, and that gastrointestinal symptoms (e.g., nausea, vomiting) can also be accompanying manifestations of anaphylaxis. It is likely that most cases of anaphylaxis can be identified using the aforementioned sets of clinical criteria. However, these criteria are based on expert opinion and have not been clinically validated [1, 2].

In evaluating suspected anaphylaxis, physicians are trained to immediately assess upper and lower airway status as well as the cardiac and hemodynamic condition of the patient. Once anaphylaxis is recognized, epinephrine is the treatment of choice and must be administered immediately, via the intramuscular (IM) route in the anterolateral thigh [3, 4]. In addition to epinephrine, other important interventions include [3]:

1. Call for emergency assistance (i.e., 911) in the absence of immediate response to IM epinephrine.
2. Position patients who are pre-syncopal, hypotensive, or syncopal in a supine position with both lower extremities elevated to increase venous return and optimize cardiac output. Allowing such patients to sit or stand can precipitate cardiac arrest [5].
3. Begin high flow oxygen (≥10 L/min) delivered via a non-rebreathing mask.
4. Maintain the airway. However, intubation should only be attempted by trained, experienced personnel.
5. In patients with persistent hypotension despite IM epinephrine treatment, obtain intravenous or intraosseus (IO) access and infuse high volumes of crystalloid fluids (i.e., normal saline).
6. If there is no reversal of hypotension after IM epinephrine and fluid challenge with normal saline, start an IV or IO infusion with a vasopressor including epinephrine, vasopressin, or dopamine at recommended doses.
7. In the event of cardiopulmonary arrest, institute resuscitative treatment as per current guidelines.

In this chapter, the pharmacologic modalities used in treatment of acute anaphylaxis will be discussed in detail in the following sequential order and according to their level of importance: (1) epinephrine; (2) oxygen; (3) intravenous fluids; (4) antihistamines; (5) corticosteroids; (6) other drugs sometimes required for patients not responding completely to epinephrine including bronchodilators, vasopressors, and glucagon; and (7) drugs recommended during cardiac arrest [6].

## 18.2 Pharmacologic Management

### *18.2.1 Epinephrine*

Epinephrine is the drug of choice and the most important agent in treating life-threatening anaphylaxis. There is evidence that epinephrine is underutilized and under-dosed in treating anaphylaxis [7]. Timely administration of epinephrine must be prioritized over all other therapeutic interventions in the management of acute anaphylaxis [2, 3]. Although there are no controlled clinical trials supporting its use in anaphylaxis, there is ample anecdotal experience demonstrating its efficacy [2]. Epinephrine is an ideal drug for treating IgE-mediated anaphylaxis due to its multiple physiologic effects including: (1) direct stimulation of alpha-adrenergic receptors resulting in peripheral vasoconstriction, reversal of hypotension, and reduction in peripheral edema; (2) stimulation of β(beta)$_2$ receptors leading to bronchodilation and inhibition of mast cell mediator release including histamine; and (3) stimulation of β(beta)$_1$ receptors thereby increasing heart rate and exerting a positive inotropic effect.

#### 18.2.1.1 Indications and Toxicity

There is consensus that all patients with life-threatening anaphylaxis should receive epinephrine [2, 3]. There is disagreement as to whether patients experiencing mild systemic allergic reactions manifested by cutaneous manifestations only (e.g., pruritus, urticaria) should receive epinephrine. An argument supporting early administration of epinephrine is the observation that cutaneous manifestations are the first features of 80% of anaphylactic reactions combined with the knowledge that early initiation of epinephrine enhances the probability of surviving [8, 9]. However, a recent guideline published by a European panel of experts recommends withholding epinephrine for cutaneous reactions until signs and symptoms of severe anaphylaxis are observed [2]. In contrast, the Joint Task Force (JTF) that published the Anaphylaxis Practice Parameter in the USA emphasized that although initial skin manifestations are not life threatening, these often progress rapidly to full-blown anaphylaxis unless treated promptly with epinephrine. With regard to the notion that treatment decisions should be individualized for each clinical scenario, the anaphylaxis parameters appropriately recognized that "treatment recommendations are subject to physician discretion and variations in sequence and performance rely on physician judgment" [3].

There are no contraindications for the use of epinephrine in the treatment of anaphylaxis [6]. Nonserious and expected adverse effects of epinephrine include tachycardia, palpitations, nausea/vomiting, pallor, tremor, dizziness, headache and anxiety; concern over these should never contraindicate its use in life-threatening anaphylaxis [6]. Physician reluctance to give epinephrine can be related to concern over rare but serious adverse cardiovascular effects (e.g., myocardial infarction, coronary spasm, and arrhythmias) associated with parenteral epinephrine especially in patients with preexisting cardiac disease. However, the risks of uncommon serious adverse reactions to epinephrine must be weighed against predictable clinical manifestations of life-threatening anaphylactic reactions likely to result from withholding epinephrine. Ironically, in patients with underlying ischemic heart disease, untreated anaphylaxis can be complicated by myocardial infarction and arrhythmias [8, 10]. On the other hand, two cases of myocardial infarction have been described after administration of very high cumulative doses of epinephrine (≥1 mg) to patients with underlying coronary disease incorrectly treated for non-anaphylactic reactions [8].

Ancillary treatments including H1 blockers, inhaled beta agonists, and systemic corticosteroids are ineffective in modifying life-threatening manifestations of severe airway obstruction and hypotension. Therefore, ancillary drugs must never be considered as primary treatment alternatives to epinephrine. Failure to give epinephrine in a timely fashion can enhance risk of fatal outcomes in patients with food-induced anaphylaxis and life-threatening allergic reactions to allergen immunotherapy injections [9, 11]. Delay or omission of epinephrine may result from failure to accurately recognize or diagnose anaphylaxis, underestimation of the severity of the reaction based on early mild clinical manifestations, and failure of a patient to carry or doctor to prescribe self-injectable epinephrine [12]. After each epinephrine injection, patients should be monitored via observation, auscultation of the airways, blood pressure, pulse as well as ECG and pulse oxymetry (if available) for therapeutic response.

#### 18.2.1.2 Route of Administration of Epinephrine

Epinephrine is best administered via the intramuscular route into the vastus lateralis muscle via the anterolateral middle third of the thigh [4]. This recommendation is based on a six-way crossover study comparing intramuscular versus subcutaneous injection of epinephrine in adult males. In this study, significantly higher plasma epinephrine levels were achieved after intramuscular (IM) injection of 0.3 mg into the anterolateral thigh via an epinephrine auto-injector device (Epipen) versus the same dose given IM or subcutaneously into the upper arm [13]. A parallel study was conducted in children with histories of food-induced anaphylaxis, comparing maximum plasma concentrations achieved after 0.3 mg IM versus subcutaneous injections of epinephrine. Although mean maximum doses achieved for the two routes were similar, the mean time to achieve maximum plasma levels was significantly more rapid via the IM route (8 min) compared with the subcutaneous route (34 min) [14]. No pharmacologic studies have been conducted in adult or pediatric patients during anaphylaxis demonstrating clinical superiority of the IM route of administration. However, given that such investigations are unlikely to be performed, it is reasonable to follow recommendations regarding IM administration based on the pharmacologic studies performed in asymptomatic volunteer subjects [13].

Because of short needle length, there is concern over the ability of commercial epinephrine auto-injector devices to reliably deliver intramuscular doses of epinephrine. A recent study in children suggests that the depth of subcutaneous tissue exceeds the 0.5 in. needle length of auto-injector devices required to reach the vastus lateralis muscle in as many as 30% of children weighing≥30 kg [15]. There is also concern raised in women in who subcutaneous tissue commonly exceeds the extended needle length of the most commonly used auto-injector device (Epipen) [16]. Therefore, to assure IM drug delivery, direct IM injection of epinephrine with a syringe and adequately sized hypodermic needle (if available) may be preferred to an auto-injector device in a clinic or hospital setting, particularly in overweight and obese patients.

Because overall rate of patient adherence to the use emergency epinephrine self-injection is very low [17], alternative routes of administration are being studied and may become available in the future. A small placebo-controlled study in children failed to show that adequate plasma epinephrine doses (comparable to the IM route) could be achieved with inhaled epinephrine given via metered dose inhaler [18]. In a rabbit model, a dissolving sublingual epinephrine tablet achieves plasma epinephrine levels comparable to IM injection [19]. To date, there is no published human data investigating sublingual epinephrine. When intravenous access cannot be achieved in intubated patients, endotracheal delivery of epinephrine can be considered, although the efficacy of this approach in anaphylaxis is unknown [6].

Intravenous epinephrine should be considered only in patients who remain hypotensive or progress to cardiopulmonary arrest, after receiving appropriate doses of IM epinephrine. A decision to initiate intravenous epinephrine must consider potential for drug-related life-threatening arrhythmias and, ideally, should be instituted in clinical settings with cardiac monitoring capabilities (i.e., in an emergency department or intensive care unit).

#### 18.2.1.3 Epinephrine Dosing

Dosing recommendations for epinephrine are listed in Table 18.1. In the USA, an initial dose range of 0.2–0.5 mg of 1:1,000 of epinephrine administered IM or subcutaneously is generally recommended for treatment of adults and 0.01 mg/kg in children (maximum dose of 0.3 mg). In a UK guidance statement, higher treatment doses are recommended than in the USA, with an initial

**Table 18.1** Dosages of epinephrine and other drugs in treating acute anaphylaxis

| | Adult patients (Joint Task Force practice parameter) | Pediatric patients (Joint Task Force practice parameter) | Adult patients (UK resuscitation council) | Pediatric patients (UK resuscitation council) |
|---|---|---|---|---|
| *IM epinephrine dosage*<br>Repeat every 5 min until response is observed (increase in blood pressure) | 0.2–0.5 mL (mg) of 1:1,000 epinephrine | 0.01 mg/kg in children (maximum 0.3 mg dosage) IM or subcutaneously every 5 min, as necessary | 0.5 mg of 1:1,000 epinephrine (0.5 mL 1:1,000) epinephrine | >12 years: 0.5 mg IM (0.5 mL of 1:1,000 epinephrine),<br>>6–12 years: 0.3 mg IM (0.3 mL)<br>>6 months–6 years: 0.15 mg IM (0.15 mL of 1:1,000 epinephrine)<br><6 months: 0.15 mg IM epinephrine (0.15 mL of 1:1,000) |
| *Intravenous dosing with epinephrine* in patients not responding to IM or subcutaneous epinephrine and fluid challenges | Epinephrine 1:1,000, 0.1–0.3 mL in 10 mL of normal saline (1:10,000 dilution), administered intravenously over several minutes<br>*or*<br>If infusion pump is available, 1:100,000 solution or dilute 1 mg in 100 mL at infusion rate of 30–100 mL/h (*5–15 μg/min*)<br>*or*<br>1 mg (1 mL) of 1:1,000 of epinephrine in 250 mL of D5W to yield a concentration of 4.0 μg/mL; infuse at *1–10 μg/min* with microdrop apparatus | 0.01 mg/kg or 0.1 mL/kg of 1:10,000 epinephrine solution; titrate to 10 μg/min; maximum dose, 0.3 mg | *Epinephrine IV bolus dose:* Prepare syringe with 10 mL of 1:10,000 of epinephrine and infuse 50 mg IV boluses of epinephrine according to clinical response<br>If repeated bolus doses are ineffective, start IV epinephrine infusion | There is no evidence on which to base a dose recommendation. The dose selected should be titrated according to response |

intramuscular (IM) dosage of 0.5 mg (or 0.5 mL of 1:1,000 epinephrine) and in patients greater than 12 years with lower doses recommended for children (0.3 mg IM for 6–12 years of age; 0.15 mg in children <6). In general, epinephrine doses are repeated every 5 min for persistent symptoms and protracted hypotension. The interval between epinephrine injections can be decreased, if clinically indicated [6].

Because no standard IV dosing protocols have been established for treating anaphylaxis, dosing regimens are borrowed from emergency cardiac resuscitation guidelines [20]. For adult patients requiring intravenous epinephrine, an epinephrine solution can be formulated with 1 mg (1 mL) of 1:1,000 epinephrine added to 250 mL of D5W (1:250,000) to yield a drug concentration of 4.0 μg/mL. The infusion rate is begun at 1 μg/min and titrated until a desired clinical response to a maximum of 10.0 μg/min. If an infusion pump is available in a hospital setting, an alternative approach is to prepare a 1:100,000 solution of epinephrine (1 mg in 100 mL saline) for intravenous infusion at 30–100 mL/h (5–15 μg/min), titrated based on clinical response or epinephrine toxic effects [6]. For children, 0.01 mg/kg (0.1 mL/kg of a 1:10,000 solution up to 10μg/min; maximum dose, 0.3 mg) is recommended.

### *18.2.2 Oxygen*

High flow oxygen should be initiated as soon as available via a rebreathing mask with an oxygen reservoir and initiated at a flow rate of≥10 L/min. Intubated patients must also be ventilated with high concentration $O_2$. Oxygen therapy is essential in patients with preexisting cardiopulmonary disorders and in patients with protracted anaphylaxis who require multiple epinephrine doses. Pulse oximetry is used to monitor response to $O_2$ therapy and titrate therapeutic $O_2$ concentrations.

### *18.2.3 Fluid Management*

Intravenous fluids should be started as soon as available for patients with hypotension and/or syncope. However, efforts to obtain intravenous access must not delay timely administration of IM epinephrine. During anaphylaxis, up to 35% of intravascular fluid can rapidly leak into the extravascular space leading to intravascular volume depletion, hypotension, and hemodynamic collapse. Profound hypotension is compounded by vasodilatation. These physiologic changes lead to compensatory vasoconstriction which combined with epinephrine, may not restore blood pressure (BP) because of intravascular volume depletion. In this scenario, volume replacement with crystalloid solutions (i.e., normal saline) is essential. A rapid IV fluid challenge with normal saline should be administered rapidly and the BP response closely monitored. It is reasonable to administer 1–2 L of normal saline to adults (5–10 mL/kg) in the first 5 min. Children can receive up to 30 mL/kg in the first hour. There is no evidence to support the use of colloids (e.g., human serum albumin) over crystalloids (e.g., normal saline) for volume resuscitation in this setting [2].

If IV access cannot be achieved or is delayed, intraosseus (IO) administration of fluid should be attempted by health-care providers experienced with this procedure. Catheters can be inserted manually but commercially available automated insertion devices are successful on first attempts. The IO route has been widely utilized in pediatric patients and increasingly in adults. Fluids and drugs can be injected under pressure into the non-collapsible venous plexus of the tibia. An anteromedial tibial approach is commonly used; the anterior femur and superior iliac crest are alternate injection sites. Fluids can be administered by the IO route for volume replacement using an infusion pump.

The procedure is safe and well tolerated with $<1\%$ of patients suffering complications [21]. Due to risk of developing infections, IO access should be maintained no longer than 72 h and replaced by venous access.

### *18.2.4 Antihistamines*

Antihistamines are considered supportive and as second-line treatment in anaphylaxis and should not be considered until after the key resuscitation measures have been implemented (i.e., maintenance of an airway, epinephrine, oxygenation, and IV fluids). Although there is little evidence defining their mechanism in anaphylaxis, antihistamines may be useful in reversing histamine-mediated cutaneous manifestations, vasodilation, and bronchoconstriction. In adults, the $H_1$ antagonist diphenhydramine (25–50 mg) can be administered IM or by slow IV infusion and 1 mg/kg in children up to 50 mg. The $H_2$ antagonist, ranitidine can be infused IV over 10–15 min at a dose of 1 mg/kg in adults, and 12.5–50 mg in children [6].

### *18.2.5 Systemic Corticosteroids*

Systemic corticosteroids, such as antihistamines, can be considered after initial key resuscitation measure has been implemented. Onset of action of systemic corticosteroids is delayed for 4–6 h and, therefore, they are not effective in the treatment of acute anaphylaxis. Second, their usefulness in modifying protracted or biphasic anaphylactic reactions have not been established [22]. Nevertheless, corticosteroids are generally used as ancillary treatment and could be most useful in treating late asthmatic reactions associated with anaphylaxis. If indicated, IV or IM methylprednisolone can be administered every 6 h or at a daily dosage of 1.0–2.0 mg $kg^{-1}$ $day^{-1}$. Alternatively, hydrocortisone 200 mg can be given IM or by slow IV infusion in patients $>12$ years of age with lesser doses recommended in younger children [2, 6].

## 18.3 Other Agents

### *18.3.1 Inhaled Albuterol*

An inhaled ß(beta) agonist such as nebulized albuterol (2.5 mg in 3 mL saline) should be considered and repeated if necessary for treating bronchospasm unresponsive to adequate doses of epinephrine [6].

### *18.3.2 Glucagon*

In patients with epinephrine refractory anaphylaxis, who are receiving regular beta-blocking agents, glucagon therapy should be considered. The pathophysiologic basis for this intervention is the ability of glucagon to bypass the β(beta)-adrenergic receptor and directly activate adenyl cyclase. The clinical evidence supporting the efficacy of IV glucagon is limited to case reports of patients on beta-blockers experiencing anaphylactic reactions to IV radiocontrast dye [23]. Intravenous glucagon 1–5 mg or 20–30 μg/kg in children (maximum childhood dose of 1 mg) is administered over 5 min and followed by IV infusion at a rate 5–15 μg/min.

### *18.3.3 Other Vasopressors*

Vasopressors should be considered in patients with persistent hypotension, despite treatment with IM epinephrine and IV fluids. Dopamine is prepared by mixing 400 mg of dopamine in 500 mL of 5% dextrose and initiated at a rate of 2–20 μg $kg^{-1}$ $min^{-1}$ and titrated to maintain systolic blood pressure greater than 90 mmHg, Vasopressin (40–50 IU by IV bolus infusion) has been reported to be effective for protracted anaphylaxis unresponsive to IV epinephrine and may considered as an effective alternative to IV infusion of epinephrine [24].

## 18.4 Persistent Anaphylaxis Unresponsive to Epinephrine

Although relatively rare if treated promptly, protracted anaphylaxis can last for up to 32 h after onset [6]. Biphasic reactions occur in 20% of cases of anaphylaxis, with a late phase occurring [25] within 72 h after the initial immediate reaction. For patients exhibited a poor or delayed response to epinephrine, an emergency response team should be called immediately for assistance. The patient should be placed in a recumbent position with legs elevated to prevent orthostasis and improve venous return and cerebral blood flow.

It is essential to establish and maintain the airway. Ventilation can be optimized initially by using a one-way valve face mask with an $O_2$ port to deliver $O_2$ at a high flow rate (≥10 L/min). In adults, a self-reinflating bag (e.g., Ambu bag) can be used to ventilate and must be greater than 700 mL to overcome anatomic dead space and provide sufficient tidal volume. If the patient cannot be ventilated (e.g., because of upper airway angioedema), endotracheal intubation or cricothyroidotomy can be attempted, but should be performed by personnel with adequate training and experience. As already mentioned, IV access should be obtained and normal saline challenge and infusions begun to restore circulating volume. High flow $O_2$, and ancillary drugs including H1 and H2 antagonists and systemic corticosteroids can be administered. Once stabilized, patients with protracted anaphylaxis (e.g., persistent hypotension) should be immediately transferred to a hospital facility for observation and treatment in a medical intensive care unit where IV epinephrine infusions or IV vasopressin can be administered intravenously, if indicated. If standard treatment of anaphylactic shock including administration of appropriate dosages of epinephrine and fluid resuscitation is unable to reverse hypotension, immediate IV infusion of arginine vasopressin (40–50 IU) has been recommended to rapidly restore blood pressure and cardiac function [24, 26, 27]. Once stabilized on emergency medications, patients should be observed for at least 8–24 h for biphasic responses.

## 18.5 Cardiac Arrest

Cardiopulmonary resuscitation and advanced cardiac life support measures should be initiated according to published guidelines [28, 29]. Prolonged resuscitation efforts are recommended considering the younger age of patients presenting with anaphylaxis than those with other causes of cardiac arrest.

Ventricular tachycardia and ventricular fibrillation are treated with immediate defibrillation followed by cardiopulmonary resuscitation (CPR) at a 30:2 compression to ventilation ratio. Absence of a normal cardiac rhythm is followed by repeat electrical defibrillation, resumption of CPR and administration of epinephrine 1 mg every 3–5 min, or vasopressin IV 40 IU in lieu of epinephrine. Failure to convert warrants repeat shock, resumption of CPR and antiarrhythmic drugs are considered including amiodarone, lidocaine, and magnesium.

However, for patients in asystole or pulseless electrical activity, electrical defibrillation is not recommended [29]. In such cases, CPR is initiated along with IV or IO administration of epinephrine or vasopressin. Atropine 1 mg IV or IO can also be considered and repeated every 3–5 min up to three doses. Patient converting to a shockable rhythm (e.g., ventricular fibrillation) should be treated as such.

## 18.6 Prevention of Anaphylaxis

Once anaphylaxis has been successfully treated either in a clinic or hospital setting, efforts should be directed at prevention of future anaphylactic events. First, patients with food-induced or drug-induced anaphylaxis must be cautioned about avoidance. Patients with anaphylactic sensitivity to foods must be instructed to carefully read labels on food products, be aware of potential risk of ingesting other foods containing cross-reactive allergens, and to be very careful about eating at restaurants where there is high likelihood of accidental oral ingestion of a food (e.g., peanuts) known to trigger anaphylaxis. Similarly, patients experiencing anaphylaxis to drugs such as beta-lactams or nonsteroidal anti-inflammatory agents must be cautious about future use of cross-reactive drugs likely to induce future events. In the case of beta-lactam agents, patient are instructed to absolutely avoid penicillins and cephalosporins and to use alternative classes of antibiotics. However, should a serious indication arise for a beta-lactam in the future, patients should be advised to consult a qualified allergist/immunologist before receiving these antibiotics.

Unfortunately, stringent compliance with avoidance measures cannot prevent exposure and anaphylaxis to causative allergens. Good examples are stinging insect anaphylaxis or accidental ingestion of an allergenic food. Patients must be educated by health-care providers with an action plan on how to self-manage future anaphylactic reactions with particular emphasis on when and how to self-administer epinephrine. The patient must be informed and educated on the necessity of carrying an epinephrine self-injector device at all times and particularly in settings where there is greater potential risk for allergen exposure (e.g., dining in a restaurant where peanuts are used commonly, camping in the woods with swarming stinging insects). A recent survey suggested that 73% of survivors of anaphylaxis reported that they failed to self-administer epinephrine during the reaction [17]. Those who failed to inject epinephrine reported using H1 blockers instead (38%) or not having received a prescription for epinephrine (28%). This experience suggests a systemic failure in communicating to patients the importance of timely self-administration of epinephrine. The high cost of epinephrine auto-injectors may account in part for low compliance rates. An alternative approach is to provide patients with pre-drawn epinephrine 0.3 mg doses in unsealed syringes. Because the drug stability is time limited, prefilled syringes should be replaced every 3 months [30].

Rapid self-administration of IM epinephrine appears to reduce the risk of fatal anaphylaxis triggered by foods and allergen injections [9, 11]. Because a significant minority of anaphylactic reactions requires more than one injection, adult patients and children>30 kg should be advised to carry sufficient epinephrine auto-injectors allowing them to self-administer at least two 0.3 mg IM injections, if necessary [31, 32]. Auto-injectors specific for children weighing 15–30 kg deliver an IM dose of 0.15 mg of epinephrine (e.g., Epipen Jr.) and achieve plasma epinephrine concentrations equivalent to 0.3 mg with lesser adverse cardiac effects than in the higher adult dose [33].

## References

1. Sampson HA, Munoz-Furlong A, Campbell RL, et al. Second symposium on the definition and management of anaphylaxis: summary report – Second National Institute of Allergy and Infectious Disease/Food Allergy and Anaphylaxis Network symposium. *J Allergy Clin Immunol.* 2006;117:391–397.
2. Soar J, Pumphrey R, Cant A, et al. Emergency treatment of anaphylactic reactions – guidelines for healthcare providers. *Resuscitation.* 2008;77:157–169.

3. The diagnosis and management of anaphylaxis: an updated practice parameter. *J Allergy Clin Immunol.* 2005;115:S483–S523.
4. Sheikh A, Shehata YA, Brown SG, Simons FE. Adrenaline for the treatment of anaphylaxis: cochrane systematic review. *Allergy.* 2009;64:204–212.
5. Pumphrey RS. Fatal posture in anaphylactic shock. *J Allergy Clin Immunol.* 2003;112:451–452.
6. The diagnosis and management of anaphylaxis practice parameter: 2010 update. *J Allergy Clin Immunol.* 2010;126(3):477–480.
7. Kemp SF, Lockey RF, Simons FE. Epinephrine: the drug of choice for anaphylaxis. A statement of the World Allergy Organization. *Allergy.* 2008;63:1061–1070.
8. Pumphrey RS. Lessons for management of anaphylaxis from a study of fatal reactions. *Clin Exp Allergy.* 2000;30:1144–1150.
9. Bernstein DI, Wanner M, Borish L, Liss GM. Twelve-year survey of fatal reactions to allergen injections and skin testing: 1990–2001. *J Allergy Clin Immunol.* 2004;113:1129–1136.
10. Simons FE, Frew AJ, Ansotegui IJ, et al. Risk assessment in anaphylaxis: current and future approaches. *J Allergy Clin Immunol.* 2007;120:S2–S24.
11. Sampson HA, Mendelson L, Rosen JP. Fatal and near-fatal anaphylactic reactions to food in children and adolescents. *N Engl J Med.* 1992;327:380–384.
12. Simons FE. Anaphylaxis: recent advances in assessment and treatment. *J Allergy Clin Immunol.* 2009;124:625–636;quiz 37–38.
13. Simons FE, Gu X, Simons KJ. Epinephrine absorption in adults: intramuscular versus subcutaneous injection. *J Allergy Clin Immunol.* 2001;108:871–873.
14. Simons FE, Roberts JR, Gu X, Simons KJ. Epinephrine absorption in children with a history of anaphylaxis. *J Allergy Clin Immunol.* 1998;101:33–37.
15. Stecher D, Bulloch B, Sales J, Schaefer C, Keahey L. Epinephrine auto-injectors: is needle length adequate for delivery of epinephrine intramuscularly? *Pediatrics.* 2009;124:65–70.
16. Song TT, Nelson MR, Chang JH, Engler RJ, Chowdhury BA. Adequacy of the epinephrine autoinjector needle length in delivering epinephrine to the intramuscular tissues. *Ann Allergy Asthma Immunol.* 2005;94:539–542.
17. Simons FE, Clark S, Camargo CA Jr. Anaphylaxis in the community: learning from the survivors. *J Allergy Clin Immunol.* 2009;124:301–306.
18. Simons FE, Gu X, Johnston LM, Simons KJ. Can epinephrine inhalations be substituted for epinephrine injection in children at risk for systemic anaphylaxis? *Pediatrics.* 2000;106:1040–1044.
19. Rawas-Qalaji MM, Simons FE, Simons KJ. Sublingual epinephrine tablets versus intramuscular injection of epinephrine: dose equivalence for potential treatment of anaphylaxis. *J Allergy Clin Immunol.* 2006;117:398–403.
20. 2005 American Heart Association Guidelines for Cardiopulmonary Resuscitation and Emergency Cardiovascular Care. *Circulation.* 2005;112:143–145.
21. Von Hoff DD, Kuhn JG, Burris HA III, Miller LJ. Does intraosseous equal intravenous? A pharmacokinetic study. *Am J Emerg Med.* 2008;26:31–38.
22. Stark BJ, Sullivan TJ. Biphasic and protracted anaphylaxis. *J Allergy Clin Immunol.* 1986;78:76–83.
23. Thomas M, Crawford I. Best evidence topic report. Glucagon infusion in refractory anaphylactic shock in patients on beta-blockers. *Emerg Med J.* 2005;22:272–273.
24. Kill C, Wranze E, Wulf H. Successful treatment of severe anaphylactic shock with vasopressin. Two case reports. *Int Arch Allergy Immunol.* 2004;134:260–261.
25. Ellis AK, Day JH. Diagnosis and management of anaphylaxis. *CMAJ.* 2003;169:307–311.
26. Meng L, Williams EL. Case report: treatment of rocuronium-induced anaphylactic shock with vasopressin. *Can J Anaesth.* 2008;55:437–440.
27. Hussain AM, Yousuf B, Khan MA, Khan FH, Khan FA. Vasopressin for the management of catecholamine-resistant anaphylactic shock. *Singapore Med J.* 2008;49:e225–e228.
28. Cummins RO, Hazinski MF. The most important changes in the international ECC and CPR guidelines 2000. *Resuscitation.* 2000;46:431–437.
29. Ali B, Zafari AM. Narrative review: cardiopulmonary resuscitation and emergency cardiovascular care: review of the current guidelines. *Ann Intern Med.* 2007;147:171–179.
30. Rawas-Qalaji M, Simons FE, Collins D, Simons KJ. Long-term stability of epinephrine dispensed in unsealed syringes for the first-aid treatment of anaphylaxis. *Ann Allergy Asthma Immunol.* 2009;102:500–503.
31. Korenblat P, Lundie MJ, Dankner RE, Day JH. A retrospective study of epinephrine administration for anaphylaxis: how many doses are needed? *Allergy Asthma Proc.* 1999;20:383–386.
32. Oren E, Banerji A, Clark S, Camargo CA Jr. Food-induced anaphylaxis and repeated epinephrine treatments. *Ann Allergy Asthma Immunol.* 2007;99:429–432.
33. Simons FE, Gu X, Silver NA, Simons KJ. EpiPen Jr versus EpiPen in young children weighing 15 to 30 kg at risk for anaphylaxis. *J Allergy Clin Immunol.* 2002;109:171–175.

# Chapter 19
# Drug Desensitizations in the Management of Allergy and Anaphylaxis to Chemotherapeutic Agents and Monoclonal Antibodies

**Aleena Banerji, Patrick Brennan, Paul Hesterberg, Eyal Oren, and F. Ida Hsu**

**Abstract** Drug desensitization is the process of safely administering a needed medication to a drug-allergic individual. The procedure involves the cautious administration of incremental doses of the drug over a period of hours to days and it is used primarily in the management of IgE-mediated drug hypersensitivity reactions. Desensitization has also safely been used for drug hypersensitivity reactions that result in mast cell degranulation that are not IgE-mediated. Desensitization is antigen-specific or drug-specific and is sustained only as long as the drug is continuously administered. The recommendation for drug desensitization should be made along with an Allergy and Immunology specialist.

While most of the desensitization protocols published in the literature have involved antibiotics, this principle, in recent years, has been applied successfully to other agents including chemotherapeutic agents, monoclonal antibodies, aspirin, allopurinol, insulin, vaccines, and other protein and small molecule therapeutics alike. In this chapter, we focus primarily on using drug desensitizations in the management of allergy to chemotherapeutic agents and monoclonal antibodies. What began as a method of administering antibiotics to sensitized individuals for the treatment of life-threatening infectious disease has now become a means of safely treating numerous cancers and rheumatologic diseases with needed chemotherapies.

**Keywords** Allergy • Drug desensitization • Hypersensitivity reactions • Drug allergy

## 19.1 Introduction

An adverse drug reaction is defined as a noxious and unintended response to a drug. Allergic drug reactions account for 5–10% of all adverse drug reactions, with cutaneous reactions being the most common form [1]. These allergic drug reactions are felt to be mediated through preformed IgE antibodies targeted against the specific drug. When the drug is recognized by these IgE molecules bound to mast cells and basophils, a cascade of allergic events transpires. The most severe form of this cascade is anaphylaxis. Allergic reactions to medications account for the majority of documented deaths from anaphylaxis each year [2].

Drug desensitization is the process of safely administering a needed medication to a drug-allergic individual. The procedure involves the cautious administration of incremental doses of the drug over a period of hours to days and it is used primarily in the management of IgE-mediated drug hypersensitivity reactions. Desensitization has also safely been used for drug hypersensitivity reactions

A. Banerji (✉)
Harvard Medical School, Brigham and Women's Hospital, Boston, MA, USA
e-mail: abanerji@partners.org

M.C. Castells (ed.), *Anaphylaxis and Hypersensitivity Reactions*,
DOI 10.1007/978-1-60327-951-2_19, 

that result in mast cell degranulation that is not IgE-mediated. The recommendation for drug desensitization should be made along with an Allergy and Immunology specialist. In our own experience, the need to offer first-line therapy for cancer and other life-threatening diseases for patients with a history of drug allergy has spurred the clinical development of drug desensitization protocols for a variety of medications.

While most of the desensitization protocols published in the literature have involved antibiotics, this principle, in recent years, has been applied successfully to other agents including chemotherapeutic agents, monoclonal antibodies, aspirin, allopurinol, insulin, vaccines, and other protein and small molecule therapeutics alike. Desensitization protocols allow patients to safely receive first-line treatments for management of life-threatening and other serious conditions. This chapter will focus primarily on using drug desensitizations in the management of allergy to chemotherapeutic agents and monoclonal antibodies.

## 19.2 Mechanism of Drug Desensitization

Drug desensitization is thought to work via the gradual introduction of a drug causing cross-linking of drug-specific IgE on the surface of mast cells in a graded fashion, thereby keeping the intracellular signal below a clinical threshold and preventing clinically significant mast cell degranulation from occurring [3, 4]. An alternative theory is that univalent drug-carrier protein molecules prevent cross-linking of surface IgE and transmission of an intracellular signal [3, 4]. Although both drug-specific IgE and IgG increase after drug desensitization, skin test reactivity has been shown to decrease [3].

Data also suggest that loss of Syk on basophils may lead to longer-term alterations in basophil function that could explain the mechanisms responsible for drug desensitization [5]. Mast cells have also been rendered unresponsive by rapid administration of suboptimal doses of antigen in the presence of calcium, similar to in vivo desensitization. However, if this same procedure is performed in STAT6-null mast cells, they cannot be desensitized [6]. This provides evidence that Syk and STAT6 are critical molecular targets in this inhibitory process during drug desensitization.

Desensitization is antigen-specific or drug-specific and is sustained only as long as the drug is continuously administered. After three half-lives elapse (i.e., at the conclusion of the course of therapy), the patient should be considered resensitized and would require repeat desensitization if further treatment with the same drug is needed.

## 19.3 Skin Testing for Drug Hypersensitivity

Various modalities are available to test for IgE-mediated allergy to selected antibiotics, anesthetic agents, and protein drugs. These include skin testing, serologic testing for specific IgE, and basophil activation testing. However, the only currently available means for predicting an IgE-mediated hypersensitivity to non-vesicant chemotherapeutic agents is skin testing, usually performed by an allergist. Although initial investigations into the use of skin testing involved only case reports with limited numbers of patients, subsequent investigation suggest skin testing has high diagnostic value [7–11].

The value of skin testing in predicting hypersensitivity reactions specifically to carboplatin has been examined. In prospective studies, the negative predictive value of carboplatin skin testing was found to be 98–99% in patients who had received multiple previous courses of carboplatin [12, 13]. Markman et al. [12] prospectively evaluated the predictive value of skin testing in 126 women with ovarian cancer and no history of hypersensitivity reactions during infusions. Of 87 skin test negative women, seven experienced a hypersensitivity reaction during subsequent infusions giving a false-negative rate of 8%.

**Table 19.1** Doses used for skin prick and intradermal testing

| | Skin prick (mg/mL) | Intradermal (mg/mL) |
|---|---|---|
| Carboplatin | 10 | 1, 5–12[a] |
| Cisplatin | 1 | 0.1, 1 |
| Oxaliplatin | 5 | 0.1, 1, 5 |
| Taxanes | Not clinically predictive | |
| Rituximab | 10 | 0.1, 1, 10 |
| Cetuximab | Not reported | |

[a]In our experience, intradermal testing with concentrations of 10 mg/mL have been noted to cause local delayed skin necrosis in a minority of subjects

Importantly, all of these reactions were classified as mild in nature. Lee et al. [14] reported their skin testing experience in 26 women with a known history of hypersensitivity reactions to carboplatin. Skin test results were positive in 81% of 108 patients tested. The rate of false-positive reactions is not well established, as the majority of patients with positive skin tests are not rechallenged, for ethical reasons, outside of a desensitization protocol.

Skin testing has also been found to be useful in diagnosis of IgE-mediated hypersensitivity to the other platinum-based chemotherapeutics including cisplatin and oxaliplatin. Concurrent skin testing with these agents may be used to determine if an individual with known hypersensitivity to one agent has a cross-reacting hypersensitivity to another. This is important, as cross-reactive hypersensitivity reactions to cisplatin have been reported in as many as 30% of patients with history of reactions to carboplatin and have even resulted in severe anaphylaxis and death [15]. If testing demonstrates a lack of cross-reactivity, this may allow effective treatment with the alternate agent [16, 17].

Less commonly, skin testing may be performed with other non-vesicant chemotherapeutic agents such as cyclophosphamide and methotrexate. As IgE-mediated reactions to 5-HT3 receptor antagonists, like ondansetron, have been reported as well, skin testing to these agents may also be considered, if the history is suggestive [18]. Because of local irritation and the risk for skin necrosis, skin testing should never be attempted with vesicant agents such as doxorubicin, although suspected IgE-mediated reactions have been reported. Skin testing has not been found to be useful for prediction of presumed non-IgE mediated hypersensitivity reactions such as those occurring with paclitaxel [19].

When skin testing, it is important to check the literature for nonirritating drug concentrations and confirm with negative results in normal control subjects. Initial testing is performed with skin prick or puncture using standardized skin testing devices. Results are assessed for development of a wheal and flare at 15–30 min that is greater than the wheal and flare seen with saline control. If negative, intradermal testing with serial dilutions of the drug may be performed, and again assessed for wheal and flare reactions greater than the saline control within 15–30 min. Examples of nonirritating intradermal concentrations for various chemotherapeutic agents are found in Table 19.1.

## 19.4 Drug Desensitization Procedures

Candidates for drug desensitization include those who present with type I hypersensitivity reactions (mast cell-mediated/IgE-dependent) including anaphylaxis. Idiosyncratic reactions including erythema multiforme, Stevens–Johnson syndrome and toxic epidermal necrolysis are not amenable to drug desensitization as any reintroduction of causal medications can be life-threatening.

Drug desensitization should be performed with the drug that is required for therapy and either the oral or intravenous route may be used. Drug desensitization protocols last several hours. Drug doses typically are doubled every 15 or 30 min, and vital signs are monitored before and throughout

| Total dose | 500 mg | Solution concentration | Total dose in each solution (mg) |
|---|---|---|---|
| Solution A | 250 ml | 0.02 mg/ml | 5.0* |
| Solution B | 250 ml | 0.20 mg/ml | 50.0* |
| Solution C | 250 ml | 2.00 mg/ml | 500.0* |

| Step | Solution | Rate (ml/h) | Time (min) | Administered dose (mg) | Cumulative dose infused (mg) |
|---|---|---|---|---|---|
| 1 | A | 2 | 15 | 0.010 | 0.010 |
| 2 | A | 5 | 15 | 0.025 | 0.035 |
| 3 | A | 10 | 15 | 0.050 | 0.085 |
| 4 | A | 20 | 15 | 0.100 | 0.185 |
| 5 | B | 5 | 15 | 0.250 | 0.435 |
| 6 | B | 10 | 15 | 0.500 | 0.935 |
| 7 | B | 20 | 15 | 1.000 | 1.935 |
| 8 | B | 40 | 15 | 2.000 | 3.935 |
| 9 | C | 10 | 15 | 5.000 | 8.935 |
| 10 | C | 20 | 15 | 10.000 | 18.935 |
| 11 | C | 40 | 15 | 20.000 | 38.935 |
| 12 | C | 75 | 184.4 | 461.065 | 500.000 |
| | | | Total time = 5.82 h | | Total dose infused = 500 mg* |

* The sum of the doses in Solutions A, B, and C equals 555 mg. Total dose infused is 500 mg.

**Fig. 19.1** 12-step drug desensitization protocol (Reproduced from [76]. With permission)

the procedure. The standard desensitization protocol used for intravenous agents at Brigham and Women's Hospital in Boston, MA, involves a 12-step dose escalation procedure. The first 11 doses are incremented every 15 min and infuse about 10% of the target treatment dose, with the last dose administering the remaining 90% over a period of about 3 h (see Fig. 19.1). The same protocol has also been used effectively for intraperitoneal therapy.

Unlike patients treated with antibiotics or aspirin, the majority of patients treated with chemotherapeutics or monoclonal antibodies require repeated drug administration at extended intervals (e.g., every 3–4 week). Since desensitization is temporary, repeated desensitization becomes necessary for each cycle of drug administration. Thus, a goal in the development of a standard protocol has been suitability for single-day outpatient treatment. At Brigham and Women's Hospital, the initial desensitization is often performed in the intensive care unit. Once the safety of the protocol has been established for a given patient, subsequent desensitizations are performed in a hospital-based outpatient infusion center. At Massachusetts General Hospital, all chemotherapeutic and monoclonal antibody drug desensitizations are performed in a specialized inpatient unit with nurses trained in drug desensitization methods.

Overall, this type of protocol is very well tolerated by the majority of patients. In a series of 413 desensitizations performed in 98 patients for various chemotherapy agents including carboplatin, cisplatin, paclitaxel, doxorubicin, and rituximab, 94% of desensitizations elicited mild (27%) or no (67%) reactions [20]. All patients received a full dose of chemotherapy. Within the 6% of desensitizations eliciting severe reactions, all were less severe than the initial presenting hypersensitivity reaction, and subsided when the infusion was paused and appropriate treatment administered. No patients required intubation, and no deaths occurred. Of note, 75% of reactions occurred during infusion of the last solution of the protocol, and 51% during the final step of the desensitization. For patients undergoing multiple desensitizations, the authors were able to adjust the protocol with subsequent cycles, and decrease the frequency and severity of reactions accordingly (Fig. 19.2).

Adjustments made to the protocol after a reaction included prolonging the step before that in which the reaction occurred, adding an additional intermediate rate step, and/or administering prophylactic medications before the step at which the patient had a reaction. The same group has also reported that pretreatment with 325 mg acetylsalicylic acid and 10 mg montelukast orally for 2 days before and on the day of desensitization reduced the severity and rate of both cutaneous and systemic reactions when compared to pretreatment with methylprednisolone. All of the patients received standard pretreatment with 25 mg diphenhydramine and 50 mg ranitidine, intravenously, 20 min prior to their infusions as well [21].

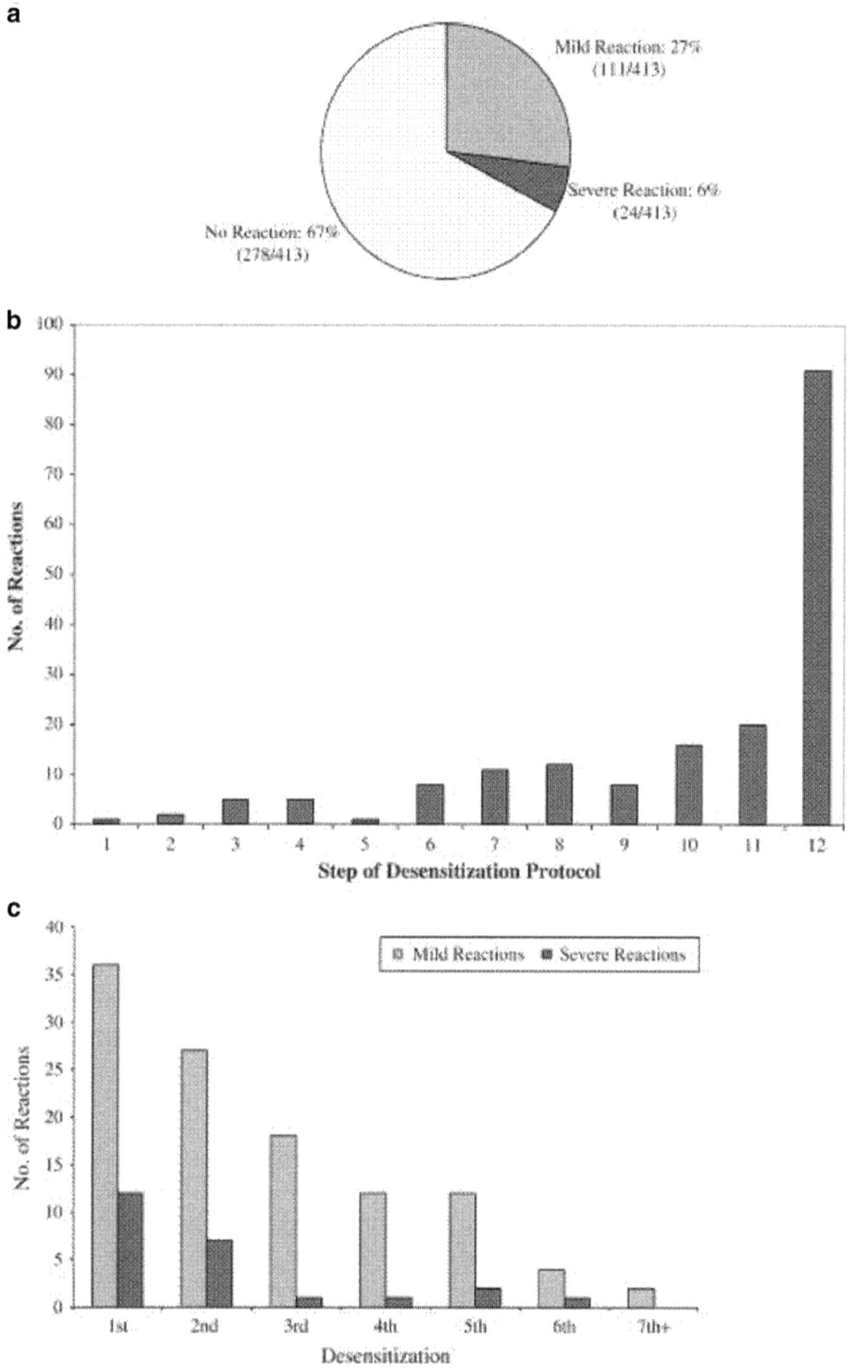


**Fig. 19.2** (**a**) Number and severity of reactions during desensitization. A mild reaction was defined as absence of chest pain, changes in blood pressure, dyspnea, oxygen, desaturation, or throat tightness. A severe reaction included one of these. (**b**) Desensitization step at which reactions occurred (total number of reactions = 180). (**c**) Desensitization course at which reactions recurred (total number of reactions = 135 [111 mild and 24 severe]) (Reproduced from [20]. With permission)

## 19.5 Hypersensitivity and Drug Desensitization to Carboplatin and Cisplatin

Carboplatin and cisplatin are platinum-based chemotherapeutic agents commonly used against ovarian, lung, head, and neck cancers. Carboplatin and cisplatin are classified as DNA alkylating agents. Carboplatin was introduced in the late 1980s and has since gained popularity in clinical treatment due to its vastly reduced side effects compared to its parent compound cisplatin.

In parallel with the increased survival of patients with ovarian cancer through the continued use of carboplatin and cisplatin, there has been an increased incidence of hypersensitivity reactions to this agent [7, 22]. A 1% incidence of hypersensitivity reactions is documented in patients receiving less than six courses of treatment, but this increases to 27% in patients receiving more than seven treatments [13]. At least 50% of the hypersensitivity reactions are described as moderately severe with symptoms of diffuse erythroderma, wheezing, facial swelling, dyspnea, and hypotension [13]. Anaphylaxis, respiratory arrest, and even death have been reported as a result of hypersensitivity reactions to platinum agents [23]. Hypersensitivity reactions to carboplatin and cisplatin often prompt their permanent discontinuation [24].

Given that a platinum-based regimen is an integral part of standard therapy for specific malignancies like ovarian cancer, eliminating platinum agents as a therapeutic option in women with a history of hypersensitivity reactions poses a significant and potentially life-shortening disadvantage for the patient. Unfortunately, despite the use of prophylactic regimens (e.g., dexamethasone, histamine-1, two receptor antagonists) the emergence of hypersensitivity reactions to platinum agents has severely limited the use of these agent. Due to the risk of hypersensitivity reactions with repeated doses of these medications, patients have been denied what is often the best systemic therapy to potentially cure their cancer.

In a recent publication from the Massachusetts General Hospital, Hesterberg et al. [25] evaluated 30 women with a history of carboplatin hypersensitivity reactions. Carboplatin skin test was positive in 20/30 patients (67%). Twenty-two of these women subsequently underwent 60 desensitizations to carboplatin. Cutaneous manifestations were the most prominent presenting symptoms of a hypersensitivity reaction (87%), with palmar involvement in 60%. Sixteen carboplatin skin test positive and six skin test negative patients were desensitized to carboplatin using continuous intravenous protocols. Six skin test positive patients (38%) developed hypersensitivity reactions during desensitization but completed the procedure with additional treatment and/or slower infusion rates. Subsequent desensitizations were tolerated with slower protocols. Two skin test negative patients (33%) had hypersensitivity reactions during the first and/or second desensitization. Both became skin test positive before the second desensitization. Both had distant hypersensitivity reaction histories. Skin testing remained negative in patients without hypersensitivity reactions during desensitization. All desensitizations were successful in administering the appropriate carboplatin dose. The same group has had similar success with cisplatin desensitization (unpublished data).

Dr. Mariana Castells, at Brigham and Women's Hospital, has published several articles regarding desensitization protocols in patients with gynecologic malignancies and hypersensitivity reactions to carboplatin and cisplatin. The first article [26] evaluated ten consecutive patients (eight with ovarian cancer) from April 2002–February 2004 with a documented hypersensitivity reaction to carboplatin requiring continued carboplatin treatment. These patients had received a median of eight courses of carboplatin before their first hypersensitivity reaction. Each patient subsequently underwent desensitization to carboplatin using a 6-h, three-solution, 12-step protocol as detailed in Fig. 19.1. All ten patients successfully completed 35 desensitizations, 31 without any adverse reactions. Four patients had symptoms during their first ($n = 3$) and third ($n = 1$) desensitization. Two of these patients had their desensitization protocols modified and all but three tolerated further courses without complications. The fourth patient was unable to receive further treatment due to progressive disease. This 6-h, 12-step protocol clearly represents a significant advance in the treatment of patients with carboplatin hypersensitivity reactions.

The second publication [26] using the same three-solution, 12-step protocol delivered as doubling drug doses in a stepwise fashion was used to treat 57 consecutive patients with a history of prior moderate to severe hypersensitivity reactions to chemotherapy. The 57 patients successfully completed 255 courses of desensitization, 127 of which were to carboplatin with a smaller number to cisplatin. Twenty-one of 26 patients (81%) with hypersensitivity reactions to carboplatin had positive skin tests to carboplatin. Eighteen patients had breakthrough symptoms over 30 courses (11.8%) that were less severe than their initial hypersensitivity reactions. After management of breakthrough symptoms, these patients finished all 30 courses and tolerated subsequent desensitizations. It is notable that these 57 patients were largely ovarian cancer patients accrued at one of the Harvard Cancer Center Institutions over a 3–4 year period highlighting the increasing frequency of referral to the allergy department for hypersensitivity reactions to chemotherapy.

Subsequent experience with 60 more patients undergoing 212 desensitizations to carboplatin was reported in a 2008 article summarizing the group's experience with 413 chemotherapy desensitizations [20]. In this series, 53 of 60 patients had positive skin test results to carboplatin. Of the seven skin test negative patients, one patient developed a delayed reaction at the site of the skin test, and was thus desensitized. Two patients with initially negative skin tests tolerated standard infusions, but subsequently developed positive skin tests and were desensitized after conversion; four patients developed reactions when treated without desensitization, and for their next cycles were desensitized without further testing. Again, cutaneous symptoms were the most prominent aspect of the initial hypersensitivity reactions, occurring in 100% of patients, with cardiovascular, gastrointestinal, and respiratory complaints affecting 57%, 42%, and 40% of patients, respectively (see Fig. 19.3). Another three patients in this series were desensitized to cisplatin, with five intravenous desensitizations, and seven desensitizations administered intraperitoneally.

Our combined experience at BWH and MGH, as shown in these studies, provides clear evidence that desensitization methods for carboplatin and cisplatin are useful, successful, and provide a well-tolerated method for patients with severe hypersensitivity reactions to receive lifesaving therapy.

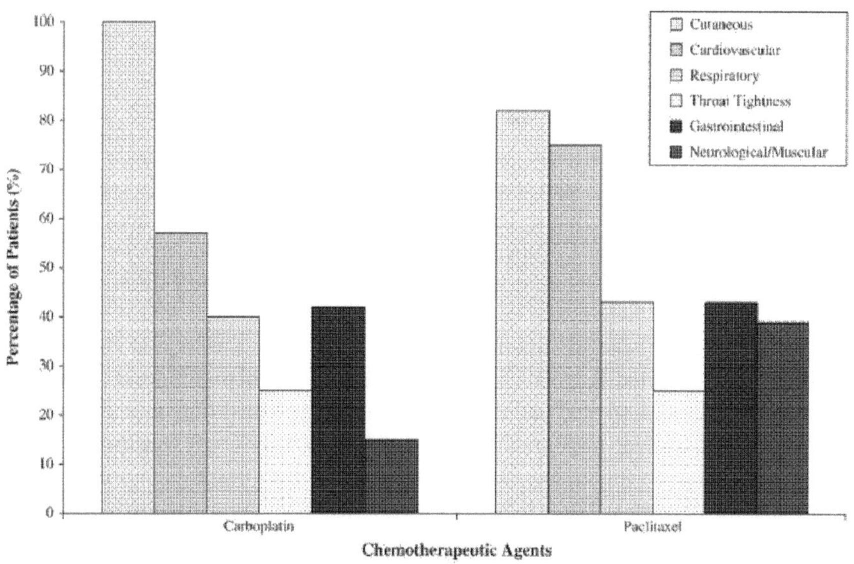


**Fig. 19.3** Frequency of signs and symptoms during initial HSRs (Reproduced with permission from [20])

## 19.6 Hypersensitivity and Drug Desensitization to Oxaliplatin

Oxaliplatin is another platinum-based chemotherapy drug in the same family as carboplatin and cisplatin and is similarly a DNA alkylating agent. It is typically administered in combination with other agents for the treatment of colorectal cancer. Colorectal cancer is the third-leading cause of cancer death in the USA. With the advent of new chemotherapy drugs like oxaliplatin, disease-free and long-term survival has improved in this patient population [27].

Initial reports of hypersensitivity reactions to oxaliplatin were low, but more recent data suggest the incidence of hypersensitivity reactions to oxaliplatin is similar to that of the earlier generation platinum agents. This rising incidence of hypersensitivity reactions to oxaliplatin is likely the result of increasing clinical use. The reported incidence of hypersensitivity reactions associated with oxaliplatin in patients with colorectal cancer is approximately 12%, with 1–2% of patients developing moderate to severe reactions [28]. The severity of the reaction can vary from mild flushing to a life-threatening anaphylactic response. For patients who have mild sensitivity to oxaliplatin, slowing the infusion rate and giving pretreatment with antihistamines and/or a steroid has been successful [29]. In the case of moderate to severe reactions to oxaliplatin, reexposure is usually not considered. With moderate to severe reactions, slowing the infusion rate and giving antihistamine pretreatment is also not a safe recommendation. Fortunately, in these cases, desensitization to oxaliplatin has been shown to be successful and safe [20, 29].

A recent review supports the success of oxaliplatin desensitization [30]. Polyzos et al. [30] retrospectively evaluated and characterized 1,224 patients exposed to an oxaliplatin-containing regimen. Three hundred and eight patients who had no previous exposure to platinum compounds developed reactions to oxaliplatin that was verified by rechallenge. The reactions occurred after the first five courses, with a median course number of 9 (range 1–24). Mild reactions occurred in 195 (63%) patients manifesting with itching and mild erythema either during treatment or within the next few hours. Severe reactions occurred in 113 (37%) patients within minutes of drug infusion manifesting with diffuse erythroderma, facial swelling, chest tightness, bronchospasm, and changes in blood pressure. Oxaliplatin withdrawal was not required in patients with a mild reaction. Patients who experienced a severe reaction could tolerate subsequent courses with appropriate premedication and oxaliplatin desensitization. This success of oxaliplatin desensitization has similarly been shown using the standard 12-step, three-bag protocol at Brigham and Women's Hospital [20] and MGH.

## 19.7 Hypersensitivity and Drug Desensitization to Taxanes

Taxanes are microtubule inhibitors that were first produced from plants. Paclitaxel (Taxol) was first derived from the Pacific yew tree while Docetaxel (Taxotere) is a semisynthetic taxane originally extracted from the needles of the European yew tree [31, 32]. Taxanes act by binding the beta-subunit of tubulin thus forming stable, nonfunctional microtubule bundles that interfere with cell mitosis [33].

Paclitaxel is approved for the treatment of ovarian and breast carcinoma, non-small cell lung cancer, as well as AIDS-related Kaposi's sarcoma. Paclitaxel has been reported to cause hypersensitivity reactions in 41% of all treated patients [31]. Severe hypersensitivity reactions were observed in 2–4% of patients receiving paclitaxel in clinical trials [31]. These reactions have included anaphylaxis manifested as dyspnea, hypotension or loss of consciousness, angioedema, and generalized urticaria. Fatal reactions have occurred despite premedication regimens. Severe reactions tended to occur within the first hour of infusion and were not observed after the third course of therapy. Other prominent symptoms commonly reported include flushing, chest tightness or pressure, hypertension, tachycardia, and severe back pain.

Docetaxel (Taxotere) is approved for the treatment of breast and non-small cell lung cancer, hormone refractory prostate cancer, gastric adenocarcinoma, as well as squamous cell carcinoma of the head and neck. Docetaxel has a reported incidence of severe hypersensitivity reactions of 2.6–9.8%, regardless of premedication regimen [32]. Elevated liver function tests have been associated with increased rate of severe hypersensitivity reactions.

Premedication regimens have reduced the incidence of severe hypersensitivity reactions to these taxanes. A 3-day regimen of dexamethasone 16 mg daily decreased the rate of severe reactions during docetaxel infusion to 2.2% among all tumor types with a more marked reduction to 0% in patients with elevated liver function tests. The premedication regimen for paclitaxel consists of dexamethasone 20 mg administered orally 12 and 6 h before infusion with additional diphenhydramine and cimetidine or rantidine given intravenously 30–60 min before the infusion [32].

As taxanes represent a clinically important class of medications for the treatment of a number of malignancies, a safe and effective method of administering these medications to patients with a history of HSR would be very useful. This was first shown to be possible in 1999 when six patients with previous paclitaxel hypersensitivity reactions were successfully desensitized to paclitaxel [34]. In 2005, Feldweg et al. [35] described a rapid three-bag, 12-step protocol that was used to desensitize 17 patients with history of severe reactions over 77 cycles of paclitaxel or docetaxel. Only four of the 17 patients developed symptoms during the desensitization protocol, and these were much less severe than their original reactions. All patients were able to complete their planned infusions, and three of the four had subsequent desensitizations without adverse reactions. This protocol was identical to that used to successfully desensitize patients to platinum-based chemotherapeutic agents, as described earlier.

Subsequent experience with 28 patients undergoing 140 intravenous and 12 intraperitoneal desensitizations to paclitaxel was included in the 2008 series by Castells et al., described above. Cutaneous and cardiovascular symptoms were reported to occur in 82% and 75% of patients' initial hypersensitivity reactions, respectively. Thirty-six percent of patients also complained of back pain during their reactions, a symptom otherwise not commonly associated with anaphylaxis (see Fig. 19.3).

The mechanism of taxane-induced hypersensitivity reactions is unknown. Paclitaxel contains Cremophor (polyoxyethylated castor oil), which may be responsible for some of the hypersensitivity reactions. Of note, a nanoparticle albumin-bound (nab)-paclitaxel formulation was recently evaluated in a phase II study of 55 patients and, despite lack of routine use of corticosteroid or antihistamine premedication, no hypersensitivity reactions were observed [36]. This formulation may provide an alternative method of administering taxanes to patients who have experienced prior hypersensitivity to these agents.

## 19.8 Hypersensitivity to Monoclonal Antibodies – General Considerations

As the use of monoclonal antibodies grows, so does the incidence of adverse reactions to these medications. Infusion-related symptoms have been reported in greater than 10% of patients being treated with monoclonal antibodies. Common symptoms experienced during infusion include diaphoresis, chills, fever, pruritus, urticaria, and dyspnea [37].

Reactions to monoclonal antibodies are diverse, and can be classified as idiosyncratic infusion reactions, serum sickness-type reactions, cutaneous reactions, and anaphylactic-type reactions [38]. As with all therapeutics, reactions to monoclonal antibodies are likely to include both on-target and off-target effects. Most monoclonal antibodies target cell surface receptors, and the rapid engagement of target receptors may lead to signaling, cytokine release, complement activation, and even cell death. It would be expected that the greater the burden of circulating target cells, the greater the potential reaction from on-target effects. Non-IgE-mediated infusion reactions to rituximab given for lymphoma, for example, are thought to correlate with disease burden [39].

Monoclonal antibodies carry unique risks with respect to hypersensitivity reactions. Because monoclonal antibodies are proteins and are relatively large molecules, they can act as both T and B cell targets. Monoclonal antibodies can act as complete antigens and do not require haptenation, as would a small molecule therapeutic. In addition, the half-lives and dosing intervals for monoclonal antibodies are generally longer than that for traditional small molecule therapeutics, and this pharmacokinetic profile is likely to elicit a different immunologic response when compared to a drug with a shorter half-life.

Therapeutic monoclonal antibodies can be divided into four subtypes, based on the method of generation, and the variable murine component. The subtypes are listed below, with the approximate percent of murine protein sequence listed in parentheses: fully murine (100%), chimeric (30%), humanized (5%), and fully human (0%). Having smaller portions of murine protein sequence is expected to decrease antigenicity, but even fully human monoclonal antibodies have complementary determining regions comprised of a nonnative sequence that can act as a foreign epitope, and thereby elicit an immunological response. The development of antibodies directed against the monoclonal-target complex, another nonnative structure, has also been demonstrated [40].

## 19.9 Hypersensitivity to Monoclonal Antibodies – Clinical Observations

Immediate hypersensitivity reactions have been reported for rituximab [41], infliximab [42–44], trastuzumab [45], omalizumab [46, 47], natalizumab [48, 49], basiliximab [50], and abciximab [51, 52]. Although there is a significant rate of adverse reactions to alemtuzumab, immediate hypersensitivity has not been reported to date.

Rituximab is a chimeric monoclonal antibody directed against CD20, a cell surface receptor present on B cells. Rituximab is commonly used for the treatment of hematologic malignancy and is also used in the treatment of rheumatologic disease thought to be driven by the production of pathologic antibodies. This monoclonal antibody was approved for use in 1997 and was the first monoclonal antibody approved for the treatment of malignancy. Infusion-related toxicity is common, and symptoms reported in more than 10% of patients include chills, nausea, asthenia, headache, angioedema, rash, pruritus, and hypotension [53]. Most of these reactions are not thought to be IgE-mediated. These standard infusion reactions correlate with disease burden, are most prominent with the first infusion, and decrease with subsequent infusions [37].

At Brigham and Women's hospital, the majority of reactions to rituximab in which a positive skin test was subsequently observed occurred on the first administration. This is unexpected, since the vast majority of the general population has not been previously exposed to monoclonal antibody therapeutics, and none of the patients who reacted on the first rituximab exposure were known to have been previously treated with monoclonal therapeutics. It is possible that the reactions observed were not IgE-mediated, and that observed positive skin testing to rituximab is nonspecific. Another potential mechanism to explain our observed reactivity pattern is xenogenic sensitization to mouse protein, and mouse-specific IgE has been demonstrated in multiple populations [54–58]. Unexpected cross-reactive epitopes may also lead to preformed IgE in the absence of drug exposure. For example, as discussed below, preexisting glycopeptide-specific IgE-mediated reactions have been described for cetuximab [60, 61].

As is seen with rituximab, infusion reactions are common with trastuzumab. Trastuzumab infusion reactions that been reported to occur in more than 10% of patients include pain, fever, nausea, chills, cough, headache, vomiting, abdominal pain, dyspnea, rash, dizziness, and throat tightness. As with rituximab, infusion-related symptoms are most prominent with the first infusion, and correlate with disease burden [60].

Side effects experienced with infliximab reported to occur in more than 10% of patients include headache, nausea, sinusitis, diarrhea, URI, and cough [43]. Compared with rituximab and trastuzumab, the incidence of acute infusion reactions is much lower with infliximab. In a study of patients with Crohn's disease, infusion reactions were reported in less than 1% of patients [61].

Interestingly, in our experience at Brigham and Women's hospital, many patients who have been referred for hypersensitivity reactions to trastuzumab and infliximab follow a similar pattern. Perhaps not surprisingly, these patients have been treated with an extended course of monoclonal antibody, and develop an immediate hypersensitivity on reintroduction after a drug hiatus. It remains to be seen whether this observation is due to referral bias or will stand as a frequent presentation history.

## 19.10 Desensitization to Monoclonal Antibodies

The basic principles of patient selection for desensitization to monoclonal antibodies are similar to selection of patients who had reactions to other medications and are described elsewhere in this book. The high rate of idiosyncratic infusion reactions to monoclonal antibodies does, however, present an additional challenge. For patient with a classic moderate to severe anaphylactic-type reaction, consisting of urticaria, airways hyperreactivity, angioedema, or hypotension, we recommend administration via desensitization. The absence of myalgias, fever, and rigors further suggests that the reaction is of the anaphylactic type. Reactions that are possibly, but not convincingly, a Gell and Coombs type I reaction present a challenge. Although the sensitivity and specificity of skin testing for monoclonal antibodies has not been reported, we rely on these tests to aid in decision making. Patients with a plausible type I hypersensitivity reaction and positive skin testing are offered desensitization. For those patients with mild reactions and negative skin testing, we recommend a standard infusion with antihistamine and/or corticosteroid premedication. We do not offer desensitization if the patient's initial reaction involved signs or symptoms of erythema multiforme, Stevens–Johnson syndrome, toxic epidermal necrolysis, or serum sickness. Similarly, we do not offer drug desensitization if the adverse reaction was limited to a delayed maculopapular rash, in the absence of positive skin testing.

Desensitization has been previously described in case reports or small series for rituximab, infliximab, trastuzumab, muromonab, cetuximab, and omalizumab [20, 46, 62–67]. Protocols that have been published vary, as does the success rate of desensitization. At Brigham and Women's hospital, we have had experience with successful desensitization to rituximab, infliximab, and trastuzumab, a manuscript describing our experience with nearly 100 desensitizations to these agents is in press (Brennan et al. 2009). For this we used the same 12-step protocol described earlier for chemotherapeutic agents [20]. Mild reactions were observed in approximately one-third of desensitizations and rates of reaction were similar for all agents. As has been observed with small molecule chemotherapeutics, reactions during desensitization mirror those seen during the initial reaction, but at a greatly reduced severity. For future desensitizations, protocols are tailored to address reactions experienced during desensitization.

### *19.10.1 Cetuximab – An Unexpected Mechanism for Hypersensitivity*

Cetuximab [68] is a recombinant human/mouse chimeric monoclonal antibody that binds to the epidermal growth factor receptor (EGFR) thereby competitively inhibiting the binding of epidermal growth factor. This interference with the binding of EGF inhibits cell growth, induces apoptosis, and decreases matrix metalloproteinase and vascular endothelial growth factor production in those cells that overexpress EGFR [68]. Cetuximab was approved for the treatment of metastatic colon cancer in 2004 and squamous cell cancer of the head and neck in 2006.

Use of cetuximab is associated with a 2–5% incidence of severe hypersensitivity reactions [68]. Reactions may include rapid onset airway obstruction (bronchospasm, stridor, hoarseness), hypotension, and/or cardiac arrest. Approximately 90% of these severe infusion reactions are noted to occur with the first infusion despite premedication with antihistamines. There have also been reports of dermatological reactions including acneiform eruptions [68]. One case of fatal toxic epidermal necrolysis was reported in 2008 [69].

A group of investigators noted a higher rate of severe hypersensitivity reactions occurring in the southeastern USA. In the states of Arkansas, Missouri, Virginia, and Tennessee, the rate of severe infusion reactions approaches 22% [59]. An analysis of pretreatment serum samples showed that 17 of 25 patients with hypersensitivity reactions during cetuximab therapy had IgE antibodies directed against cetuximab. Only one of 51 patients who tolerated their cetuximab infusions without a reaction had similar IgE antibodies. A detailed evaluation of the epitope bound by this anti-cetuximab IgE antibody revealed a specificity for the oligosaccharide galactose-alpha-1,3-galactose, which is present on the Fab portion of the cetuximab heavy chain, as well as other non-primate mammalian proteins. The overall prevalence of IgE antibodies directed against galactose-alpha-1,3-galactose was found to be higher in the southeastern USA, thus explaining the increased rate of severe hypersensitivity reactions to cetuximab in this area. The reason for the increased production of this particular antibody in this population has not been elucidated to date, but has also been reported to be associated with delayed anaphylaxis after consumption of red meat [70].

A desensitization protocol for cetuximab administration was described in a case report in 2009 [65]. The patient did have detectable IgE antibodies against cetuximab and was successfully desensitized using a 3-h intravenous protocol. Of note, she was challenged with cetuximab 1 week later and tolerated this infusion without need for repeat desensitization.

An alternative to desensitization is substitution with panitumumab, which is a fully humanized monoclonal antibody directed against EGFR and indicated to treat metastatic colorectal carcinoma. Panitumumab is produced in a different cell line from cetuximab and does not have the same glycosylation pattern. Therefore, it would not be expected to contain the galactose-alpha-1,3-galactose epitope [59]. There have been at least ten cases of successful use of panitumumab in patients who experienced hypersensitivity reactions to cetuximab [71–74].

## 19.11 Summary

For as long as humans have been using medications in the treatment of disease, sensitization to these medications has occurred. This was true of the earliest antibiotics and remains so with the newest monoclonal and chemotherapeutic agents. The mechanism underlying sensitization to chemotherapeutics is largely unknown but, as with the case of cetuximab, small parts of that story are starting to be revealed.

Almost since the first cases of allergy to medications were reported, successful drug desensitization protocols have been developed [75]. What began as a method of administering antibiotics to sensitized individuals for the treatment of life-threatening infectious disease has now become a means of safely treating numerous cancers and rheumatologic diseases with needed chemotherapies.

In this chapter, we have sought to review the fundamental aspects of skin testing and desensitization procedures as well as lay the foundation for how to safely administer these medications to sensitized individuals. Drawing on the extensive experience of the physicians of the Massachusetts

General Hospital and Brigham and Women's Hospital, we have illustrated the safety and efficacy of a 12-step drug desensitization procedure that can be used in other institutions. By instituting such a desensitization program under the direction of allergists, drug-allergic individuals will be able to safely receive otherwise restricted lifesaving chemotherapeutics and monoclonal antibodies.

## References


1. American Academy of Allergy, Asthma and Immunology. *The Allergy Report.* Vol 3. Conditions that may have an allergic component. Milwaukee:AAAAI; 2000.2.
2. Bochner BS, Lichtenstein LM. Anaphylaxis. *N Engl J Med.* 1991;324(25):1785–1790.
3. Solensky R. Drug desensitization. *Immunol Allergy Clin North Am.* 2004;24(3):425–443, vi.
4. Chisholm-Burns MA,Wells B, Schwinghammer T, et al. *Pharmacotherapy principles and practice.* Australia/ New Zealand: McGraw-Hill; 2007.
5. Macglashan D, Miura K. Loss of syk kinase during IgE-mediated stimulation of human basophils. *J Allergy Clin Immunol.* 2004;114(6):1317–1324.
6. Morales AR, Shah N, Castells M. Antigen-IgE desensitization in signal transducer and activator of transcription 6-deficient mast cells by suboptimal doses of antigen. *Ann Allergy Asthma Immunol.* 2005;94(5):575–580.
7. Weidmann B, Mulleneisen N, Bojko P, Niederle N. Hypersensitivity reactions to carboplatin. Report of two patients, review of the literature, and discussion of diagnostic procedures and management. *Cancer.* 1994;73(8):2218–2222.
8. Sood AK, Gelder MS, Huang SW, Morgan LS. Anaphylaxis to carboplatin following multiple previous uncomplicated courses. *Gynecol Oncol.* 1995;57(1):131–132.
9. Windom HH, McGuire WP3rd, Hamilton RG, Adkinson NF Jr. Anaphylaxis to carboplatin – a new platinum chemotherapeutic agent. *J Allergy Clin Immunol.* 1992;90(4Pt 1):681–683.
10. Broome CB, Schiff RI, Friedman HS. Successful desensitization to carboplatin in patients with systemic hypersensitivity reactions. *Med Pediatr Oncol.* 1996;26(2):105–110.
11. Goldberg A, Confino-Cohen R, Fishman A, Beyth Y, Altaras M. A modified, prolonged desensitization protocol in carboplatin allergy. *J Allergy Clin Immunol.* 1996;98(4):841–843.
12. Markman M, Zanotti K, Peterson G, Kulp B, Webster K, Belinson J. Expanded experience with an intradermal skin test to predict for the presence or absence of carboplatin hypersensitivity. *J Clin Oncol.* 2003;21(24):4611–4614.
13. Zanotti KM, Rybicki LA, Kennedy AW, et al. Carboplatin skin testing: A skin-testing protocol for predicting hypersensitivity to carboplatin chemotherapy. *J Clin Oncol.* 2001;19(12):3126–3129.
14. Lee CW, Matulonis UA, Castells MC. Rapid inpatient/outpatient desensitization for chemotherapy hypersensitivity: Standard protocol effective in 57 patients for 255 courses. *Gynecol Oncol.* 2005;99(2):393–399.
15. Dizon DS, Sabbatini PJ, Aghajanian C, Hensley ML, Spriggs DR. Analysis of patients with epithelial ovarian cancer or fallopian tube carcinoma retreated with cisplatin after the development of a carboplatin allergy. *Gynecol Oncol.* 2002;84(3):378–382.
16. Enrique E, Malek T, Castello JV, de Mateo JA. Usefulness of skin testing with platinum salts to demonstrate lack of cross-reactivity between carboplatin and cisplatin. *Ann Allergy Asthma Immunol.* 2008;100(1):86.
17. Leguy-Seguin V, Jolimoy G, Coudert B, et al. Diagnostic and predictive value of skin testing in platinum salt hypersensitivity. *J Allergy Clin Immunol.* 2007;119(3):726–730.
18. Fernando SL, Broadfoot AJ. Ondansetron anaphylaxis: A case report and protocol for skin testing. *Br J Anaesth.* 2009;102(2):285–286.
19. Weiss RB, Donehower RC, Wiernik PH, et al. Hypersensitivity reactions from taxol. *J Clin Oncol.* 1990;8(7):1263–1268.
20. Castells MC, Tennant NM, Sloane DE, et al. Hypersensitivity reactions to chemotherapy: Outcomes and safety of rapid desensitization in 413 cases. *J Allergy Clin Immunol.* 2008;122(3):574–580.
21. Breslow RG, Caiado J, Castells MC. Acetylsalicylic acid and montelukast block mast cell mediator-related symptoms during rapid desensitization. *Ann Allergy Asthma Immunol.* 2009;102(2):155–160.
22. Markman M, Kennedy A, Webster K, et al. Clinical features of hypersensitivity reactions to carboplatin. *J Clin Oncol.* 1999;17(4):1141.
23. Zweizig S, Roman LD, Muderspach LI. Death from anaphylaxis to cisplatin: A case report. *Gynecol Oncol.* 1994;53(1):121–122.
24. Robinson JB, Singh D, Bodurka-Bevers DC, Wharton JT, Gershenson DM, Wolf JK. Hypersensitivity reactions and the utility of oral and intravenous desensitization in patients with gynecologic malignancies. *Gynecol Oncol.* 2001;82(3):550–558.

25. Hesterberg PE, Banerji A, Oren E, et al. Risk stratification for desensitization of patients with carboplatin hypersensitivity: Clinical presentation and management. *J Allergy Clin Immunol.* 2009;123(6):1262–1267, e1.
26. Lee CW, Matulonis UA, Castells MC. Carboplatin hypersensitivity: A 6-h 12-step protocol effective in 35 desensitizations in patients with gynecological malignancies and mast cell/IgE-mediated reactions. *Gynecol Oncol.* 2004;95(2):370–376.
27. Bonosky K, Miller R. Hypersensitivity reactions to oxaliplatin: What nurses need to know. *Clin J Oncol Nurs.* 2005;9(3):325–330.
28. Saif MW. Hypersensitivity reactions associated with oxaliplatin. *Expert Opin Drug Saf.* 2006;5(5):687–694.
29. Gammon D, Bhargava P, McCormick MJ. Hypersensitivity reactions to oxaliplatin and the application of a desensitization protocol. *Oncologist.* 2004;9(5):546–549.
30. Polyzos A, Tsavaris N, Gogas H, et al. Clinical features of hypersensitivity reactions to oxaliplatin: A 10-year experience. *Oncology.* 2009;76(1):36–41.
31. Paclitaxel [package insert]. Princeton, NJ: Bristol-myers Squibb Company; 2007.
32. Docetaxel [package insert]. Bridgewater, NJ: Aventis Pharmaceuticals; 2003.
33. Crown J, O'Leary M. The taxanes: an update. *Lancet.* 2000;355(9210):1176–1178.
34. Fishman A, Gold T, Goldberg A, et al. Effective desensitization protocol to paclitaxel following hypersensitivity reaction. *Int J Gynecol Cancer.* 1999;9(2):156–159.
35. Feldweg AM, Lee CW, Matulonis UA, Castells M. Rapid desensitization for hypersensitivity reactions to paclitaxel and docetaxel: A new standard protocol used in 77 successful treatments. *Gynecol Oncol.* 2005;96(3):824–829.
36. Roy V, LaPlant BR, Gross GG, Bane CL, Palmieri FM, North Central Cancer Treatment Group. Phase II trial of weekly nab (nanoparticle albumin-bound)-paclitaxel (nab-paclitaxel) (abraxane) in combination with gemcitabine in patients with metastatic breast cancer (N0531). *Ann Oncol.* 2009;20(3):449–453.
37. Dillman RO. Infusion reactions associated with the therapeutic use of monoclonal antibodies in the treatment of malignancy. *Cancer Metastasis Rev.* 1999;18(4):465–471.
38. Calogiuri G, Ventura MT, Mason L, et al. Hypersensitivity reactions to last generation chimeric, umanized and human recombinant monoclonal antibodies for therapeutic use. *Curr Pharm Des.* 2008;14(27):2883–2891.
39. Byrd JC, Waselenko JK, Maneatis TJ, et al. Rituximab therapy in hematologic malignancy patients with circulating blood tumor cells: Association with increased infusion-related side effects and rapid blood tumor clearance. *J Clin Oncol.* 1999;17(3):791–795.
40. Curtis BR, Swyers J, Divgi A, McFarland JG, Aster RH. Thrombocytopenia after second exposure to abciximab is caused by antibodies that recognize abciximab-coated platelets. *Blood.* 2002;99(6):2054–2059.
41. Grillo-Lopez AJ, White CA, Varns C, et al. Overview of the clinical development of rituximab: First monoclonal antibody approved for the treatment of lymphoma. *Semin Oncol.* 1999;26(5 Suppl 14):66–73.
42. Baert F, Noman M, Vermeire S, et al. Influence of immunogenicity on the long-term efficacy of infliximab in crohn's disease. *N Engl J Med.* 2003;348(7):601–608.
43. Maini R, St Clair EW, Breedveld F, et al. Infliximab (chimeric anti-tumour necrosis factor alpha monoclonal antibody) versus placebo in rheumatoid arthritis patients receiving concomitant methotrexate: A randomised phase III trial. ATTRACT Study Group. *Lancet.* 1999;354(9194):1932–1939.
44. Soykan I, Ertan C, Ozden A. Severe anaphylactic reaction to infliximab: Report of a case. *Am J Gastroenterol.* 2000;95(9):2395–2396.
45. Cook-Bruns N. Retrospective analysis of the safety of herceptin immunotherapy in metastatic breast cancer. *Oncology.* 2001;61(Suppl 2):58–66.
46. Dreyfus DH, Randolph CC. Characterization of an anaphylactoid reaction to omalizumab. *Ann Allergy Asthma Immunol.* 2006;96(4):624–627.
47. Price KS, Hamilton RG. Anaphylactoid reactions in two patients after omalizumab administration after successful long-term therapy. *Allergy Asthma Proc.* 2007;28(3):313–319.
48. Polman CH, O'Connor PW, Havrdova E, et al. A randomized, placebo-controlled trial of natalizumab for relapsing multiple sclerosis. *N Engl J Med.* 2006;354(9):899–910.
49. Leonard PA, Woodside KJ, Gugliuzza KK, Sur S, Daller JA. Safe administration of a humanized murine antibody after anaphylaxis to a chimeric murine antibody. *Transplantation.* 2002;74(12):1697–1700.
50. Baudouin V, Crusiaux A, Haddad E, et al. Anaphylactic shock caused by immunoglobulin E sensitization after retreatment with the chimeric anti-interleukin-2 receptor monoclonal antibody basiliximab. *Transplantation.* 2003;76(3):459–463.
51. Hawkins C, Gatenby P, McGill D. Severe hypotension complicating primary angioplasty: Allergy to abciximab. *Allergy.* 2003;58(7):688–689.
52. Pharand C, Palisaitis DA, Hamel D. Potential anaphylactic shock with abciximab readministration. *Pharmacotherapy.* 2002;22(3):380–383.
53. Rituximab [product insert]. San Francisco, CA: Genentech; 2008.
54. Bush RK, Wood RA, Eggleston PA. Laboratory animal allergy. *J Allergy Clin Immunol.* 1998;102(1):99–112.

55. Park A, Edwards M, Donaldson M, Ghatei M, Meeran K. Lesson of the week: Interfering antibodies affecting immunoassays in woman with pet rabbits. *BMJ.* 2003;326(7388):541–542.
56. Platts-Mills TA, Satinover SM, Naccara L, et al. Prevalence and titer of IgE antibodies to mouse allergens. *J Allergy Clin Immunol.* 2007;120(5):1058–1064.
57. Matsui EC, Simons E, Rand C, et al. Airborne mouse allergen in the homes of inner-city children with asthma. *J Allergy Clin Immunol.* 2005;115(2):358–363.
58. Matsui EC, Wood RA, Rand C, Kanchanaraksa S, Swartz L, Eggleston PA. Mouse allergen exposure and mouse skin test sensitivity in suburban, middle-class children with asthma. *J Allergy Clin Immunol.* 2004;113(5):910–915.
59. Chung CH, Mirakhur B, Chan E, et al. Cetuximab-induced anaphylaxis and IgE specific for galactose-alpha-1,3-galactose. *N Engl J Med.* 2008;358(11):1109–1117.
60. Tratuzumab [product insert]. San Francisco, CA: Genentech; 2008.
61. Colombel JF, Loftus EV Jr, Tremaine WJ, et al. The safety profile of infliximab in patients with crohn's disease: The Mayo Clinic experience in 500 patients. *Gastroenterology.* 2004;126(1):19–31.
62. Duburque C, Lelong J, Iacob R, et al. Successful induction of tolerance to infliximab in patients with Crohn's disease and prior severe infusion reactions. *Aliment Pharmacol Ther.* 2006;24(5):851–858.
63. Georgitis JW, Browning MC, Steiner D, Lorentz WB. Anaphylaxis and desensitization to the murine monoclonal antibody used for renal graft rejection. *Ann Allergy.* 1991;66(4):343–347.
64. Lelong J, Duburque C, Fournier C, et al. Desensitisation to infliximab in patients with crohn's disease. *Rev Mal Respir.* 2005;22(2 Pt 1):239–246.
65. Jerath MR, Kwan M, Kannarkat M, et al. A desensitization protocol for the mAb cetuximab. *J Allergy Clin Immunol.* 2009;123(1):260–262.
66. Melamed J, Stahlman JE. Rapid desensitization and rush immunotherapy to trastuzumab (herceptin). *J Allergy Clin Immunol.* 2002;110(5):813–814.
67. Puchner TC, Kugathasan S, Kelly KJ, Binion DG. Successful desensitization and therapeutic use of infliximab in adult and pediatric Crohn's disease patients with prior anaphylactic reaction. *Inflamm Bowel Dis.* 2001;7(1):34–37.
68. Cetuximab [product insert]. Princeton, NJ: Bristol Myers Squibb; 2004.
69. Lin WL, Lin WC, Yang JY, et al. Fatal toxic epidermal necrolysis associated with cetuximab in a patient with colon cancer. *J Clin Oncol.* 2008;26(16):2779–2780.
70. Commins SP, Satinover SM, Hosen J, et al. Delayed anaphylaxis, angioedema, or urticaria after consumption of red meat in patients with IgE antibodies specific for galactose-alpha-1,3-galactose. *J Allergy Clin Immunol.* 2009;123(2):426–433.
71. Helbling D, Borner M. Successful challenge with the fully human EGFR antibody panitumumab following an infusion reaction with the chimeric EGFR antibody cetuximab. *Ann Oncol.* 2007;18(5):963–964.
72. Heun J, Holen K. Treatment with panitumumab after a severe infusion reaction to cetuximab in a patient with metastatic colorectal cancer: A case report. *Clin Colorectal Cancer.* 2007;6(7):529–531.
73. Nielsen DL, Pfeiffer P, Jensen BV. Six cases of treatment with panitumumab in patients with severe hypersensitivity reactions to cetuximab. *Ann Oncol.* 2009;20(4):798.
74. Saif MW, Peccerillo J, Potter V. Successful re-challenge with panitumumab in patients who developed hypersensitivity reactions to cetuximab: Report of three cases and review of literature. *Cancer Chemother Pharmacol.* 2009;63(6):1017–1022.
75. Garai F. Successful desensitization to penicillin. *J Am Med Assoc.* 1949;141(1):25.
76. Lee C-W, Matulonis UA, Castells MC. *Gynecologic oncology.* Carboplatin sensitivity: A 6-h 12-step protocol effective in 35 desensitiztions in patients with gynecological malignancies and mast-cell/IgE-mediated reactions. Salem, MA: Elsevier; 2004.

# Chapter 20
# Rapid Desensitizations for Antibiotic-Induced Hypersensitivity Reactions and Anaphylaxis

**Tito Rodriguez Bouza, Ross I. Palis, Henry J. Legere III, and Mariana C. Castells**

**Abstract** Drug-induced anaphylaxis prevents the utilization of antibiotic drugs to patients in need of first-line therapy, including those with cystic fibrosis. Avoidance of antibiotic therapy may be limited by the severity of the infection and the microbial sensitivity. Rapid desensitization for antibiotic-induced drug allergies is the induction of temporary clinical unresponsiveness to antibiotics by gradual reintroduction of small doses of antibiotic until the full antibiotic dose is delivered. Clinical unresponsiveness can be maintained until completion of the antibiotic course by regular administration of the antibiotic allowing safe administration of first-line medications to patients who have presented with hypersensitivity reactions to those medications, including anaphylaxis.

Principles, indications, targets and management of rapid desensitization procedures, including IgE- and non-IgE-dependent hypersensitivity reactions for the most relevant groups of antibiotics, antifungals and antivirals will be reviewed, and rapid desensitization protocols will be addressed for each group.

**Keywords** Anaphylaxis • Desensitization • Drug allergy • Drug hypersensitivity • Antibiotics • Hypersensitivity reactions • Penicillin • Beta-lactams

## 20.1 Introduction

Serious adverse drug reactions have been reported in 6.7% of hospitalized patients, and adverse drug reactions are the fourth to sixth leading cause of death in such patients [1]. Rapid intravenous desensitization for antibiotic-induced drug allergies allows for the safe administration of first-line medications to patients who have presented with IgE- and non-IgE-mediated reactions to those medications during prior administrations.

Drug-induced type I hypersensitivity reactions (HSRs), including anaphylaxis, result from the cross-linking of IgE on mast cells and basophils by drug antigens. This results in the activation of IgE-sensitized cells with subsequent release of allergic and inflammatory mediators. These mediators can cause limited skin reactions (flushing, pruritus, urticaria, angioedema) and/or multi-organ system involvement (sneezing, sinus and nasal congestion, cough, shortness of breath, wheezing, abdominal pain, nausea, vomiting, diarrhea) with hypotension and cardiovascular collapse during anaphylaxis.

Non-IgE-mediated HSRs can present with similar constellations of symptoms as type I HSRs without involving prior sensitization to the offending drug. Examples include vancomycin-induced

M.C. Castells (✉)
Harvard Medical School, Brigham and Women's Hospital, Boston, MA, USA
e-mail: mcastells@partners.org

M.C. Castells (ed.), *Anaphylaxis and Hypersensitivity Reactions*,
DOI 10.1007/978-1-60327-951-2_20, © Springer Science+Business Media, LLC 2011

red man syndrome, so-called anaphylactoid reactions to intravenous contrast dyes or reactions associated with the infusion of taxanes chemotherapy.

## 20.2 Definition of Rapid Intravenous Desensitization

Rapid intravenous desensitization is the induction of temporary immune tolerance to drug antigens in a relatively short time, typically 4 to12 h. It allows patients to be treated safely with medications to which they have presented with mast cell-mediated symptoms. The technique of rapid desensitization has been successful using different protocols at various institutions [2–6]. Protocols introduce small amounts of drug antigens that are escalated up to the full therapeutic dose. Nearly all rapid desensitization protocols are empiric and based on trial and error. A recent protocol developed at the Harvard Medical School teaching hospital, Brigham and Women's Hospital (BWH), is based on an *in vitro* model of precise escalating doses of antigen, which drives mast cells to unresponsiveness [7].

Desensitization is a temporary phenomenon that can be maintained as long as the antibiotic is given at regular therapeutic intervals based on the pharmacokinetics and half-life of the desensitizing antibiotic. An early report indicated that a nurse who was successfully desensitized to penicillin experienced urticaria when maintenance doses were changed and therapeutic blood levels were not maintained. Successful maintenance of desensitization was achieved when therapeutic blood levels were reinstituted [8].

## 20.3 Indications for Desensitization

### *20.3.1 Inclusion Criteria for Desensitization*

All type I HSRs, mediated by IgE antibodies leading to mast cell and basophil degranulation, are amenable to rapid desensitization. Type I HSRs to antibiotics are clinically defined as those occurring during or shortly after an antibiotic infusion and characterized by the following symptoms and signs grouped by organ system: cutaneous (flushing, pruritus, urticaria, angioedema), cardiovascular (chest pain, tachycardia, sense of impending doom, presyncope, syncope, hypertension, hypotension), respiratory (sneezing, nasal congestion, dyspnea, coughing, wheezing, oxygen desaturation), throat tightness, gastrointestinal (nausea, vomiting, abdominal pain, diarrhea, bloating) and neuromuscular (disorientation, hallucination, vision disturbances, ringing/pounding in ears, unusual taste, back pain, numbness/weakness). Generalized HSRs, including anaphylaxis, can be graded as mild (1), moderate (2), or severe (3) (Table 20.1) [9].

### *20.3.2 Type I HSRs (IgE-Mediated)*

Drug-induced type I HSRs result from the release of mediators from IgE-sensitized mast cells or basophils and can affect all organ systems, potentially leading to anaphylaxis and death. Disseminated intravascular coagulation and seizure-like activity are rare complications of anaphylaxis [10]. Retrospectively, finding an elevated tryptase in serum [11] and histamine in urine [12] can support the diagnosis. Epinephrine is the only treatment that can reverse anaphylaxis [13, 14].

Drug antigens can sensitize patients after multiple courses, and repeated exposures are needed for the development of specific IgE [15]. Sensitizing drugs can act as complete antigens, such as

**Table 20.1** Clinical features and severity grading of anaphylaxis (Adapted from [9])

| Grading system for generalized hypersensitivity reactions | |
|---|---|
| Grade 1, Mild[a]: Skin and subcutaneous tissues | Generalized erythema, urticaria, periorbital edema, or angioedema |
| Grade 2, Moderate: Respiratory, cardiovascular, or gastrointestinal involvement | Dyspnea, stridor, wheeze, nausea, vomiting, dizziness (presyncope), diaphoresis, or abdominal pain |
| Grade 3, Severe: Hypoxia, hypotension, or neurologic compromise | Cyanosis or $SpO2 \leq 92\%$ at any stage, hypotension ($SBP < 90$ mmHg in adults), confusion, collapse, LOC, or incontinence |

*SBP* systolic blood pressure, *LOC* loss of consciousness
[a]Mild reactions can be further subclassified into those with and without angioedema

insulin, or as haptens, which are coupled to a carrier protein, such as penicillin coupled to albumin [16]. Cross-linking of specific IgE bound to high-affinity IgE receptors, FcεRI (on mast cells or basophils), induce the activation of these cells with the subsequent release of membrane and granule mediators. Some of these mediators include vasoactive amines such as histamine, proteases such as tryptase, and proinflammatory and vasoactive prostaglandins and leukotrienes [17].

The diagnosis of type I HSRs to drugs relies on the demonstration of *in vivo* or *in vitro* drug-specific IgE. Skin testing to drug antigens, such as penicillin, has a very high negative predictive value, as only 1.8 to 3% of patients with negative skin tests developed reactions that were mild and limited to the skin on drug re-exposure in series evaluated in the United States [18–20]. Recent European data indicated that 17.4% of patients with negative skin testing to beta-lactam reagents reacted on oral challenge [21].Positive predictive values of beta-lactam skin testing ranges from 50 to 70% in patients with a clinical history of type I HSR to this class of antibiotics [22, 23].

### *20.3.3 HSRs – Non-IgE-Mediated*

HSRs induced by drug antigens on initial exposure, without prior sensitization and with a similar clinical presentation to IgE-mediated HSRs reactions (including anaphylaxis) are considered non-IgE-mediated HSRs. Such adverse reactions respond to epinephrine and antihistamines in the same fashion as IgE-mediated HSRs, indicating that mast cells and/or basophil mediators are responsible for most of the acute symptomatology. Classic examples include adverse reactions to hyperosmolar preparations of iodinated radiocontrast media [24] and vancomycin-induced "red man syndrome" [25].

### *20.3.4 Adverse Reactions Not Amenable to Desensitization*

Patients with adverse reactions to antibiotics manifested as erythema multiforme, Stevens – Johnson syndrome (SJS), toxic epidermal necrolysis (TEN), exfoliative dermatitis, hemolytic anemias, interstitial nephritis or DRESS (drug rash with eosinophilia and systemic symptoms) syndrome are not amenable to desensitization. Only a few case reports of desensitization to antiretroviral, antitubercular, and antifungal medications in patients presenting with serum-sickness-like HSRs have been published and have shown variable success [26–30]. Some patients with type IV (cell-mediated) HSRs have undergone successful desensitization using long protocols lasting several days to weeks, for which the mechanism is unknown.

#### 20.3.4.1 Cellular and Molecular Targets

Mast cells and/or basophils are thought to be the major cellular targets of desensitization, since suboptimal doses of antigen administered prior to an optimal dose renders those cells unresponsive to antigen but not to other activating stimuli [7, 31]. Suboptimal doses can provide excessive monomeric antigen incapable of cross-linking surface FcεRI receptors [32] or can induce rapid internalization of antigen cross-linked receptors, thereby depleting the cell surface of these receptors [33]. Basophils can be desensitized *in vitro* to penicillin, but basophils isolated from a patient desensitized to penicillin were activated *in vitro* by penicillin antigens [34], indicating that the continued presence of antigens is critical to maintaining the state of desensitization.

*In vitro* rapid desensitization of human mast cells induces decreased levels of signal-transducing molecules, such as syk, because of ubiquitination and degradation [35, 36]. Naturally occurring syk-deficient basophils are unresponsive to drug antigens, indicating that syk is critical for activation [37]. In recent studies, STAT-6, which is responsible for the transcription of IL-4 and IL-13, has been shown to be important in the mechanism of rapid desensitization. STAT-6-deficient mast cells are capable of releasing mediators during the early phase of IgE-mediated mast cell activation but cannot release late-phase cytokines, such as TNF-α and IL-6, and cannot be desensitized to antigens [7, 38].

#### 20.3.4.2 Principles and Protocols of Rapid Desensitization

The goal of rapid desensitization is to induce tolerization with few or no side effects while escalating to the therapeutic dose. Although nearly all desensitization protocols are empiric and based on trial-and-error clinical experiences, *in vitro* desensitization of mast cells and basophils has provided some understanding of the mechanisms underlying successful *in vivo* desensitizations. An initial dose is established based on the predetermined target dose, followed by incremental dose escalations delivered at fixed time intervals (typically between 10 and 30 min) until the target dose is attained. Based on *in vitro* observations, twofold or threefold dose escalations at each time interval has been more successful at reducing side effects than tenfold dose escalation [7, 39].

Tolerization is maintained only if drug antigens are administered at regular intervals [8]. Pharmacokinetics of each antibiotic dictates the intervals, and if two interval half-lives are exceeded, the patient may require repeat desensitization.

#### 20.3.4.3 Symptoms During the Desensitization and Their Management

Signs and symptoms of a type I HSR that may occur during rapid antibiotic desensitization range in their magnitude of severity. Most reactions are limited to isolated cutaneous signs and symptoms, such as flushing, pruritus, urticaria, and/or angioedema. However, these findings may be accompanied by (or present solely as) extracutaneous systemic manifestations involving the cardiovascular (chest pain, tachycardia, bradycardia, sense of impending doom, presyncope, syncope, hypertension, hypotension), respiratory (sneezing, nasal congestion, coughing, throat tightness, dysphonia), gastrointestinal (nausea, vomiting, abdominal cramping, diarrhea), and/or neuromuscular (disorientation, hallucination, vision disturbances, ringing/pounding in ears, unusual taste, back pain, numbness/weakness) systems.

If the patient develops any of these signs or symptoms during the desensitization procedure, the protocol should be temporarily halted until the patient has been treated appropriately and the symptoms have resolved. Typically, this involves turning off the intravenous infusion pump for a period of approximately 20–30 min while antihistamines (sometimes in combination with corticosteroids) are administered to curtail the symptoms. Although rare, epinephrine may be required to treat a severe systemic reaction occurring during rapid desensitization. Careful attention should be paid to the specific protocol step(s) during which the reaction occurred and all medical interventions performed, and this information should be documented in the clinical record for retrospective review. Once the symptoms have resolved and the patient is clinically stable, the protocol can be resumed safely. Some clinicians resume the protocol at the step prior to which the reaction occurred or at the beginning of the step during which the reaction occurred. Others, including those at our institution, resume at the exact point where the infusion was stopped. In nearly all cases, rapid intravenous desensitization protocols are completed, thereby allowing patients to receive the full dose of the intended medication [2, 5].

Should the patient require a future administration of the antibiotic, his or her desensitization reaction history is reviewed and the next protocol will be modified in order to minimize the risk of further HSRs by adding premedications and/or insert extra steps prior to the step during which the reaction previously occurred.

#### 20.3.4.4 Safety Measures

Rapid intravenous desensitization should only be performed by board-certified allergists familiar with the procedure and with the recognition and treatment of anaphylaxis. Medications and equipment for cardiopulmonary resuscitation and the treatment of anaphylaxis should always be present at the bedside. The patient should have one-to-one nursing, and vital signs should be checked at regular intervals. A physician should be present for the initiation of the procedure and be closely available should any reactions occur during the desensitization. The patient usually undergoes the initial procedure in an intensive-care setting; however, subsequent protocols on the same patient using the same antibiotic can be safely performed in an outpatient setting or, in special cases, by way of home infusion pump. We were unable to identify any reported fatalities in patients undergoing intravenous desensitizations to penicillins or non-penicillin beta-lactam antibiotics [2, 5].

Ideally, patients should be stable prior to initiation of a rapid intravenous desensitization procedure, but in patients with cystic fibrosis (CF) complicated by severe obstructive lung disease and/or imminent lung transplantation, successful antibiotic desensitizations have been well tolerated [5]. Additionally, clinicians should exercise caution if a patient being evaluated for desensitization is taking beta-adrenergic receptor antagonists, and these medications should be discontinued if possible. Pretreatment with systemic corticosteroids is not advised during the initial desensitization procedure unless the patient has an underlying illness that necessitates its administration. However, if the patient has repeatedly required corticosteroids during past desensitizations, they may be administered prospectively to curtail anticipated reactions. Regarding antihistamines, there is controversy as to whether or not premedication is initially warranted. On the one hand, there is legitimate concern that antihistamines may mask the early, cutaneous symptoms of an eventual systemic and potentially life-threatening reaction. On the other hand, evidence taken from subcutaneous immunotherapy suggests that pre-administration of antihistamines can decrease systemic reactions and could make patients more comfortable during their desensitization procedure.

#### 20.3.4.5 Beta-Lactams

The incidence of self-reported penicillin allergy is as high as 10% of the population of the United States [40]. However, as low as 1% of these self-reported cases demonstrate objective evidence of IgE-mediated hypersensitivity via penicillin skin testing [41].

Penicillin skin testing, performed by epicutaneous and intradermal methods, should ideally include both the major (benzylpenicilloyl) and minor determinants (penicillin G and/or minor determinant mix [MDM]). Standardized penicillin major determinant skin testing reagents have not been commercially available in the United States from 2004 through the time of this review, and MDMs have never been standardized but have been used in large penicillin trials. Previous studies have determined the positive predictive value of penicillin skin testing to be 50–70% [22, 23] while the negative predictive value ranges from 97% to 99% in the United States to 82.6% in a recent European study using different reagents [21–23, 40].

Additionally, specific IgE measurement detecting major determinants in serum is available, with positive predictive values of 45.5% and negative predictive values of 77.1% using the CAP system [42]. Sensitivity and specificity of this *in vitro* testing method has been determined to be 38–54% and 87–100%, respectively [43, 44] . If both skin testing and CAP testing are negative, it is very likely that the patient in question can safely receive penicillin; however, an oral medication challenge is strongly recommended to confirm the lack of reactivity [45]. Patients who are truly allergic to penicillin are at risk for a type I HSR to cephalosporin antibiotics, with a reported reaction rate of 4–11%. In most cases, this has been attributed to the common beta-lactam ring structure, especially in the case of first- and second-generation cephalosporins. Specific IgE antibodies can also be directed against the side chains of cephalosporins rather than the beta-lactam ring, which poses a far less risk of adverse reaction in penicillin-allergic patients. Interestingly, both the monobactams and carbapenem [46] classes of antibiotics also contain beta-lactam rings but exhibit no significant cross-reactivity with penicillin. However, patients with an allergy to ceftazidime (a third-generation cephalosporin) are at risk for HSR to aztreonam (a monobactam), as both antibiotics share a common side chain.

Patients with a clinical history suggestive of IgE-mediated hypersensitivity to penicillin and positive skin and/or blood testing to the major and/or minor penicillin determinants are good candidates for drug desensitization if a beta-lactam antibiotic is determined to be a first-line treatment for their infection.

The decision regarding whether or not a patient requires desensitization to a non-penicillin beta-lactam antibiotic is based primarily on the clinical history. The non-irritating concentrations for cephalosporins have been published but not standardized [47] and the positive and negative predictive values of these tests have not been validated. Recent recommendations by the American Academy of Allergy, Asthma and Immunology (AAAAI) Adverse Reactions to Drugs, Biologicals, and Latex Committee have been released [47]. In those cases where readministration of the antibiotic is warranted and the patient has a convincing history suggesting a type I HSR, he or she should undergo rapid intravenous desensitization.

A typical protocol for desensitization starts at 1/10,000 to 1/100 of the target dose, and doubling doses are delivered every 15–20 min over the course of several hours until reaching the target dose [6, 48, 49]. Protocols for oral and intravenous penicillin desensitization are shown in Tables 20.2 and 20.3.

Ceftazidime desensitization was done in seven cystic fibrosis patients to treat IgE-mediated HSRs with no major systemic reactions during desensitization [50]. Cefotaxime desensitization was done in a 51-year-old man with bacterial spondylitis, and the treatment was continued for 4 weeks with no adverse events [51]. Eight patients with positive skin tests to penicillin and cephalosporins (cefepime, ceftriaxone, cefazolin) were desensitized to beta-lactam antibiotics using a 2 h 15 min protocol, during which threefold escalating doses were administered every 15 min without major side effects [52]. An imipenem-allergic patient was desensitized to intravenous imipenem for multidrug resistant *Acinetobacter pneumoniae* and the treatment was continued for 21 days without adverse events [53].

Beta-lactam antibiotic hypersensitivity and the consequent need for rapid desensitization pose a unique problem in patients with CF, as over 30% of this population develops HSRs to this class of

**Table 20.2** Oral penicillin V desensitization (Adapted from [6])

| Step | Penicillin concentration (Units/mL) | Units | Cumulative dose (units) |
|---|---|---|---|
| 1. | 1,000 | 100 | 100 |
| 2. | 1,000 | 200 | 300 |
| 3. | 1,000 | 400 | 700 |
| 4. | 1,000 | 800 | 1,500 |
| 5. | 1,000 | 1,600 | 3,100 |
| 6. | 1,000 | 3,200 | 6,300 |
| 7. | 1,000 | 6,400 | 12,700 |
| 8. | 10,000 | 12,000 | 24,700 |
| 9. | 10,000 | 24,000 | 48,700 |
| 10. | 10,000 | 48,000 | 96,700 |
| 11. | 80,000 | 80,000 | 176,700 |
| 12. | 80,000 | 160,000 | 336,700 |
| 13. | 80,000 | 320,000 | 656,700 |
| 14. | 80,000 | 640,000 | 1,296,700 |

Interval between doses: 15 min

**Table 20.3** Intravenous penicillin desensitization (Adapted from [48])

| Step | Penicillin concentration (mg/mL) | Flow rate (mL/h) | Amount (mg) | Cumulative dose (mg) |
|---|---|---|---|---|
| 1. | 0.01 | 6 | 0.015 | 0.015 |
| 2. | 0.01 | 12 | 0.03 | 0.045 |
| 3. | 0.01 | 24 | 0.06 | 0.105 |
| 4. | 0.1 | 5 | 0.125 | 0.23 |
| 5. | 0.1 | 10 | 0.25 | 0.48 |
| 6. | 0.1 | 20 | 0.5 | 1 |
| 7. | 0.1 | 40 | 1 | 2 |
| 8. | 0.1 | 80 | 2 | 4 |
| 9. | 0.1 | 160 | 4 | 8 |
| 10. | 10 | 3 | 7.5 | 15 |
| 11. | 10 | 6 | 15 | 30 |
| 12. | 10 | 12 | 30 | 60 |
| 13. | 10 | 25 | 62.5 | 123 |
| 14. | 10 | 50 | 125 | 250 |
| 15. | 10 | 100 | 250 | 500 |
| 16. | 10 | 200 | 500 | 1,000 |

Interval between doses: 15 min

antibiotics, particularly antipseudomonal penicillin derivatives and cephalosporins, due to repeated exposures. Rapid antibiotic desensitization in this patient population has also proven to be challenging, with approximate 25% desensitization failure rates reported in previous case series using empiric protocols [54, 55]. We recently evaluated a case series of 15 CF patients with clinical histories of type I HSRs to antibiotics undergoing 52 antibiotic desensitizations, 44 (85%) to beta-lactams, using a standardized protocol modeled after the BWH three-solution, 12-step chemotherapy desensitization protocol [2] and reported a 100% protocol completion rate [5]. Of note, a subset of patients who tolerated the desensitization procedure without complications subsequently developed signs and symptoms of HSRs during administration of full-strength antibiotic doses. This observation led us to modify subsequent protocols by adjusting the concentration (hence the bag volume) of the strongest solution (Solution 3 in most cases) to match the concentration typically administered to nonallergic patients (see Table 20.4a, b, c). This modification resulted in improved tolerability of full-strength antibiotic doses in these patients following desensitization and has since been implemented successfully in non-CF patients with antibiotic hypersensitivity (Table 20.4).

**Table 20.4** Cephalosporin desensitization (Adapted from [5])

(a) 12-Step protocol using solution volumes of 250 mL

| Name of medication: Ceftazidime | | | | | Total mg/bag | Amount of bag infused (mL) |
|---|---|---|---|---|---|---|
| Solution 1 | 250 mL of 0.080 mg/mL | | | | 20.00 | 9.25 |
| Solution 2 | 250 mL of 0.800 mg/mL | | | | 200.00 | 18.75 |
| Solution 3 | 250 mL of 7.937 mg/mL | | | | 1,984.26 | 250.00 |
| Step | Solution | Rate (mL/h) | Time (min) | Volume infused per step ( mL) | Dose administered with this step (mg) | Cumulative dose (mg) |
| 1. | 1 | 2.0 | 15 | 0.50 | 0.040 | 0.040 |
| 2. | 1 | 5.0 | 15 | 1.25 | 0.100 | 0.140 |
| 3. | 1 | 10.0 | 15 | 2.50 | 0.200 | 0.340 |
| 4. | 1 | 20.0 | 15 | 5.00 | 0.400 | 0.740 |
| 5. | 2 | 5.0 | 15 | 1.25 | 1.000 | 1.740 |
| 6. | 2 | 10.0 | 15 | 2.50 | 2.000 | 3.740 |
| 7. | 2 | 20.0 | 15 | 5.00 | 4.000 | 7.740 |
| 8. | 2 | 40.0 | 15 | 10.00 | 8.000 | 15.740 |
| 9. | 3 | 10.0 | 15 | 2.50 | 19.843 | 35.583 |
| 10. | 3 | 20.0 | 15 | 5.00 | 39.685 | 75.268 |
| 11. | 3 | 40.0 | 15 | 10.00 | 79.370 | 154.638 |
| 12. | 3 | 80.0 | 174.375 | 232.50 | 1,845.362 | 2,000.000 |

(b) 12-Step protocol using solution volumes of 100 mL

| Name of medication: Ceftazidime | | | | | Total mg/bag | Amount of bag infused (mL) |
|---|---|---|---|---|---|---|
| Solution 1 | 100 mL of 0.200 mg/mL | | | | 20.00 | 9.25 |
| Solution 2 | 100 mL of 2.000 mg/mL | | | | 200.00 | 18.75 |
| Solution 3 | 100 mL of 19.607 mg/mL | | | | 1,960.65 | 250.00 |
| Step | Solution | Rate (mL/h) | Time (min) | Volume infused per step (mL) | Dose administered with this step (mg) | Cumulative dose (mg) |
| 1 . | 1 | 2.0 | 15 | 0.50 | 0.100 | 0.100 |
| 2 . | 1 | 5.0 | 15 | 1.25 | 0.250 | 0.350 |
| 3 . | 1 | 10.0 | 15 | 2.50 | 0.500 | 0.850 |
| 4 . | 1 | 20.0 | 15 | 5.00 | 1.000 | 1.850 |
| 5 . | 2 | 5.0 | 15 | 1.25 | 2.500 | 4.350 |
| 6 . | 2 | 10.0 | 15 | 2.50 | 5.000 | 9.350 |
| 7 . | 2 | 20.0 | 15 | 5.00 | 10.000 | 19.350 |
| 8 . | 2 | 40.0 | 15 | 10.00 | 20.000 | 39.350 |
| 9 . | 3 | 10.0 | 15 | 2.50 | 49.016 | 88.366 |
| 10 . | 3 | 20.0 | 15 | 5.00 | 98.0325 | 186.399 |
| 11 . | 3 | 40.0 | 15 | 10.00 | 196.065 | 382.464 |
| 12 . | 3 | 80.0 | 61.87 | 82.50 | 1,617.536 | 2,000.00 |

(continued)

**Table 20.4** (continued)

(c) 16-Step protocol using solution volumes of 20 mL

| Name of medication: Cefepime | | | | | Total mg/bag | Amount of bag infused (mL) |
|---|---|---|---|---|---|---|
| Solution 1 | | 20 mL of 0.100 mg/mL | | | 2.00 | 1.87 |
| Solution 2 | | 20 mL of 1.000 mg/mL | | | 20.00 | 3.75 |
| Solution 3 | | 20 mL of 10.000 mg/mL | | | 200.30 | 7.50 |
| Solution 4 | | 20 mL of 96.053 mg/mL | | | 1,921.30 | 20.00 |
| Step | Solution | Rate (mL/h) | Time (min) | Volume infused per step (mL) | Dose administered with this step (mg) | Cumulative dose (mg) |
| 1. | 1 | 0.5 | 15 | 0.12 | 0.013 | 0.013 |
| 2. | 1 | 1 | 15 | 0.25 | 0.025 | 0.038 |
| 3. | 1 | 2 | 15 | 0.50 | 0.050 | 0.088 |
| 4. | 1 | 4 | 15 | 1.00 | 0.100 | 0.188 |
| 5. | 2 | 1 | 15 | 0.25 | 0.250 | 0.438 |
| 6. | 2 | 2 | 15 | 0.50 | 0.500 | 0.938 |
| 7. | 2 | 4 | 15 | 1.00 | 1.000 | 1.938 |
| 8. | 2 | 8 | 15 | 2.00 | 2.000 | 3.938 |
| 9. | 3 | 2 | 15 | 0.50 | 5.000 | 8.938 |
| 10. | 3 | 4 | 15 | 1.00 | 10.000 | 18.938 |
| 11. | 3 | 8 | 15 | 2.00 | 20.000 | 38.938 |
| 12. | 3 | 16 | 15 | 4.00 | 40.000 | 78.938 |
| 13. | 4 | 4 | 15 | 1.00 | 96.053 | 174.991 |
| 14. | 4 | 10 | 15 | 2.50 | 240.133 | 415.123 |
| 15. | 4 | 20 | 15 | 5.00 | 480.266 | 895.389 |
| 16. | 4 | 40 | 17.25 | 11.50 | 1,104.611 | 2,000.000 |

(a) Total time = 339.37 min (5 h 39 min)
(b) Total time = 226.875 min (3 h 46 min)
(c) Total time = 242.25 min (4 h 2 min)

#### 20.3.4.6 Glycopeptides

Vancomycin is an antimicrobial agent that is often used as an alternative treatment for serious staphylococcal and streptococcal infections in patients with HSRs to beta-lactam antibiotics or whose infection failed to respond to beta-lactam antibiotics.

The incidence of adverse reactions has been reported to be in the range of 5–14% in adults, with the most common manifestation as the red man syndrome (RMS), thought to be due to nonspecific histamine release [56]. Skin testing to vancomycin will likely produce false positive results due to direct degranulation of mast cells on intracutaneous administration [57], making it difficult to identify truly IgE-mediated reactions. Due to this direct release of histamine, an increased risk for an adverse reaction to vancomycin has been reported with the concurrent use of narcotics, some of which can also directly result in the degranulation of mast cells [58].

As such, desensitization should be considered in the cases of severe RMS reactions, which present with systemic life-threatening symptoms and are resistant to slow infusion rates.

Seven patients with serious staphylococcal infections resistant to beta-lactam antibiotics underwent a rapid continuous intravenous protocol described by Wong et al. (Table 20.5) without major side effects [58].

Slow desensitization protocols have been successfully administered on the next day after failure of single-day, short-course rapid desensitization protocols [59], although it is unclear if such success was achieved due to depletion of mast cells after the prior unsuccessful attempt or due to the protocol itself. Moreover, slow desensitization would require several days for serum concentrations to reach therapeutic levels and thus would increase the risk of emergence of vancomycin-resistant bacteria.

**Table 20.5** Vancomycin desensitization (Adapted from [58])

| Step | Vancomycin concentration (mg/mL) | Infusion rate (mL/min) | Cumulative dose (mg) |
|---|---|---|---|
| 1. | 0.0001 | 1.0 | 0 |
| 2. | 0.001 | 0.33 | 0.001 |
| 3. | 0.001 | 1.0 | 0.0043 |
| 4. | 0.01 | 0.33 | 0.0143 |
| 5. | 0.01 | 1.0 | 0.047 |
| 6. | 0.1 | 0.33 | 0.147 |
| 7. | 0.1 | 1.0 | 0.48 |
| 8. | 1.0 | 0.33 | 1.48 |
| 9. | 1.0 | 1.0 | 4.78 |
| 10. | 10.0 | 0.22 | 14.8 |
| 11. | 10.0 | 0.44 | 37 |

Interval between doses: 10 min
Intravenous administration

#### 20.3.4.7 Quinolones

Skin testing in quinolone hypersensitivity has not been standardized and positive predictive values are not available when using concentrations ranging from 0.02 to 0.000001 mg/mL [60–62]; therefore, challenge is the only reliable test to confirm the diagnosis. Quinolones share a common core structure across their class leading to evidence of clinical [63] and *in vitro* [64] IgE-mediated cross-reactivity among quinolones. A 35-year-old woman with chronic granulomatous disease and *Burkholderia cepacia* infection who twice developed immediate urticaria to intravenous ciprofloxacin was intravenously desensitized with no side effects, allowing an uneventful 4 weeks treatment (Table 20.6) [65]. A 15-year-old girl with CF and pulmonary infection with decline in pulmonary function developed urticaria over her scalp, face, and arms on the second day of her second course of ciprofloxacin and was successfully desensitized using an oral protocol [66]. A 28-month-old girl who developed an immediate reaction after ciprofloxacin administration, consisting of atypical symptoms including trembling, headache, tachycardia, flushing, fever (102.3 °F) and vomiting with positive intradermal test at 0.004 mg/mL was also successfully desensitized [62].

#### 20.3.4.8 Aminoglycosides

Tobramycin is used for the treatment of gram-negative infections, either via systemic infusion or topically, as in the case of nebulized aerosol for CF patients. Two case reports have been published regarding tobramycin desensitization, both in CF patients with type I HSRs and positive skin tests at non-irritating concentrations (Table 20.7) [67–69].

#### 20.3.4.9 Macrolides

The mechanism of HSRs to macrolide antibiotics remains unknown, and macrolide skin testing is negative in most cases [69]. A 68-year-old female with giant cell arteritis presented with a nodular cellulitis involving the lower extremities with *Mycobacterium chelonae* cultured from skin biopsy specimens. Clarithromycin is the treatment of choice for *M. chelonae* infection [70], but she reported anaphylaxis to erythromycin 20 years ago and bronchospasm with roxitromycin 5 years

**Table 20.6** Ciprofloxacin desensitization (Adapted from [65])

| Step | Ciprofloxacin concentration (mg/mL) | Volume (mL) | Amount (mg) | Cumulative dose (mg) |
|---|---|---|---|---|
| 1. | 0.1 | 0.1 | 0.01 | 0.01 |
| 2. | 0.1 | 0.2 | 0.02 | 0.03 |
| 3. | 0.1 | 0.4 | 0.04 | 0.07 |
| 4. | 0.1 | 0.8 | 0.08 | 0.15 |
| 5. | 1 | 0.16 | 0.16 | 0.31 |
| 6. | 1 | 0.32 | 0.32 | 0.63 |
| 7. | 1 | 0.64 | 0.64 | 1.27 |
| 8. | 2 | 0.6 | 1.2 | 2.47 |
| 9. | 2 | 1.2 | 2.4 | 4.87 |
| 10. | 2 | 2.4 | 4.8 | 9.67 |
| 11. | 2 | 5 | 10 | 19.67 |
| 12. | 2 | 10 | 20 | 39.67 |
| 13. | 2 | 20 | 40 | 79.67 |
| 14. | 2 | 40 | 80 | 159.67 |
| 15. | 2 | 120 | 240 | 399.67 |

Interval between doses: 15 min
Intravenous administration

**Table 20.7** Tobramycin desensitization (Adapted from [68])

| Step | Amount (mg) | Cumulative dose (mg) |
|---|---|---|
| 1. | 0.001 | 0.001 |
| 2. | 0.002 | 0.003 |
| 3. | 0.004 | 0.007 |
| 4. | 0.008 | 0.015 |
| 5. | 0.016 | 0.031 |
| 6. | 0.032 | 0.063 |
| 7. | 0.064 | 0.127 |
| 8. | 0.128 | 0.255 |
| 9. | 0.256 | 0.511 |
| 10. | 0.512 | 1.023 |
| 11. | 1 | 2.023 |
| 12. | 2 | 4.023 |
| 13. | 4 | 8.023 |
| 14. | 8 | 16.023 |
| 15. | 16 | 32.023 |
| 16. | 32 | 64.023 |
| 17. | 16 | 80.023 |

Interval between doses: 30 min
Intravenous administration

ago. Due to treatment resistance from alternative antibiotic combination therapy, she was successfully desensitized to clarithromycin using a rapid oral protocol (Table 20.8) [71].

#### 20.3.4.10 Linezolid

Linezolid is a member of the oxazolidinone class and is used for the treatment of serious infections caused by Gram-positive bacteria including streptococci, vancomycin-resistant enterococci, and methicillin-resistant *Staphylococcus aureus*. A 41-year-old woman who developed immediate generalized urticaria, flushing and facial swelling after re-exposure to linezolid was successfully desensitized with

**Table 20.8** Clarithromycin desensitization (Adapted from [71])

| Step | Clarithromycin suspension (mg/mL) | Volume (mL) | Amount (mg) | Cumulative dose (mg) |
|---|---|---|---|---|
| 1. | 0.05 | 0.1 | 0.005 | 0 |
| 2. | 0.05 | 0.2 | 0.01 | 0 |
| 3. | 0.05 | 0.4 | 0.02 | 0 |
| 4. | 0.05 | 1 | 0.05 | 0.1 |
| 5. | 0.05 | 2 | 0.1 | 0.2 |
| 6. | 0.05 | 4 | 0.2 | 0.4 |
| 7. | 0.5 | 0.8 | 0.4 | 0.8 |
| 8. | 0.5 | 1.6 | 0.8 | 1.6 |
| 9. | 0.5 | 3.2 | 1.6 | 3.2 |
| 10. | 0.5 | 6.4 | 3.2 | 6.4 |
| 11. | 5 | 1.2 | 6 | 12.4 |
| 12. | 5 | 2.4 | 12 | 24.4 |
| 13. | 5 | 4.8 | 24 | 48.4 |
| 14. | 50 | 1 | 50 | 98.4 |
| 15. | 50 | 2 | 100 | 198.4 |
| 16. | 50 | 4 | 200 | 398.4 |
| 17. | 50 | 8 | 400 | 798.4 |
| 18. | 50 | 10 | 500 | 1,298.4 |

Interval between doses: 15 min
Oral administration

**Table 20.9** Linezolid desensitization (Adapted from [72])

| Step | Linezolid concentration (mg/mL) | Volume (mL) | Amount (mg) | Cumulative dose (mg) |
|---|---|---|---|---|
| 1. | 0.0183 | 2 | 0.0366 | 0.0366 |
| 2. | 0.0549 | 2 | 0.0732 | 0.1098 |
| 3. | 0.1279 | 2 | 0.146 | 0.2558 |
| 4. | 0.2744 | 2 | 0.293 | 0.5488 |
| 5. | 0.5674 | 2 | 0.586 | 1.1348 |
| 6. | 1.1524 | 2 | 1.17 | 2.3048 |
| 7. | 1.548267 | 3 | 2.34 | 4.6448 |
| 8. | 1.86696 | 5 | 4.69 | 9.3348 |
| 9. | 1.87148 | 10 | 9.38 | 18.7148 |
| 10. | 2.500987 | 15 | 18.8 | 37.5148 |
| 11. | 3.000592 | 25 | 37.5 | 75.0148 |
| 12. | 3.000296 | 50 | 75 | 150.0148 |
| 13. | n/a | Tablet | 200 | 350.0148 |
| 14. | n/a | Tablet | 400 | 750.0148 |

Interval between doses: 20 min
Oral administration
Doses 1–12 compounded from intravenous solution of linezolid at 2 mg/mL

only mild cutaneous symptoms using an oral protocol with the intravenous solution, providing the 100% oral bioavailability of linezolid and followed by a successful 6-week treatment course (Table 20.9) [72].

#### 20.3.4.11 Antivirals (Including Antiretroviral Agents)

Reports on desensitization to antivirals have been described to enfuvirtide and acyclovir. The mechanism of HSRs to those agents is not well understood, but IgE has not been demonstrated.

**Table 20.10** Acyclovir desensitization (Adapted from [74])

| Step | Amount (mg) | Cumulative dose (mg) |
|---|---|---|
| 1. | 0.05 | 0.05 |
| 2. | 0.1 | 0.15 |
| 3. | 0.2 | 0.35 |
| 4. | 0.4 | 0.75 |
| 5. | 0.8 | 1.55 |
| 6. | 1.6 | 3.15 |
| 7. | 3.2 | 6.35 |
| 8. | 6.0 | 12.35 |
| 9. | 12.0 | 24.35 |
| 10. | 24.0 | 48.35 |
| 11. | 50.0 | 98.35 |
| 12. | 100.0 | 198.35 |
| 13. | 200.0 | 398.35 |
| 14. | 400.0 | 798.35 |

Interval between doses: 15 min
Oral administration

A 38-year-old woman with AIDS developed an erythematous maculopapular rash while on several antiretroviral medication regimens, including enfuvirtide in combination therapy. All medications were discontinued until her rash resolved and she subsequently developed an acute maculopapular rash following her next two doses of enfuvirtide. The patient was successfully desensitized [73].

A 65-year-old woman with AIDS complicated by recurrent mucocutaneous herpes simplex virus (HSV) infections developed acute swelling of the face and extremities, ocular pruritus, nausea, vomiting, and diarrhea following administration of her second course of oral acyclovir therapy. On rechallenge, cutaneous symptoms reappeared along with dysphagia, dysphonia, and wheezing. She was successfully desensitized using the following protocol (Table 20.10) [74].

#### 20.3.4.12 Antitubercular Drugs

Anaphylactic reactions to rifampin have been described, but the most common adverse event is a non-IgE-mediated "flu-like" syndrome that usually develops 1–4 h after exposure and is promoted by high-dose, intermitent and long intervals between doses [75]. Patients presenting with clinical histories consistent with type I HSRs and positive skin tests after determination of non-irritant concentrations to rifampin were successfully desensitized using a slow oral 7-day protocol [30]. A 45-year-old patient presented with urticaria, angioedema, and shortness of breath that required epinephrine and several hours later developed fever, chills, and arthralgias after rifampin re-exposure. The same patient presented with urticaria, angioedema, and chest heaviness after exposure to isoniazid with generalized pruritus on subsequent challenge. The patient was "double desensitized" to rifampin and isoniazid [29].

#### 20.3.4.13 Sulfonamides

Currently, the most frequently encountered sulfonamide antibiotic is the combination of trimethoprim and sulfamethoxazole (TMP-SMX). In patients with AIDS, where TMP-SMX is used as first-line therapy for the prophylaxis and treatment of *Pneumocystis jirovecii (carinii)* infection, cutaneous drug reactions to sulfonamides and sulfones (i.e. dapsone) are even more frequent than to penicillins, typically resulting in discontinuation of preferred therapy [76]. Sulfonamide metabolism via cytochrome P450 N-oxidation leads to N4-sulfonamidoyl haptenization, as well as to sulfonamide hydroxylamines and nitrososulfonamides, which are thought to be major haptenic antigens for allergic reactions to these drugs [48]. It is believed that HIV infection leads to impaired acetylation and/or glutathione deficiency states, thereby increasing the likelihood of this process [77]. HIV infection alone or infection with opportunistic organisms may also stimulate the activity of cytochrome P450 enzymes and lead to an increased rate of oxidation and production of reactive metabolites. Additionally, viral infections stimulate production of interferon-gamma, which causes increased expression of major histocompatibility complex (MHC) class I and class II cell surface molecules, including those on keratinocytes. This condition would favor the presentation of processed drug antigens on MHC molecules to drug-specific CD4+ and CD8+ T cells, resulting in delayed skin eruptions [48]. The typical TMP-SMX-induced reaction in HIV-positive patients occurs during the second week of treatment and consists of a generalized maculopapular eruption that is usually accompanied by fever and pruritus. The lack of a diagnostic skin or *in vitro* testing for TMP-SMX hypersensitivity in HIV-positive patients makes critical analysis of desensitizations difficult. As such, among a typical group of patients who undergo TMP-SMX desensitization, some individuals would not be truly allergic [48, 78]. Patients with more recent clinical histories of sulfonamide hypersensitivity are more likely to fail desensitization than those with remote histories of adverse reactions [79].

In a study performed in Italy utilizing a 36-h protocol, 79.5% of desensitized patients compared to 72% of rechallenged patients were able to tolerate treatment to TMP-SMX [78]. Among the limitations to this study was the exclusion of 14 of the 73 patients who reacted to TMP alone before rechallenge or desensitization. A more recent study in the United States was terminated prematurely by the Data and Safety Monitoring Board after observing rates of treatment success of 73% for the desensitization group (utilizing a 6-day dose escalation protocol) and only 54% for the rechallenge group [80]. Some researchers have found that low CD4+ counts are predictive of successful desensitization [81, 82], whereas others have found no such correlation [78, 83]. There have been no attempts to standardize TMP-SMX desensitization protocols, so no clear data support the selection of any single TMP-SMX desensitization protocol as being the most effective (Table 20.13). Moreover, comparison among protocols is difficult due to the different variables and populations among the studies undertaken (Tables 20.11–20.13) [84].

#### 20.3.4.14 Antifungals

Fluconazole and itraconazole have been reported to induce type I HSR-like reactions and successful desensitizations have been described. A 36-year-old male presented with a pruritic rash on day 4 of fluconazole therapy that reappeared on re-exposure. Due to treatment failure on itraconazole, desensitization was successfully performed utilizing a 15-day protocol. The previously described rash reappeared on days 4–6 of the desensitization protocol and disappeared when the dose was increased (Table 20.14) [87].

**Table 20.11** Trimethoprim-sulfamethoxazole desensitization (Adapted from [85])

| Step | TMP-SMX (mg of SMX/mL) | Amount (mL) | Dose (mg) |
|---|---|---|---|
| 1. | 4 | 0.25 | 1 |
| 2. | 4 | 1.0 | 4 |
| 3. | 40 | 0.5 | 20 |
| 4. | 40 | 2.0 | 80 |
| 5. | n/a | 1 tablet | 400 |

Interval between dose: 30 min
Oral administration

**Table 20.12** Trimethoprim-sulfamethoxazole desensitization (Adapted from [86])

| Day | TMP (mg) | SMX (mg) | Form |
|---|---|---|---|
| 1–3 | 20 | 100 | Liquid |
| 4–6 | 40 | 200 | Liquid |
| 7–9 | 60 | 300 | Liquid |
| 10–12 | 80 | 400 | Tablet |
| 13–15 | 120 | 600 | Tablet |
| 16–22 | 160 | 800 | Tablet |
| 23–25 | 240 | 1,200 | Tablet |
| 26–continue | 320 | 1,600 | Tablet |

Oral administration

**Table 20.13** Comparison of published Trimethoprim-sulfamethoxazole desensitization protocols (Adapted from [48])

| Study | Number of patients | Initial dose (SMX) | Number of steps | Total duration | Rate of success (%) |
|---|---|---|---|---|---|
| Absar et al. (1994 | 27 | 2 mg | 10 | 10 days | 85 |
| Gluckstein and Ruskin (1995) | 21 | 0.02 mg | 5 | 5 h | 71 |
| Nguyen et al. [1][a] | 45 | 10 ng | 40 | 36 h | 60 |
| Belchi-Hernandez et al. (1996, 1996) | 34 | 1 mg | 21 | 11 days | 79 |
| Kalanadhabhatta et al. (1996) | 13 | 20 ng | 37 | 27 h | 100 |
| Caumes et al. (1997) | 48 | 4 mg | 8 | 3 days | 77 |
| Rich et al. (1997) | 22 | 20 ng | 24 | 8 days | 86 |
| Ryan et al. (1998) | 14 | 2 mg | 33 | 33 days | 69 |
| Demoly et al. (1998) | 44 | 1 μg | 12 | 6 h | 95 |
| Bonfanti et al. [2][a] | 34 | 10 ng | 40 | 36 h | 79 |
| Yoshizawa et al. (2000) | 17 | 2 mg | 10 | 5 days | 88 |

[a]Same protocol used

**Table 20.14** Fluconazole desensitization (Adapted from [87])

| Step | Fluconazole concentration (mg/mL) | Dose | Amount (mg) |
|---|---|---|---|
| 1. | 1 | 0.2 mL | 0.2 |
| 2. | 1 | 0.4 mL | 0.4 |
| 3. | 1 | 0.8 mL | 0.8 |
| 4. | 1 | 1.6 mL | 1.6 |
| 5. | 1 | 3.2 mL | 3.2 |
| 6. | 1 | 6.4 mL | 6.4 |
| 7. | 10 | 1.0 mL | 10 |
| 8. | 10 | 2.0 mL | 20 |
| 9. | 10 | 4.0 mL | 40 |
| 10. | 50 mg | 1 tablet | 50 |
| 11. | 50 mg | 1 tablet | 100 |
| 12. | 50 mg | 3 tablet | 150 |
| 13. | 200 mg | 1 tablet | 200 |
| 14. | 100 mg | 3 tablet | 300 |
| 15. | 200 mg | 2 tablet | 400 |

Interval between doses: 24 h
Oral administration

A 30-year-old woman presented with a confluent, erythematous rash during a 1-week course of itraconazole, with skin clearance on discontinuation of the medication and reappearance of the lesions hours after reintroduction of the drug. Desensitization was successfully achieved following a 4.5-h protocol [88, 89].

## 20.4 Conclusions

Oral and intravenous rapid desensitization protocols are available to patients who develop IgE- and non-IgE-dependent HSRs to antibiotics, including anaphylaxis. The review outlined in this chapter demonstrates the myriad antibiotic classes to which desensitization protocols have been utilized – penicillins, non-penicillin beta-lactams (especially cephalosporins), glycopeptides, macrolides, quinolones, aminoglycosides, oxazolidinones, antivirals, antituberculars, antifungals and sulfonamides. Typical HSR signs and symptoms amenable to rapid desensitization include pruritus, flushing, urticaria, angioedema, respiratory and gastrointestinal distress and changes in blood pressure, with severe cases leading to hypotension and shock.

During rapid desensitization, drug antigens are reintroduced in an incremental fashion, allowing for full therapeutic doses to be delivered with minor or no side effects. When the antibiotic leading to these symptoms is penicillin or a cephalosporin, the mechanism is often IgE-mediated; however, other classes of antibiotics such as glycopeptides (e.g. vancomycin) can produce these symptoms in a non-IgE-dependent manner, and these reactions are also amenable to rapid desensitization. Temporary tolerization is achieved in hours and can be maintained if drug antigens are administered at regular intervals, depending on pharmacokinetic parameters.

Desensitization should only be done in settings with one-on-one nurse–patient care and where resuscitation personnel and resources are readily available. After a successful desensitization, repeated desensitizations can be done in outpatient or inpatient settings with similar conditions for patients on chemotherapy or monoclonal antibody therapies. This provides flexibility and allows patients to remain in clinical studies. Breakthrough symptoms during desensitization procedures are generally less severe than the initial HSR, and deaths have not been reported in the last 10 years due to a reaction during a desensitization procedure.

Managing breakthrough symptoms with antihistamines and steroids and decelerating the dose escalation with intermediate infusion steps successfully improves the tolerability of desensitization protocols. Blocking leukotrienes and prostaglandins has improved side effects.

Delayed, non-mast cell-mediated reactions occurring days to weeks after drug treatment, such as serum sickness, erythema multiforme, Stevens-Johnson syndrome and toxic epidermal necrolysis are not amenable for desensitization, and these drugs should generally not be reintroduced to the patient except in the most dire of circumstances where absolutely no alternative therapeutic options exist.

Education of nurses, pharmacists and oncology and allergy specialists will lead to the judicious use of desensitization protocols for patients with HSRs in need of first-line therapy. Basic research is needed to uncover the cellular and molecular mechanisms underlying the temporary tolerization induced by desensitization so that pharmacologic interventions can improve its safety and efficacy.

## References

1. Lazarou J, Pomeranz BH, Corey PN. Incidence of adverse drug reactions inhospitalized patients. *JAMA*. 279;1998:1200–1205.
2. Castells MC, Tennant NM, Sloane DE, et al. Hypersensitivity reactions to chemotherapy: outcomes and safety of rapid desensitization in 413 cases. *J Allergy Clin Immunol*. 2008;122(3):574–580.

3. Sullivan TJ, Yecies LD, Shatz GS, Parker CW, Wedner HJ. Desensitization of patients allergic to penicillin using orally administered beta-lactam antibiotics. *J Allergy Clin Immunol.* 1982;69(3):275–282.
4. Hesterberg PE, Banerji A, Oren E, et al. Risk stratification for desensitization of patients with carboplatin hypersensitivity: clinical presentation and management. *J Allergy Clin Immunol.* 2009;123(6):1262–1267, e1.
5. Legere HJ III, Palis RI, Bouza TR, Uluer AZ, Castells MC. A safe protocol for rapid desensitization in patients with cystic fibrosis and antibiotic hypersensitivity. *J Cyst Fibros.* 2009;8(6):418–424.
6. Wendel GD Jr, Stark BJ, Jamison RB, Molina RD, Sullivan TJ. Penicillin allergy and desensitization in serious infections during pregnancy. *N Engl J Med.* 1985;312(19):1229–1232.
7. Morales AR, Shah N, Castells M. Antigen-IgE desensitization in signal transducer and activator of transcription 6-deficient mast cells by suboptimal doses of antigen. *Ann Allergy Asthma Immunol.* 2005;94(5):575–580.
8. Naclerio R, Mizrahi EA, Adkinson NF Jr. Immunologic observations during desensitization and maintenance of clinical tolerance to penicillin. *J Allergy and Clin Immunol.* 1983;71(3):294–301.
9. Brown SG. Clinical features and severity grading of anaphylaxis. *J Allergy Clin Immunol.* 2004; 114(2):371–376.
10. Simons FE. Anaphylaxis. *J Allergy and Clin Immunol.* 2008;121(2 Suppl):S402-S407.
11. Schwartz LB, Metcalfe DD, Miller JS, Earl H, Sullivan T. Tryptase levels as an indicator of mast-cell activation in systemic anaphylaxis and mastocytosis. *N Engl J Med.* 1987;316(26):1622–1626.
12. Torres MJ, Blanca M, Fernandez J, et al. Selective allergic reaction to oral cloxacillin. *Clin Exper Allergy.* 1996;26(1):108–111.
13. Kemp SF, Lockey RF, Simons FE. Epinephrine: the drug of choice for anaphylaxis. A statement of the World Allergy Organization. *Allergy.* 2008;63(8):1061–1070.
14. Sampson HA, Munoz-Furlong A, Campbell RL, et al. Second symposium on the definition and management of anaphylaxis: summary report. Second National Institute of Allergy and Infectious Disease/Food Allergy and Anaphylaxis Network symposium. *J Allergy Clin Immunol.* 2006;117(2):391–397.
15. Solensky R. Drug hypersensitivity. *Med Clin NA.* 2006;90(1):233–260.
16. Zhao Y, Qiao H. Detection of specific IgE antibodies to major and minor antigenic determinants in sera of penicillin allergic patients. *Chin Med J (Engl).* 2003;116(12):1904–1910.
17. Castells M. Update on mast cells and mast cell precursors and hypersensitivity responses. *Allergy Asthma Proc.* 1997;18(5):287–292.
18. Pichichero ME, Pichichero DM. Diagnosis of penicillin, amoxicillin, and cephalosporin allergy: reliability of examination assessed by skin testing and oral challenge. *J Pediatr.* 1998;132(1):137–143.
19. Macy E, Burchette RJ. Oral antibiotic adverse reactions after penicillin skin testing: multi-year follow-up. *Allergy.* 2002;57(12):1151–1158.
20. Macy E, Mangat R, Burchette RJ. Penicillin skin testing in advance of need: multiyear follow-up in 568 test result-negative subjects exposed to oral penicillins. *J Allergy Clin Immunol.* 2003;111(5):1111–1115.
21. Bousquet PJ, Pipet A, Bousquet-Rouanet L, Demoly P. Oral challenges are needed in the diagnosis of beta-lactam hypersensitivity. *Clin Exp Allergy.* 2008;38(1):185–190.
22. Weiss ME, Adkinson NF. Immediate hypersensitivity reactions to penicillin and related antibiotics. *Clin Allergy.* 1988;18(6):515–540.
23. Solley GO, Gleich GJ, Van Dellen RG. Penicillin allergy: clinical experience with a battery of skin-test reagents. *J Allergy Clin Immunol.* 1982;69(2):238–244.
24. Sicherer SH. Risk of severe allergic reactions from the use of potassium iodide for radiation emergencies. *J Allergy Clin Immunol.* 2004;114(6):1395–1397.
25. Luskin AT, Luskin SS. Anaphylaxis and anaphylactoid reactions: diagnosis and management. *Am J Ther.* 1996;3(7):515–520.
26. DeSimone JA, Ojha A, Pathak R, Cohn J. Successful desensitization to enfuvirtide after a hypersensitivity reaction in an HIV-1-infected man. *Clin Infect Dis.* 2004;39(10):e110–112.
27. Dutau H, Saadjian M, Bonneau V, Charpin D. Unsuccessful rapid intravenous desensitization to rifampicin. *Allergy.* 2000;55(8):778–779.
28. Takahashi T, Hitani A, Yamada H, Nakamura T, Iwamoto A. Desenitization to fluconazole in an AIDS patient. *Ann Pharmacother.* 2001;35(5):642–643.
29. Holland CL, Malasky C, Ogunkoya A, Bielory L. Rapid oral desensitization to isoniazid and rifampin. *Chest.* 1990;98(6):1518–1519.
30. Buergin S, Scherer K, Hausermann P, Bircher AJ. Immediate hypersensitivity to rifampicin in 3 patients: diagnostic procedures and induction of clinical tolerance. *Int Arch Allergy Immunol.* 2006;140(1):20–26.
31. Pruzansky JJ, Patterson R. Desensitization of human basophils with suboptimal concentrations of agonist. Evidence for reversible and irreversible desensitization. *Immunology.* 1988;65(3):443–447.
32. Paolini R, Numerof R, Kinet JP. Phosphorylation/dephosphorylation of high-affinity IgE receptors: a mechanism for coupling/uncoupling a large signaling complex. *Proc Natl Acad Sci USA.* 1992;89(22):10733–10737.
33. Rubinchik E, Shalit M, Levi-Schaffer F. Responsiveness of human skin mast cells to repeated activation: an *in vitro* study. *Allergy.* 1998;53(1):14–19.

34. Pienkowski MM, Kazmier WJ, Adkinson NF Jr. Basophil histamine release remains unaffected by clinical desensitization to penicillin. *J Allergy Clin Immunol.* 1988;82(2):171–178.
35. Macglashan D, Miura K. Loss of syk kinase during IgE-mediated stimulation of human basophils. *J Allergy Clin Immunol.* 2004;114(6):1317–1324.
36. Odom S, Gomez G, Kovarova M, et al. Negative regulation of immunoglobulin E-dependent allergic responses by Lyn kinase. *J Exp Med.* 2004;199(11):1491–1502.
37. Kepley CL. Antigen-induced reduction in mast cell and basophil functional responses due to reduced Syk protein levels. *Int Arch Allergy Immunol.* 2005;138(1):29–39.
38. Malaviya R, Uckun FM. Role of STAT6 in IgE receptor/FcepsilonRI-mediated late phase allergic responses of mast cells. *J Immunol.* 2002;168(1):421–426.
39. Shalit M, Levi-Schaffer F. Challenge of mast cells with increasing amounts of antigen induces desensitization. *Clin Exp Allergy.* 1995;25(9):896–902.
40. Executive summary of disease management of drug hypersensitivity: a practice parameter. Joint Task Force on Practice Parameters, the American Academy of Allergy, Asthma and Immunology, the American Academy of Allergy, Asthma and Immunology, and the Joint Council of Allergy, Asthma and Immunology. *Ann Allergy Asthma Immunol.* 1999; 83(6Pt3):665–700.
41. Simpson AB, Murphy AW, Yousef E. The acceptability of a four-part protocol for penicillin allergy testing by practicing allergists. *Allergy Asthma Proc.* 2009;30(2):192–201.
42. Fontaine C, Mayorga C, Bousquet PJ, et al. Relevance of the determination of serum-specific IgE antibodies in the diagnosis of immediate beta-lactam allergy. *Allergy.* 2007;62(1):47–52.
43. Sanz ML, Gamboa PM, Antepara I, et al. Flow cytometric basophil activation test by detection of CD63 expression in patients with immediate-type reactions to betalactam antibiotics. *Clin Exp Allergy.* 2002;32(2):277–286.
44. Blanca M, Mayorga C, Torres MJ, et al. Clinical evaluation of Pharmacia CAP System RAST FEIA amoxicilloyl and benzylpenicilloyl in patients with penicillin allergy. *Allergy.* 2001;56(9):862–870.
45. Blanca M, Romano A, Torres MJ, et al. Update on the evaluation of hypersensitivity reactions to betalactams. *Allergy.* 2009;64(2):183–193.
46. Atanaskovic-Markovic M, Gaeta F, Gavrovic-Jankulovic M, Velickovic TC, Valluzzi RL, Romano A. Tolerability of imipenem in children with IgE-mediated hypersensitivity to penicillins. *J Allergy Clin Immunol.* 2009;124(1):167–169.
47. Solensky R. Bloomberg GR, Castells MC, et al. Cephalosporin Administration to Patients With a History of Penicillin Allergy. *Immunology.* AAoAA ed, 2009.
48. Solensky R. Drug desensitization. *Immunol Allergy Clin North Am.* 2004;24(3):425–443,vi.
49. Madaan A, Li JT. Cephalosporin allergy. *Immunol Allergy Clin NA.* 2004;24(3):463–476, vi-vii.
50. Ghosal S, Taylor CJ. Intravenous desensitization to ceftazidime in cystic fibrosis patients. *J Antimicrobial Chemother.* 1997;39(4):556–557.
51. Papakonstantinou G, Bogner JR, Hofmeister F, Hehlmann R. Cefotaxime desensitization. *Clin Invest.* 1993;71(2):165–167.
52. Win PH, Brown H, Zankar A, Ballas ZK, Hussain I. Rapid intravenous cephalosporin desensitization. *J Allergy Clin Immunol.* 2005;116(1):225–228.
53. Gorman SK, Zed PJ, Dhingra VK, Ronco JJ. Rapid imipenem/cilastatin desensitization for multidrug-resistant Acinetobacter pneumonia. *Ann Pharmacother.* 2003;37(4):513–516.
54. Burrows JA, Toon M, Bell SC. Antibiotic desensitization in adults with cystic fibrosis. *Respirology.* 2003;8(3):359–364.
55. Turvey SE, Cronin B, Arnold AD, Dioun AF. Antibiotic desensitization for the allergic patient: 5 years of experience and practice. *Ann Allergy Asthma Immunol.* 2004;92(4):426–432.
56. Lin RY. Desensitization in the management of vancomycin hypersensitivity. *Arch Intern Med.* 1990;150(10):2197–2198.
57. Polk RE, Israel D, Wang J, Venitz J, Miller J, Stotka J. Vancomycin skin tests and prediction of "red man syndrome" in healthy volunteers. *Antimicrob Agents Chemother.* 1993;37(10):2139–2143.
58. Wong JT, Ripple RE, Maclean JA, Marks DR, Bloch KJ. Vancomycin hypersensitivity: synergism with narcotics and "desensitization" by a rapid continuous intravenous protocol. *J Allergy Clin Immunol.* 1994;94(2Pt1):189–194.
59. Kitazawa T, Ota Y, Kada N, et al. Successful vancomycin desensitization with a combination of rapid and slow infusion methods. *Intern Med.* 2006;45(5):317–321.
60. Scherer K, Bircher AJ. Hypersensitivity reactions to fluoroquinolones. *Curr Allergy Asthma Rep.* 2005;5(1):15–21.
61. Venturini Diaz M, Lobera Labairu T, del Pozo Gil MD, Blasco Sarramian A, Gonzalez Mahave I. In vivo diagnostic tests in adverse reactions to quinolones. *J Investig Allergol Clin Immunol.* 2007;17(6):393–398.
62. Erdem G, Staat MA, Connelly BL, Assa'ad A. Anaphylactic reaction to ciprofloxacin in a toddler: successful desensitization. *Pediatr Infect Dis J.* 1999;18(6):563–564.
63. Davila I, Diez ML, Quirce S, Fraj J, De La Hoz B, Lazaro M. Cross-reactivity between quinolones. Report of three cases. *Allergy.* 1993;48(5):388–390.

64. Manfredi M, Severino M, Testi S, et al. Detection of specific IgE to quinolones. *J Allergy Clin Immunol.* 2004;113(1):155–160.
65. Gea-Banacloche JC, Metcalfe DD. Ciprofloxacin desensitization. *J Allergy Clin Immunol.* 1996;97(6):1426–1427.
66. Lantner RR. Ciprofloxacin desensitization in a patient with cystic fibrosis. *J Allergy Clin Immunol.* 1995;96(6Pt1):1001–1002.
67. Schretlen-Doherty JS, Troutman WG. Tobramycin-induced hypersensitivity reaction. *Ann Pharmacother.* 1995;29(7–8):704–706.
68. Earl HS, Sullivan TJ. Acute desensitization of a patient with cystic fibrosis allergic to both beta-lactam and aminoglycoside antibiotics. *J Allergy Clin Immunol.* 1987;79(3):477–483.
69. Araujo L, Demoly P. Macrolides allergy. *Curr Pharm Des.* 2008;14(27):2840–2862.
70. Brown-Elliott BA, Wallace RJ Jr. Clinical and taxonomic status of pathogenic nonpigmented or late-pigmenting rapidly growing mycobacteria. *Clin Microbiol Rev.* 2002;15(4):716–746.
71. Holmes NE, Hodgkinson M, Dendle C, Korman TM. Report of oral clarithromycin desensitization. *Br J Clin Pharmacol.* 2008; 66(2):323–324.
72. Cawley MJ, Lipka O. Intravenous linezolid administered orally: a novel desensitization strategy. *Pharmacotherapy.* 2006;26(4):563–568.
73. Shahar E, Moar C, Pollack S. Successful desensitization of enfuvirtide-induced skin hypersensitivity reaction. *AIDS.* 2005;19(4):451–452.
74. Henry RE, Wegmann JA, Hartle JE, Christopher GW. Successful oral acyclovir desensitization. *Ann Allergy.* 1993;70(5):386–388.
75. Martinez E, Collazos J, Mayo J. Hypersensitivity reactions to rifampin. Pathogenetic mechanisms, clinical manifestations, management strategies, and review of the anaphylactic-like reactions. *Medicine* (Baltimore). 1999;78(6):361–369.
76. Coopman SA, Johnson RA, Platt R, Stern RS. Cutaneous disease and drug reactions in HIV infection. *N Engl J Med.* 1993;328(23):1670–1674.
77. Dibbern DA Jr, Montanaro A. Allergies to sulfonamide antibiotics and sulfur-containing drugs. *Ann Allergy Asthma Immunol.* 2008;100(2):91–100; quiz 3,11.
78. Bonfanti P, Pusterla L, Parazzini F, et al. The effectiveness of desensitization versus rechallenge treatment in HIV-positive patients with previous hypersensitivity to TMP-SMX: a randomized multicentric study. C.I.S.A.I. Group. *Biomed Pharmacother.* 2000;54(1):45–49.
79. Choquet-Kastylevsky G, Vial T, Descotes J. Allergic adverse reactions to sulfonamides. *Curr Allergy Asthma Rep.* 2002;2(1):16–25.
80. Leoung GS, Stanford JF, Giordano MF, et al. Trimethoprim-sulfamethoxazole (TMP-SMZ) dose escalation versus direct rechallenge for Pneumocystis Carinii pneumonia prophylaxis in human immunodeficiency virus-infected patients with previous adverse reaction to TMP-SMZ. *J Infect Dis.* 2001;184(8):992–997.
81. Caumes E, Guermonprez G, Lecomte C, Katlama C, Bricaire F. Efficacy and safety of desensitization with sulfamethoxazole and trimethoprim in 48 previously hypersensitive patients infected with human immunodeficiency virus. *Arch Dermatol.* 1997;133(4):465–469.
82. Carr A, Penny R, Cooper DA. Efficacy and safety of rechallenge with low-dose trimethoprim-sulphamethoxazole in previously hypersensitive HIV-infected patients. *AIDS.* 1993;7(1):65–71.
83. Nguyen MT, Weiss PJ, Wallace MR. Two-day oral desensitization to trimethoprim-sulfamethoxazole in HIV-infected patients. *AIDS.* 1995;9(6):573–575.
84. Solensky R. Drug desensitization. *Immunol Allergy Clin NA.* 2004;24(3):425–443,vi.
85. Demoly P, Messaad D, Sahla H, et al. Six-hour trimethoprim-sulfamethoxazole-graded challenge in HIV-infected patients. *J Allergy Clin Immunol.* 1998;102(6Pt1):1033–1036.
86. White MV, Haddad ZH, Brunner E, Sainz C. Desensitization to trimethoprim sulfamethoxazole in patients with acquired immune deficiency syndrome and Pneumocystis carinii pneumonia. *Ann Allergy.* 1989;62(3):177–179.
87. Craig TJ, Peralta F, Boggavarapu J. Desensitization for fluconazole hypersensitivity. *J Allergy Clin Immunol.* 1996;98(4):845–846.
88. Douglas R, Spelman D, Czarny D, O'Hehir R. Desensitization to itraconazole. *J Allergy Clin Immunol.* 1997;99(2):269.
89. Bittleman DB, Stapleton J, Casale TB. Report of successful desensitization to itraconazole. *J Allergy Clin Immunol.* 1994;94(2Pt1):270–271.

# Chapter 21
# Induction of Tolerance for Food-Induced Anaphylaxis

**A. Wesley Burks and Pooja Varshney**

**Abstract** Anaphylaxis is the most severe manifestation of IgE-mediated food allergy, which has been linked to a loss of oral tolerance or a failure in the induction of tolerance. Oral tolerance is the physiologic mechanism by which immune responses to an antigen are suppressed by prior administration of the antigen by the oral route. This normal process is crucial in allowing a wide array of dietary proteins access to the body without activating harmful immune responses. A growing understanding of the factors involved in the development of oral tolerance has spurred recent studies investigating potential therapies targeting these pathways. Further work is necessary to define the molecular mechanisms involved in oral tolerance induction and to identify specific targets for immunomodulatory treatments. Definitive therapies for food allergy and food-induced anaphylaxis are on the horizon and will soon expand the treatment options available to individuals living with these diseases.

**Keywords** Anaphylaxis • Food allergy • Oral tolerance • Peanut allergy • Food-induced anaphylaxis

## 21.1 Introduction

Food allergy is the leading cause of anaphylaxis treated in emergency departments in Europe, Asia, and North America [1–3]. Studies have reported an increase in hospital admissions for food-related anaphylaxis, particularly in young children [4, 5]. Anaphylaxis is the most severe manifestation of IgE-mediated food allergy, which has been linked to a loss of oral tolerance or a failure in the induction of tolerance. Oral tolerance is the physiologic mechanism by which immune responses to an antigen are suppressed by prior administration of the antigen by the oral route [6, 7]. This normal process results in tolerance to the wide array of food antigens encountered in the lumen of the gastrointestinal tract while allowing the mucosal immune system to defend against harmful pathogens [7].

Oral tolerance presumably evolved as an analog of self-tolerance to prevent potentially dangerous hypersensitivity reactions to harmless food proteins and commensal gut flora. The lumen of the

A.W. Burks (✉)
Duke University Medical Center, Durham, NC, USA
e-mail: titorodriguezbouza@gmail.com

M.C. Castells (ed.), *Anaphylaxis and Hypersensitivity Reactions*,
DOI 10.1007/978-1-60327-951-2_21, © Springer Science+Business Media, LLC 2011

gastrointestinal tract, the largest immunologic organ in the body, is continually exposed to numerous dietary proteins. Here, antigen-presenting cells encounter food proteins and subsequently activate regulatory T lymphocytes that reside in the loose connective tissue beneath the gastrointestinal epithelium [8]. These cells then suppress cellular and humoral immune responses to the protein. In non-allergic hosts, the majority of food proteins are absorbed without provoking injurious local or systemic immune responses [9]. The pathologic cellular and humoral immune responses that characterize food allergy and resultant anaphylaxis most likely result from either a failure in establishing tolerance or a breakdown in the existing tolerance [8].

## 21.2 Immunology and Oral Tolerance

The area of the mucosal surface of the gastrointestinal tract exceeds by several folds that of the skin [9]. The gastrointestinal mucosa is also more permeable to antigens than intact skin and, therefore, represents the major site of contact with foreign antigenic materials. Approximately 130–190 g of food protein are absorbed daily in the gut [10]. The gut microbiota is an additional source of natural antigenic stimulation, with approximately 10 [12] microorganisms per gram of stool [11]. The gut also lodges the most abundant lymphoid tissue in the body, with $10^{12}$ lymphoid cells per meter of human small intestine as well as a population of immunoglobulin-secreting cells that exceeds by several fold the total number found in all other lymphoid organs [12].

Antigen exposure in the gut normally results in several major immunologic responses. The production of noninflammatory secretory IgA is the initial response to antigen encounter in the gastrointestinal tract. Antigens stimulate B cells residing in the organized mucosal lymphoid tissue, which then migrate to distant mucosal and glandular sites and differentiate into polymeric-IgA-producing plasma cells [13]. Polymeric IgA crosslinks luminal antigens on subsequent exposure, thereby preventing their interaction with gut epithelial cells. Priming of the systemic immune system may also occur, resulting in activation of humoral and cellular immunity to protect against the offending pathogen on future encounters [9].

In contrast to the above processes, exposure to dietary proteins and commensal bacteria normally leads to a state of systemic and/or local immunologic tolerance, which allows these exogenous antigens to gain access to the body without activating a potentially damaging immune response [9]. Studies in the mid-twentieth century demonstrated that oral feeding of an antigen induces T cell-mediated inhibition of subsequent immune responses, thus illustrating the principle of oral tolerance [6]. Mice that are immunized and then boosted subcutaneously with an antigen produce strong in vitro cellular and humoral responses to the antigen on re-exposure. In contrast, mice fed the antigen orally and then immunized subcutaneously exhibit greatly reduced in vitro immune responses to the antigen, demonstrating oral tolerance. Transferring T cells from antigen-fed "tolerant" mice to naïve mice also results in suppression of in vitro immune responses to subcutaneous immunization.

Though they normally do not activate harmful immune responses, both food proteins and commensal gut flora exert a stimulatory effect on the developing immune system [10]. Adult mice reared on a balanced diet containing amino acids but no intact food proteins have poorly developed gut-associated lymphoid tissue resembling suckling mice, with low levels of secretory IgA and reduced numbers of intraepithelial lymphocytes [14]. They also have a predominantly Th2 cytokine profile, with high concentrations of interleukin (IL)-10 and IL-4 and a low concentration of interferon-gamma (IFN-gamma). The presence of microbiota in the murine gut has been shown to drive the expansion of B and T cells in Peyer's patches and mesenteric lymph nodes, demonstrating the importance of commensal microorganisms in the normal development of mucosal immunity [15].

## 21.3 Antigen Processing in the Gastrointestinal Tract

The journey for a dietary protein involves multiple steps before tolerance or hypersensitivity is established. Ingested dietary proteins are degraded by gastric acid and luminal enzymes, resulting in the destruction of immunogenic epitopes [8]. The digestion of intact proteins to amino acid chains less than eight amino acids long renders them nonreactive with structures responsible for antigen recognition and thereby immunologically ignored; in this manner, digestion of proteins is an important step in oral tolerance induction [16].

Disruption of the enzymatic digestion process has been shown to impair tolerance in both animal and human models, leading to hypersensitivity [17]. A peptic digest of bovine serum albumin (BSA) is tolerogenic when administered orally or directly injected into the mouse ileum [18]. In contrast, untreated BSA is immunogenic when administered to mice by ileal injection; it is, however, tolerogenic when administered orally, most likely due to degradation in the digestive tract. Human studies have also demonstrated the importance of enzymatic digestion in the induction of oral tolerance. Suppression of gastric acid secretion by anti-ulcer medications has been shown to lead to increased food-specific IgE production in patients; impaired peptic digestion of proteins may render harmless digestion-labile food proteins into potent sensitizers [19].

Proteins that are not degraded by gastric and intestinal enzymes encounter the intestinal epithelium and the lymphoid tissue beneath it in various ways (see Fig. 21.1) [7]. Dendritic cells extend processes through the epithelium to sample luminal antigens. M cells are specialized epithelial cells overlying Peyer's patches that take up particulate antigens and deliver them to subepithelial dendritic cells. Dendritic cells in turn present antigens to B cells in Peyer's patches. Soluble antigens, which are not efficiently taken up by M cells, cross the epithelium by transcellular or paracellular routes to the lamina propria, where they encounter T cells or macrophages. Intestinal epithelial cells act as nonprofessional antigen-presenting cells and can present antigens to primed T cells.

## 21.4 Mechanisms of Oral Tolerance

Oral tolerance is induced through two primary effector mechanisms – active suppression by regulatory T (Treg) cells and clonal anergy or deletion (see Fig. 21.2). The dose of the antigen is the primary factor that determines which will take place [20]. Low doses of antigen induce Treg cells that produce immunosuppressive cytokines such as transforming growth factor (TGF) beta and IL-10. Treg cells were initially characterized by the stable expression of the high-affinity component of the IL-2 receptor, CD25 [21]. Recent studies have shown that they express the transcription factor forkhead box P3 (FOXP3), which has been shown to be the key regulatory gene in the development of the Treg subset from naïve CD4+T cells [22] (see Fig. 21.3). CD4+CD25+Treg cells migrate to lymphoid organs and suppress CD4+CD25- effector cells through cell–cell interaction involving surface-bound TGF-beta [23], although their suppressor function has also been shown to occur independently of TGF-beta [24]. Regulatory T cells also migrate to target organs, where they inhibit disease by releasing nonantigen-specific cytokines [9].

Defective regulatory T cell development has been shown to play a key role in the development of food allergy. Mutations in the gene encoding FOXP3 can lead to immune dysregulation, as seen in Immune Dysregulation, Polyendocrinopathy, Enteropathy, X-linked (IPEX) Syndrome, which is characterized by autoaggressive lymphocyte clones due to failure in Treg development [25]. Recently, an IPEX variant characterized by severe allergic as well as autoimmune manifestations has been described [26]. A mutation in a noncoding region of the FOXP3 gene results in a disorder characterized by severe food allergy, atopic dermatitis, elevated serum IgE, and eosinophilia in addition to enteropathy.

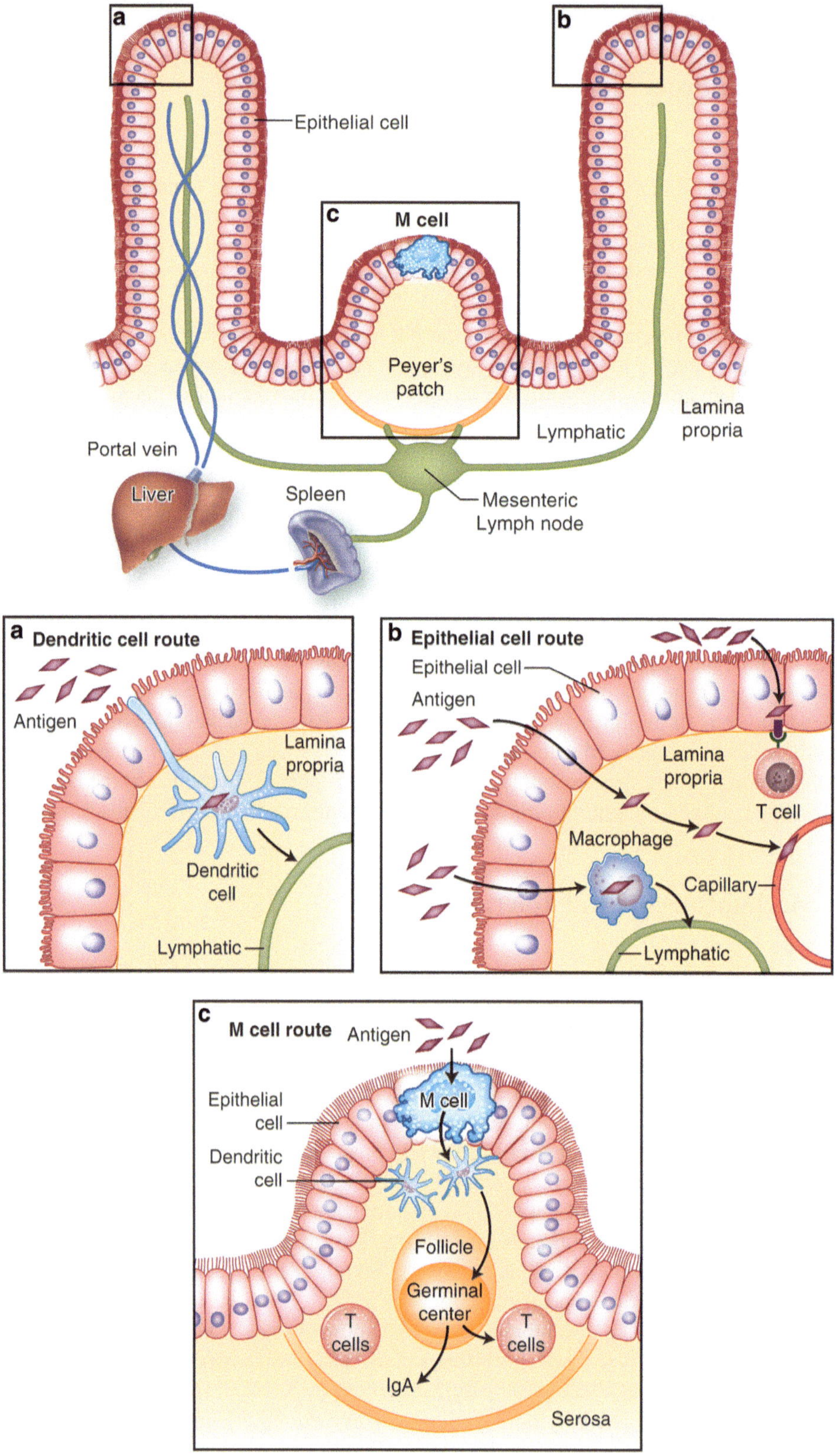


**Fig. 21.1** Sites of antigen uptake in the gut. (**a**) Antigen can be sampled by dendritic cells that extend processes into the lumen. (**b**) M cells overlying Peyer's patches take up particulate antigens and then deliver them to dendritic cells in the subepithelial region and then to underlying B-cell follicles, where IgA commitment occurs. (**c**) Soluble antigens can cross the epithelium through transcellular or paracellular routes to then encounter T cells or macrophages in the lamina propria (Adapted from [7]. With permission)

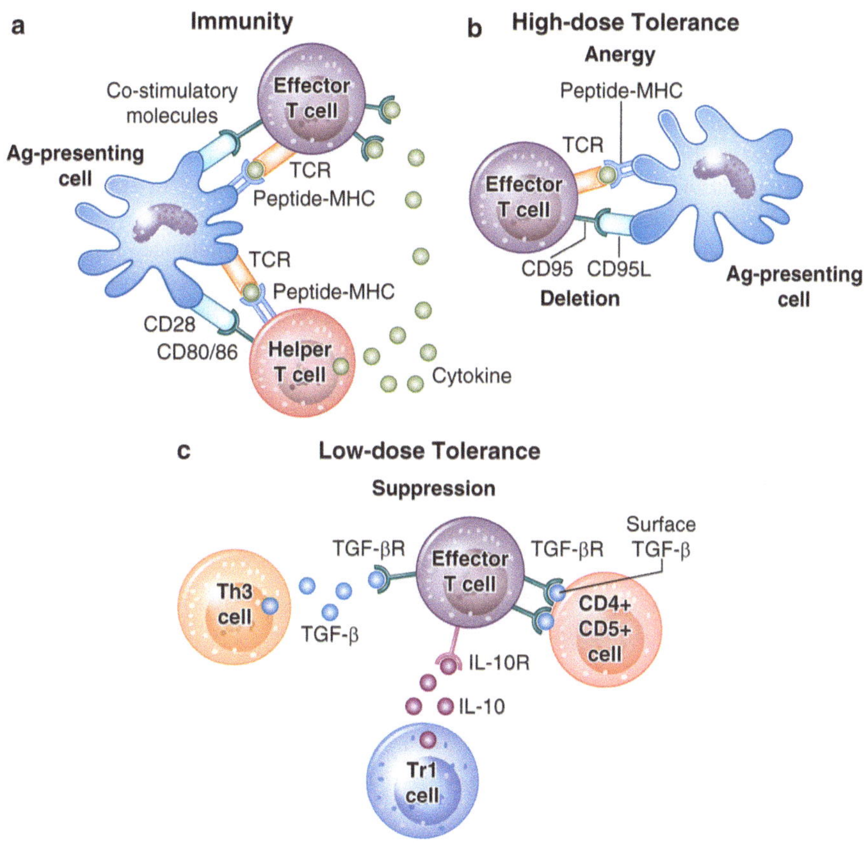


**Fig. 21.2** Mechanisms of oral tolerance. (**a**) Generation of an immune response requires T-cell receptor ligation with peptide-MHC complexes in the presence of appropriate costimulatory molecules (CD80 and CD86) and cytokines. (**b**) High-dose tolerance is induced by T-cell receptor cross-linking in the absence of costimulation or in the presence of inhibitory ligands (CD95 and CD95 ligand), leading to anergy or deletion, respectively. (**c**) Low doses of oral antigen lead to the activation of regulatory CD4+CD25+T cells, which suppress immune responses through soluble or cell surface-associated cytokines (IL-10 and TGF-β(beta)). *L* Ligand, *R* Receptor (Adapted from [7]. With permission)

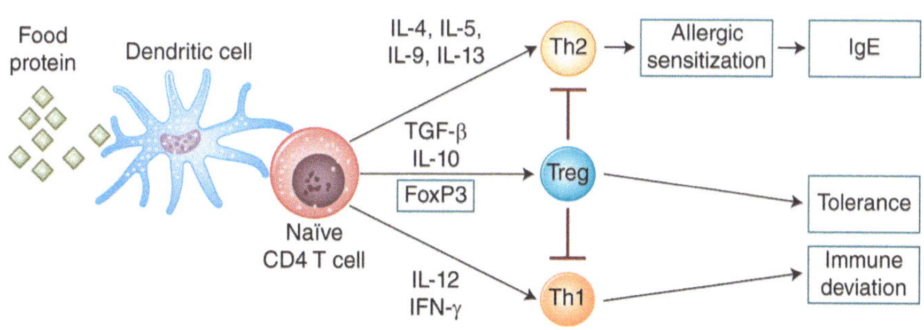


**Fig. 21.3** Allergic sensitization versus oral tolerance. Food antigen exposure in the gastrointestinal mucosal immune system can result in oral tolerance induction or allergic sensitization (Adapted from [63]. With permission). *FoxP3* fork-head box P3, *IFN* interferon, *IL* interleukin, *TGF* transforming growth factor, *Th* T-helper cell, *Treg* T-regulatory cell

Furthermore, the appearance of circulating CD4+CD25+T cells has been associated with development of tolerance in children with non-IgE-mediated milk allergy [27]. Subjects who outgrew their allergy had higher frequencies of circulating CD4+CD25+T cells and decreased in vitro peripheral blood mononuclear cell proliferative responses to bovine-lactoglobulin than those with persistent milk allergy. Depletion of CD25+ cells led to increased in vitro proliferation against beta-lactoglobulin, suggesting that regulatory T cells are capable of suppressing effector T cells and herald the induction of mucosal tolerance against dietary antigens.

Whereas low doses of antigen favor regulatory T cell-driven tolerance, high doses induce tolerance via lymphocyte anergy or clonal deletion. Anergy can be induced through binding of a peptide antigen in the absence of costimulatory signals provided either by soluble cytokines such as IL-2 or by interactions between receptors on T cells (CD28) and counterreceptors on antigen-presenting cells (CD80 and CD86) [28]. High antigen doses induce deletion by means of apoptosis; in mice transgenic for ovalbumin-specific T-cell receptor genes, oral antigen administration was found to result in the deletion of antigen-specific T cells in Peyer's patches [29].

It is quite likely that features of both low- and high-dose tolerance overlap in vivo and may not be mutually exclusive. Despite the fact that cytotoxic T lymphocyte-associated antigen (CTLA-4) was first described in a pathway of anergy induction, its binding leads to CD4+ T cell production of TGF-beta, which may counterbalance CD28-costimulation of T cell activation [30]. Macrophages take up apoptotic cells, and the phagocytosis of these dying cells results in the downregulation of pro-inflammatory cytokines and the induction of TGF-beta, a known immunosuppressive cytokine [31]. These events contribute to an immunosuppressive milieu favoring tolerance.

## 21.5 Factors Influencing Development of Tolerance

Several major factors influence the development of oral tolerance, including antigen properties, route of exposure, age of the host, genetic factors, and gut flora (see Fig. 21.3). Soluble antigens tend to be more tolerogenic than particulate antigens, although most food allergens are soluble proteins. Solubility can change during food preparation and heat treatment. For example, roasting has been shown to progressively decrease the solubility of peanut proteins, thereby increasing the capacity of peanut-specific IgE to bind the proteins encountered in the gut [32]. Other characteristics of dietary proteins render them allergenic, including certain innate immunostimulatory properties. The mammalian immune system recognizes microbial proteins in association with pathogen-associated molecular patterns that induce either Th1 or Th2 responses. Likewise, other motifs on dietary proteins may be recognized and result in a Th2 response in genetically susceptible individuals [33].

Route of allergen exposure also plays a role in the development of allergy or tolerance. As mentioned previously, oral administration of an antigen followed by subcutaneous immunization results in greatly reduced in vitro immune responses to the antigen, demonstrating oral tolerance [6]. Food antigen exposure by means other than ingestion can result in hypersensitivity. Murine studies have demonstrated that epicutaneous exposure to peanut protein can induce a potent Th2 immune response with high levels of IL-4 and serum IgE production, potentially preventing the subsequent induction of oral tolerance [34]. Epicutaneous allergen exposure in mice has also been shown to prime for marked esophageal eosinophilic inflammation in a Th2-dependent manner [35]. A retrospective study of factors associated with the development of peanut allergy in children demonstrated a link with the use of skin preparations containing peanut oil, an area warranting further study [36].

Host factors also play a central role in the determination of allergy or oral tolerance. Food allergy has been shown to have a significant heritable component, and a recent study demonstrated a strong familial aggregation of food allergy and sensitization to food allergens [37]. An individual's genetic make-up plays an important role in whether exposure to a given protein results in sensitization or tolerance. In a study of peanut allergen gene immunization, mice were immunized with plasmid DNA encoding Ara h 2, one of the major peanut allergens [38]. Subsequent injection with peanut protein resulted in anaphylaxis in all of the C3H/HeSn mice but none of the AKR/J or BALB/c mice, illustrating that immune responses were strain-dependent. In another study of murine susceptibility to food allergy and anaphylaxis, C3H/HeJ and BALB/c mice were sensitized to cow's milk or peanut protein by intragastric administration [39]. When challenged, 87% of the milk-sensitized C3H/HeJ mice developed anaphylactic symptoms with milk exposure, and 100% of peanut-sensitized C3H/HeJ mice developed anaphylaxis with peanut exposure. In contrast, none of the BALB/c mice experienced anaphylaxis with food challenge. Splenocytes from C3H/HeJ mice exhibited increased IL-4 and IL-10 secretion, whereas those from BALB/c mice demonstrated increased IFN-gamma secretion. These differential immune responses (Th2 versus Th1, respectively) may explain the strain-dependent susceptibility to food allergy.

The host's age is another factor influencing the development of oral tolerance to a given dietary protein. Immaturity of the immunologic and gastrointestinal systems predisposes infants to impaired tolerance and resultant food allergy [40]. Infants and young children have an immature mucosal surface, with increased intestinal permeability, decreased gastric acidity, and decreased intestinal and pancreatic enzyme production. As a result, intact allergenic proteins are more likely to be absorbed into the bloodstream, subsequently stimulating the immune system and resulting in IgE production [40]. In addition, infants' immature immune systems are skewed towards Th2 responsiveness [41]. These responses are rapidly suppressed during the first year of life in nonatopic children but persist in atopic children.

In addition to sensitization via the gastrointestinal tract, skin permeability to mucosal antigens is most likely an important event in the pathogenesis of food allergy [42]. Individuals with atopic dermatitis have impaired epithelial barrier function, which may result in sensitization to allergens encountered through the epicutaneous route [34]. In addition to allergen exposure, individuals with atopic dermatitis are also frequently colonized by toxin-producing Staphylococcus aureus strains. Murine studies have shown that epicutaneous sensitization with staphylococcal enterotoxin B (SEB) can result in allergic skin inflammation with Th2 skewing and increased IgE synthesis [43]. Additionally, staphylococcal toxins have been shown to enhance murine Th2 immune responses when administered with food antigens, resulting in anaphylaxis on oral challenge [44]. Impaired oral tolerance is evidenced by decreased expression of TGF-beta and diminished regulatory T cell function, illustrating that sensitization may occur due to a breakdown in oral tolerance mechanisms.

The normal flora of the gastrointestinal tract also plays an important role in the development of oral tolerance. The maturation of the gastrointestinal immune system is dependent on the presence of commensal microorganisms [15]. Mice raised in germ-free environments maintain Th2-mediated immune responses after administration of an oral tolerogen, while Th1 responses are diminished [45]. Reconstitution of the intestinal tract with *Bifidobacterium infantis,* predominant gut bacteria, allowed the induction of oral tolerance, though only if performed in the neonatal period, demonstrating the shared roles of intestinal flora as well as age of exposure in the development of tolerance. The presence of gut microbiota also drives the expansion of Foxp3-expressing CD4+ T cells in mesenteric lymph nodes and stimulates the production of IL-10 and interferon-gamma [15].

## 21.6 Potential Therapeutic Strategies

An increasing understanding of the role of oral tolerance in food allergy and anaphylaxis has led to the identification of potential therapeutic targets and prevention strategies. IL-10 is an important regulator of oral tolerance, which is modulated in part by local IgA production in the gut [46].

Recent murine studies have shown that pretreatment with *Lactococcus lactis* transfected with the gene for recombinant murine IL-10 protected mice from anaphylaxis after oral antigen challenge by attenuating the Th2 immune response [47]. This protection was mediated by the induction of oral tolerance, as evidenced by inhibition of antigen-specific IgE and production of antigen-specific IgA in addition to the production of IL-10.

Probiotic bacteria have been studied for their immunomodulatory properties, including their potential use in the prevention of food hypersensitivity. Oral administration of a probiotic mixture was shown to reduce both systemic and local anaphylactic symptoms in mice challenged with shrimp tropomyosin [48]. However, at present, there is insufficient evidence in humans to recommend the administration of probiotics to infants for the prevention of food allergy [49]. The Chinese herbal formula FAHF-2 (food allergy herbal formula-2) has been found to completely block anaphylactic reactions to peanut in sensitized mice [50]. The induction of tolerance was associated with increased numbers of IFN-gamma-producing CD8+ cells and decreased levels of IL-4 and IL-5. Human safety trials of FAHF-2 are currently underway.

Allergen immunotherapy is a potential modality for specific oral tolerance induction. Subcutaneous peanut immunotherapy has been studied but was found to be associated with a high rate of recurrent systemic reactions [51]. Several alternatives, including sublingual, oral, and recombinant allergen immunotherapy, are currently being investigated in highly supervised research settings. In a placebo-controlled study of hazelnut sublingual immunotherapy, the mean quantity of hazelnut triggering allergic symptoms significantly increased in the active treatment group, while those receiving placebo had no significant change in allergen threshold [52]. Subjects in the hazelnut treatment group also had significant increases in IgG4 and IL-10 levels, changes not seen in those receiving placebo. Of note, over half of the subjects had oral allergy symptoms at entry challenge. Sublingual immunotherapy has not yet been shown to be effective in food allergies associated with systemic symptoms, such as milk, egg, and peanut.

Several trials of oral immunotherapy for food allergy have been undertaken, including studies in milk-, egg-, and peanut-allergic subjects (see Table 21.1 [8]).

Nine (36%) of 25 subjects in a milk or egg oral immunotherapy protocol achieved permanent tolerance after 2 months off treatment versus 7 (35%) of 20 in the elimination diet control group [56]. Both groups experienced significant decreases in allergen-specific IgE levels, supporting the investigators' clinical observation that specific oral immunotherapy may not alter natural course of tolerance development. However, 3 (12%) of 25 subjects responded with regular intake and 4 (16%) of 25 were partial responders, suggesting that the desensitized state could be maintained by regular allergen exposure.

A study of oral immunotherapy in children with severe milk allergy revealed that a significantly higher number of subjects in the treatment group could tolerate an entire serving of milk after the 1-year protocol [57]. All subjects who followed an elimination diet failed a double-blind, placebo-controlled food challenge at the end of the study. A recent double-blind, placebo-controlled study of milk oral immunotherapy resulted in a significant increase in the median cumulative threshold dose inducing a reaction in the active treatment group when compared with placebo (5,140 vs 40 mg, $p=0.0003$) [60]. Although milk-specific IgE levels did not change in either group, milk-specific IgG4 levels increased significantly in the active treatment group. Peanut oral immunotherapy resulted in clinical desensitization in 27 of 29 children after 4–22 months of treatment [59]. Titrated skin prick tests and basophil activation showed a significant decrease by 6 months into treatment. Peanut-specific $IgG_4$ increased with treatment, and peanut-specific IgE increased initially and then decreased after 12–18 months on therapy. Double-blind, placebo-controlled studies of peanut OIT are currently underway.

Thus far, most studies of food allergen immunotherapy have assessed *desensitization*, which refers to a temporary state of reduced sensitivity to an allergen that is contingent on regular exposure to the agent. In contrast, tolerance refers a long-term change in the immune response to a

**Table 21.1** Selected oral immunotherapy studies (Adapted from [8])

| | Allergen (number of subjects) | Length of therapy (months) | Outcome |
|---|---|---|---|
| Patriarca et al. [53] | Cow's milk (24) | 3–12 | Desensitization successful in 45 (83%) of 54 treatments |
| | Whole egg (13) | | |
| | Albumin (3) | | |
| | Fish (10) | | |
| | Orange (2) | | |
| | Peanut (1) | | |
| | Corn (1) | | |
| | Peach (1) | | |
| | Apple (1) | | |
| | Lettuce (1) | | |
| | Beans (1) | | |
| Meglio et al. [54] | Cow's milk (21) | 6 | 15 (71%) of 21 achieved intake of 200 mL/day; 3 tolerated 40–80 mL/day |
| Buchanan et al. [55] | Egg (7) | 24 | All subjects tolerated more egg protein at study conclusion than during initial rush; 4 (57%) passed an 8 g challenge at conclusion |
| Staden et al. [56] | Cow's milk or egg (45) | 11–59 | Nine (36%) of 25 on treatment achieved tolerance; 7 (35%) of 20 on elimination diet achieved tolerance |
| Longo et al. [57] | Cow's milk (30) | 12 mo | Eleven (36%) of 30 achieved daily intake of 150 mL/day; 16 (54%) of 30 ingested 5–150 mL/day |
| Skripak et al. [58] | Cow's milk (19) | 3–4 | Increased cumulative threshold dose in treatment group (5,140 mg versus 40 mg in placebo group, $p=0.0003$) |
| Jones et al. [59] | Peanut (29) | 4–22 | 27/29 (93%) successfully desensitized |

protein that persists once immunotherapy is stopped. Six subjects in an open peanut oral immunotherapy pilot study recently demonstrated clinical tolerance by passing a food challenge 4 weeks after stopping treatment [61]. Over the course of treatment, peanut-specific IgE levels decreased significantly while peanut-specific IgG4 levels increased. Cytokine and cellular analyses done on a larger group of enrolled subjects suggest that IL-10 secretion and the induction Foxp3 positive regulatory T cells are important mediators in the development of tolerance [59]. Randomized, placebo-controlled studies are needed to establish whether food allergen immunotherapy can induce long-lasting tolerance.

Recombinant allergen immunotherapy is a strategy that has been effective in murine studies. Researchers have engineered peanut protein allergens with altered epitope-binding sites [62]. These recombinant proteins were administered rectally to peanut-allergic C3H/HeJ mice weekly for 3 weeks. Those receiving the highest dose of protein demonstrated persistent protection from anaphylaxis during food challenges 10 weeks later, suggesting the induction of long-term tolerance. Downregulated Th2 cytokine production and increased IFN-gamma and TGF-beta production provided laboratory evidence of tolerance. Human studies are beginning with this form of immunotherapy. Other forms of tolerance induction under investigation include peptide immunotherapy, DNA immunization, and immunostimulatory sequences [63].

An important area of oral tolerance research involves the prevention of allergic disease. A central question addresses whether early exposure to common allergenic food proteins favors the development of tolerance over allergy. Interestingly, rates of peanut allergy are relatively lower in countries that have peanut snacks that are safe for infants, such as Israel [64]. To explore the impact of early peanut consumption, a recent study compared the rate of peanut allergy among Jewish children living in the United Kingdom and Israel [65]. The prevalence of peanut allergy was found to be more than tenfold higher in the United Kingdom, a difference that could not be accounted for by differences in atopy, social class, or genetic background. A survey of feeding practices revealed that Israeli infants consume peanut in larger quantities and at an earlier age than their British counterparts, raising the question of whether early peanut introduction facilitates oral tolerance induction.

The principle of early feeding to promote oral tolerance remains unproven, and as such, cannot be implemented in clinical practice [66]. The American Academy of Pediatrics recently revised its recommendations for early infant feeding due to mixed evidence relating the timing of complementary food introduction and the development of allergy [67]. At this time, exclusive breastfeeding as well as delaying the introduction of solid foods for at least 4–6 months is the only recommendation that has been shown to prevent atopic dermatitis, cow milk allergy, and wheezing in early childhood. The LEAP Study (Learning Early About Peanut Allergy, http://www.leapstudy.co.uk) is designed to further address the question of early introduction versus allergen avoidance. High-risk infants aged 4–10 months are randomized to receive an age-appropriate peanut snack or avoid peanut consumption. The rates of developing peanut allergy by age 5 years will be compared.

## 21.7 Conclusions

Oral tolerance is crucial in allowing a wide array of dietary proteins access to the body without activating harmful immune responses. A breakdown in oral tolerance mechanisms or a failure to establish tolerance can result in food allergy and anaphylaxis. A growing understanding of the factors involved in the development of oral tolerance has spurred recent work investigating potential therapies targeting these pathways. Further work is necessary to define the molecular mechanisms involved in oral tolerance induction and to identify specific targets for immunomodulatory treatments. Definitive therapies for food allergy and food-induced anaphylaxis are on the horizon and will soon expand the treatment options available to individuals living with these diseases.

## References

1. Mehl A, Wahn U, Niggemann B. Anaphylactic reactions in children – a questionnaire-based survey in Germany. *Allergy.* 2005;60(11):1440–1445.
2. Smit DV, Cameron PA, Rainer TH. Anaphylaxis presentations to an emergency department in Hong Kong: incidence and predictors of biphasic reactions. *J Emerg Med.* 2005;28(4):381–388.
3. Yocum MW, Butterfield JH, Klein JS, Volcheck GW, Schroeder DR, Silverstein MD. Epidemiology of anaphylaxis in Olmsted County: a population-based study. *J Allergy Clin Immunol.* 1999;104(2Pt1):452–456.
4. Liew WK, Williamson E, Tang ML. Anaphylaxis fatalities and admissions in Australia. *J Allergy Clin Immunol.* 2009;123(2):434–442.
5. Poulos LM, Waters AM, Correll PK, Loblay RH, Marks GB. Trends in hospitalizations for anaphylaxis, angioedema, and urticaria in Australia, 1993–1994 to 2004–2005. *J Allergy Clin Immunol.* 2007;120(4):878–884.
6. Chase M. Inhibition of experimental drug allergy by prior feeding of the sensitizing agent. *Proc Soc Exp Biol Med.* 1946;61:257–259.
7. Chehade M, Mayer L. Oral tolerance and its relation to food hypersensitivities. *J Allergy Clin Immunol.* 2005;115(1):3–12;quiz3.
8. Burks AW, Laubach S, Jones SM. Oral tolerance, food allergy, and immunotherapy: implications for future treatment. *J Allergy Clin Immunol.* 2008;121(6):1344–1350.
9. Faria AM, Weiner HL. Oral tolerance. *Immunol Rev.* 2005;206:232–259.
10. Brandtzaeg P. Development and basic mechanisms of human gut immunity. *Nutr Rev.* 1998;56(1Pt2):S5-S18.

11. Macfarlane GT, Macfarlane S. Human colonic microbiota: ecology, physiology and metabolic potential of intestinal bacteria. *Scand J Gastroenterol Suppl.* 1997;222:3–9.
12. Mestecky J, McGhee JR. Immunoglobulin A (IgA): molecular and cellular interactions involved in IgA biosynthesis and immune response. *Adv Immunol.* 1987;40:153–245.
13. Kraehenbuhl JP, Neutra MR. Transepithelial transport and mucosal defence II: secretion of IgA. *Trends Cell Biol.* 1992;2(6):170–174.
14. Menezes Jda S, Mucida DS, Cara DC, et al. Stimulation by food proteins plays a critical role in the maturation of the immune system. *Int Immunol.* 2003;15(3):447–455.
15. Hrncir T, Stepankova R, Kozakova H, Hudcovic T, Tlaskalova-Hogenova H. Gut microbiota and lipopolysaccharide content of the diet influence development of regulatory T cells: studies in germ-free mice. *BMC Immunol.* 2008;9:65.
16. Aalberse RC. Structural biology of allergens. *J Allergy Clin Immunol.* 2000;106(2):228–238.
17. Untersmayr E, Jensen-Jarolim E. The role of protein digestibility and antacids on food allergy outcomes. *J Allergy Clin Immunol.* 2008;121(6):1301–1318;quiz9–10.
18. Michael JG. The role of digestive enzymes in orally induced immune tolerance. *Immunol Invest.* 1989;18(9–10):1049–1054.
19. Untersmayr E, Bakos N, Scholl I, et al. Anti-ulcer drugs promote IgE formation toward dietary antigens in adult patients. *FASEB J.* 2005;19(6):656–658.
20. Friedman A, Weiner HL. Induction of anergy or active suppression following oral tolerance is determined by antigen dosage. *Proc Natl Acad Sci USA.* 1994;91(14):6688–6692.
21. Sakaguchi S, Sakaguchi N, Asano M, Itoh M, Toda M. Immunologic self-tolerance maintained by activated T cells expressing IL-2 receptor alpha-chains (CD25). Breakdown of a single mechanism of self-tolerance causes various autoimmune diseases. *J Immunol.* 1995;155(3):1151–1164.
22. Hori S, Nomura T, Sakaguchi S. Control of regulatory T cell development by the transcription factor Foxp3. *Science.* 2003;299(5609):1057–1061.
23. Nakamura K, Kitani A, Strober W. Cell contact-dependent immunosuppression by CD4(+)CD25(+) regulatory T cells is mediated by cell surface-bound transforming growth factor beta. *J Exp Med.* 2001;194(5):629–644.
24. Piccirillo CA, Letterio JJ, Thornton AM, et al. CD4(+)CD25(+) regulatory T cells can mediate suppressor function in the absence of transforming growth factor beta1 production and responsiveness. *J Exp Med.* 2002;196(2):237–246.
25. Ochs HD, Gambineri E, Torgerson TR. IPEX, FOXP3 and regulatory T-cells: a model for autoimmunity. *Immunol Res.* 2007;38(1–3):112–121.
26. Torgerson TR, Linane A, Moes N, et al. Severe food allergy as a variant of IPEX syndrome caused by a deletion in a noncoding region of the FOXP3 gene. *Gastroenterology.* 2007;132(5):1705–1717.
27. Karlsson MR, Rugtveit J, Brandtzaeg P. Allergen-responsive CD4+CD25+ regulatory T cells in children who have outgrown cow's milk allergy. *J Exp Med.* 2004;199(12):1679–1688.
28. Appleman LJ, Boussiotis VA. T cell anergy and costimulation. *Immunol Rev.* 2003;192:161–180.
29. Chen Y, Inobe J, Marks R, Gonnella P, Kuchroo VK, Weiner HL. Peripheral deletion of antigen-reactive T cells in oral tolerance. *Nature.* 1995;376(6536):177–180.
30. Chen W, Jin W, Wahl SM. Engagement of cytotoxic T lymphocyte-associated antigen 4 (CTLA-4) induces transforming growth factor beta (TGF-beta) production by murine CD4(+) T cells. J *Exp Med.* 1998;188(10):1849–1857.
31. Freire-de-Lima CG, Nascimento DO, Soares MB, et al. Uptake of apoptotic cells drives the growth of a pathogenic trypanosome in macrophages. *Nature.* 2000;403(6766):199–203.
32. Kopper RA, Odum NJ, Sen M, Helm RM, Stanley JS, Burks AW. Peanut protein allergens: the effect of roasting on solubility and allergenicity. *Int Arch Allergy Immunol.* 2005;136(1):16–22.
33. Shreffler WG, Castro RR, Kucuk ZY, et al. The major glycoprotein allergen from Arachis hypogaea, Ara h 1, is a ligand of dendritic cell-specific ICAM-grabbing nonintegrin and acts as a Th2 adjuvant in vitro. *J Immunol.* 2006;177(6):3677–3685.
34. Strid J, Hourihane J, Kimber I, Callard R, Strobel S. Epicutaneous exposure to peanut protein prevents oral tolerance and enhances allergic sensitization. *Clin Exp Allergy.* 2005;35(6):757–766.
35. Akei HS, Mishra A, Blanchard C, Rothenberg ME. Epicutaneous antigen exposure primes for experimental eosinophilic esophagitis in mice. *Gastroenterology.* 2005;129(3):985–994.
36. Lack G, Fox D, Northstone K, Golding J. Factors associated with the development of peanut allergy in childhood. *N Engl J Med.* 2003;348(11):977–985.
37. Tsai HJ, Kumar R, Pongracic J, et al. Familial aggregation of food allergy and sensitization to food allergens: a family-based study. *Clin Exp Allergy.* 2009;39(1):101–109.
38. Li X, Huang CK, Schofield BH, et al. Strain-dependent induction of allergic sensitization caused by peanut allergen DNA immunization in mice. *J Immunol.* 1999;162(5):3045–3052.
39. Morafo V, Srivastava K, Huang CK, et al. Genetic susceptibility to food allergy is linked to differential TH2-TH1 responses in C3H/HeJ and BALB/c mice. *J Allergy Clin Immunol.* 2003;111(5):1122–1128.

40. Nowak-Wegrzyn A, Sampson HA. Adverse reactions to foods. *Med Clin North Am.* 2006;90(1):97–127.
41. Prescott SL, Macaubas C, Smallacombe T, Holt BJ, Sly PD, Holt PG. Development of allergen-specific T-cell memory in atopic and normal children. *Lancet.* 1999;353(9148):196–200.
42. Brandtzaeg P. History of oral tolerance and mucosal immunity. *Ann N Y Acad Sci.* 1996;778:1–27.
43. Laouini D, Kawamoto S, Yalcindag A, et al. Epicutaneous sensitization with superantigen induces allergic skin inflammation. *J Allergy Clin Immunol.* 2003;112(5):981–987.
44. Ganeshan K, Neilsen CV, Hadsaitong A, Schleimer RP, Luo X, Bryce PJ. Impairing oral tolerance promotes allergy and anaphylaxis: a new murine food allergy model. *J Allergy Clin Immunol.* 2009;123(1):231–238,e4.
45. Sudo N, Sawamura S, Tanaka K, Aiba Y, Kubo C, Koga Y. The requirement of intestinal bacterial flora for the development of an IgE production system fully susceptible to oral tolerance induction. *J Immunol.* 1997;159(4):1739–1745.
46. Frossard CP, Tropia L, Hauser C, Eigenmann PA. Lymphocytes in Peyer patches regulate clinical tolerance in a murine model of food allergy. *J Allergy Clin Immunol.* 2004;113(5):958–964.
47. Frossard CP, Steidler L, Eigenmann PA. Oral administration of an IL-10-secreting Lactococcus lactis strain prevents food-induced IgE sensitization. *J Allergy Clin Immunol.* 2007;119(4):952–959.
48. Di Felice G, Barletta B, Butteroni C, et al. Use of probiotic bacteria for prevention and therapy of allergic diseases: studies in mouse model of allergic sensitization. *J Clin Gastroenterol.* 2008;42Suppl3Pt1:S130-S132.
49. Osborn DA, Sinn JK. Probiotics in infants for prevention of allergic disease and food hypersensitivity. *Cochrane Database Syst Rev.* 2007(4):CD006475.
50. Qu C, Srivastava K, Ko J, Zhang TF, Sampson HA, Li XM. Induction of tolerance after establishment of peanut allergy by the food allergy herbal formula-2 is associated with up-regulation of interferon-gamma. *Clin Exp Allergy.* 2007;37(6):846–855.
51. Nelson HS, Lahr J, Rule R, Bock A, Leung D. Treatment of anaphylactic sensitivity to peanuts by immunotherapy with injections of aqueous peanut extract. *J Allergy Clin Immunol.* 1997;99(6Pt1):744–751.
52. Enrique E, Pineda F, Malek T, et al. Sublingual immunotherapy for hazelnut food allergy: a randomized, double-blind, placebo-controlled study with a standardized hazelnut extract. *J Allergy Clin Immunol.* 2005;116(5):1073–1079.
53. Patriarca G, Nucera E, Roncallo C, et al. Oral desensitizing treatment in food allergy: clinical and immunological results. *Aliment Pharmacol Ther.* 2003;17(3):459–465.
54. Meglio P, Bartone E, Plantamura M, Arabito E, Giampietro PG. A protocol for oral desensitization in children with IgE-mediated cow's milk allergy. *Allergy.* 2004;59(9):980–987.
55. Buchanan AD, Green TD, Jones SM, et al. Egg oral immunotherapy in nonanaphylactic children with egg allergy. *J Allergy Clin Immunol.* 2007;119(1):199–205.
56. Staden U, Rolinck-Werninghaus C, Brewe F, Wahn U, Niggemann B, Beyer K. Specific oral tolerance induction in food allergy in children: efficacy and clinical patterns of reaction. *Allergy.* 2007;62(11):1261–1269.
57. Longo G, Barbi E, Berti I, et al. Specific oral tolerance induction in children with very severe cow's milk-induced reactions. *J Allergy Clin Immunol.* 2008;121(2):343–347.
58. Skripak JM, Nash SD, Rowley H, et al. A randomized, double-blind, placebo-controlled study of milk oral immunotherapy for cow's milk allergy. *J Allergy Clin Immunol.* 2008;122(6):1154–1160.
59. Jones SM, Pons L, Roberts JL, et al. Clinical efficacy and immune regulation with peanut oral immunotherapy. *J Allergy Clin Immunol.* 2009;124(2):292–300,e1–97.
60. Skripak JM, Nash SD, Rowley H, et al. A randomized, double-blind, placebo-controlled study of milk oral immunotherapy for cow's milk allergy. *J Allergy Clin Immunol.* 2008;122(6):1154–1160.
61. Varshney P, Jones SM, Pons L, et al. Oral immunotherapy (oit) induces clinical tolerance in peanut-allergic children. *J Allergy Clin Immunol.* 2009;123(2, Suppl 1):S174.
62. Li X-M, Srivastava K, Grishin A, et al. Persistent protective effect of heat-killed *Escherichia coli* producing "engineered," recombinant peanut proteins in a murine model of peanut allergy. *J Allergy Clin Immunol.* 2003;112(1):159–167.
63. Scurlock AM, Burks AW, Jones SM. Oral immunotherapy for food allergy. *Curr Allergy Asthma Rep.* 2009;9(3):186–193.
64. Levy Y, Broides A, Segal N, Danon YL. Peanut and tree nut allergy in children: role of peanut snacks in Israel? *Allergy.* 2003;58(11):1206–1207.
65. Du Toit G, Katz Y, Sasieni P, et al. Early consumption of peanuts in infancy is associated with a low prevalence of peanut allergy. *J Allergy Clin Immunol.* 2008;122(5):984–991.
66. Burks AW. Early peanut consumption: postpone or promote? *J Allergy Clin Immunol.* 2009;123(2):424–425.
67. Greer FR, Sicherer SH, Burks AW, and the Committee on N, Section on A, Immunology. Effects of early nutritional interventions on the development of atopic disease in infants and children: the role of maternal dietary restriction, breastfeeding, timing of introduction of complementary foods, and hydrolyzed formulas. *Pediatrics.* 2008;121(1):183–191.

# Chapter 22
# Management of Anaphylaxis: Relevance of Causes and Future Trends in Treatment

**Scott P. Commins and Thomas A.E. Platts-Mills**

**Abstract** Establishing the etiology of recurrent anaphylaxis is a critical aspect of treatment, as the identification of causal allergens allows the use of either avoidance or immunotherapy in the management. Assigning etiology is limited, however, by the number of known antigenic exposures associated with anaphylaxis. Given that anaphylaxis is a severe allergic reaction that can be rapid and occasionally fatal, identification of novel agents that can cause anaphylaxis provides an important step forward in diagnosis and management. The discovery of IgE antibodies to the oligosaccharide alpha-gal has made it possible to investigate several novel aspects of allergic disease, including the role of glycosylation in creating a risk for severe hypersensitivity reactions. The recombinant anti-IgE antibody, omalizumab, has the potential to inhibit allergen-induced mast cell activation regardless of the allergen specificity of the IgE molecules. The mechanisms of action of omalizumab are discussed with specific attention to the role that this monoclonal antibody may have in treating anaphylactic events. In addition to omalizumab, other potential treatments for anaphylaxis may include molecules that can induce tolerance without causing degranulation/secretion of allergic mediators. Certainly the preference of patients and providers alike is the ability to avoid triggering allergens; hence, the continued search for targets of specific IgE remains critical to recommending appropriate avoidance.

**Keywords** Anaphylaxis • Allergens • Alpha-gal • Omalizumab • Glycosylation • IgE • CCD

## 22.1 Introduction

Immunoglobulin E (IgE) was originally identified by Dr. Ishizaka in 1966 when he demonstrated that IgE was the substance responsible for mediating immediate hypersensitivity reactions in the skin, and by implication, anaphylactic reactions [1]. Years of subsequent publications have confirmed that allergen-specific IgE has a central role in allergen-induced anaphylaxis. The clinical signs and symptoms of anaphylaxis develop when IgE-Fcε(epsilon) RI complexes on the mast cell surface are cross-linked by a multivalent allergen leading to receptor aggregation. This is followed rapidly by mast cell degranulation, release of histamine, and the synthesis of lipid mediators. The high-affinity receptor for IgE, Fcε(epsilon) RI, is expressed as an α(alpha)β(beta)γ(gamma)2-tetramer on mast cells and basophils and as an α(alpha)β(beta)2-trimer on human antigen-presenting cells, eosinophils, monocytes, smooth muscle cells, and platelets. The extracellular domain of the α(alpha)-chain

S.P. Commins (✉)
University of Virginia Health System, Charlottesville, VA, USA
e-mail: spc7w@virginia.edu

M.C. Castells (ed.), *Anaphylaxis and Hypersensitivity Reactions*,
DOI 10.1007/978-1-60327-951-2_22, © Springer Science+Business Media, LLC 2011

contains the IgE binding site, whereas the intracellular portion of the β(beta)- and γ(gamma)-chains contain the immunoreceptor tyrosine-based activation motifs (ITAMs). After cross-linking of the IgE-Fcε(epsilon)RI complexes, phosphorylation of the ITAMs by src kinases, Lyn and Fyn, leads to recruitment and further activation of downstream kinases and molecules, such as Syk and ZAP-70 [2]. The signaling cascade leads to immediate release of preformed mediators (e.g., histamine, proteases) followed by release of newly synthesized mediators (e.g., cysteinyl leukotrienes). This process underlies the clinical signs and symptoms of anaphylaxis: generalized urticaria, laryngeal edema, lower-airway obstruction, gastrointestinal symptoms, and hypotension.

## 22.2 Relevance of Causes

Establishing the etiology of recurrent anaphylaxis is a critical aspect of treatment, as the identification of causal allergens allows the use of either avoidance or immunotherapy in the management. Assigning etiology is limited, however, by the number of known antigenic exposures associated with anaphylaxis. The most frequent allergens involved in anaphylactic reactions are proteins found in peanuts, tree nuts, fish, shellfish, bee and wasp venoms, as well as drug haptens and latex. In cases of idiopathic anaphylaxis Fcε(epsilon) RI receptors may be aggregated by an antigen not yet identified [3], or the signal cascade may be activated by a mutated surface membrane receptor tyrosine kinase c-kit (D816V) [4], yet the current approach to treatment is based largely on the frequency of episodes: short-term treatment of the acute episodes is considered reasonable for infrequent attacks, whereas prophylactic therapy with oral corticosteroids may be necessary for patients with frequent events [5]. Given that anaphylaxis is a severe allergic reaction that can be rapid and occasionally fatal and that establishing the etiology is pivotal to long-term management, identification of novel causative agents can provide an important step forward in facilitating new, allergen-specific approaches to management.

### *22.2.1 Established Causes and Their Treatment*

The diagnosis of anaphylaxis, laboratory testing available to support the clinical diagnosis, and the specific tests used to establish allergen sensitization are reviewed in detail elsewhere [3] and briefly summarized in Table 22.1. In general, *Hymenoptera* sting-triggered anaphylaxis requires evaluation

**Table 22.1** Treatment options in anaphylaxis: relevance of the cause

| Cause | Treatment/management |
|---|---|
| Hymenoptera venom | Immunotherapy,[a] avoidance |
| Fire ant | Immunotherapy, avoidance |
| Radiocontrast material | Premedication |
| Food | Avoidance, oral immunotherapy |
| Medication | Desensitization, avoidance, premedication |
| Idiopathic | Symptomatic treatment (infrequent episodes), prophylaxis (frequent episodes) |

[a]Practice parameter guidelines recommend venom immunotherapy only in patients ≥16 years old

by an allergy/immunology specialist as venom immunotherapy is well established in the treatment of adults [6]. Biting insects that do not produce venom can also produce immediate anaphylactic and large hypersensitivity reactions and this has been reported with fire ants [7], many species of ticks [8], jumper ants [9], and kissing bugs [10]. For food-induced anaphylaxis, the clinical history is coupled with results of skin, in vitro and/or food challenge testing to devise an appropriate avoidance diet, provide education, and recommend appropriate medications. In certain centers, oral immunotherapy may be available through ongoing studies or provider-based decisions. In addition, many medications can trigger anaphylaxis; so it is important to establish whether IgE is involved as therapeutic considerations often include desensitization protocols. Alternatively, if the process appears to be non-IgE-mediated or the antigenic determinants have not been established, then treatment is generally restricted to premedication regimens (e.g., for radio-contrast material) [11] or avoidance (e.g., mucocutaneous hypersensitivity reactions such as Stevens–Johnson Syndrome or toxic epidermal necrolysis, which are not reported to cause anaphylaxis). Recognition of mast cell activation syndromes and mastocytosis can be done by measurement of tryptase levels, bone marrow biopsy, and c-kit D816V mutation evaluation.

## 22.2.2 *Novel Causes of Anaphylaxis*

Identification of novel agents that can cause anaphylaxis provides an important step forward in diagnosis and management. In contrast to the view that carbohydrate-directed IgE has minimal, if any, clinical significance, recent data suggest that IgE antibodies to carbohydrate epitopes can be an important factor in some cases of anaphylaxis that previously appeared to be idiopathic [12]. Specifically, IgE antibodies to the carbohydrate galactose-α(alpha)-1,3-galactose (alpha-gal) were found to be capable of eliciting serious, even fatal, reactions to the monoclonal antibody (ab) cetuximab [12]. Moreover, alpha-gal has recently been identified as a novel food allergen [13]. These patients have a consistent history of urticarial or anaphylactic reactions which start 3–6 h after eating beef, pork, or lamb [13]. Strikingly, the patients are specific that the reactions occur with beef, pork, or lamb but not with chicken, turkey, or fish, which accurately mirrors the specificity of the IgE antibodies in their serum [13]. It is important to recognize that many of the patients have severe reactions with documented fall in blood pressure even when they do not experience any symptoms for the first 3 or more hours [13]. Screening serum samples from multiple geographic locales has revealed a distinct regional distribution of IgE antibodies to alpha-gal. To date, we have found patients in Virginia, North Carolina, South Carolina, Georgia, Tennessee, Arkansas, Texas, Oklahoma, Maryland, and Missouri, a distribution that roughly correlates with the higher incidence of cetuximab hypersensitivity reactions [14] and the endemic area of the *Amblyomma americanum* (Lone Star tick) [15].

### 22.2.2.1 Overview of Cross Reactive Carbohydrate Determinants

The presence of IgE antibodies to carbohydrate antigens was first identified from in vitro experiments looking at cross-reactivity between different plant-derived antigens [16]. In part because of this approach, the carbohydrate epitopes identified were generally, or exclusively, cross-reactive, which led to the designation cross reactive carbohydrate determinants (CCD). The best recognized of the CCDs is $MUXF^3$, which is present on many different plant proteins but was first defined on a protein derived from pineapple stem bromelain [17]. This protein is not a significant allergen in its own right, so that IgE antibodies binding to bromelain are almost always specific for $MUXF^3$.

This is an important principle because these oligosaccharide epitopes may be better presented on a parent molecule than on an artificial carrier. However, it is important to remember that the relationship to the parent molecule may alter the antigenicity of the sugars, just as the presence of an oligosaccharide may alter the antigenicity of an associated peptide [18, 19]. More relevant here, there are no reports of anaphylaxis occurring when patients with serum IgE antibodies to $MUXF^3$ eat plant foods carrying this epitope.

Several different syndromes involving mammalian cross-reactivity have been described. The pork-cat syndrome can cause anaphylactic responses on eating pork [20]. However, the cross-reactive IgE antibodies in these cases are specific for protein epitopes on albumin [20, 21]. On the other hand, Mamikoglu reported a series of patients in Arkansas who had IgE antibodies to beef, pork, and lamb, which could well have been cases with IgE antibodies to a mammalian CCD such as alpha-gal [22].

It is not difficult to argue that oligosaccharides are immunogenic, the A and B antigens of red blood cells are an excellent example [23]. In addition, it has been extensively recognized that all immunocompetent humans have serum IgG antibodies specific for alpha-gal [24, 25]. Thus, the question is why do some individuals produce IgE responses against oligosaccharides? IgE antibody responses to plant-derived carbohydrate epitopes such as $MUXF^3$ appear to be a common feature of IgE antibody responses to many pollens. For these, there do not appear to be obvious regional or other features that selectively enhance the responses to this CCD [26]. On the other hand, there is extensive evidence that the stings of bees and other venomous insects can induce IgE antibody responses to CCDs that cross-react with plant glycoproteins [16]. In the case of developing an IgE antibody that recognizes alpha-gal, it may be that such a response is induced by a tick or insect protein where the glycosylation is acting as a hapten and there may not be an associated T-cell response (Fig. 22.1). Another relevant example is that of latex allergy: the glycan epitopes present in a latex extract can bind carbohydrate-directed IgE present in the serum of a pollen-allergic patient not originally sensitized to latex, resulting in a positive in vitro assay for IgE to latex [27]. Additionally, if a patient is sensitized to the allergen tested by immunoassay, the presence of carbohydrate-directed IgE plus anti-peptide IgE can result in a higher quantitative result, suggesting a more severe sensitization than is actually the case. A final example is the high occurrence of clinically irrelevant results for peanut sIgE in patients sensitized to grass pollen who have no symptoms related to peanuts [28].

Although not related to CCDs, similar cross-reactivity has been well described for IgE directed against protein epitopes in the oral allergy syndrome [29]. The obvious example is birch pollen exposure giving rise to IgE antibodies to Bet v 1, which cross-reacts with the closely related proteins

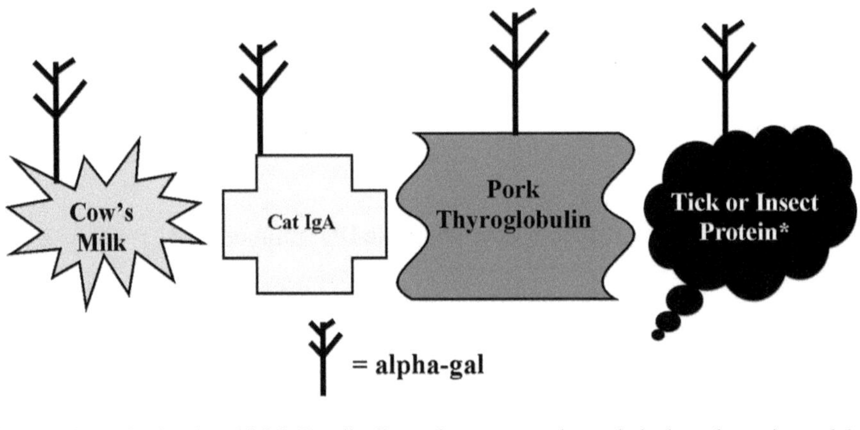


**Fig. 22.1** Possible mechanism by which IgE antibodies to the cross-reactive carbohydrate determinant alpha-gal may develop. In this model, the IgE response is induced by a yet unknown tick or insect protein where glycosylation is acting as a hapten and there may not be an associated T cell response

of apple, hazelnut, or the cherry-derived allergen Pru a 1. In this instance, the epitope recognized by the IgE antibody is important since linear (amino acid) epitopes are unlikely to be altered by cooking/heating. If the IgE response is to a conformational epitope, however, cooking may alter the epitope enough to allow a patient to consume the food when it is cooked without provocation of symptoms [30].

#### 22.2.2.2 Implications for Recombinant Therapeutics

The finding of functional IgE to carbohydrates derived from mammals as well as plants has major implications for the recombinant protein industry. Specifically, the cell type used for expression of a recombinant therapeutic glycoprotein has significant implications for the presence, number, and diversity of protein-linked oligosaccharides attached during the synthesis and secretion of the molecule. From a pharmacological perspective, the potential for changes in glycosylation to adversely affect the activity, serum half-life, or immunogenicity of the recombinant protein is a well-known cause for concern. Studies have shown, for example, that variations exist in the glycosylation pattern of tissue plasminogen activator isolated from different cell lines [31]. The most commonly used production cell lines for monoclonal antibodies are CHO, NS0, and Sp2/0 and each of these can add sugar residues that are not present in normal serum-derived IgG [32]. As recent studies have shown [12], a particular concern is the addition of galactose in an α(alpha)(1→3) linkage by NS0 and Sp2/0 cells such that galactose-α(alpha)-1,3-galactose (alpha-gal) is formed. In humans and higher primates, the gene encoding alpha-1,3-galactosyltransferase produces an inactive enzyme, so these species cannot produce alpha-gal; in contrast, this group of animals make IgG antibodies specific for this oligosaccharide [33]. The implication of antibodies directed against the monoclonal antibody is that the response to treatment may be influenced by accelerated clearance of the molecule or of sensitization potentially causing reactions on re-exposure. In the case of cetuximab, which carries alpha-gal, the patients who reacted had specific IgE to this oligosaccharide prior to the exposure and anaphylaxis occurred during the first infusion [12].

In addition to alpha-gal, the main production cell lines can add an α(alpha)(2→3) linked N-glycol neuraminic acid that is not present in humans and may have immunogenic properties. In particular, CHO cells can add *N*-acetylneuraminic acid in α(alpha)(2→3) linkage rather than the α(2→6) linkage found in humans [32] Moreover, there is new evidence that fucose residues (or the absence of such sugars) on IgG Fc may influence activation of Fcγ(gamma)RIIa and Fcγ(gamma) RIIIa. The Fc gamma receptors may have different glycosylation patterns themselves. Thus, knowledge and awareness of the oligosaccharides present on all recombinant molecules (not only monoclonal antibodies) is critical to understanding the etiology of infusion reactions. While glycosylation of the Fc portion of the molecule (Asn 297) is known to play a significant role in Fc binding and the activation of antibody-dependent cellular cytotoxicity (ADCC), it is not clear that the same is true for glycosylation on the Fab side. Although current knowledge limits the ability to change glycosylation patterns, if a glycosylation site is present it is relatively easy to engineer the amino acid sequence so that the glycosylation site(s) on the Fab are no longer present.

## 22.3 Future Trends in Treatment: Anti-IgE

### *22.3.1 Mechanism of Action*

Omalizumab is a monoclonal antibody with a human IgG1 framework and a complementarity-determining region from a murine anti-IgE antibody. Omalizumab recognizes the Cε(epsilon)3 domain of the heavy chain of free human IgE and its binding prevents IgE from interacting with

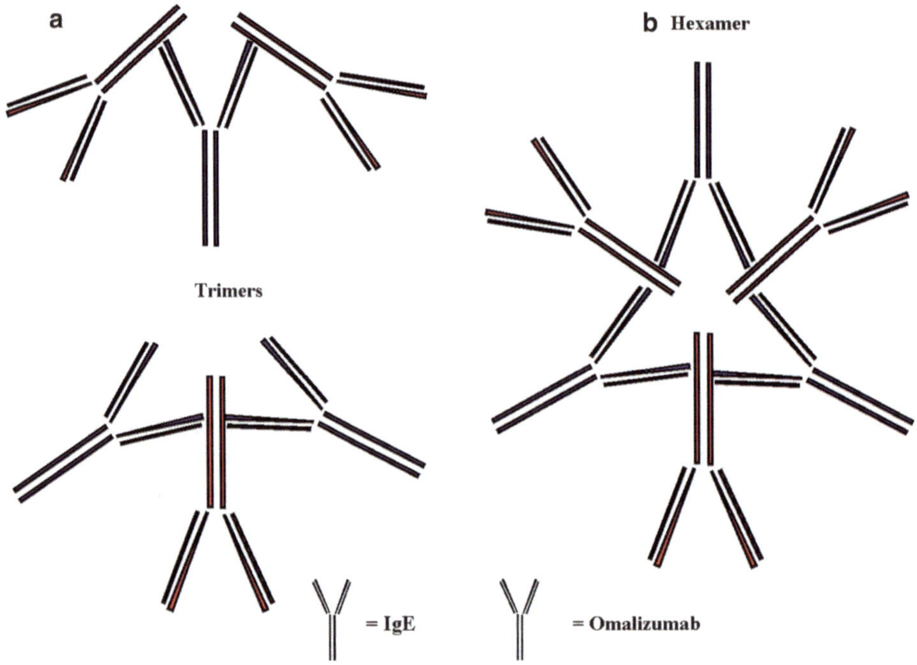


**Fig. 22.2** Representative immune complexes formed between omalizumab (blue) and IgE (red) in sera. The hexamer (**b**) predominates when components are present in a 1:1 M ratio; the trimers (**a**) predominate when one of the components is in excess of the other

**Table 22.2** Proposed mechanisms of action of omalizumab

| |
|---|
| Rapidly reduces the level of free IgE in serum |
| Effectively reduces the level of Fcε(epsilon) receptors on mast cell and basophils |
| Inhibits IgE binding to high- and low-affinity Fcε(epsilon) receptors |
| Reduces basophil responsiveness to allergen stimulation |
| Reduction in presentation of allergen by dendritic cells (DCs) to T cells via: |
| 1. Blocking IgE binding to Fcε(epsilon) receptors on DCs, or |
| 2. By downregulation of IgE receptors on circulating precursor DCs |
| Stabilization of mast cells |

high- or low-affinity IgE receptors [34, 35]. The Cε(epsilon)3 domain is the same site that binds Fcε(epsilon)RIα(alpha) and Fcε(epsilon)RII receptors; hence, omalizumab cannot bind receptor-bound IgE and cannot directly induce mast cell or basophil degranulation or anaphylaxis [34–36]. The binding of omalizumab to circulating IgE results in a rapid decrease in the levels of circulating free IgE [37] and exists in serum as immune complexes of either trimers or hexamers (Fig. 22.2). Omalizumab functions not only to block IgE binding to Fcε(epsilon)RI but also to downregulate Fcε(epsilon)RI expression on circulating basophils [38]. The reduction in receptor density was accompanied by reduced basophil responsiveness to stimulation by allergen of approximately 90% [38]. This indicates that Fcε(epsilon)RI-receptor density is regulated by circulating levels of free IgE and that reducing free IgE with omalizumab is very effective in decreasing Fcε(epsilon)RI expression [39]. Thus, omalizumab has the potential to inhibit allergen-induced mast cell activation regardless of the allergen specificity of the IgE molecules. The mechanisms of action of omalizumab (see Table 22.2) might also include reduced presentation of allergen by dendritic cells (DCs) to T-cells by blocking IgE binding to Fcε(epsilon)RI receptors on dendritic cells [40] or by down-regulation of IgE receptors on circulating precursor dendritic cells [41].

### 22.3.2 *Evidence for a (Broader) Role in Allergic Diseases*

Omalizumab was approved in the United States in July 2003 for the treatment of patients over 12 years old with moderate to severe asthma who have a positive skin test or in vitro test for an aeroallergen with poor control using inhaled corticosteroids and have a total IgE between 30 and 700 IU/mL [42]. The efficacy of omalizumab as add-on therapy in poorly controlled asthma was confirmed in an open-label study of patients with moderate to severe asthma lacking control despite current best standard care [43]. Positive therapeutic effects with omalizumab have also been seen in other IgE-mediated allergic disorders, including atopic dermatitis [44, 45], cold urticaria [46], chronic urticaria [47–49], seasonal and perennial allergic rhinitis [50] as well as idiopathic angioedema [51]. In addition, a small study reported efficacy of omalizumab in the treatment of latex allergy [52]. While there have been no published studies of omalizumab in cases of IgE-mediated food allergy, there has been a study using a different anti-IgE molecule that demonstrated increased tolerance of peanuts in patients with anaphylactic reactions to the food [53]. Given the central role of IgE in anaphylaxis, it has been suggested [54] and now reported [55] that omalizumab has efficacy in treating anaphylactic events. A role for omalizumab in anaphylaxis is further supported by the report of two patients with systemic mastocytosis who had spontaneous episodes of anaphylaxis on numerous occasions. These patients were placed on omalizumab therapy and no subsequent anaphylactic events were reported at 5 and 24 months [56]. Interestingly, the ability of omalizumab to decrease the frequency of episodes of anaphylaxis in these two patients occurred within a short time and, therefore, did not appear to rely on the ability of omalizumab to decrease mast cell numbers. The authors hypothesized that the downregulation of receptors is accompanied by an ability to resist spontaneous degranulation (i.e., there is an increase in the threshold required to trigger degranulation) [56]. While the exact mechanism by which omalizumab decreased the episodes of spontaneous anaphylaxis is unknown, it may relate more to a stabilization of mast cells with a concomitant decrease in surface IgE and associated decreases in receptor (Fcε(epsilon)RI) number [56].

### 22.3.3 *Safety and Efficacy*

In preclinical testing, omalizumab was shown to be safe, having side effects comparable to placebo. It was also clear that antibodies against the monoclonal were not produced [57]. Although reported, anaphylactic reactions with omalizumab are rare and most occurred with the first dose (39%) and within 30 min (35%) [58]. Dosing is calculated using body weight and total IgE (0.016 mg/kg/level of total IgE in IU/mL) for efficacy. Although it may take up to 12–16 weeks for the clinical effect to be observed in asthma, total free IgE levels in serum drop significantly in more than 95% of patients 1 h after administration [59, 60]. The effect of omalizumab correlated with total free IgE dropping to below 50 ng/mL. The goal of treatment is to obtain an omalizumab dose sufficient to reduce the level of total free IgE to roughly 25 ng/mL [59]. Similar dosing for treatment of asthma has been applied to the protocols for anaphylaxis and these calculations have produced consistent decreases in free total IgE to date.

## 22.4 Conclusion

Anaphylaxis that occurs without an immediate cause is a significant medical problem. Recurrent cases cause severe anxiety to the patients and their families, as well as carrying a real risk of morbidity and mortality. The discovery of IgE antibodies to the oligosaccharide alpha-gal has made it possible to investigate several novel aspects of allergic disease. One obvious issue is that the glycosylation of therapeutic recombinant molecules, particularly monoclonal antibodies, can create a risk for severe hypersensitivity reactions. While it is anticipated that the use of omalizumab will continue to expand for patients with recurrent anaphylaxis, the current treatment for acute episodes continues to be epinephrine. Certainly, the preference of patients and providers alike is the ability to avoid triggering allergens; hence, the continued search for targets of specific IgE remains critical to recommending appropriate avoidance. In addition to omalizumab, other potential treatments for anaphylaxis may include molecules that can induce tolerance without causing degranulation/secretion of allergic mediators (e.g., a targeted spleen tyrosine kinase (syk) inhibitor [61]) or via the inhibitory receptor superfamily (IRS) [62]. Potential targets within the IRS family include Fcγ(gamma)RIIB and Siglec-8 [62], both of which build on an emerging theme of immunoreceptor tyrosine-based inhibitory motif (ITIM)-containing inhibitory receptors in mast cells [64, 65]. Targeting such receptors and molecules with inhibitory effects may eventually lead to the development of novel therapeutics for the management of anaphylaxis.

## References


1. Ishizaka K, Ishizaka T, Hornbrook MM. Physicochemical properties of reaginic antibody. V. Correlation of reaginic activity with gamma-E-globulin antibody. *J Immunol.* 1966;97(6):840–853.
2. Kambayashi T, Koretzky GA. Proximal signaling events in Fc epsilon RI-mediated mast cell activation. *J Allergy Clin Immunol.* 2007;119(3):544–552; quiz 553–544.
3. Simons FE. 9. Anaphylaxis. *J Allergy Clin Immunol.* 2008;121(2 Suppl):S402–S407; quiz S420.
4. Akin C. Molecular diagnosis of mast cell disorders. *J Mol Diagn.* 2006;8:412–419.
5. Greenberger PA. Idiopathic anaphylaxis. *Immunol Allergy Clin North Am.* 2007;27(2):273–293, vii–viii.
6. Golden DB. Insect sting allergy and venom immunotherapy: a model and a mystery. *J Allergy Clin Immunol.* 2005;115(3):439–447; quiz 448.
7. Caplan EL, Ford JL, Young PF, Ownby DR. Fire ants represent an important risk for anaphylaxis among residents of an endemic region. *J Allergy Clin Immunol.* 2003;111(6):1274–1277.
8. Gauci M, Loh RK, Stone BF, Thong YH. Allergic reactions to the Australian paralysis tick, Ixodes holocyclus: diagnostic evaluation by skin test and radioimmunoassay. *Clin Exp Allergy.* 1989;19(3):279–283.
9. Solley GO. Stinging and biting insect allergy: an Australian experience. *Ann Allergy Asthma Immunol.* 2004;93(6):532–537.
10. Montgomery RW. Anaphylaxis to kissing bugs. *West J Med.* 1979;130(3):268–269.
11. Lieberman P, Siegle RL, Treadwell G. Radiocontrast reactions. *Clin Rev Allergy.* 1986;4(2):229–245.
12. Chung CH, Mirakhur B, Chan E, et al. Cetuximab-induced anaphylaxis and IgE specific for galactose-alpha-1,3-galactose. *N Engl J Med.* 2008;358(11):1109–1117.
13. Commins SP, Satinover SM, Hosen J, et al. Delayed anaphylaxis, angioedema, or urticaria after consumption of red meat in patients with IgE antibodies specific for galactose-alpha-1,3-galactose. *J Allergy Clin Immunol.* 2009;123(2):426–433.
14. O'Neil BH, Allen R, Spigel DR, et al. High incidence of cetuximab-related infusion reactions in Tennessee and North Carolina and the association with atopic history. *J Clin Oncol.* 2007;25(24):3644–3648.
15. Commins SP, Platts-Mills TA. Anaphylaxis syndromes related to a new mammalian cross-reactive carbohydrate determinant. *J Allergy Clin Immunol.* 2009;124(4):652–657.
16. Aalberse RC, Koshte V, Clemens JG. Immunoglobulin E antibodies that crossreact with vegetable foods, pollen, and Hymenoptera venom. *J Allergy Clin Immunol.* 1981;68(5):356–364.
17. Ishihara H, Takahashi N, Oguri S, Tejima S. Complete structure of the carbohydrate moiety of stem bromelain. An application of the almond glycopeptidase for structural studies of glycopeptides. *J Biol Chem.* 1979;254(21):10715–10719.
18. Huang X, Barchi JJ Jr, Lung FD, et al. Glycosylation affects both the three-dimensional structure and antibody binding properties of the HIV-1IIIB GP120 peptide RP135. *Biochemistry.* 1997;36(36):10846–10856.
19. Sandrin MS, Fodor WL, Mouhtouris E, et al. Enzymatic remodeling of the carbohydrate surface of a xenogenic cell substantially reduces human antibody binding and complement-mediated cytolysis. *Nat Med.* 1995;1(12):1261–1267.

20. Fuentes Aparicio V, Sanchez Marcen I, Perez Montero A, Baeza ML, de Barrio Fernandez M. Allergy to mammal's meat in adult life: immunologic and follow-up study. *J Investig Allergol Clin Immunol.* 2005;15(3):228–231.
21. Jacquenet S, Moneret-Vautrin DA, Bihain BE. Mammalian meat-induced anaphylaxis: clinical relevance of anti-galactose-alpha-1,3-galactose IgE confirmed by means of skin tests to cetuximab. *J Allergy Clin Immunol.* 2009;124(3):603–605.
22. Mamikoglu B. Beef, pork, and milk allergy (cross reactivity with each other and pet allergies). *Otolaryngol Head Neck Surg.* 2005;133(4):534–537.
23. Galili U, Buehler J, Shohet SB, Macher BA. The human natural anti-Gal IgG. III. The subtlety of immune tolerance in man as demonstrated by crossreactivity between natural anti-Gal and anti-B antibodies. *J Exp Med.* 1987;165(3):693–704.
24. Galili U, Rachmilewitz EA, Peleg A, Flechner I. A unique natural human IgG antibody with anti-alpha-galactosyl specificity. *J Exp Med.* 1984;160(5):1519–1531.
25. Macher BA, Galili U. The Galalpha1,3Galbeta1,4GlcNAc-R (alpha-Gal) epitope: a carbohydrate of unique evolution and clinical relevance. *Biochim Biophys Acta.* 2008;1780(2):75–88.
26. Mari A. IgE to cross-reactive carbohydrate determinants: analysis of the distribution and appraisal of the in vivo and in vitro reactivity. *Int Arch Allergy Immunol.* 2002;129(4):286–295.
27. Foetisch K, Westphal S, Lauer I, et al. Biological activity of IgE specific for cross-reactive carbohydrate determinants. *J Allergy Clin Immunol.* 2003;111(4):889–896.
28. Guilloux L, Morisset M, Codreanu F, Parisot L, Moneret-Vautrin DA. Peanut allergy diagnosis in the context of grass pollen sensitization for 125 patients: roles of peanut and cross-reactive carbohydrate determinants specific IgE. *Int Arch Allergy Immunol.* 2009;149(2):91–97.
29. Ortolani C, Ispano M, Pastorello E, Bigi A, Ansaloni R. The oral allergy syndrome. *Ann Allergy.* 1988;61 (6 Pt 2):47–52.
30. Bohle B, Zwolfer B, Heratizadeh A, et al. Cooking birch pollen-related food: divergent consequences for IgE- and T cell-mediated reactivity in vitro and in vivo. *J Allergy Clin Immunol.* 2006;118(1):242–249.
31. Buelens K, Hillmayer K, Compernolle G, Declerck PJ, Gils A. Biochemical importance of glycosylation in thrombin activatable fibrinolysis inhibitor. *Circ Res.* 2008;102(3):295–301.
32. Jefferis R. Glycosylation as a strategy to improve antibody-based therapeutics. *Nat Rev Drug Discov.* 2009;8(3):226–234.
33. Galili U. The alpha-gal epitope and the anti-Gal antibody in xenotransplantation and in cancer immunotherapy. *Immunol Cell Biol.* 2005;83(6):674–686.
34. Shields RL, Werther WR, Zioncheck K, et al. Anti-IgE monoclonal antibodies that inhibit allergen-specific histamine release. *Int Arch Allergy Immunol.* 1995;107(1–3):412–413.
35. Shields RL, Whether WR, Zioncheck K, et al. Inhibition of allergic reactions with antibodies to IgE. *Int Arch Allergy Immunol.* 1995;107(1–3):308–312.
36. Presta LG, Lahr SJ, Shields RL, et al. Humanization of an antibody directed against IgE. *J Immunol.* 1993;151(5):2623–2632.
37. Casale TB, Bernstein IL, Busse WW, et al. Use of an anti-IgE humanized monoclonal antibody in ragweed-induced allergic rhinitis. *J Allergy Clin Immunol.* 1997;100(1):110–121.
38. MacGlashan DW Jr, Bochner BS, Adelman DC, et al. Down-regulation of Fc(epsilon)RI expression on human basophils during in vivo treatment of atopic patients with anti-IgE antibody. *J Immunol.* 1997;158(3):1438–1445.
39. Lin H, Boesel KM, Griffith DT, et al. Omalizumab rapidly decreases nasal allergic response and Fcε(epsilon)RI on basophils. *J Allergy Clin Immunol.* 2004;113(2):297–302.
40. Maurer D, Ebner C, Reininger B, et al. The high affinity IgE receptor (Fcε(epsilon) RI) mediates IgE-dependent allergen presentation. *J Immunol.* 1995;154(12):6285–6290.
41. Prussin C, Griffith DT, Boesel KM, Lin H, Foster B, Casale TB. Omalizumab treatment downregulates dendritic cell Fcε(epsilon)RI expression. *J Allergy Clin Immunol.* 2003;112(6):1147–1154.
42. Holgate S, Casale T, Wenzel S, Bousquet J, Deniz Y, Reisner C. The anti-inflammatory effects of omalizumab confirm the central role of IgE in allergic inflammation. *J Allergy Clin Immunol.* 2005;115(3):459–465.
43. Ayres JG, Higgins B, Chilvers ER, Ayre G, Blogg M, Fox H. Efficacy and tolerability of anti-immunoglobulin E therapy with omalizumab in patients with poorly controlled (moderate-to-severe) allergic asthma. *Allergy.* 2004;59(7):701–708.
44. Lane JE, Cheyney JM, Lane TN, Kent DE, Cohen DJ. Treatment of recalcitrant atopic dermatitis with omalizumab. *J Am Acad Dermatol.* 2006;54(1):68–72.
45. Vigo PG, Girgis KR, Pfuetze BL, Critchlow ME, Fisher J, Hussain I. Efficacy of anti-IgE therapy in patients with atopic dermatitis. *J Am Acad Dermatol.* 2006;55(1):168–170.
46. Boyce JA. Successful treatment of cold-induced urticaria/anaphylaxis with anti-IgE. *J Allergy Clin Immunol.* 2006;117(6):1415–1418.

47. Spector SL, Tan RA. Effect of omalizumab on patients with chronic urticaria. *Ann Allergy Asthma Immunol.* 2007;99(2):190–193.
48. Spector SL, Tan RA. Therapeutic alternatives for chronic urticaria: additional reports on omalizumab. *Ann Allergy Asthma Immunol.* 2008;101(6):647.
49. Spector SL, Tan RA. Omalizumab also successful in chronic urticaria. *J Allergy Clin Immunol.* 2008;121(3):784.
50. Casale TB, Stokes JR. Immunomodulators for allergic respiratory disorders. *J Allergy Clin Immunol.* 2008;121(2):288–296.
51. Sands MF, Blume JW, Schwartz SA. Successful treatment of 3 patients with recurrent idiopathic angioedema with omalizumab. *J Allergy Clin Immunol.* 2007;120(4):979–981.
52. Leynadier F, Doudou O, Gaouar H, et al. Effect of omalizumab in health care workers with occupational latex allergy. *J Allergy Clin Immunol.* 2004;113(2):360–361.
53. Leung DY, Sampson HA, Yunginger JW, et al. Effect of anti-IgE therapy in patients with peanut allergy. *N Engl J Med.* 2003;348(11):986–993.
54. Chang TW, Shiung YY. Anti-IgE as a mast cell-stabilizing therapeutic agent. *J Allergy Clin Immunol.* 2006;117(6):1203–1212; quiz 1213.
55. Warrier P, Casale TB. Omalizumab in idiopathic anaphylaxis. *Ann Allergy Asthma Immunol.* 2009;102(3):257–258.
56. Carter MC, Robyn JA, Bressler PB, Walker JC, Shapiro GG, Metcalfe DD. Omalizumab for the treatment of unprovoked anaphylaxis in patients with systemic mastocytosis. *J Allergy Clin Immunol.* 2007;119(6):1550–1551.
57. Wagelie-Steffen AL, Kavanaugh AF, Wasserman SI. Biologic therapies for the treatment of asthma. *Clin Chest Med.* 2006;27(1):133–147, vii.
58. Corren J, Casale TB, Lanier B, Buhl R, Holgate S, Jimenez P. Safety and tolerability of omalizumab. *Clin Exp Allergy.* 2009;39(6):788–797.
59. Hochhaus G, Brookman L, Fox H, et al. Pharmacodynamics of omalizumab: implications for optimised dosing strategies and clinical efficacy in the treatment of allergic asthma. *Curr Med Res Opin.* 2003;19(6):491–498.
60. Milgrom H, Fick RB, Jr., Su JQ, et al. Treatment of allergic asthma with monoclonal anti-IgE antibody. rhuMAb-E25 Study Group. *N Engl J Med.* 1999;341(26):1966–1973.
61. MacGlashan D Jr, Undem BJ. Inducing an anergic state in mast cells and basophils without secretion. *J Allergy Clin Immunol.* 2008;121(6):1500–1506, 1506 e1501–1504.
62. Li L, Yao Z. Mast cell and immune inhibitory receptors. *Cell Mol Immunol.* 2004;1(6):408–415.
63. Yokoi H, Choi OH, Hubbard W, et al. Inhibition of Fcε(epsilon)RI-dependent mediator release and calcium flux from human mast cells by sialic acid-binding immunoglobulin-like lectin 8 engagement. *J Allergy Clin Immunol.* 2008;121(2):499–505, e491.
64. Saxon A, Zhu D, Zhang K, Allen LC, Kepley CL. Genetically engineered negative signaling molecules in the immunomodulation of allergic diseases. *Curr Opin Allergy Clin Immunol.* 2004;4(6):563–568.
65. Zhu D, Kepley CL, Zhang K, Terada T, Yamada T, Saxon A. A chimeric human-cat fusion protein blocks cat-induced allergy. *Nat Med.* 2005;11(4):446–449.

# Index



M.C. Castells (ed.), *Anaphylaxis and Hypersensitivity Reactions*,
DOI 10.1007/978-1-60327-951-2, © Springer Science+Business Media, LLC 2011

MIX
Papier aus verantwortungsvollen Quellen
Paper from responsible sources
FSC® C105338

If you have any concerns about our products,
you can contact us on
**ProductSafety@springernature.com**

In case Publisher is established outside the EU,
the EU authorized representative is:
**Springer Nature Customer Service Center GmbH**
**Europaplatz 3, 69115 Heidelberg, Germany**

Printed by Libri Plureos GmbH
in Hamburg, Germany